BROWSE'S
INTRODUCTION TO
THE SYMPTOMS & SIGNS OF SURGICAL DISEASE

FIFTH EDITION

Kevin G Burnand MS FRCS MBBS
Honorary Consultant Surgeon, Guy's and St Thomas' Hospitals NHS Foundation Trust, UK
Emeritus Professor of Surgery, King's College London (St Thomas' campus), UK
Former Court of Examiners of the Royal College of Surgeons of England, UK

John Black MD FRCS FRCP
Honorary Consultant Surgeon, Worcestershire Royal Hospital, UK
Past-President, Royal College of Surgeons of England, UK
Former Examiner, Intercollegiate Board in General Surgery, UK

Steven A Corbett BSc PhD FRCS FRCS(Tr&Orth)
Consultant Orthopaedic Surgeon and Clinical Lead, Guy's and St Thomas' Hospitals NHS Foundation Trust,
London, UK

William EG Thomas MS FRCS
Consultant Surgeon Emeritus and former Clinical Director of Sheffield Teaching Hospitals NHS Foundation
   Trust, Sheffield, UK
Honorary Senior Lecturer in Surgery, University of Sheffield, UK
Past Vice President and Member of Council, Royal College of Surgeons of England, UK
Former Court of Examiners of the Royal College of Surgeons of England, UK
Former Examiner, Intercollegiate Board in General Surgery, UK

Emeritus Editor
Norman L Browse Kt MD FRCS FRCP
Professor of Surgery, Emeritus, University of London
Hon. Consulting Surgeon, St Thomas' Hospital, London
Past-President, Royal College of Surgeons of England, UK

CRC Press
Taylor & Francis Group
Boca Raton London New York

CRC Press is an imprint of the
Taylor & Francis Group, an **informa** business

CRC Press
Taylor & Francis Group
6000 Broken Sound Parkway NW, Suite 300
Boca Raton, FL 33487-2742

© 2015 by Taylor & Francis Group, LLC
CRC Press is an imprint of Taylor & Francis Group, an Informa business

Printed and bound in India by Replika Press Pvt. Ltd.

No claim to original U.S. Government works

Printed on acid-free paper
Version Date: 20140722

International Standard Book Number-13: 978-1-4441-4603-5 (Pack - Book and Ebook) 978-1-4441-4605-9 (Paperback)

Visit the Taylor & Francis Web site at
http://www.taylorandfrancis.com

and the CRC Press Web site at
http://www.crcpress.com

Contents

Preface to the First Edition

I believe that the main object of basic medical education is to train the student to talk to and to examine a patient in such a way that he can discover the full history of the patient's illness, elicit the abnormal physical signs, make a differential diagnosis and suggest likely methods of treatment. The object of further medical training is to amplify these capabilities in range and depth through practical experience and specialist training.

It is surprising, but a fact, that some students present themselves for their qualifying examination unable to take a history or to conduct a physical examination in a way that is likely to detect all the abnormal symptoms and signs. Even more are unable to interpret and integrate the facts they do elicit. I think there are two reasons for these deficiencies. First, and most important, students do not spend enough time seeing patients and practising the art of history taking and clinical examination. It is essential for them to realize at the beginning of their training that the major part of medical education is an **apprenticeship**, an old but well-proven system whereby the apprentice watches and listens to someone more experienced than himself and then tries it himself under supervision. The second reason is the lack of books which describe how to examine a patient and explain how the presence or absence of particular symptoms and signs lead the clinician to the correct diagnosis.

In this book I have attempted to describe, in detail, the relevant features of the history and physical signs of the common surgical diseases in a way which emphasizes the importance of the routine application of the techniques of history taking and examining.

The details of these techniques are fully described, and headings such as age, sex, symptoms, position, site, shape and surface are constantly repeated in an unobtrusive way. I hope that when you have finished reading the book you will have these headings so deeply imprinted in your mind that you will never forget them. If so, I will consider that the book has succeeded, for you will always take a proper history and perform a correct and complete examination.

Because the main object of the book is to emphasize the proper techniques of history taking and clinical examination, I have described only the common conditions that you are likely to see in a surgical clinic. Indeed the whole book is presented in a manner similar to that used by most teachers when they are in the presence of the patient. Special investigations and treatment are completely excluded because neither can be applied sensibly if you get the history and physical signs wrong.

To make the book useful for revision, I have put a number of the lists and classifications in special Revision Panels. The photographs are close to the relevant text but their legends contain enough information to make the picture-plus-legend a useful revision piece.

I hope this book will be more of a **teach-book** than a **text-book**, which will be read many times during your basic and higher medical training. There is a well-known saying 'A bad workman always blames his tools'. The doctor cannot make this excuse because his basic tools are his five senses. If he has not trained his senses properly in the manner described in this book and kept them finely honed by constant practice, he will practise bad medicine but he will have only himself to blame.

Norman Browse
1978

Preface to the Third Edition

The disease and abnormalities described in this book have not changed for many thousands of years, nor have their symptoms and signs. Why then produce a third edition? The main reason is to improve and modernize the presentation of the information within the book in the belief that better presentation facilitates and improves learning.

Whereas the symptoms and signs of surgical disease have not changed in the past 20 years, methods of printing and publishing have. Computer graphics and colour printing now enable publishers to produce books of superb design, with infinite varieties of colour, at acceptable costs. The main changes in this new edition are therefore the introduction of colour into the general presentation and design, and the conversion of all 'blackboard-style' line drawings into coloured illustrations – still simple – but giving them the added impact on the memory provided by colour.

At the same time I have tried to illustrate all the clinical conditions with colour photographs – except for the few rare conditions, worthy of presentation, for which modern colour photographers are difficult to obtain. Unfortunately, the current trend is for patients to be unwilling to be photographed for illustrations to be used in books for teaching, thus making the compilation of a comprehensive library of clinical photographs far more difficult than it used to be.

I have also added a considerable number of new Revision panels, now on a blue background, as students find them particularly helpful.

To remind students of their importance, the illustrations of methods of clinical examination (mostly black-and-white photographs) are outlined in Revision Panel blue.

I hope this revised presentation will give the book a new modern appearance and that is will continue to be attractive to new readers in the same way that it has been to the gratifyingly larger number of students who have acquired it for their libraries over the past 20 years.

Sir Norman Browse
1997

Preface to the Fourth Edition

The first edition of this book was written, 25 years ago, to help medical students develop their bedside clinical skills, namely, their ability to take full clinical history and to conduct a complete clinical examination – the prime purpose of medical education.

Although the symptoms and signs of the common 'surgical' diseases have not changed for centuries, the style in which they are presented in textbooks and our understanding of the underlying pathological processes and, in some instances, their classification have. These changes have prompted the production of this fourth edition.

The past 25 years have also seen changes in the style and methods of medical education, especially in the UK, with the term 'problem-orientated medicine' purporting to describe the current popular approach. This is not a new approach. Students beginning their medical training have always been taught to begin the taking of a history by asking the patient 'What are you complaining of?'. To me, this is and always has been a problem-orientated approach.

Having asked all the questions about the patient's main complaint, together with those concerning all the other bodily systems, the student's growing knowledge of the symptoms and signs of individual diseases inevitably begins to guide them to those further questions which are likely to illuminate the cause of the main complaint. This is why it is helpful to learn the symptoms and signs of the common diseases from a book at the same time as acquiring that knowledge through growing clinical experience. This book seeks to expedite that learning.

I firmly believe that what some criticize as dogmatic teaching – following a strict ritual when taking a history and performing an examination – must remain a vital part of clinical education because it accelerates diagnosis and helps avoid errors and omissions.

Medical students know and appreciate this. The continuing success of this book indicates that it helps to fill the deficit that exists in those new courses of medical education that have mistakenly reduced the apprenticeship aspects of learning medicine.

Having retired from clinical practice, I felt it was important to ask three surgical colleagues with an approach to clinical teaching similar to my own, but who are still clinically active, to join me as editors. They have combined Chapters 2 and 3 and Chapters 13 and 15 of the third edition into single chapters (now Chapters 3 and 14) and added a new chapter on the symptoms and signs of trauma (Chapter 2).

In this edition, John Black has revised Chapters 8, 12, 13, 14, 16 and 17; Kevin Burnand has revised Chapters 1, 3, 7 and 15 and written the new Chapter 2; and William Thomas has revised Chapters 4, 5, 6, 9, 10 and 11. I have collated and edited their revisions to ensure that the book's original systematic approach and style of presentation were maintained. I am most grateful for their hard work and willing co-operation. When the fifth edition is needed, in 5–8 years' time, I know it will be in excellent hands.

I hope this edition retains its style as a ward-round 'teach-book' aimed directly at the individual student rather than a library-shelf textbook. Whenever possible, the illustrations have been kept on the same page as the relevant text, as have many of the revision panels. All are there to help you reinforce those vital items of knowledge which must be in your mind when sitting in front of a patient – not hidden somewhere in the memory of a computer.

Note. Throughout the book, whenever a particular complaint is more common in one sex, the patient has been referred to as 'he' and 'she' accordingly. If there is no sexual predominance, 'they' has been used in the singular sense.

Sir Norman Browse
2005

Preface to the Fifth Edition

The first edition of this book was written 36 years ago by Sir Norman Browse to help medical students develop their bedside clinical skills by learning how to take a full history and to conduct a full clinical examination. The preface to the first edition lays down the principles of the book, namely detailed, systematic working through the standard headings, without which valuable clues to the diagnosis can be missed. Although the book was illustrated profusely with clinical photographs and diagrams, investigations and management were excluded specifically. The idea of a companion volume covering these was first suggested in 1980, but *Browse's Introduction to the Investigation and Management of Surgical Disease* did not appear until 2010, with the same four editors as the present volume.

Although the diseases themselves remain the same, their pattern of presentation, relative frequency and classification is changing constantly. Peptic ulceration in first world countries is now treated so swiftly and effectively that it rarely presents to surgeons, while diseases associated with obesity are far more common. Some formerly common conditions such as the complications of syphilis are now rare, while the introduction of screening has altered the profile of, for example, breast cancer. This is one reason for another edition.

A second reason is demand to include the full range of surgical conditions. Although the original book was aimed at medical students, its systematic and highly detailed approach with stress on basic principles has made it attractive to trainee surgeons preparing for postgraduate examinations. The four editors have revised those chapters in their individual areas of expertise, but there are now many more authors, whose details are listed in full and against the relevant chapters in the Table of Contents. The sections on orthopaedics and trauma have been expanded massively and there are new chapters on cardiothoracic and neurological surgery. Investigation and management remain by and large excluded but are mentioned occasionally and briefly where they form part of clinical assessment, as for example with major trauma. The book now covers all areas of surgical disease except for otorhinolaryngology and ophthalmology.

All of the line diagrams have been redrawn and there are some new clinical photographs of higher quality than before. The popular revision panels have been retained.

It is ironic that Sir Norman's single author purposefully didactic clinically orientated book now requires four editors and multiple authors. The reader may be reassured that the original approach has not changed. Even today most diagnoses can be made by taking a careful history and carrying out a full examination, and this book is intended to help the student to acquire these basic skills.

Citations throughout the text to *Investigation and Management* are to the companion volume: Browse N et al. *Browse's Introduction to the Investigation and Management of Surgical Disease*; ISBN 9780340945742; Boca Raton: CRC Press, 2010.

The Editors
2015

Contributors

Timothy JP Batchelor MBChB BSc(Hons) MSc FRCS(CTh)
Consultant Thoracic Surgeon
University Hospitals Bristol NHS Foundation Trust
Bristol, UK

Diane L Back FRCS Ed Orth
Consultant Trauma and Orthopaedic Surgeon
Guy's and St Thomas' Hospitals NHS
    Foundation Trust
London, UK

Peter Bullock FRCS MRCP
Consultant Neurosurgeon
King's College Hospital
Honorary Neurosurgeon
Guy's and St Thomas' Hospitals NHS Foundation
    Trust and The Maudsley Hospital
London, UK

Matthew Bultitude MBBS MRCS MSc FRCS(Urol)
Consultant Urological Surgeon
Guy's and St. Thomas' Hospitals NHS
    Foundation Trust
London, UK

Tom Carrell MA MChir FRCS
Consultant Vascular Surgeon
Guy's and St Thomas' Hospitals NHS
    Foundation Trust
London, UK

Ben Challacombe MS FRCS(Urol)
Consultant Urological Surgeon and Honorary
    Senior Lecturer
Guy's and St Thomas' Hospitals NHS Foundation
    Trust and King's College London
London, UK

James A Gossage BSc(Hons) MS FRCS
Consultant Oesophagogastric and General Surgeon
Guy's and St Thomas' Hospitals NHS
    Foundation Trust
Senior Lecturer
King's College London
London, UK

Jonathan Lucas MBBS FRCS(Eng) FRCS(Orth&Tr)
Lead Clinician for Spinal Surgery and Consultant
    Spinal Surgeon
Guy's and St Thomas' Hospitals NHS
    Foundation Trust
London, UK

Mark McGurk MD BDS FRCS FDSRCS DLO
Professor of Oral and Maxillofacial Surgery
King's College London and Guy's and St Thomas'
    Hospitals NHS Foundation Trust
London, UK

Ruth McKee MD FRCS
Consultant Colorectal Surgeon
Glasgow Royal Infirmary
Glasgow, UK

Bijan Modarai PhD, FRCS
Senior Lecturer in Vascular Surgery and Honorary
    Consultant Vascular Surgeon
King's College London and Guy's and St Thomas'
    Hospitals NHS Foundation Trust
London, UK

Pari-Naz Mohanna MBBS(Hons) BSc(Hons)
MD(Hons) FRCS(Plast)
Department of Plastic and Reconstructive Surgery
Guy's and St Thomas' Hospitals NHS Foundation
    Trust
London, UK

Samer Saour MB BCh BAO MRCS FRCS(Plast)
Specialist Registrar in Plastic Surgery
Department of Plastic and Reconstructive Surgery
Guy's and St Thomas' Hospitals NHS Foundation
  Trust
London, UK

Sam Singh MA MRCS Msc FRCS(Orth)
Consultant Orthopaedic Surgeon
Guy's and St Thomas' Hospitals NHS
  Foundation Trust
London, UK

Jay D Smith MBBS, BSc, MRCS, FRCS(Tr & Orth)
Consultant Orthopaedic Surgeon
Hillingdon Hospital NHS Foundation Trust
Uxbridge, UK

Leandros-Vassilios Vassiliou DDS MD MRCS
Specialty Registrar Oral and Maxillofacial Surgery
King's College London and Guy's and St Thomas'
  Hospitals NHS Foundation Trust
London, UK

Acknowledgements

The editors are grateful to the many specialist authors who contributed to this book and to the editorial team at CRC Press led by Jo Koster and Stephen Clausard.

Thanks are due to Kate Burnand MRCS who redrew many of the diagrams, and to Kate Nardoni and Susan Tyler who turned them into professional art work. We also thank Carrie Walker, Paul Bennett and Ruth Maxwell for their work on the final appearance of the book.

History-taking and clinical examination

You must be alert from the moment you first see the patient. Employ your eyes, ears, nose and hands in a systematic fashion to collect information from which you can deduce the diagnosis. The ability to appreciate an unusual comment or minor abnormality can lead you to the correct diagnosis. This skill only develops from the diligent and frequent practice of the routines outlined in this chapter. **Always give the patient your whole attention and never take short cuts.**

In the outpatient clinic, have patients walk into the consulting room to meet you, rather than finding them lying undressed on a couch in a cubicle. General malaise and debility, breathlessness, cyanosis and difficulty with particular movements or an abnormal gait are much more obvious during exercise.

Patients like to know to whom they are talking. They are probably expecting to see a specific doctor. You should tell patients your name, and explain why you are seeing them. This is particularly important for trainee surgeons and medical students.

A parent, spouse or friend who is accompanying the patient can often provide valuable information about changes in health and behaviour not noticed by the patient. Remember, however, that many patients are inhibited from discussing their problems in front of a third person. It can also be difficult if the relative or friend, with the best of intentions, constantly replies on behalf of the patient. When the time comes for the examination, the friend or relative can be asked to leave and further questions can then be asked in private. It is also often helpful if a chaperone is present.

Talk with patients or, better still, let them talk to you. At first, guide the conversation, but do not dictate it. Treat patients as rational, intelligent human beings. They know what worries them better than you do, but they are visiting a doctor to obtain a diagnosis and if necessary receive treatment. **At all stages, explain what you are doing, and why you are doing it.**

All questions should be put in simple plain language, **avoiding medical terms and jargon**, and using lay expressions as much as possible. When a patient is not fluent in English, an interpreter is required. When conducting an interview through an interpreter, keep your questions short and simple, and have them translated and answered one at a time.

You should not use leading questions. Allow patients to choose their own answers. Do not say, 'Did the pain move to the right-hand side?' This is a leading question because it implies that it should have moved in that direction, and an obliging patient will sometimes answer yes just to please you. The patient should be asked whether the pain ever moves. When the answer is yes, the supplementary question is 'Where does it go to?' If, however, patients fail to understand the question, a number of possible answers may have to be proposed, which can then be confirmed or rejected.

Remember that a question that you do not think is leading the patient may be interpreted incorrectly if they do not realize that there is more than one answer. For example, 'Has the pain changed?' can be a bad question, as there are a variety of ways in which the pain can change. It can alter in severity, nature, site, etc., but the patient may be so disturbed by the intensity of the pain that they think only of its severity and forget the other features that have altered. In such situations, it often helps to include possible answers to the question, for example, 'Has the pain moved to the top, bottom, or side of your abdomen or anywhere else?', 'Has the pain got worse, better or stayed the same?' or 'Can you walk as far, less far or the same distance that you could a year ago?'

The patient should provide the correct answer providing you ask the question correctly. Do not be overconcerned about the questions – worry about the answers, and accept that it will sometimes take a long time and a great deal of patience and perseverance to get a good history.

At some stage, you will read the referral letter, which may suggest a diagnosis. It is often better to read this after you have taken your own history as it can bias your independent opinion.

HOW TO TAKE THE HISTORY

The history should be taken in the order described below and in Revision panel 1.1. **Try not to write and talk to the patient at the same time.** It is however, important to document dates and times and drug history and dosage accurately, which you may not recall after you have finished the examination and left the room. Brief notes as you talk to the patient are therefore essential.

Always make sure you know and record, the patient's name and address, age, sex and occupation. Whenever you write a note about a patient, whether it is a short progress report or a full history, make sure that you write down the date and time that the patient was seen.

The present complaint/problem

Start by asking the patient what is their main complaint and record the answer. Ask the patient to use their own words to describe exactly what it is that they have found to be wrong with themselves, and not what they have been told is wrong, perhaps by another doctor. It is also worth asking 'What is the problem that you want me (e.g. the surgeon) to sort out?' If you ask 'What is the matter?', the patient will often tell you what they think is their diagnosis, or what they have been told by others. It is better not to know what the patient thinks is the diagnosis, or

the diagnoses given by other doctors (see the point about referral letters above), because neither may be correct. Try to tease out the patient's complaints and problems and come to your own conclusions!

Complaints should be listed in order of severity, with a record of precisely when and how they started. Whenever possible, it should be noted why the patient is more concerned with one complaint than another.

History of the present complaint

The full history of the main complaint or complaints must be recorded in detail, with precise dates. It is important to get right back to the beginning of the problem. For example, a patient may complain of a recent sudden attack of indigestion. When further questioning reveals that similar symptoms occurred some years previously, their description should be included in this section.

Remaining questions about the affected system

When a patient complains of indigestion, for example, it is sensible, after recording the history of the indigestion, to move on at this point to other questions about the alimentary system.

Systematic direct questions

These are direct questions that every patient should be asked, because the answers may amplify your knowledge about the main complaint and will often reveal the presence of other disorders of which the patient was unaware, or thought irrelevant. An absence of associated symptoms is often just as important as positive answers. The standard set of direct and important supplementary questions is described in detail below because they are so important. **It is essential to know them by heart because it is very easy to forget to ask some of them.** When you have to go back to the patient to ask a forgotten question, the answer often proves to be very important.

The only way to memorize this list is by practice, which means taking as many histories as possible and writing them out in full. The answers to every question must be recorded.

Synopsis of a History (Revision Panel 1.1)

Revision panel 1.1

Synopsis of a history

Names. Age and date of birth. Sex.
Marital status. Occupation. Ethnic group.
Hospital or practice record number

Present complaints or problems (PC, CO)

Preferably in the patient's own words

History of the present complaint (HPC)

Include the answers to the direct questions
concerning the system of the presenting complaint

Systematic direct questions

(a) Alimentary system and abdomen

Appetite. Diet. Weight. Nausea. Dysphagia.
Regurgitation. Flatulence. Heartburn. Vomiting.
Haematemesis. Indigestion pain. Abdominal pain.
Jaundice. Abdominal distension. Bowel habit.
Nature of stool. Rectal bleeding. Mucus. Slime.
Prolapse. Incontinence. Tenesmus

(b) Respiratory system

Cough. Sputum. Haemoptysis. Dyspnoea.
Hoarseness. Wheezing. Chest pain. Exercise
tolerance

(c) Cardiovascular system

Dyspnoea. Paroxysmal nocturnal dyspnoea.
Orthopnoea. Chest pain. Palpitations. Ankle
swelling. Dizziness. Limb pain. Walking distance.
Colour changes in hands and feet

(d) Urogenital system

Loin pain. Frequency of micturition including
nocturnal frequency. Poor stream. Dribbling.
Hesitancy. Dysuria. Urgency. Precipitancy.
Painful micturition. Polyuria. Thirst. Haematuria.
Incontinence

In males: Problems with sexual intercourse and
impotence

In females: Date of menarche or menopause.
Frequency. Quantity and duration of menstruation.
Vaginal discharge. Dysmenorrhoea. Dyspareunia.
Previous pregnancies and their complications.
Prolapse. Urinary incontinence. Breast pain. Nipple
discharge. Lumps. Skin changes

(e) Nervous system

Changes of behaviour or psyche. Depression.
Memory loss. Delusions. Anxiety. Tremor. Syncopal
attacks. Loss of consciousness. Fits. Muscle
weakness. Paralysis. Sensory disturbances.
Paraesthesias. Dizziness. Changes of smell, vision
or hearing. Tinnitus. Headaches

(f) Musculoskeletal system

Aches or pains in muscles, bones or joints. Swelling
joints. Limitation of joint movements. Locking.
Weakness. Disturbances of gait

Previous history (PH)

Previous illnesses. Operations or accidents.
Diabetes. Rheumatic fever. Diphtheria. Bleeding
tendencies. Asthma. Hay fever. Allergies.
Tuberculosis. Sexually transmitted diseases.
Tropical diseases

Drug history

Insulin. Steroids. Antidepressants and the
contraceptive pill. Drug abuse

Immunizations

BCG. Diphtheria. Tetanus. Typhoid. Whooping
cough. Measles

Family history (FH)

Causes of death of close relatives. Familial illnesses
in siblings and offspring

Social history (SH)

Marital status. Sexual habits. Living
accommodation. Occupation. Exposure to
industrial hazards. Travel abroad. Leisure
activities

Habits

Smoking. Drinking. Number of cigarettes smoked
per day. Units of alcohol drunk per week

The alimentary system (see Chapters 15 and 16)

Appetite Has the appetite increased, decreased, or remained the same? If it has decreased, is this caused by a loss of appetite, or is it because of apprehension as eating always causes pain?

Diet What type of food and when does the patient eat? Are they vegetarian, or do they avoid any particular foods?

Weight Has the patient's weight changed, and if so, by how much and over how long a time? Many patients never weigh themselves, but they usually notice if their clothes have got tighter or looser, and friends may have told them of a change in physical appearance.

Teeth and taste Can they chew their food? Do they have their own teeth? Do they get odd tastes and sensations in their mouth? Are there any symptoms of water brash or acid brash? (This is the sudden filling of the mouth with watery or acid-tasting fluid – saliva and gastric acid, respectively.)

Swallowing Do they have any difficulty in swallowing (dysphagia)? If so, ask about the type of food that causes difficulty, for example solids, liquids or both, and the level at which they feel the food sticking. Also ask about the duration and progression of these symptoms, and whether swallowing is painful.

Regurgitation Do they regurgitate? This means the effortless return of food into the mouth. It is quite different from vomiting, which is associated with a powerful involuntary contraction of the abdominal wall. If they do regurgitate, what comes up? Is it fluid or solid? Regurgitated food is either digested, or recognizable and undigested?

How often does regurgitation occur and does anything, such as bending over, stooping or straining, precipitate it?

Flatulence Does the patient belch frequently? Does this relate to any other symptoms?

Heartburn This is a burning sensation experienced behind the sternum, caused by the reflux of acid into the oesophagus. Patients may not realize that this symptom comes from the alimentary tract, which is why it must be specifically asked about. If patients do experience heartburn, how often does it happen and does anything precipitate it, such as lying flat or bending over?

Vomiting This is the forcible ejection of stomach or intestinal contents through the mouth as the result of involuntary spasms of the oesophagus, stomach and abdominal wall. If patients do vomit, how often do they do so? Is the vomiting preceded by nausea? What is the nature and volume of the vomit? Is it recognizable food from previous meals, digested food, clear acidic (burning) fluid or bile-stained fluid (bitter-tasting)?

Is the vomiting preceded by another symptom such as indigestion pain, headache or giddiness? Does it follow eating, and what is its relationship to food? Is it effortless?

Haematemesis This is defined as the vomiting of blood. Always ask if patients have ever vomited blood because it is such an important symptom. Old, altered blood looks like **coffee grounds**.

Some patients have difficulty in differentiating between vomited or regurgitated blood and coughed-up blood – *haemoptysis* (see Chapter 2). Haemoptysis is usually pale pink and frothy.

When patients have had a haematemesis, always ask whether they have had a recent nose bleed. They may be vomiting swallowed blood.

Patients are rarely able to make useful guesses at the amount of blood vomited up, and the addition of gastric juice makes questions on the volume of blood vomited of little value. Associated collapse and/or faintness suggests major blood loss has occurred.

Indigestion or abdominal pain (dyspepsia) This is correctly defined as difficulty in digesting food and is usually accompanied by discomfort or abdominal pain and often by heartburn and belching (see above). Some patients call all abdominal pains indigestion; the difference between a discomfort after eating and a pain after eating may be very small.

It is therefore better to concentrate on elucidating the important features of the pain or discomfort, its site, time of onset, severity, nature, progression, duration, radiation, course and precipitating, exacerbating and relieving factors.

Jaundice This is a yellow colouration of the tissues as a consequence of excessive quantities of bile pigments accumulating in the blood (see Chapter 15).

Have the patient's skin or eyes ever turned yellow? When did this happen, and how long did it last? Were there any accompanying symptoms such as fever, abdominal pain or loss of appetite? Did the skin itch?

Did the faeces or urine change colour?

Have they had any recent injections, drugs or blood transfusions?

Have they been abroad, and what immunizations have they had?

Abdominal distension Have they noticed that their abdomen has become swollen (distended)? What brought this to their attention? When did it begin, and how has it progressed? Is it constant or variable?

What factors are associated with any variation in the distension?

Is it painful or accompanied by pain? Does it affect their breathing?

Is it relieved by belching, vomiting, passing flatus or defaecation?

Have they lost weight or had any urinary problems?

If female, could they be pregnant, and when was their last period?

Defaecation This is the act of discharging bowel contents though the anus (see Chapter 16) How often does the patient defaecate per day? Are the actions regular or irregular?

What are the physical characteristics of the stool?:

- *Colour*: brown, black, pale yellow, white, silver, bloody (see below)?
- *Consistency*: hard, soft, frothy or watery?
- *Size*: bulky, pellets, string- or tape-like?
- *Specific gravity*: does it float or sink?
- *Smell?*: is it particularly foul?

Beware of the terms '**diarrhoea**' (a frequent and copious discharge of liquid faeces) and '**constipation**' (an infrequent or difficult bowel evacuation of hard faeces). These terms are often misinterpreted by the patient, and should not be written in the notes without also recording the frequency of bowel action and the consistency of the faeces (see Chapter 16).

Rectal bleeding Has the patient ever passed any blood in the stool?

Was it **bright or dark**? Were the amounts large or small, and on how many occasions did it occur?

Was it mixed in with or on the surface of the stool, or did it appear only after the stool had been passed?

Flatus or mucus passage per rectum Is the patient passing more gas (flatus) than usual, or has it ceased?

Has the patient ever passed mucus (slime) or pus (yellow/green opaque liquid)?

Pain on defaecation Does this occur? If so, when does the pain begin – before, during, after or at times unrelated to defecation? Are there any other aggravating or relieving factors?

Prolapse and incontinence Does anything come out of the anus on straining? Does it return spontaneously or have to be pushed back?

Is the patient continent of faeces and flatus? If not, does anything cause incontinence, such as standing or coughing? Are they aware that they are being incontinent, and is it associated with a severe urge to pass stool?

Have they had any injuries or anal operations in the past?

If they are female, what is their obstetric history?

Tenesmus Do they experience a constant and urgent desire to pass stool (see Chapter 16).

The respiratory system (see Chapter 2)

Cough This is the abrupt/explosive expulsion of air from the lungs through partially closed vocal cords, causing a characteristic noise and often producing mucus (sputum; see below).

How long have they had a cough, and how often do they cough? Does the coughing come in bouts?

Does anything, such as a change of posture, precipitate or relieve the coughing?

Is it a dry or a productive cough (with sputum; see below)?

Sputum This is the mucus/pus that is coughed up. What is the quantity (teaspoon, dessertspoon, etc.) and the colour (white, clear or yellow) of the sputum?

Some patients only produce sputum in the morning or when they are in a particular position.

Haemoptysis This is coughed-up blood (see Chapter 2).

Has the patient noticed it? Was it frothy and pink, which is suggestive of heart failure? Were there red streaks in the mucus, or clots of blood?

What quantity was produced? How often does the haemoptysis occur?

Shortness of breath/dyspnoea (see Chapter 2)
Do they become breathless? Is dyspnoea present at rest? Do they wheeze (make a rasping or whistling sound, which suggests asthma)?

How many stairs can they climb? How far can they walk on a level surface before the dyspnoea interferes with this or stops them? Can they walk and talk at the same time?

Is it present when sitting, or made worse by lying down? Dyspnoea on lying flat is called *orthopnoea*. How many pillows do they need at night?

Does the breathlessness wake them up at night – this is called paroxysmal nocturnal dyspnoea – or get worse if they slip off their pillows?

Severity of dyspnoea can be graded numerically (see Chapter 2).

Is the dyspnoea induced or exacerbated by external factors such as allergy to animals, pollen or dust? Does the difficulty with breathing occur on breathing out or in?

Pain in the chest (see Chapter 2) Ascertain the site, severity and nature of the pain. Chest pains can be continuous, pleuritic (made worse by inspiration), constricting (see below) or stabbing.

The cardiovascular system (see Chapter 2)

Cardiac symptoms

Breathlessness/dyspnoea These are defined by the same questions as those described above.

Orthopnoea and paroxysmal nocturnal dyspnoea These symptoms are particularly associated with heart failure (see Chapter 2).

Pain Cardiac pain typically begins in the midline behind the sternum (retrosternal), but may occasionally be experienced in the epigastrium. It is often described as constricting or band-like. The patient should be asked if the pain radiates to the neck or to the left arm, and whether it is exacerbated by exercise or excitement and relieved by rest (all suggestive of cardiac pain).

Palpitations These are episodes when the patient becomes aware of a sudden fluttering or thumping of the heart in the chest. These symptoms are indicative of an arrhythmia but can be caused by extrasystoles.

Ankle swelling/oedema Do either the ankles or legs swell? When do they swell? What is the effect on the swelling of bed rest and/or elevation of the leg?

It is important to consider cardiac failure in patients with ankle oedema, although there are a number of other causes of ankle swelling (see Chapters 2 and 10).

Dizziness, headache and blurred vision These are some of the symptoms associated with hypertension and postural hypotension. They can also be caused by neurological, vestibular or ocular disorders (see Chapter 3).

Peripheral vascular symptoms (see Chapter 10)

Does the patient get pain in the leg muscles on exercise, which interferes with walking (intermittent claudication)? Does it occur in the thigh, buttocks, calf or foot? How far can the patient walk before the pain begins? Is the pain so bad that they have to stop walking? How long does the pain take to wear off? Can the same distance be walked again?

In a man, a recent loss of penile erections in association with buttock claudication suggests occlusion of the abdominal aorta or internal iliac artery (Leriche's syndrome).

Is there any pain in the limb at rest? Which part of the limb is painful (typically, this is the foot)? Does the pain interfere with sleep? What positions relieve the pain (typically, hanging the foot over the side of the bed or getting up and walking around). Do analgesic drugs provide any relief?

Are the extremities of the limbs cold? Are there colour changes in the hands, particularly in response to cold, classically from white, to blue, before turning red? Raynaud's phenomenon (see Chapter 10) is rarely associated with all the typical changes in colour.

Does the patient experience any paraesthesias in the limb (tingling or numbness) which indicates critical ischaemia and a limb at risk?

Has the patient experienced any transient weakness of the limbs (transient ischaemic attack), loss of vision (amaurosis fugax, or fleeting blindness) or difficulty with speech. These symptoms may presage a full-blown stroke (see Chapter 10).

The urogenital system (see Chapters 17 and 18)

Urinary tract symptoms

Pain Has there been any pain in the loin (*kidney*), groin or suprapubic region (*bladder*)? What is its nature and severity? Does it radiate to the groin or scrotum, suggesting a ureteric calculus?

Micturition How frequently does the patient pass urine, and how many times by day and by night?

Is the volume and frequency excessive (**polyuria**)? Is the patient thirsty? Do they drink excessive volumes of water, suggesting diabetes?

Is micturition painful (**dysuria**)? What is the nature and site of the pain?

Is there any difficulty with micturition, such as a need to strain or to wait to get started? How is the stream? Can it be stopped at will? Is there any dribbling at the end of micturition? These symptoms suggest prostatism.

Does the bladder feel empty at the end of micturition, or do they have to pass urine a second time (**double micturition**; see Chapter 17)?

Haematuria (blood in the urine) Has the patient ever experienced this? Where in the stream and how often did it occur? Was there any associated pain?

Pneumaturia The patient may notice bubbles in the urine, suggesting a fistula between bladder and bowel.

Incontinence of urine Does this occur with urgency or on coughing and straining (**stress incontinence**)? Does it occur continuously without awareness (true), or is it associated with discomfort and a full bladder (overflow)? In females, is there any history of prolapse with stress incontinence?

Genital tract symptoms – male

Scrotum, penis and urethra Has the patient any pain in the penis or urethra during micturition or on intercourse? Is there any difficulty with retraction of the foreskin, or has there been any purulent urethral discharge now or in the past (sexually transmitted infections)?

Has the patient noticed any pain or swelling of the scrotum, and can he achieve an erection and satisfactory ejaculation? Is the patient fertile?

Genital tract symptoms – female

Menstruation When did menstruation begin (the menarche)? When did it end (the menopause)? What is the duration and quantity of the menses? Is menstruation associated with pain (dysmenorrhoea)? What is the nature and severity of the pain? Is there any abdominal pain midway between the periods (mittelschmerz)? Has the patient noticed any pain on intercourse (dyspareunia)?

Has the patient had any vaginal discharge? What is its character and amount? Has she noticed any prolapse of the vaginal wall or cervix or any urinary incontinence, especially when straining or coughing (stress incontinence)?

Pregnancies Record details of the patient's pregnancies – number, dates and complications.

Breasts (see Chapter 13) Do the breasts change during the menstrual cycle? Are they ever painful or tender, and does this occur premenstrually (cyclical breast pain)?

Has the patient noticed any swellings or lumps in the breasts? Did she breast-feed her children? Has there been any nipple discharge or bleeding? Has she noticed any skin changes over the breasts, or any change in contour?

The nervous system (see Chapter 3)

Mental state Is the patient placid or nervous? Has the patient noticed any changes in their behaviour or reactions to others? Patients will often not appreciate such changes themselves, and these questions may have to be asked of close relatives.

Does the patient get depressed and withdrawn, or are they excitable and extroverted?

Brain and cranial nerves Does the patient ever lose consciousness or have fits (epilepsy)? What happens during a fit? It is often necessary to ask a relative or a bystander to describe the fit. Did the patient lie still or jerk about, bite their tongue or pass urine? Was the patient sleepy after the fit? Was there any sense (an **aura**) that the fit was about to develop? Has there been any subsequent change in the senses of smell, vision and hearing?

Is there a history of headache? Where is it experienced? How long has it been occurring, and when does it occur? Are the headaches associated with any visual symptoms (migraine, hypertension, tension and raised intracranial pressure)?

Has the face ever become weak or paralysed? Have any of the limbs been paralysed (strokes or demyelinating disease), or has the patient ever experienced pins and needles in a limb (paraesthesias)?

Has there ever been any buzzing in the ears, or dizziness (vestibular symptoms)?

Has there ever been any loss of speech (**aphasia**)? Can the patient speak clearly and use words properly? Do they know what they want to say but cannot express it (**expressive dysphasia**)?

Peripheral nerves Are any limbs or part of a limb weak or paralysed? Is there ever any loss of skin sensation? Does the patient experience any tingling or pins and needles in the limbs (paraesthesias), suggestive of peripheral neuropathy or nerve compression?

The musculoskeletal system

Ask if the patient suffers from pain, swelling or limitation of the movement of any joint. What precipitates or relieves these symptoms? What time of day does this occur? Are any limbs or groups of muscles weak or painful?

Can the patient walk normally?

Are there any known congenital musculoskeletal deformities?

Previous history of other illnesses, accidents or operations

Record, with dates, the history of any conditions that are not directly related to the present complaint.

Ask specifically about a previous diagnosis of tuberculosis, diabetes, rheumatic fever, tropical diseases and bleeding tendencies. The likelihood of intimate contact with carriers of the human immunodeficiency virus and of other sexually transmitted infections should be explored, especially if the patient's lifestyle is considered to be high risk.

Drug history

Ask whether the patient is taking any drugs. Specifically, enquire about insulin, steroids, antidepressants, diuretics, antihypertensives, hormone replacement therapy and the contraceptive pill.

Patients usually remember about drugs they are taking which have been prescribed by a doctor, but often forget about self-prescribed drugs.

History of allergies

Patients should be specifically questioned on their known allergies to drugs, especially penicillin and other antibiotics, and also to adhesive plaster. A history of hay fever, asthma and eczema is worth noting as is any previous episodes of anaphylaxis.

Write all the patient's known allergies in large letters on the front of their notes.

Immunizations

Most children are immunized against diphtheria, tetanus, whooping cough, measles, mumps, rubella and poliomyelitis. Ask about these, as well as about smallpox, typhoid and tuberculosis vaccination.

Many individuals, especially medical staff, will also have been immunized against viral hepatitis, and this is worth recording.

Family history

Enquire about the health and age, or cause of death, of the patient's parents, grandparents and any brothers and sisters who have died or have familial diseases.

Also ask about any children who may have died or developed specific diseases.

Draw a family tree if there is an obvious familial disorder (e.g. neurofibromatosis).

You will need information about the mother's pregnancy if the patient is a child. Did she take any drugs during pregnancy? What was the birth weight? Were there any difficulties during delivery? Was the physical and mental development normal in early life?

Social history

Record the patient's marital status, and the type and place of their dwelling (e.g. lives in a hostel or of no fixed abode).

Ask about the patient's sexual orientation and their occupation, with special regard to contact with hazards such as dusts, asbestos and chemicals.

What are the patient's leisure activities?

Has the patient travelled extensively or lived abroad? List the countries and the dates if these appear to be relevant.

Habits

Does the patient smoke? If so, what do they smoke – cigarettes, cigars or a pipe? Record the frequency, quantity and duration of their smoking habit.

Does the patient drink alcohol? Record the type and quantity consumed (in units/week) and the duration of the habit. 1 unit = a very small glass of whisky, half a small glass of wine or a half/third of a pint of beer.

Does the patient have any unusual eating habit (e.g. are they a vegan)?

AN EXAMPLE OF HOW TO TAKE A DETAILED HISTORY OF PAIN

The method of taking a history from a patient with 'pain' is now used as an example of how to take a detailed history.

Pain is an unpleasant sensation of varying intensity. We have all experienced pain. It is one of nature's ways of warning us that something is going wrong in our body. It can come from any of the body's systems, but there are certain features common to all pains that should always be recorded.

Tenderness is pain induced by a stimulus, such as pressure from the doctor's hand, or forced movement. Remember that **the patient feels pain – the doctor elicits tenderness.** It is possible for a patient to be lying still without pain and yet have an area of tenderness. Patients may complain of tenderness if they happen to have pressed their fingers on a painful area or have discovered a tender spot by accident. Thus, tenderness can be both a symptom and a physical sign.

A careful history of 'a pain' frequently provides the diagnosis, so you must question the patient closely about each of the following features.

Site

Many factors may indicate the source of the pain, but the most valuable indicator is its site.

It is of little value to describe a pain as 'abdominal pain'; you must try to be more specific. Although patients do not describe the site of their pain in anatomical terms, they can normally point to the site of maximum intensity, which you should convert into an exact anatomical description.

When the pain is indistinct in nature and spreads diffusely over a large area, you must illustrate the area in which the pain is felt and the point (as indicated by the patient) of maximum discomfort.

It is also worthwhile asking about the depth of the pain. Patients can often tell you whether the pain is near to the skin or deep inside. **Splanchnic pain** from an organ, which is experienced through the autonomic system, is poorly localized to the midline, while **somatic pain** from the body's surface layers is well localized.

Time and mode of onset

It may be possible to pinpoint the onset of the pain very precisely, but if this cannot be done, the part of the day or night when the pain began should be recorded. Ask if the pain began gradually or suddenly.

When pain has a truly acute/sudden onset, patients often remember the time precisely, or exactly what they were doing at the time. This occurs when a viscus perforates or a blood vessel splits (dissects) or ruptures.

Inflammation, infarction or obstruction of a hollow viscus all produce a pain of more insidious onset.

You should record the calendar dates on which the pain occurred, but it is also very useful to add in brackets the time interval between each episode and the current examination, because it is these intervals, rather than the actual dates, that are more relevant to the problems of diagnosis.

For example, write, 'Sudden onset of severe epigastric pain on 16th September, 2013, at 11.00 a.m. (3 days ago)'; remember that such comments are useless if you forget to record the date and time of the examination.

Severity

Individuals react differently to pain. What is a 'severe pain' to one person might be described as a 'dull ache' by another. Avoid adjectives used by a patient to describe the severity of their pain. A far better indication of severity is the effect of the pain on the patient's life:

- Did it stop the patient going to work?
- Did it make the patient go to bed?
- Did they try proprietary analgesics?
- Did they have to call their doctor?
- Did it wake the patient up at night, or stop them going to sleep?
- Was the pain better lying still, or did it make them roll around?

The answers to these questions provide a better indication of the severity of a pain than words such as mild, severe, agonizing or terrible. Your assessment of the way the patient responds to their pain, formed while you are taking the history, may influence your diagnosis.

CHAPTER 1 | HISTORY-TAKING AND CLINICAL EXAMINATION

Nature or character of the pain

Patients often find it difficult to describe the nature of their pain, but some of the adjectives that are commonly used, such as aching, stabbing, burning, throbbing, constricting, distending, gripping or colicky, are clearly recognized by most people.

'**Burning and throbbing**' sensations are within everyone's experience. Almost everyone has experienced a burning sensation in the skin following contact with intense heat, so when a patient spontaneously states that their pain is 'burning' in nature, it is likely to be so. Most have experienced a throbbing sensation at some time in their life from an inflammatory process such as toothache, so this description is also usually accurate.

A '**stabbing pain**' is sudden, severe, sharp and short-lived. Hopefully, few of us have experienced a real stabbing!

The adjective '**constricting**' suggests a pain that encircles the relevant part (chest, abdomen, head or limb) and compresses it from all directions. A pain that feels like an iron band tightening around the chest is typical of angina pectoris, and is almost diagnostic of this.

When patients speak of '**tightness**' in their chest or limb, do not immediately assume that they have a constricting pain. They may be describing a tightness caused by distension, which may occur in any structure that has an encircling and restricting wall, such as the bowel, bladder, an encapsulated tumour or a fascial compartment. Tension in the containing wall may cause a pain that the patient may describe as 'distension', 'tightness' or a 'bursting feeling'.

A '**colicky pain**' comes and goes like a sine wave. It feels like a migrating constriction in the wall of a hollow tube that is attempting to force the contents of the tube forwards. It is not a word that many patients use, and it is dangerous to ask them if their pain is 'colicky' without giving an example. This is not difficult, because most of us have experienced intestinal colic during an episode of diarrhoea, and many females have suffered colicky pains with their periods or in labour. Remember that not all recurring, intermittent pain is necessarily colic; it should also have a gripping nature.

'**Just a pain, doctor.**' Many pains have none of the features mentioned above and defy description! They may vary in severity from a mild discomfort or ache, to an agonizing pain that makes the patient think they are about to die. When a patient cannot describe the nature of their pain, do not press the point. You will only make them try to fit their description to your suggestions, which may be misleading.

Progression of the pain

Once it has started, a pain may progress in a variety of ways:

- It may begin at its maximum intensity and remain at this level until it disappears.
- It may increase steadily until it reaches a peak or a plateau, or conversely it may begin at its peak and decline slowly.
- The severity may fluctuate. The intensity of the pain at the peaks and troughs of the fluctuations, and the rate of development and regression of each peak, may vary.
- The pain may disappear completely between each exacerbation.
- The time between the peaks of an abdominal colic indicates the likely site of a bowel obstruction. In upper small bowel obstruction, the frequency of the colic is approximately every 1–2 minutes, whereas in the ileum it is every 20 minutes, and in the large bowel every 30–60 minutes.
- It is essential to find out how the pain has progressed and ascertain the timing of any fluctuations before its nature can be determined.

End of the pain

A pain may end spontaneously, or as a result of some action taken by the patient or doctor. The end of a pain is either sudden or gradual. The way in which a pain ends may give a clue to the diagnosis, or indicate the development of a new problem.

Patients always think that an improvement in their pain means that they are getting better. They are usually right, but sometimes their condition may have become worse, for example an intestinal perforation relieving the colic but causing peritonitis and septicaemia.

Duration of the pain

The duration of a pain will be apparent from the time of its onset and end, but it is nevertheless worthwhile stating the duration of the pain in your notes. The length of any periods of exacerbation or remission should also be recorded.

Factors that relieve the pain

Position, movement, a hot-water bottle, aspirins and other analgesics, food or antacids may all relieve the pain. The natural response to a pain is to search for relief. Sometimes patients try the most bizarre remedies, and many convince themselves that these help, so accept some of their replies to this question with caution.

Factors that exacerbate the pain

Anything that makes the pain worse, such as movement, eating or opening the bowels, is also likely to be known to the patient.

The type of stimulus that exacerbates a pain will depend on the organ from which it emanates and on its cause. For example, intestinal pains may be made worse by eating particular types of food, while musculoskeletal pains are affected by joint movements, muscle exercise and posture. If the initial description has indicated the source of the pain, you can ask direct questions about these potential triggers.

Radiation and referral

You should always ask if the pain is experienced anywhere else or has moved from its initial site.

Radiation This is the extension of the pain to another site while the initial pain persists. For example, patients with a posterior penetrating duodenal ulcer usually have a persistent pain in the epigastrium, but the pain may also spread through to the back. The extended pain usually has the same character as the initial pain.

A pain that occurs in one site and then disappears before reappearing in another site is not radiation: it is a new pain in another place.

Referred pain This is pain that is felt at a distance from its source. For example, inflammation of the diaphragm causes a pain experienced only at the tip of the shoulder (Fig. 1.1). Referred pain is caused by the inability of the central nervous system to distinguish between visceral and somatic sensory impulses.

Cause

It is often worthwhile asking patients what they think is the cause of their pain. Even if they are

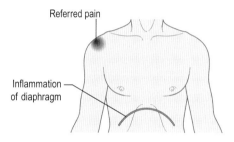

Referred pain

Inflammation of diaphragm

Fig. 1.1 Pain referral.

hopelessly wrong, you may get some important insight into their worries.

A patient will sometimes appear obsessed with the cause of their condition. Careful questioning may reveal that compensation will be gained or lost as a consequence of your opinion! Nevertheless, always listen to the patient's views with care and tolerance.

Psychogenic cause

Beware of patients whose mental attitude to their pain symptoms seems out of proportion – either over-responding to them or ignoring them. The patient whose symptoms do not fit any known pattern who tells you with a big smile that they have 'terrible' pain, or who, while complaining of severe pain, appears quite unconcerned ('*la belle indifférence*') may well be neurotic, hysterical or fabricating their symptoms and even physical signs (Munchausen's syndrome, see Chapter 15).

A diagnosis of Munchausen's syndrome or psychogenic cause should only be made when all possible organic causes for the patient's symptoms have been excluded. In this situation, your clinical experience is your greatest help.

Revision panel 1.2

The features of a pain that must be elicited and recorded

Site

Time and mode of onset

Record the time and date of onset, and the way the pain began – suddenly or gradually

Severity

Assess the severity of the pain by its effect on the patient

CHAPTER 1 | HISTORY-TAKING AND CLINICAL EXAMINATION

Revision panel 1.2 (continued)

Nature/character

Aching, burning, stabbing, constricting, throbbing, distending, colicky

Progression

Describe the progression of the pain. Did it change or alter?

The end of the pain

Describe how the pain ended. Was the end spontaneous, or brought about by some action by the patient or doctor?

Duration

Record the duration of the pain

Relieving and exacerbating factors

Radiation

Record the time and direction of any radiation of the pain; remember to ask if the nature of the pain changed at the time it moved

Referral

Was the pain experienced anywhere else?

Cause

Note the patient's opinion of the cause of the pain

THE CLINICAL EXAMINATION

The following chapters of this book each deal with a specific region of the body and its surgical diseases. The methods of examination peculiar to each region are described in detail in the relevant chapter.

The emphasis to date in this introductory chapter has been on the importance of taking a precise and full history, but it now moves on to a description of the basic plan of a physical examination.

Your ability to perform a thorough clinical examination can only be improved by frequent bedside practice. Examine as many patients, as you can as this experience increases fluency. Repetition is the secret of learning. This axiom applies as much to the doctor as it does to the sportsman or the concert pianist. Your visual, tactile and aural appreciation of the patient's physical signs will improve by repeatedly exercising these senses.

Experienced clinicians usually begin the routine physical examination with a **provisional or differential diagnosis** in mind that has been gleaned from the history. The full impartial systematized examination is then often modified to look for specific signs that confirm or refute the working diagnosis. When, however, a sign is elicited that refutes this, the astute clinician returns to the textbook routine.

Students and trainees must not follow this method. Although it is understandable and practical when used by an experienced consultant surgeon in a busy clinic, it is inherently dangerous! Students must discipline themselves to use the standard textbook routine for every physical examination if mistakes are to be avoided. When this is abandoned, some parts of the examination will be omitted, which can have serious consequences.

The easiest way to ensure that your examination is complete is to learn the routine by heart and repeat it to yourself during the examination. While looking at a lump, say to yourself 'site, size, shape, …'. If you do not do this, you will find, when you come to present the case or write the notes, that you have forgotten to elicit some of the lump's physical features, necessitating a re-examination of the patient.

Always maintain the basic pattern of looking, feeling, tapping and listening:

- Inspection.
- Palpation.
- Percussion.
- Auscultation.

In the musculoskeletal system, percussion and auscultation are replaced by moving the joint (look, feel, move).

Note **It is often best to examine initially the part of body that is the source of the patient's complaint, before completing the full examination of all other systems.**

GENERAL ASSESSMENT

The first part of the physical examination is performed when taking the history. While you are talking to the patient, you can observe the patient's general demeanour, and their attitudes to their disease. These observations will inevitably affect the manner in which you conduct the examination.

Your instructions will need to be extremely simple if the patient appears slow, or coaxing and gentle if the patient is shy or embarrassed.

The patient's general mental state, their memory and their use of words should be noted. A number of terms are used to describe various speech and communication disorders (see Chapter 3). When a patient has been admitted as an emergency, especially if they have been injured, it is important to record their level of consciousness using the Glasgow Coma Scale (see Chapters 3 and 5).

You can also observe a number of physical characteristics when taking the history, such as posture, mobility, weight, colour of the skin, facial appearance and general body build. These should be looked at in detail and recorded at the start of the examination.

GENERAL APPEARANCE

Colour

One of the first things to observe is the colour of the patient's skin, not their racial colour, although it is important to record their racial origin, but changes from what you would expect to be their normal colour. Although minor colour variations are easier to appreciate in fair-skinned people, they are also visible on careful perusal in dark-skinned races.

The skin may be pale or tinged blue, yellow or brown.

Pallor/anaemia

Normal skin colour varies depending upon the thickness of the skin, the state of the skin circulation and the degree and type of pigmentation. Pallor of the skin usually indicates anaemia providing the skin thickness and circulation appear to be normal (Fig. 1.2a, b).

Anaemia is best detected by looking at the colour of the mucous membranes:

- Look at the colour of the conjunctiva on the inner side of the lower eyelid.
- Look at the colour of the buccal mucous membrane.
- Stretch the skin of the palm and look at the colour of the palmar creases; then compare the colour of the patient's palm against your own palm (assuming your haemoglobin level is normal!).

(a) The patient is very pale.

(b) The conjunctiva is also pale.

Fig. 1.2 ANAEMIA

Cyanosis

Cyanosis is the purple–blue colour imparted to the skin and mucus membranes by deoxygenated blood within them. It is most apparent in areas with thin skin and a rich blood supply, such as the lips, tongue, fingernails and ear lobes. Cyanosis is difficult to see in black skin and also hard to detect when the patient is anaemic.

There are two categories of cyanosis:

- **central cyanosis**, when the defect lies in the cardiopulmonary circulation (see Chapter 2);
- **peripheral cyanosis**, when poor tissue perfusion causes excessive deoxygenation in the peripheral tissues (see Chapter 10).

The cyanosis is central if it is caused by cardiopulmonary disease, and the patient's extremities are usually warm. It is best appreciated by inspecting the inner aspect of the lips (Fig. 1.3.) When the cyanosis is caused by a peripheral abnormality, the extremities such as the fingers, toes and nose are blue and cold, but the central organs such as the lips and tongue remain pink.

Fig. 1.3 A child with central cyanosis and blue lips.

Polycythaemia

An excess of circulating red blood cells gives the patient a purple–red, florid appearance (Fig. 1.4).

Fig. 1.4 A patient with polycythaemia. Note: florid purple–red appearance.

Polycythaemia may be mistaken for cyanosis, from which it differs, in that **the colour of all the skin is heightened**, especially the colour of the cheeks, the neck and the backs of the hands and feet. The discolouration of peripheral cyanosis is usually limited to the tips of the hands, feet and nose.

Jaundice

Jaundice is a yellow discolouration of the skin caused by an excess of bilirubin (bile pigment), a breakdown product of haemoglobin, in the plasma.

The yellow colour is first visible in the white background of the sclerae (Fig.1.5), but as the jaundice increases, the whole skin turns yellow.

Fig. 1.5 Jaundice. The sclerae have yellow discolouration.

With the onset of jaundice, white skin first turns a pale lemon yellow. As the bilirubin level increases, the skin becomes yellow–orange and sometimes almost brown. The skin eventually turns a yellow–grey–green colour in patients with primary biliary cirrhosis, when severe jaundice has existed for many years.

Jaundice can be caused by:

- excessive haemolysis – prehepatic jaundice;
- by liver malfunction – hepatic jaundice;
- by obstruction of the bile ducts – posthepatic jaundice.

The symptoms, signs and cause of jaundice are discussed in much more detail in Chapter 15.

Brown pigmentation

An increase in the natural brown pigmentation of the skin (melanin) can be generalized or localized. The causes of this are discussed in more detail in Chapter 4.

THE PATIENT'S SIZE, SHAPE AND PHYSICAL CHARACTERISTICS

When you look at a patient, you will subconsciously put them into one of four categories: their body will look normal, wasted or overweight, or have some skeletal or sexual characteristics that look out of proportion.

The principal conditions that cause these changes in body build are now briefly discussed.

Wasting/cachexia

There are many causes of wasting. Almost all serious diseases cause some loss of appetite and weight, so only the common conditions are listed in Revision panel 1.3.

The degree of wasting is apparent from the way in which the skeleton, particularly around the shoulder girdle, becomes visible. Folds of loose skin may be present on the arms, trunk and buttocks.

Severe wasting of the upper half of the body with oedema of the lower half, commonly seen in the elderly, is usually caused by advanced carcinoma that has either destroyed the liver and caused hypoproteinaemia, or formed large intra-abdominal masses that have obstructed the vena cava or iliac veins. This clinical picture can also be caused by the combination of two diseases: for example a disease that causes wasting, such as a carcinoma, in combination with congestive heart failure. Although you should always try to make one diagnosis wherever possible, many elderly people have more than one disease.

Overweight

Patients with normal skeletal and sexual proportions whose bodies are bigger than they should be are most likely to be obese from overeating (Fig. 1.6)! Three important medical disorders are known to cause an increase in weight that can easily be mistaken for

---

Revision panel 1.3

The common causes of wasting

In children
Severe gastroenteritis
Malabsorption syndromes

In young adults
Tuberculosis
Reticuloses
Anorexia nervosa

In middle age
Diabetes
Thyrotoxicosis
Carcinoma

In old age
Carcinoma
Senility
Gross cardiorespiratory disease

All age groups
Starvation

Fig. 1.6 Gross obesity usually affects the whole body, but may, as in this patient, be predominantly confined to the buttocks and thighs.

HISTORY-TAKING AND CLINICAL EXAMINATION

CHAPTER 1 |

> ## Revision panel 1.4
>
> ### The common causes of an increase in weight
>
> Obesity
>
> Pregnancy
>
> Interstitial fluid retention (renal, cardiac or hepatic failure)
>
> Localized fluid retention (massive ovarian cysts, ascites)
>
> Myxoedema
>
> Cushing's syndrome

Fig. 1.7 Facies of a patient with myxoedema.

obesity. These are water retention, myxoedema and Cushing's syndrome (Revision panel 1.4).

Water retention

Chronic glomerular nephritis, hypoproteinaemia, hepatic failure and cardiac failure all cause an increase in body weight as a consequence of 'fluid retention'. The whole body swells, but the swelling is most noticeable in the dependent parts.

These patients have oedema of the ankles and legs, or the sacral region if they have been confined to bed, and also in the loose tissues of the face, especially in the skin below the eyes. The swelling around the eyes is often the first symptom and is present when the patient wakes up.

Ankle oedema and sacral oedema 'pit', which is an indentation in the subcutaneous tissue produced by prolonged digital pressure.

Myxoedema

This is caused by a deficiency of thyroid hormone, usually as a result of autoimmune destruction of the thyroid gland (see Chapter 12). Patients with the condition develop a puffy face with a 'peaches and cream' complexion (Fig. 1.7), a generalized, non-pitting increase in the subcutaneous tissues of the trunk and limbs and a dulling of thought, speech and action

Cushing's syndrome

Cushing's syndrome is caused by an excess of adrenal glucocorticoids. The iatrogenic prescription of corticosteroids as a medical treatment is the most common cause. The majority of patients with endogenous Cushing's syndrome have a pituitary adenoma that secretes adrenocorticotrophic hormone (ACTH), and the rest have adrenal adenomas, adrenal hyperplasia, neurofibromas or a paraneoplastic syndrome with exogenous ACTH production, from, for instance, a carcinoma of bronchus.

The patient puts on weight, particularly on the face, neck and trunk, while the arms and legs stay thin. The face becomes 'moon shaped' (Fig. 1.8a),

(a) An increase of fat on the trunk and shoulders but thin arms and legs. Red striae can be seen on the abdomen and breasts.

(b) A round 'moon' face, some early hypertrichosis and an unusually florid acneiform rash.

Fig. 1.8 CUSHING'S SYNDROME

and the rounded, thickened shoulders are often described as a 'buffalo hump'.

There is excess of lanugo hair, and an increase in skin pigmentation with thinning leading to red–purple striae in the skin that has been stretched, particularly in the skin of the abdomen (Fig. 1.8a). Back pain from osteoporosis, hypertension and oedema are common.

Bodily disproportion

A variety of skeletal abnormalities and a few rare disorders of general body development are usually associated with chromosomal abnormalities that will be apparent from your initial general inspection (Figs. 1.9–1.11). The common conditions are shown in Revision panel 1.5 and some are discussed in more detail in other chapters in the book.

Fig. 1.9 Acromegaly. A heavy head with a prominent nose, chin and lips. These patients also have long arms and large hands and feet.

CHAPTER 1 | HISTORY-TAKING AND CLINICAL EXAMINATION

(a) The patient is tall and slim with long arms.

Fig. 1.10 MARFAN'S SYNDROME

(b) The long spindly fingers of a person with Marfan's syndrome.

(c) The high-arched palate of Marfan's syndrome.

Revision panel 1.5

Diagnoses made on initial general inspection

Paget's disease (osteitis deformans) (see Chapter 6)

Acromegaly

Marfan's syndrome

Kleinfelter's syndrome (see Chapter 18)

Turner's syndrome

Dwarfism:

    Achondroplasia
    Renal dwarfism
    'Cretinism'
    Pituitary insufficiency

(a)   (b)

Fig. 1.11 DWARFISM
(a, b) An achondroplastic child standing beside a normal child of the same age. The facial and skeletal abnormalities are all obvious. Note that the umbilicus of the achondroplastic child is below the mid-point of the vertical height.

Diseases affecting the facial appearance and head shape

This section deals with diseases that particularly affect facial expression and appearance.

Bell's palsy

Bell's palsy is an idiopathic lower motor paralysis of the facial nerve affecting the muscles of facial expression (Fig. 1.12). The absence of tone in the facial muscles makes the affected side of the face look smooth and sloppy. The corner of the mouth droops, the nasolabial creases become asymmetrical and less noticeable, and the lower eyelid droops. The asymmetry of the mouth can be increased by asking the patient to bare their teeth. The lids fail to close on the affected side when they attempt to shut their eyes.

Scleroderma

This is an autoimmune collagen disease that causes progressive thickening of the skin of the face. This reduces the patient's ability to use their

Fig. 1.12 Bell's palsy. Right-sided facial weakness.

(a) Note the tight skin, small mouth, fine wrinkles around the eyes and small telangiectases.

(b) The spindle-shaped fingers of scleroderma.

Fig. 1.13 SCLERODERMA

muscles of facial expression. The thick skin has a pale, waxy appearance. The mouth is constricted (microstomia), and jaw movements become restricted (Fig. 1.13).

Telangiectases appear on the cheeks, around the mouth and across the nose, and fine, white, horizontal scars appear on the neck. Difficulty with swallowing may be experienced (see Chapters 4, 10 and 15).

Down's syndrome

Down's syndrome is a congenital abnormality usually associated with an extra chromosome 21 (trisomy 21). It affects approximately 1 infant in 700. Males and females of all races are equally affected.

The dominant facial characteristic is that the outer ends of the palpebral fissures slant upwards and

(a) The short stature, floppiness and typical facial features of Down's syndrome.

(b) Prominent epicanthic folds (arrow).

(c) Face and nasal bridge flattened.

Fig. 1.14 DOWN'S SYNDROME

there are prominent epicanthic folds (mongoloid appearance). (Fig. 1.14) The face and nasal bridge are flattened, and the tongue protrudes. Affected children often have a squint and one-third have congenital heart disease.

Mental retardation, floppiness and a short stature are the dominant features. A Down's baby is distinguishable from a 'cretin' because their skin and hair are smooth and fine, not coarse and thick, and they are not slow and sluggish.

Abnormal skull shape including hydrocephalus

Abnormalities of the shape of the skull are described in Chapter 3.

Hydrocephalus (Fig. 1.15)

The baby may be born with a large head, often now detected by prenatal ultrasound, or the head may become enlarged after delivery if adequate drainage is not provided. There may be an associated meningomyocele (Fig. 1.16).

Fig. 1.15 Congenital hydrocephalus. The bright light behind the baby's head reveals the thinness of the bones of the skull.

Fig. 1.16 A meningo-myelocele of the spine.

Fig. 1.17 Koilonychia.

- *Pits and furrows* are associated with skin diseases such as psoriasis.
- *Bitten nails* may indicate nervousness and anxiety.

Temperature Observe the temperature of the hands – but remember that it will be affected by the air and room temperatures.

Moisture Are the patient's palms sweating excessively?

Colour Pallor of the skin of the hands, especially in the skin creases of the palm and in the nail beds, suggests anaemia. Reddish-blue hands occur in polycythaemia.

The fingers may be stained with nicotine.

Callosities The position of any callosities may reflect the patient's occupation.

Examination of the head and neck

Eyes

Look for any asymmetry of the position, size or colour of the eyes, and especially for any abnormality in the width of the palpebral fissures. This can be caused by **ptosis** (droopy eyelids) or **proptosis** (exophthalmos) when the eyeball is pushed forwards, pushing the lids apart.

The **size** and equality of the two pupils should be recorded (dilated, constricted or unequal).

The **reaction** of the pupil to light is checked by shining a bright light off and on the pupil.

THE EXAMINATION

The hands

Make early physical contact with the patient in the examination by holding their hand and counting the pulse. The physical contact that is essential for the clinical examination forges a bond between you and the patient. It is an extraordinary privilege granted to you by the patient and must never be abused.

The features that can be observed by examining the hands are as follows:

Pulse See below.

Nails Look at the colour and shape of the nails.

- *Spoon-shaped nails (koilonychia)* are associated with anaemia (Fig. 1.17).
- *Clubbing* of the nails occurs in pulmonary and cardiopulmonary disease and various gastrointestinal disorders (Fig. 1.18).
- *Splinter haemorrhages* under the nails are caused by small arterial emboli (Fig. 1.19).

Normal nail/nailfold angle

Acute angle caused by a curved nail, **not** clubbing

Nail/nailfold angle greater than 180° = **clubbing**

(a) Normal and abnormal nail/nailfold angles.

(d) Clubbing of all the fingers. Note the swelling of the terminal phalanges.

Fig. 1.18 CLUBBING

(b) A normal finger.

(c) A nail/nailfold angle of greater than 180° denotes clubbing.

Fig. 1.19 Splinter haemorrhages caused by small arterial emboli.

The pupil's reaction to accommodation is assessed by asking the patient to look into the distance and then to refocus on a finger held close to their eye.

The **eye movements** are examined by fixing the patient's head with one hand while asking them to watch your finger as it travels upwards and downwards and inwards and outwards to the full extremes of movement. Patients should be asked if they experience any **double vision (diplopia)** in any particular position. While the eye movements are being tested, the presence of any **strabismus (squint)** can usually be easily seen, which may be **concomitant (divergent or convergent)** or **paralytic**.

Look for the presence of **nystagmus** (oscillations of the eye characterized by a slow drift and a rapid jerk back) at the inward and outward extremes of movement.

Inspect the lids, conjunctiva, cornea and lens. **Styes, Meibomian cysts** and **blepharitis** may inflame the lids or cause a swelling. The edges of the eyelids may be everted or inverted **(ectropion or entropion)** and the eye may water (epiphora) if the tear duct or lacrimal sac is blocked.

A painful red eye may be caused by **acute conjunctivitis** (when there is usually an associated discharge), **acute iritis** (when the anterior chamber of the eye is inflamed), **acute glaucoma** (which is associated with severe pain and a misty cornea), **acute keratitis** (from a corneal ulcer, seen as a cloudy opacity) or an inflamed sclera in **episcleritis**.

When an elderly patient has a gradual loss of eyesight, they are likely to have a **cataract** (which can be confirmed by finding a loss of part or the whole of the 'red-reflex' when a powerful light is shone on the pupil).

Other possible causes of gradual loss of vision including **optic nerve or retinal damage**, can only be detected by inspecting the retina through an ophthalmoscope. This requires practice, and you should take every opportunity to use the ophthalmoscope by inspecting the retinas of all the patients you examine.

Ophthalmoscopy is best carried out in a darkened room to ensure that the pupils are dilated. The ophthalmoscope is an illuminated lens system that can be focused on the retina. Patients are asked to stare fixedly at a point on the wall behind the examiner. The instrument is switched on and held by its handle in the right hand. The examiner then places his right eye against the lens opening and his left hand on the patient's forehead above their right eye. He then looks through the aperture of the ophthalmoscope, and brings the instrument very close to the patient's right pupil by placing his forehead against his left hand on the patient's forehead.

The light can be watched illuminating the fundus through the pupil, as the instrument and the patient's eye are brought close together. The approach should be slightly from the temporal side, at an angle of 10–15° to the direct line, to avoid noses colliding! When the pupils are level, this approach usually ensures that the optic nerve disc is the first part of the fundus to come into view. If the disc is not seen, a retinal artery should be followed back until the edge of the pale yellow disc is seen.

The optic disc is 'cupped' by chronic glaucoma and swollen by papilloedema (Fig. 1.20).

Other abnormalities that can be detected by careful fundoscopy of the rest of the retina include haemorrhages and exudates (in diabetes and hypertension), retinal emboli and infarcts and occasionally retinal detachment. At the end of the examination, the patient should be asked to look directly at the light of the ophthalmoscope in order to inspect the macula.

Fig. 1.20 Papilloedema, a diagnostic sign of a chronically raised intracranial pressure, most often caused by a space-occupying intracranial tumour or a chronic subdural haematoma. (Courtesy of Dr E. Graham.)

A few common disorders of the eyes

Arcus senilis

This is a white rim around the outer edge of the iris caused by sclerosis and cholesterol deposition in the edge of the cornea (Fig. 1.21). It is common in the elderly. It may be associated with hyperlipoproteinaemia and often coexists with generalized atherosclerosis (see Chapter 10).

Fig. 1.21 Arcus senilis: a thin white rim around the iris (arrow). It is a common abnormality and does not indicate advanced arterial disease. Note that the patient also has a basal cell carcinoma (arrowhead) (BCC).

Xanthelasma

(Xanthoma)

These are painless opaque yellow 'fatty' plaques in the skin of the eyelids (Fig. 1.22). One or two on the eyelids do not necessarily indicate any underlying disease, but they are known to be associated with hyperlipidaemia and arterial disease.

Fig. 1.22 Xanthelasma of the upper eyelid (arrows).

Exophthalmos

(Proptosis)

This is the forward protrusion of the eye from its normal position in the orbit. In the normal eye, the lower eyelid just touches the lower edge of the iris (the inferior limbus), provided the lower lid is normal, while the upper lid crosses the eye midway between the pupil and the superior limbus. The first sign of exophthalmos is the appearance of

sclera below the inferior limbus. The proptosis has to be considerable before sclera is visible above the superior limbus (Fig. 1.23).

The position of the upper eyelid is also altered by the tone of the levator palpebrae superioris muscle. Retraction of the upper eyelid reveals sclera above the superior limbus. You will not mistake this for exophthalmos if you remember to check the position of the lower eyelid.

When the eye is pushed forwards, four secondary physical signs appear:

1. The patient can look up without wrinkling the forehead.
2. Convergence is restricted.
3. The patient blinks less often than normal.
4. The patient may not be able to close their eyes, and corneal ulceration may develop.

The conjunctiva becomes oedematous if the protrusion interferes with the venous and lymphatic drainage of the conjunctiva. This is called **chemosis**.

The causes of exophthalmos are listed in Revision panel 1.6, and the rare pulsating exophthalmos in Revision panel 1.7.

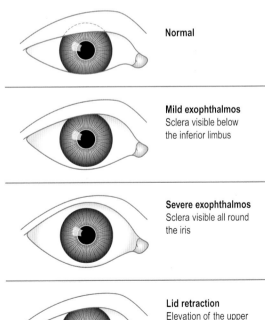

Normal

Mild exophthalmos
Sclera visible below the inferior limbus

Severe exophthalmos
Sclera visible all round the iris

Lid retraction
Elevation of the upper eyelid

Fig. 1.23 Exopthalmos/proptosis: the relations of the eyelids to the iris.

CHAPTER 1 | HISTORY-TAKING AND CLINICAL EXAMINATION

Revision panel 1.6
The causes of exophthalmos

Endocrine

Thyrotoxicosis (before, during and after its onset)

Cushing's syndrome (rare)

Non-endocrine

Congenital deformities of the skull (craniostenosis, oxycephaly, hypertelorism)

Orbital or periorbital tumours

Periorbital meningioma

Optic nerve glioma

Orbital haemangioma

Lymphoma

Osteoma

Pseudotumour (granuloma)

Carcinoma of the antrum

Neuroblastoma

Inflammation

Orbital cellulitis

Ethmoid or frontal sinusitis

Vascular causes

Cavernous sinus arterio-venous fistula

Eye disease

Severe myopia

Severe glaucoma (buphthalmos)

Revision panel 1.7
The causes of pulsating exophthalmos

Carotid artery–cavernous sinus arterio-venous fistula

Aneurysm of the ophthalmic artery

Vascular neoplasm in the orbit

Cavernous sinus thrombosis

Ectropion

In this deformity, the eyelids are everted (Fig. 1.24) because of atonia or weakness of the obicularis oculi muscles, or scarring and contracture of the lids. When the eyelid becomes everted, the tear duct is separated from the conjunctiva, which causes **epiphora** (weeping), conjunctival inflammation and exposure keratitis.

Fig. 1.24 Ectropion: eversion of the lower eyelid.

Entropion

This is present when the eyelid inverts. It is usually caused by traumatic scarring or trachoma. It causes pain, irritation and epiphora.

Subconjunctival haemorrhage

This is a bleed occurring between the conjunctiva and the sclera. It is usually spontaneous and harmless, but can be associated with a fractured base of skull, hypertension, blood dyscrasia, anticoagulation, choking (asphyxia) or scurvy.

Horner's syndrome

This is the set of physical signs that follow interruption of the sympathetic nerve supply to the head and neck arising from the first and second thoracic segments of the spinal cord (Revision panel 1.8). The sympathetic nerves pass to the three cervical ganglia, before synapsing with postganglionic nerves to the structures of the head and neck. These nerves can be interrupted by trauma or disease anywhere along this pathway.

Absence of sympathetic tone causes **miosis** (narrowing of the pupil), **ptosis** (drooping of the eyelid), **vasodilatation** and **anhidrosis** (absence of sweating) over the cheek and eye (Fig. 1.25). The condition is considered further in Chapter 2.

Fig. 1.25 Horner's syndrome.

Revision panel 1.8

Horner's syndrome

A small pupil (*myosis*)

Drooping of the upper eyelid (*ptosis*)

A warm, pink cheek (*vasodilatation*)

Absence of sweating (*anhidrosis*)

Nasal congestion (*nasal vasodilatation*)

Apparent enophthalmos

The causes of Horner's syndrome, with the common cause in bold, are:

- brain lesions – posterior inferior cerebellar artery thrombosis;
- spinal cord lesions – syringomyelia, tumours;
- injuries to the lower roots of the brachial plexus;
- surgical excision of the inferior cervical ganglion (cervical sympathectomy);
- tumours in the apex of the lung (**Pancoast tumour**);
- tumours in the neck;
- aneurysm and dissection of the carotid artery.

Ptosis

Horner's syndrome, myasthenia gravis (Fig. 1.26) and any cause of paralysis of the IIIrd cranial

nerve can cause ptosis (see Chapter 3). Some cases are congenital and many are idiopathic, listed in Revision panel 1.9.

Revision panel 1.9

The causes of ptosis

Inflammation

Tumours

Excess eyelid skin

Muscle weakness (myopathies, myasthenia) (Fig. 1.26)

IIIrd cranial nerve palsy

Fig. 1.26 Ptosis in myasthenia gravis. The heavy, dropping eyelid is much worse on the patient's left side. The eye signs of generalized diseases are often asymmetrical and sometimes even unilateral.

The ears and nose

These must be examined after the eyes. This is often forgotten during routine examination. Do not forget to look into the ears, and also remember to look up the nose. Examination of these structures is especially important if there is any possibility of disease in the head and neck

Clinical examination of the ear requires an **auroscope**. This instrument directs a beam of light down a conical metal speculum; the ear is then viewed through a lens. The speculum should be gently inserted into the external auditory meatus, while the ear is retracted upwards and backwards to straighten the external auditory canal. Wax may be present and must be removed before the tympanic membrane can be seen. The whole of the tympanic membrane can only be seen if the angle of the speculum is altered.

Normal tympanic membranes vary in colour, translucency and shape – so you should look at as many normal tympanic membranes as possible.

The external auditory canal may contain **wax** or **foreign bodies**. You may see **otitis externa** (dermatitis), **blood** or **pus**.

The tympanic membrane may be normal, torn by **injury**, bulging and inflamed (**acute otitis media**), or perforated (**chronic otitis media**).

A few common disorders of the ear and nose

Bat ears

These are ears that jut out from the side of the head rather than lying flat against it (Fig. 1.27). Cup-shaped ears that protrude from the side of the skull are a feature of Down's syndrome.

Fig. 1.27 Bat ears.

Cauliflower ears

Cauliflower ears are ears distorted by multiple subperichondral haematomas caused by repeated trauma (Fig. 1.28). They occur in boxers, wrestlers and rugby players (especially front row forwards).

Fig. 1.28 A 'cauliflower ear'. The swelling is a subperichondral haematoma and is almost blocking the external auditory meatus.

Keloid nodules

Many females and males have their ears pierced. The scar tissue may overgrow and produce a large nodule inside the lobe of the ear, especially if the hole becomes infected or the patient has any 'keloid' tendency. The nodule is firm and spherical, and may become pedunculated (Fig. 1.29).

Fig. 1.29 Keloid scars at the site of ear piercing. The mass of scar tissue usually protrudes from the posterior aspect of the ear lobe. Keloid scars are more common in black-skinned races.

Accessory auricles

These are small pieces of skin-covered cartilage separate from the pinna. They are found on the side of the face just in front of the tragus (Fig. 1.30). They are present from birth and cause no symptoms.

Fig. 1.30 An accessory auricle.

Saddle nose

The bridge of the nose is depressed and widened due to congenital abnormalities such as achondroplasia, hypertelorism (wide-set eyes) or destruction of the nasal cartilages caused by leprosy, cutaneous leishmaniasis or congenital syphilis.

Rhinophyma

This is a thickening of the skin over the tip of the nose caused by hypertrophy and adenomatous changes in its sebaceous glands (Fig. 1.31). It is not

Fig. 1.31 Rhinophyma.

caused by an excessive intake of alcohol, but can be exacerbated by it.

The mouth (see Chapter 11)

Note the colour and state of the lips. Ask to see the patient's tongue; observe its movement, symmetry and surface. Look at the teeth and gums. Use a spatula to inspect the soft palate, tonsils and posterior wall of the oropharynx.

The neck (see Chapter 12)

The important features to examine in the neck are the jugular veins, the trachea, the thyroid and the lymph glands.

Examination of the chest wall and lungs (see Chapter 2)

Inspection

Cyanosis caused by cardiopulmonary disease is most easily appreciated by inspecting the inner aspect of the lips (see pages 13, 14).

Count the rate of respiration and notice the rhythm A slow respiratory rate occurs in patients with cerebral compression or damage, while rapid respiration is often seen in patients with ventilation–perfusion mismatch.

A fluctuating respiratory rate and volume, interspersed with periods of **apnoea** (cessation of breathing) and episodes of **tachypnoea** (rapid breathing), is called **Cheyne–Stokes** or periodic respiration. It is caused by variations in the sensitivity of the respiratory centre to normal stimuli, and occurs commonly in patients with heart failure and severe cerebrovascular accidents.

Compare the duration of inspiration and expiration and note whether respiration seems to require extra voluntary effort. Watch the chest during inspiration to see if there is any inward (paradoxical) movement of the intercostal spaces. This is usually caused by obstruction to the inflow of air into the lungs, but in an injured patient may indicate instability of a segment of the chest wall (e.g. two sets of rib fractures).

Record any abnormality in the shape of the chest. The two common deformities are *funnel chest* (pectus excavatum) and *pigeon chest* (pectus carinatum) (see Chapter 2).

Palpation

Trachea Check that the trachea is in a central position at the suprasternal notch (Fig. 1.32). The trachea is deviated *away from* a 'tension' pneumothorax and *towards* a collapsed lung.

Chest expansion Spread your hands around the patient's chest so that your thumbs just meet in the midline. Ask the patient to take a deep breath. Your thumbs should be dragged apart to a distance roughly equivalent to half the chest expansion. When the expansion is asymmetrical, it will be felt and seen.

Chest expansion is the difference between the circumference of the chest at full inspiration and full expiration, measured at the level of the nipples (T4). Unilateral changes in expansion are associated with lung collapse, consolidation and interstitial lung disease (see Chapter 2).

Apex beat The apex beat is the lowest and most lateral point of the cardiac impulse. It is situated in the fifth intercostal space in the mid-clavicular line (Fig. 1.33). It is shifted laterally if the heart enlarges, and moves medially or laterally when the mediastinum changes position. The mediastinum moves to one side if it is pulled over by a collapsed, contracted lung, or pushed over by air or fluid in the opposite pleural cavity (tension pneumothorax or pleural effusion).

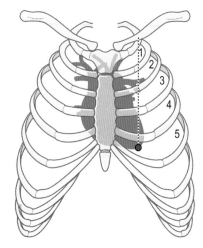

Fig. 1.33 The apex beat is normally felt in the fifth intercostal space in the mid-clavicular line.

Tactile vocal fremitus To detect this, place your whole hand firmly on the chest and ask the patient to say '99'. The vibrations that you can feel with your hand are called the **vocal fremitus**. Compare the strength of these vibrations on either side of the chest, front and back, and over the apical, middle and basal zones of the lung.

A blocked bronchus leading to lung collapse or a layer of fluid or air between the visceral and parietal layers of the pleura (pleural effusion) suppresses the

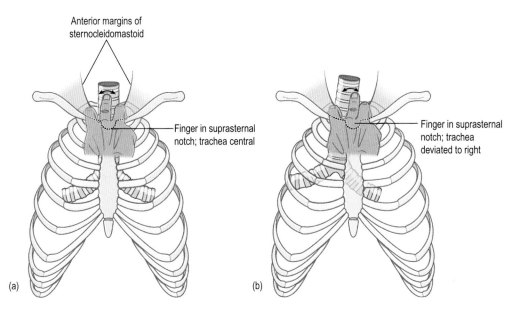

Fig. 1.32 (a) Central trachea. (b) Deviated trachea.

conduction of sound waves and reduces the intensity of the palpable fremitus.

Regional lymph nodes The axillary and supraclavicular lymph nodes may be enlarged by infection (e.g. tuberculosis or malignant lung tumours [metastases]).

Percussion

The whole of the surface of both lungs must be percussed. The surface markings of the lungs are shown in Fig. 1.34.

Place the left hand flat on the chest wall, keeping the middle finger, which you intend to strike, straight and firmly applied to the underlying skin. Tap the centre of the middle phalanx of this middle finger with the tip of the middle finger of the right hand by forcibly flexing the right wrist (Fig. 1.35).

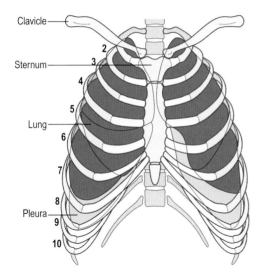

Fig. 1.34 The surface markings of the lungs.

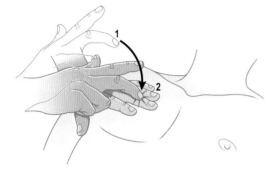

Fig. 1.35 Percussion (see text above).

Listen carefully to the sound and compare it with the sound produced by percussing the same area on the other side of the chest.

Percuss over the whole of the front and back of both lung fields. The two areas most often forgotten are the lateral zones high in the axillae and the anterior aspect of the lung apices behind the clavicles. Percuss the latter area by striking the clavicle directly with the percussing finger.

The normal chest gives a resonant sound when percussed, a sound that is, to some extent, felt by the percussing finger as well as being heard. Anything solid in the pleural space or in the substance of the lungs decreases the resonance and makes the sound dull. Any extra air, whether in the pleural space (a pneumothorax) or in the lung substance (an emphysematous bulla or multiple bullae), makes the sound more resonant (hyper-resonance).

Auscultation

The normal sounds of breathing can be heard all over the chest except over the heart and spine. A longer 'rustling' inspiratory sound is followed immediately by a shorter, softer, expiratory sound. There is no gap between the two phases. This noise is known as **vesicular breathing**' and is caused by the movement of air in and out of the smaller bronchioles and alveoli. It produces a rustling noise, which is similar to the sound of gas being blown down plastic tubing.

The sound of air moving in the larger bronchioles and main bronchi is heard over the lung fields when the periphery of the lung has been solidified by pneumonia or collapse (*atelectasis*). This sound is harsher and louder than the low rustle of vesicular breathing. The inspiratory and expiratory phases are of equal length and separated by a short, silent gap. This is called **bronchial breathing**. The quality of the sound and the presence of the gap are the two distinguishing features.

When the lung alveoli are full of fluid, exudate or pus (**consolidation**) but the air passages remain patent, the thickened lung transmits the sound from the larger bronchi, and bronchial breathing indicates an area of consolidated lung.

Absent breath sounds

Breath sounds are abolished or diminished by any process that reduces the normal conduction of sound through the lung substance and chest wall. The common causes are bronchial obstruction (producing collapse of the distal part of the lung), pleural effusion and pneumothorax.

Added sounds

There are two varieties of added sounds: referred to as **wheezes** and **crackles.**

Wheezes These are the unmistakable whistling sounds made by air passing through narrowed air passages. They are commonly heard in patients with asthma or chronic bronchitis. Their pitch depends upon the velocity of airflow and the diameter of the bronchioles from which they originate.

Crackles These caused by air passing through bronchioles containing water, mucus or pus. They may be coarse or fine.

Pleural rub The visceral and parietal layers of the pleura normally slide easily over one another without causing any sound. If the pleura is inflamed, the roughened pleural surfaces rubbing together during inspiration and expiration can produce a noise that is similar to the sound heard when a finger is pressed hard onto a pane of glass and then slid across it. It is a mixture of grating and squeaking sounds. The patient often complains of pleuritic pain over the area where the rub can be heard.

Examination of the heart and circulation (see Chapters 2 and 10)

It is common practice to feel the pulse when you take the patient's hand at the beginning of the examination (see above). Any abnormalities detected at this stage require reassessment by further careful palpation of the radial pulse.

The pulse

The following features should be observed and recorded.

The rate Count for 15 seconds or longer, especially if the pulse feels irregular, and express the rate in beats/minute.

The rhythm The pulse beat may be regular or irregular. When the pulse is irregular, it may have a regular recurring pattern or be totally irregular. The latter is sometimes called an **irregularly irregular** pulse and indicates **atrial fibrillation** (Fig. 1.36).

The volume The examining fingers can appreciate the expansion of the artery with each beat, and consequently get an impression of the amount of blood passing through the artery. Patients with a high cardiac output have a strong pulse. Patients in haemorrhagic (hypovolaemic) shock have a weak, thin, 'thready' pulse.

The nature of the pressure wave Every pressure wave has definable characteristics such as the rate of increase and decrease of pressure, and the height of the pressure. The shape of the pulse wave can be appreciated more easily over the carotid than the radial artery.

A steep rise followed by a rapid fall, with a large pulse pressure (high peak), is called a **collapsing or water-hammer pulse** and is typical of **aortic regurgitation**. Conversely, a **tight aortic stenosis** causes a slow rise and fall, called an **anacrotic pulse** (Fig. 1.37).

Compare the pulses of both wrists This should always be done because a stenosis or occlusion of the subclavian artery, or an aortic dissection, can produce asymmetrical pulses.

Rhythm and volume irregularly irregular

Fig. 1.36 Atrial fibrillation.

Flattened
Slow rise and fall, called anacrotic, caused by aortic stenosis

Fig. 1.37 An anacrotic pulse.

Measure the blood pressure

The blood pressure is usually measured in the brachial artery with a sphygmomanometer. The cuff, which must fit snugly and be at least 10 cm wide (as a narrow cuff gives false readings), should be firmly wrapped around the middle of the upper arm and inflated above the systolic pressure (250–300 mmHg). It should then be slowly deflated until the start of blood flow is detected by listening over the brachial artery at the elbow with a stethoscope or by palpating the pulse at the wrist. This pressure is the **systolic blood pressure**.

The sounds that indicate the commencement of flow in the brachial artery below the cuff are caused by turbulent blood flow. They were first described by Korotkoff and are known as *Korotkoff sounds*.

The cuff is further deflated until the Korotkoff sounds suddenly diminish or, more often, disappear. This is the **diastolic pressure**.

It is worth repeating both measurements on several occasions with the patient sitting and lying down and again at the end of the examination when the patient is more relaxed. Remember that the readings from a very fat arm will be falsely high by as much as 10 mmHg.

Note **Whenever there is the possibility of disease of the aorta and its branches, the blood pressure should be measured in both arms (see 'Compare the pulses of both wrists', above).**

Inspect the head and neck again

The signs particularly indicative of cardiovascular disease are cyanosis, plethora, xanthomata, arcus senilis and dyspnoea (see above).

Jugular venous pressure

The pressure in the great veins is slightly greater than the pressure in the right atrium. The pressure in the right atrium is one of the most important indicators and influences of cardiac activity. An increase in the right atrial pressure increases cardiac output by stimulating an increase of cardiac contractility and rate.

The pressure in the right atrium can be estimated clinically from the pressure in the internal jugular veins. In a normal person reclining at 45°, the great veins in the neck are collapsed, and there should be no visible venous pulsations above the level of the

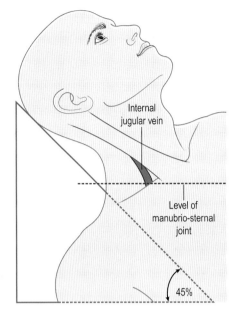

Fig. 1.38 Measurement of jugular venous pressure.

manubrio-sternal joint. When the patient is reclining at 45°, this is at the same level as the mid-point of the clavicles (Fig. 1.38). The venous pulse is seen as a double pulse wave followed by a pause, and may be elevated or visualized by compressing over the liver to increase the venous return.

The right atrial pressure is raised if there are visible pulsations in the internal jugular veins when the patient is reclining at 45°. The vertical distance between the upper limit of the venous distension and the level of the clavicle should be estimated by eye and expressed and recorded in centimetres.

Obstruction of the great veins in the superior mediastinum will also cause distension of the neck veins, but there is no visible venous pulse wave within the distended veins.

Neck arteries

The carotid, subclavian and superficial temporal pulses should be palpated in the head and neck. The whole length of the subclavian and carotid arteries should be auscultated, especially over the sternoclavicular joints, in the supraclavicular fossae and at the level of the hyoid bone just below the angle of the jaw. These sites correspond to the origins of the subclavian, vertebral and internal carotid arteries, respectively (Fig. 1.39).

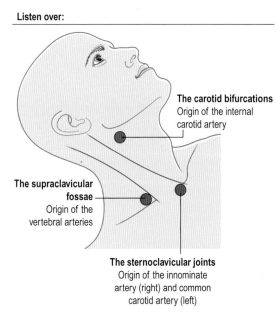

Listen over:

The carotid bifurcations
Origin of the internal carotid artery

The supraclavicular fossae
Origin of the vertebral arteries

The sternoclavicular joints
Origin of the innominate artery (right) and common carotid artery (left)

Fig. 1.39 The sites of auscultation for vascular bruits on the neck.

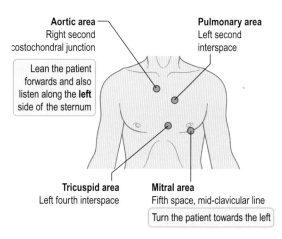

Aortic area
Right second costochondral junction

Pulmonary area
Left second interspace

Lean the patient forwards and also listen along the **left** side of the sternum

Tricuspid area
Left fourth interspace

Mitral area
Fifth space, mid-clavicular line

Turn the patient towards the left

Fig. 1.40 Areas of cardiac auscultation.

Examination of the heart (see Chapter 2)

Inspection The heart may be seen to be beating rapidly or to be heaving up the chest wall with each beat.

Palpation Place your whole hand firmly on the chest wall, just below the left nipple, and ascertain the strength of the cardiac impulse. It may be weak, normal or heaving in nature.

The **apex beat** is the lowest and most lateral point at which the cardiac impulse can be felt (and seen; see above). It should be in the fifth intercostal space, in the mid-clavicular line (an imaginary vertical line that passes through the middle of the clavicle). The apex beat moves laterally and may be felt in the mid-axillary line if the heart is enlarged.

It may also be possible to feel vibrations, called **thrills**, which correspond to audible heart murmurs. Thrills may be felt during systole, during diastole or throughout the whole cardiac cycle.

Remember to palpate the back of the chest. Thrills from abnormalities of the aorta, such as a **patent ductus arteriosus** or a **coarctation of the aorta**, are conducted posteriorly as well as anteriorly.

Percussion The area of cardiac dullness should be delineated by percussion.

Auscultation The whole of the anterior aspect of the heart must be examined with the stethoscope, but the areas where the sounds from the four valves are best heard are shown in Fig. 1.40.

Begin by listening at the apex of the heart (the mitral area) before listening over the aortic, pulmonary and tricuspid areas. Identify the **first and second heart sounds**.

The heart sounds are traditionally described as sounding like the words **lub-dub**; that is to say, the first sound is slightly longer and softer than the second sound. As this is not always the case, it is wise to confirm that the sound you believe to be the first sound corresponds to the beginning of the cardiac impulse or coincides with the subclavian or carotid pulse.

Having decided which sound is which, listen carefully to the **second sound**. It may be sharper and shorter than usual – almost a **click** – or it may be **split**. A double, or split, second sound occurs when the aortic and pulmonary valves close asynchronously. A double sound can be heard when the sounds are 0.2 or more seconds apart and indicates **pulmonary hypertension**.

Next, listen carefully to the intervals between the two main sounds, and between diastole and systole, for any **additional heart sounds or murmurs**.

Murmurs are caused by turbulent flow and the vibration of parts of the heart. They may vary in nature from a low-pitched rumble to a high-toned swish. Try to decide whether the murmur occupies the whole or part of diastole or systole and whether its intensity changes.

Think of the way you are going to record your findings (Fig. 1.41), two blocks for the main heart sounds (M and T, and A and P) and a zig-zag line for the murmur. Imagine your drawing as you listen to the sound and you will find it easier to define the timing of the murmur.

The sounds at the apex, from the mitral valve, can be made louder by asking the patient to turn over onto their left side; the aortic valve sounds can be amplified by asking the patient to lean forwards.

Always listen to the heart sounds at the back of the chest. The murmur of a patent ductus or coarctation can often be heard over the aorta, posteriorly, just to the left of the midline.

Test for oedema

Oedema commonly appears first in the feet and ankles, but may be more apparent in the sacral and buttock regions if the patient has been bedridden for some time. Cardiac oedema is very soft and 'pits' easily. The common causes of ankle oedema are listed in Revision panel 1.10.

Examination of the abdomen

Examination of the abdomen is described in detail in Chapter 15. A large number of patients with surgical disease have intra-abdominal pathology, so a good technique for abdominal examination is essential.

Examination of the abdomen follows the standard pattern:

- Inspection for asymmetry, distension, masses, visible peristalsis and skin discolouration.
- Palpation for superficial and deep tenderness, the normal viscera (liver, spleen and kidneys) and any abnormal masses.
- Percussion of the liver and splenic areas and any other masses.
- Auscultation for bowel sounds and vascular bruits.
- Rectal examination and vaginal examination.

Mitral incompetence

M&T   A&P

Pansystolic murmur
Soft first sound
May be a short mid-diastolic murmur preceded by a third sound

Mitral stenosis

o.s.   M&T   A&P

Diastolic murmur with a presystolic crescendo preceded by an opening snap (o.s.)
Loud first sound

Aortic incompetence

M&T   A&P

Early diastolic mumur
May be a soft mid-diastolic murmur

Aortic stenosis

M&T   A&P

Systolic murmur preceded by an ejection click (e)
Split second sound

Patent ductus arteriosus

M&T   A&P

'Machinery' murmur
Continuous throughout systole and diastole

Fig. 1.41 The sounds of some common cardiac abnormalities. M and T, first heart sound; A and P, second heart sound.

There are four things that should always be remembered:

1. Palpate the supraclavicular lymph glands.
2. Palpate the hernial orifices.
3. Feel the femoral pulses.
4. Examine the genitalia.

Note **Always remember to listen to the abdomen, and always carry out a rectal examination.**

Examination of the limbs

There are four main tissues to be examined in a limb:

- the bones and joints (see Chapters 6, 7 and 8);
- the muscles and soft tissues (Chapters 6, 7 and 8);
- the arteries and veins (Chapter 10);
- the nerves (Chapter 3).

The examination of these structures is covered elsewhere in the book as indicated.

Test the urine, faeces and sputum

It is important to note the colour and smell of the urine before using the modern simple dipstick methods for testing it for sugar, blood, acetone and protein. Do not forget to measure the specific gravity of the urine, and to inspect any precipitate under the microscope.

Look at the faeces if the patient complains that they are abnormal. This can be inspected on the glove used for rectal examination (see Chapter 16).

Look at the sputum if the patient is producing any.

HISTORY AND EXAMINATION OF A LUMP

History

Most patients with a lump feel it frequently and should be able to answer the following (Revision panel 1.11).

1. **When was the lump first noticed?**
   It is important to be precise with dates and terminology. Do not write 'the lump first

---

Revision panel 1.11

The history of a lump or an ulcer

Duration
When was it first noticed?

First symptom
What brought it to the patient's notice?

Other symptoms
What symptoms does it cause?

Progression
How has it changed since it was first noticed?

Persistence
Has it ever disappeared or healed?

Multiplicity
Has (or had) the patient any other lumps or ulcers?

Cause
What does the patient think caused it?

---

appeared 6 months ago', when you mean 'the lump was first noticed 6 months ago'.

Many lumps may exist for months, even years, before the patient notices them.

2. **What made the patient notice the lump?**
   There are four common answers to this question:
   - 'I felt or saw it when washing.'
   - 'I had a pain and found the lump when I felt the painful area.'
   - 'Someone else noticed it and told me about it.'
   - 'I found it on self examination', for example a breast lump in a female.

3. **What are the symptoms of the lump?**
   The lump may be painful, and if it is, you must take a careful history of the pain, as described earlier in this chapter (see page 9). The presence or absence of pain may in itself be important, particularly if it is the presenting feature. Pain is usually associated with inflammation, not neoplastic change. Many patients expect cancer to be painful and

therefore often ignore a malignant lump just because it does not hurt.

The characteristic feature of pain associated with acute infection is its throbbing nature.

A lump may be disfiguring or interfere with movement, respiration or swallowing. Describe the history of each symptom carefully.

4. **Has the lump changed since it was first noticed?**

   The patient should be able to tell you if the lump has got bigger or smaller, or has fluctuated in size and when they noticed a change in size.

   They may also have appreciated other changes in the nature of the lump that they can tell you about.

5. **Does the lump ever disappear?**

   A lump may disappear on lying down, or during exercise, and yet be irreducible at the time of your examination.

   The patient should always be asked if the lump ever disappears completely, because this physical characteristic is peculiar to only a few types of lump.

6. **Has the patient ever had any other lumps?**

   You must ask this question because it might not have occurred to the patient that there could be any connection between their present lump and a previous lump, or even a coexisting one (e.g. neurofibromas or lipomas).

7. **What does the patient think caused the lump?**

   Lumps occasionally follow injuries or systemic illnesses known only to the patient.

Examination (Revision panel 1.12)

Site/position The location of a lump must be described in exact anatomical terms, using distances measured from bony points. Do not guess distances; use a tape measure.

Colour and texture of the overlying skin The skin over a lump may be discoloured, may be inflamed or may have become smooth and shiny, or thick and rough.

Shape Remember that lumps have three dimensions. You cannot have a circular lump because a circle is a plane figure. Many lumps are not spherical, elliptical or hemispherical, but have an asymmetrical outline. In these circumstances, it is permissible to use descriptive terms such as **dumb-bell shaped**, **pear shaped** or **kidney shaped**.

Size Once the shape has been established, it is possible to measure its dimensions.

Remember that all solid objects have at least three dimensions: width, length and height or depth, although the latter may be impossible to measure clinically. Asymmetrical lumps will need more measurements to describe them accurately, and sometimes a diagram will clarify your written description.

Surface The first feature of the lump that you will feel will be its surface. It may be **smooth or irregular**. An irregular surface may be covered with smooth bumps, rather like cobblestones, which can be called **bosselated**, or may be irregular or rough.

There may be a mixture of surfaces if the lump is large.

Temperature Is the lump hot or of normal temperature? Assess the skin temperature with the dorsal surfaces of your fingers, because they are usually dry (free of sweat) and cool.

Tenderness Is the lump tender? If so, is the whole lump tender? Always try to feel the non-tender part before feeling the tender area, and watch the patient's face to ensure that you are not causing discomfort as you palpate.

Edge The edge of a lump may be **clearly defined or indistinct**. It may have a definite pattern.

Composition Any lump must be composed of one or more of the following:

- calcified tissues such as bone, which make it '**bony-hard**';
- tightly packed cells, which make it '**solid' or 'firm' or 'rubbery**' depending on the tissue of origin and the individual's stromal response;
- extravascular fluid, such as urine, serum, cerebrospinal fluid, synovial fluid or extravascular blood, which make the lump '**soft and cystic**';
- **gas,** which makes it soft and compressible;
- **intravascular blood,** which makes it pulsatile.

The physical signs that help you decide the composition of a lump are: consistency, fluctuation, a fluid thrill, translucency, resonance, pulsatility, compressibility and bruits.

CHAPTER 1 | HISTORY-TAKING AND CLINICAL EXAMINATION

Consistency The consistency of a lump may vary from very soft to very hard. As it is difficult to describe hardness, it is common practice to compare the consistency of a lump to well-known objects.

A simple scale for consistency is as follows:

- Stony hard: not indentable – usually bone or calcification.
- Firm: hard but not as hard as bone – similar to an unripe apple or pear.
- Rubbery but slightly squashable – similar to a rubber ball.
- Spongy: soft and very squashable, but still with some resilience, like a sponge.
- Soft: squashable and with no resilience, like a balloon.

The consistency of a lump is dependent not only upon its structure, but also on the tension within the lump. **Some fluid-filled lumps feel hard, some solid lumps are soft;** therefore, the final decision about composition of a lump (i.e. whether it is fluid or solid) rarely depends solely upon an assessment of the consistency.

Fluctuation Pressure on one side of a fluid-filled cavity makes all the other surfaces protrude (Fig. 1.42). This is because an increase of pressure within a cavity is transmitted equally and at right angles to all parts of its wall. When you press on one aspect of a solid lump, it may or may not bulge out in another direction, but it will not bulge outwards in every other direction.

Fig. 1.42 Fluctuation.

Fluctuation is elicited by feeling at least two other areas of the lump between the thumb and index finger of the left hand while pressing on a third central point with the index finger of the right hand (Fig. 1.42). The lump fluctuates and contains fluid if two areas on opposite aspects of the lump bulge out when a third area is pressed in. This examination should be carried out in two planes, the second at right angles to the first.

Fluid thrill A percussion wave is easily conducted across a large fluid collection or cyst but not across a solid mass. The presence of a fluid thrill is detected by tapping one side of the lump, by flicking the middle finger of the right hand against the thumb, and feeling the transmitted vibration when it reaches the other side, where the second detecting left hand is placed (Fig. 1.43). When it is present, a fluid thrill is a diagnostic and extremely valuable physical sign.

Fig. 1.43 Fluid thrill.

Beware – a percussion wave can be transmitted along the wall of a large swelling. This is prevented by placing the edge of the patient's or an assistant's hand on the lump midway between the percussing and palpating hands. Percussion waves cannot be felt across small fluid-filled lumps because the wave moves so quickly that the time gap cannot be appreciated or distinguished from the mechanical shaking of the tissue caused by the percussion.

Translucency (transillumination) Light passes easily through clear fluids but does not pass through solid tissues. A lump that transilluminates must contain water, serum, lymph or plasma. Highly refractile light can also appear to transilluminate through a large lipoma (see page 146), while blood and other opaque fluids do not transmit light.

Transillumination requires a bright pinpoint light source and a darkened room. The light should be placed on one side of the lump, not directly on top of it. Transillumination is present when the whole lump glows at a distance from the light source (Fig. 1.44).

Attempts at transillumination with a poor-quality flashlight in a bright room are bound to fail and mislead. The room must be really dark!

Resonance Solid and fluid-filled lumps sound dull when percussed. A gas-filled lump, such as a hernial sac containing bowel, sounds hollow and resonant.

Pulsatility Lumps may pulsate because they are near to an artery and are moved by its pulsations (**transmitted pulsation**) or because they are connected with the heart or arterial system (**expansile pulsation**). The most common cause of expansile pulsation is an aneurysm, with, rarely, very vascular tumours.

Always let your hand rest still for a few seconds on every lump to discover if it is pulsating. When a lump pulsates, you must find out whether the pulsations are transmitted or are expansile. Place a finger (or fingers if the lump is large) of each hand on opposite sides of the lump and feel if they are pushed **outwards and upwards**. When they are,

Fig. 1.44 Transillumination of a ganglion of the thumb.
Note: Light is visible beyond the site of application.

Fig. 1.45 Transmitted versus expansile pulsation.

the lump has an *expansile* pulsation. When they are pushed only **upwards,** the lump has a *transmitted* pulsation (Fig. 1.45).

Compressibility Some fluid-filled lumps can be compressed until they disappear. When the compressing hand is removed, the lump re-forms. This finding is a common feature of **vascular malformations and fluid collections** that can be pushed back into a cavity, a joint or a cistern (see Chapter 10). **Compressibility should not be confused with reducibility** (see below). A lump that is reducible – such as a hernia – can be pushed away into another place but will often not reappear spontaneously without the stimulus of coughing or gravity.

Reducibility You should always see if a lump is reducible (disappears) by gently compressing it. A reducible lump becomes smaller and then moves to another place as it is compressed. It may disappear quite suddenly after appropriate pressure has been applied. The lump may return, when you ask the patient to cough, expanding as it does so. This is called a **cough impulse and is a feature of hernias** and some vascular lumps. The reduction can be maintained by pressing over the point at which the lump finally disappeared.

In some ways, the differences between compressibility (see above) and reducibility are semantic.

Bruits Always listen to a lump. A systolic bruit or a machinery murmur (throughout both systole and diastole) may be audible over vascular lumps that contain an arteriovenous fistula. Audible bowel sounds can be heard over a hernia containing bowel.

Relations to surrounding structures By careful palpation, it is usually possible to decide which structure contains the lump, and what its relation is to the overlying and deeper tissues. The attachment of skin and other superficial structures to a lump can easily be determined because both are readily accessible to the examiner and any limitation of their movement easily felt. The lump should be gently moved while the skin is inspected for movement or 'puckering'.

Attachment to deeper structures is more difficult to determine. **The underlying muscles must be tensed** to see if this reduces the mobility of an overlying lump or makes it easier or more difficult to feel (Fig. 1.46). The former indicates that the lump is attached to the fascia covering the superficial surface of the muscle or to the muscle itself; the latter that the lump is within or deep to the muscles.

Lumps that are attached to bone move very little, if at all!

Lumps that are attached to or arising from vessels or nerves may be moved from side to side across the length of the vessel or nerve, but not up and down along their length.

Lumps in the abdomen that are freely mobile usually arise from the intestine, its mesentery or the omentum (see Chapter 15).

Movement   No movement

Fig. 1.46 Attachment of lumps to the skin and deep tissue.

State of the regional lymph glands Never forget to palpate the lymph glands that would normally drain lymph from the region occupied by the lump:

- the skin, muscles and bones of the limbs and trunk drain to the axillary and inguinal glands;
- the head and neck to the cervical glands;
- and the intra-abdominal structures to the preaortic and para-aortic glands.

Local tissues It is important to examine the overlying and nearby skin, subcutaneous tissues, muscles and bones, and the local circulation and nerve supply of adjacent tissues. This is more relevant when examining an ulcer, but some lumps are associated with a local vascular or neurological abnormality, so this part of the examination must not be forgotten, as for example skin ulceration can occur over a locally advanced breast cancer.

General examination It is often tempting to examine only the lump about which the patient is complaining. This will cause you to make innumerable misdiagnoses.

Note **You must always examine the whole patient.**

Revision panel 1.12

The examination of a lump or ulcer

Local examination

Site

Size

Shape

Surface

Depth

Colour

Temperature

Tenderness

Edge

Composition:
  Consistency
  Fluctuation
  Fluid thrill
  Translucency
  Resonance
  Pulsatility
  Compressibility
  Bruit

Reducibility

Relations to surrounding structures – mobility/fixity

Regional lymph glands

State of local tissues:
  Arteries
  Nerves
  Bones and joints

General examination

HISTORY AND EXAMINATION OF AN ULCER

An ulcer is 'a dissolution of the continuity of an epithelium' (i.e. an epithelial defect, not a wound). Unless their ulcers are painless or in an inaccessible part of the body, patients notice ulcers from the moment they begin, and can describe most of their clinical features.

HISTORY

The questions to be asked concerning an ulcer follow a pattern similar to those asked about a lump.

1. **When was the ulcer first noticed?**
   Ask the patient when the ulcer began and whether it could have been present for some time before it was noticed. The latter often occurs with neurotrophic ulcers on the sole of the foot.
2. **What drew the patient's attention to the ulcer?**
   The most common reason is pain, but the 'sore' or defect may be visible. Occasionally, the presenting feature is bleeding, or a purulent discharge, which may be foul smelling.
3. **What are the symptoms of the ulcer?**
   The ulcer may be painful. It may interfere with daily activities such as walking, eating or defaecation.
   Record the history of each symptom.
4. **How has the ulcer changed since it first appeared?**
   The patient's observations about changes in size, shape, discharge and pain are likely to be accurate. If the ulcer has healed and broken down, record the features of each episode.
5. **Has the patient ever had a similar ulcer on the same site, or elsewhere?**
   Obtain a complete history of any previous ulcer.
6. **What does the patient think caused the ulcer?**
   Many patients believe they know the cause of their ulcer, and they are often right. In many cases, it is trauma. When possible, the severity and type of injury should be assessed. A large ulcer following a minor injury suggests that the skin was abnormal before the injury, which is then the final cause of breakdown in an already damaged epithelium.

EXAMINATION

The examination of an ulcer follows the same pattern as the examination of a lump. When an ulcer has an irregular shape that is difficult to describe, draw it in your notes and add the dimensions. When an exact record of size and shape is needed, place a thin sheet of sterile transparent plastic sheet over the ulcer and trace around its edge with a felt-tipped pen.

After recording the site, size and shape of the ulcer, you must examine the base (surface), edge, depth, discharge and surrounding tissues, the state of the local tissues and local lymph glands and complete the general examination.

Base

The base, or floor, of an ulcer usually consists of slough or granulation tissue (capillaries, collagen, fibroblasts, bacteria and inflammatory cells – pus), but recognizable structures such as tendon or bone may be visible. The nature of the floor occasionally gives some indication of the cause of the ulcer:

- Solid brown or grey dead tissue indicates full-thickness skin death.
- Syphilitic ulcers (nowadays rare) have a slough that looks like a yellow–grey wash-leather.
- Tuberculous ulcers have a base of bluish unhealthy granulation tissue.
- Ischaemic ulcers often contain poor granulation tissue, and tendons and other structures may lie bare in their base.

The redness of the granulation tissue reflects its underlying vascularity and indicates the ability of the ulcer to heal. Healing epidermis is seen as a pale layer extending in over the granulation tissue from the edge of the ulcer.

Edge

There are five types of edge (Fig. 1.47).

A flat, gently sloping edge This indicates that the ulcer is shallow, and this type of ulcer is usually relatively superficial. Venous ulcers usually have this

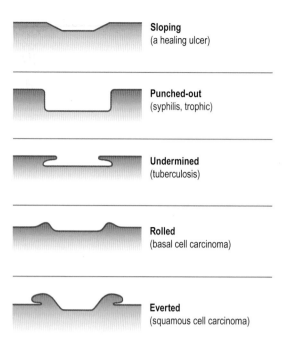

Sloping
(a healing ulcer)

Punched-out
(syphilis, trophic)

Undermined
(tuberculosis)

Rolled
(basal cell carcinoma)

Everted
(squamous cell carcinoma)

Fig. 1.47 The varieties of ulcer edge.

type of edge, but so do many other types of ulcer. The new skin growing in around the edge of a healing ulcer is pale pink and almost transparent.

A square-cut or punched-out edge This follows the rapid death and loss of the whole thickness of the skin without much attempt at repair of the defect. This form of ulcer is most often seen in the foot where pressure has occurred on an insensitive piece of skin, i.e. a **trophic ulcer** secondary to a neurological defect. The classic textbook example of a punched-out ulcer is the ulcer of **tertiary syphilis**, but these lesions are rare today in Europe. Most of the punched-out ulcers that are now seen are caused by the neuropathy of **diabetes and peripheral arterial ischaemia** or, outside Europe and North America, **leprosy**.

An undermined edge When an infection in an ulcer affects the subcutaneous tissues more than the skin, the edge becomes undermined. This type of ulcer is commonly seen in the buttock as a result of **pressure necrosis**, because the subcutaneous fat is more susceptible to pressure than the skin; however, the classic textbook example is the **tuberculous**

ulcer – which is now uncommon in Europe and North America.

A rolled edge This develops when there is slow growth of tissue in the edge of the ulcer. The edge looks like the heaped-up mound around an ancient Roman earthwork. A rolled edge is typical, and almost diagnostic, of a **basal cell carcinoma (rodent ulcer)**. The edge is usually pale pink or white, with clumps and clusters of cells visible through the paper-thin superficial covering of squamous cells. Telangiectases are commonly seen in the pearly edge.

An everted edge This develops when the tissue in the edge of the ulcer is growing so rapidly that it spills out of the ulcer to overlap the normal skin. An everted edge is **typical of a carcinoma** and is seen in the skin, in the bowel, in the bladder and in the respiratory tract.

Depth

Record the depth of the ulcer in millimetres, and anatomically by describing the structures it has penetrated or reached.

Discharge

The discharge from an ulcer may be serous, sanguineous, serosanguinous or purulent. There may be a considerable quantity of discharge, which is easily visible, or it may only be apparent from inspection of the patient's dressings.

You may be unable to see the features of the ulcer if it is covered with coagulated discharge (a scab). This may have to be removed to examine the ulcer properly. Students should not do this without the permission of the doctor in charge of the patient.

Relations

Describe the relations of the ulcer to its surrounding tissues, particularly those deep to it. It is important to know if the ulcer is adherent or invading deep structures such as tendons, periosteum and bone – which may indicate the presence of osteomyelitis.

The local lymph glands must be carefully examined. They may be enlarged because of secondary infection or secondary tumour deposits, and they may be tender.

State of the local tissues

Pay particular attention to the local blood supply and innervation of the adjacent skin. Many ulcers in the lower limbs are secondary to vascular and neurological disease. There may also be evidence of previous ulcers that have healed.

General examination

This is very important because many systemic diseases as well as many skin diseases present with 'ulcers'. Examine the whole patient with care, looking especially at their hands and facies, which can supply important clues to the diagnosis (see above).

Revision panel 1.13

The four basic techniques

Inspection

Palpation

Percussion

Auscultation

And with a joint

Look

Feel

Move

Revision panel 1.14

A classification of the aetiology of disease

Congenital

Genetic

Sporadic

Acquired

Traumatic

Inflammatory:

Physical
Chemical
Infection:
    Viral
    Bacterial
    Rickettsial
    Spirochaetal
    Protozoal
    Fungal
    Helminthic
    Mycoplasm
    Prions

Neoplastic:
    Benign
    Malignant
    Primary:
        Carcinoma
        Sarcoma
        Others
Secondary

Degenerative

Autoimmune

Proliferative

Metabolic

Hormonal

Mechanical

Vascular

Self-induced

Psychosomatic

Iatrogenic

2 The heart, lungs and pleura

INTRODUCTION

The chest is an airtight cage. Its movements and pressure changes enable ventilation of the lungs, while the bony chest wall protects the lungs, trachea, heart, great vessels, thymus and oesophagus.

The history-taking and physical examination pertinent to disorders of the chest are described in Chapter 1.

The main symptoms of chest disease – chest pain, cough and shortness of breath – are common to a number of disorders affecting the heart, lungs, pleura, chest wall and mediastinum. There is also a considerable overlap in the clinical signs of heart and lung disorders.

Some diseases of the chest may be without symptoms and clinical signs. For example, the first presentation of ischaemic heart disease can be a fatal episode of ventricular fibrillation, while a lung cancer may be detected only incidentally when a chest X-ray is performed for a completely different reason (see *Investigation and Management*, Chapter 14).

BREATHLESSNESS

Breathlessness is usually the result of lung or heart disease, although it can be caused by severe anaemia (see Chapter 1). The causes are summarized in Revision panel 2.1.

Dyspnoea is the sensation of breathlessness experienced by patients. It is usually first felt during exercise, such as climbing hills and stairs. As symptoms become more severe, patients may be breathless on minimal exertion (e.g. dressing or brushing their teeth) or even at rest.

Characteristics of breathlessness

Onset and duration

Dyspnoea of acute onset is usually noticed at rest. Development over a few minutes suggests an inhaled foreign body, a pneumothorax, severe acute asthma, a pulmonary embolism or pulmonary oedema (usually as a consequence of an acute myocardial infarction or decompensation of pre-existing heart failure).

Development over a slightly longer period – typically hours to days – is more characteristic of pneumonia, acute asthma, acute bronchitis, retained secretions, a haemothorax, an empyema or pulmonary haemorrhage.

Chronic breathlessness is often first noticed on exercise and increases with time. In airway obstruction secondary to an endobronchial tumour, a pleural effusion, a pericardial effusion or anaemia, symptoms come on over weeks and months.

The onset of breathlessness can be much more insidious, perhaps over several years, with many patients attributing their symptoms to 'old age'. Conditions that present like this include interstitial lung disease, chronic obstructive pulmonary disease (COPD) and emphysema. Mediastinal masses, hyperthyroidism and cardiac disorders (including ischaemic heart disease, valvular heart disease and the cardiomyopathies) also develop slowly.

Severity

The severity of chronic breathlessness from lung disease is graded according to the Medical Research Council Dyspnoea Scale, a useful measure of disability (Revision panel 2.2).

Revision panel 2.1

The causes of breathlessness

Airways

Asthma

Chronic obstructive pulmonary disease (COPD)

Obstruction of the airways (e.g. tumour of the trachea or major bronchi, inhaled foreign body, sputum retention)

Tracheomalacia

Lung parenchyma

Pulmonary embolus

Pneumonia

Pulmonary oedema

Interstitial lung disease

COPD/emphysema/bullous lung disease

Pulmonary contusion

Pulmonary haemorrhage

Pleural space

Pleural effusion

Pneumothorax

Pleural tumour (e.g. mesothelioma)

Haemothorax

Empyema

Heart

Valvular heart disease

Ischaemic heart disease

Cardiomyopathies

Arrhythmias

Pericardial effusion

Cyanotic congenital heart disease

Chest wall and diaphragm

Trauma (fractured ribs) with associated pain

Flail chest

Diaphragmatic hernia

Diaphragmatic paralysis

Mediastinum

Mediastinal lymphadenopathy

Large mediastinal mass

Other

Anaemia

Hyperthyroidism

Revision panel 2.2

The Medical Research Council Dyspnoea Scale

1. Not troubled by breathlessness except on strenuous exercise
2. Short of breath when hurrying or walking up a slight hill
3. Walks slower than contemporaries on level ground because of breathlessness, or has to stop for breath when walking at own pace
4. Stops for breath after walking about 100 m or after a few minutes on level ground
5. Too breathless to leave the house, or breathless when dressing or undressing

The equivalent scale for heart disease is the New York Heart Association (NYHA) Functional Classification (Revision panel 2.3). A higher NYHA class is associated with a worse prognosis.

Effect of posture

Orthopnoea is the sensation or worsening of breathlessness when lying flat. It is a symptom of pulmonary oedema secondary to heart failure. Patients often sleep with several pillows or in an upright position.

Trepopnoea is breathlessness experienced while lying on one side, but not on the other. It is a symptom of unilateral chest disease (such as a collapsed lung

Revision panel 2.3

NYHA Functional Classification

1. Cardiac disease present, but no symptoms and no limitation in ordinary physical activity, such as walking and climbing stairs
2. Mild symptoms (mild shortness of breath and/or angina) and slight limitation during ordinary activity
3. Marked limitation in activity caused by symptoms, even during ordinary activity such as walking short distances (20–100 m). Comfortable only at rest
4. Severe limitations, with symptoms even at rest. Mostly bedbound

secondary to endobronchial obstruction). The patient tends to lie with the diseased side upwards, as this eases symptoms by increasing perfusion to the good lung.

Nocturnal breathlessness

Paroxysmal nocturnal dyspnoea (PND) occurs in patients with heart failure and is a consequence of enhanced renal reabsorption at night, which leads to increased circulatory volume. After several hours' sleep, the patient wakes with a frightening sensation of suffocation. The symptoms usually subside after half an hour, and are relieved by sitting upright.

Associated symptoms

Fatigue and lethargy are commonly associated with chronic dyspnoea. Patients report a progressive reduction in exercise tolerance. Anorexia and weight loss may also occur.

PNEUMOTHORAX

A pneumothorax is a collection of air within the pleural space resulting in lung collapse. It can cause respiratory and eventually haemodynamic distress, depending on the size and type of pneumothorax (Fig. 2.1).

Primary spontaneous pneumothoraces are caused by a ruptured apical subpleural bleb or bulla. Secondary spontaneous pneumothoraces are the result of underlying lung disease. The most common cause is a ruptured bulla on a background of emphysema. Other causes are listed in Revision panel 2.4.

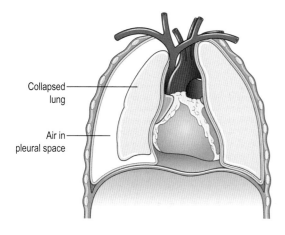

Fig. 2.1 Pneumothorax.

Collapsed lung

Air in pleural space

> ### Revision panel 2.4
> ## Causes of pneumothorax
> **Primary**
> Apical bleb or bulla
>
> **Secondary**
> COPD and emphysema
> Cystic fibrosis
> Cavitating infections and tumours (e.g. tuberculosis)
> *Pneumocystis jiroveci (carinii)* pneumonia in AIDS patients
> Alpha-1 antitrypsin deficiency
> Connective tissue disorders
> Catamenial pneumothorax (associated with menstruation)
> Trauma (blunt or penetrating)

History

Age Primary spontaneous pneumothoraces occur in young adults (peak age 16–30 years). Secondary pneumothoraces tend to occur in late middle and old age.

Symptoms The two main symptoms are shortness of breath and pleuritic chest pain localized to the side of the pneumothorax. The onset is usually sudden. There may have been similar episodes before, but the first episode is often very frightening for the patient.

Previous history

In primary spontaneous pneumothorax, there are no predisposing factors. Smoking is only a risk factor for recurrence. A history of chronic lung disease, particularly COPD and emphysema as a result of smoking, will almost certainly be present in middle-aged and elderly patients with a secondary pneumothorax. Marfan's syndrome (see Chapter 1) is associated with an increased incidence of pneumothorax in younger people.

Examination

General appearance Patients who present with a primary pneumothorax are typically tall and thin.

The stigmata of the underlying chest disease may be present in patients with a secondary pneumothorax. Patients with COPD may have a barrel-shaped chest and pursed-lip breathing.

CHAPTER 2 | THE HEART, LUNGS AND PLEURA

Inspection Tachypnoea (a respiratory rate of more than 20 breaths per minute) is often present. Respiratory rates may be significantly higher with a large pneumothorax or when there is severe underlying chest disease. Tachycardia is common, but evidence of shock indicates a tension pneumothorax (see below). In severe cases, there may be central cyanosis but surgical emphysema is uncommon (Fig. 2.2).

Palpation The trachea is usually central in the case of a simple pneumothorax. Deviation to the contralateral side occurs in tension pneumothorax. Surgical emphysema is sometimes palpable just beneath the skin covering the anterior chest wall and neck.

Percussion Classically, a hyper-resonant, or *tympanic*, percussion note is detected on the ipsilateral side.

Auscultation Air entry on the ipsilateral side is quiet or absent, while breath sounds and air entry on the contralateral side should be normal. A crackling sound will be heard as the stethoscope compresses the skin if surgical emphysema is present.

Fig. 2.2 Gross surgical emphysema in a patient with a drained pneumothorax and ongoing air leak.

Tension pneumothorax

This uncommon but dangerous condition occurs if a breach in the visceral pleura covering the lung acts as a one-way valve between the lung and the pleural space. The volume and pressure of air in the pleural space increase with every breath, causing movement of the mediastinum away from the pneumothorax, reduced venous return to the heart and eventually shock (Fig. 2.3).

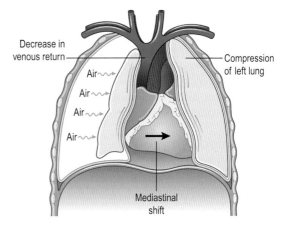

Decrease in venous return

Compression of left lung

Air

Air

Air

Air

Mediastinal shift

Fig. 2.3 Tension pneumothorax.

Examination

On examination, there will be distended neck veins, deviation of the trachea to the contralateral side and signs of shock if left untreated. Urgent measures are needed (see *Investigation and Management*, Chapter 14).

PLEURAL EFFUSION

This is defined as fluid in the pleural space, formed when the rate of pleural fluid production is greater than the rate of resorption (Fig. 2.4). Increased

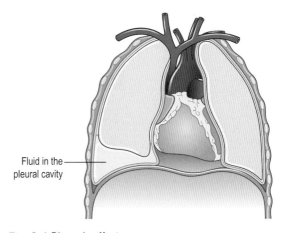

Fluid in the pleural cavity

Fig. 2.4 Pleural effusion.

production of fluid occurs in diseases causing pleural inflammation or in heart failure, while reduced fluid resorption can be caused by tumour deposits.

Bilateral effusions tend to be transudates, characterized by a protein content of less than 30 g/L, occurring in heart failure, hypoalbuminaemia, liver failure, renal failure or hypothyroidism.

Unilateral effusions tend to be exudates with a higher protein content. The many causes are shown in Revision panel 2.5. Pleural infection and malignancy are most common.

Revision panel 2.5

Causes of a pleural exudate

Chest
Pneumonia (may lead to empyema)

Other infections (e.g. tuberculosis)

Malignancy (e.g. mesothelioma, lung cancer, metastatic disease)

Pulmonary embolus

Trapped lung, where the lung cannot expand because of a constricting coat caused by infection or tumour

Haemothorax

Chylothorax

Gastrointestinal tract, abdomen and pelvis
Acute pancreatitis

Subphrenic abscess

Oesophageal perforation

Meig's syndrome (associated ovarian tumour)

Iatrogenic
Radiation therapy

Post surgery (e.g. coronary artery bypass, liver transplant)

Collagen vascular disease
Rheumatoid arthritis

Systemic lupus erythematosus

Granulomatosis with polyangiitis

Idiopathic

History

Age Patients with pleural effusions are usually elderly because the underlying diseases are more common in this age group.

Symptoms Shortness of breath and chest discomfort are the two main symptoms. There is usually a progressive increase in the severity of symptoms over several months. In patients with pneumonia, this may be days or weeks, and after an oesophageal rupture the effusion is immediate (see Chapter 15).

Occasionally, chest pain is severe, especially with pleural malignancy. The pain is usually pleuritic in nature. However, invasion of the chest wall can cause deep-seated pain.

Weight loss and general malaise may also occur.

Previous history

Occupational exposure to asbestos makes mesothelioma more likely (see below). A history of previously treated malignancy, particularly cancers of the lung or breast or a cancer of gynaecological origin, may indicate a metastatic relapse.

Examination

Effusions of more than 300 mL are usually detectable clinically at the lung bases.

General appearance There may be stigmata of the underlying cause, such as rheumatoid arthritis, systemic lupus erythematosus or heart failure. Wasting and cachexia are present in advanced metastatic malignancy.

Inspection A high respiratory rate indicates a large effusion, bilateral effusions or a patient with little respiratory reserve.

Reduced chest wall movement is sometimes seen on the side of the effusion.

Palpation The trachea is usually central, except with massive effusions, when it may be deviated away from the affected side.

Tactile vocal fremitus is reduced over the effusion.

Percussion The percussion note over the fluid is described as *stony dull*.

Auscultation Air entry is reduced or absent under the fluid. Sometimes bronchial breathing can be heard in the collapsed lung just above the fluid level. Vocal resonance is reduced, differentiating the effusion from consolidation.

Chylothorax produces physical signs identical to those of a pleural effusion. Half of the cases are caused by trauma, most commonly iatrogenic damage to the thoracic duct during chest surgery. Malignancy (lymphoma or metastatic disease) accounts for the bulk of the remaining cases.

MESOTHELIOMA

Mesotheliomas are rare malignant tumours arising from the mesothelial layer of the pleura. In almost all cases, the cause is asbestos exposure, typically 30–40 years earlier. The incidence in the UK is around 2000 cases per year, and is expected to increase for another 10 or 15 years.

History

Dyspnoea results from either the presence of a pleural effusion or the mass effect of the pleural tumour. The underlying lung may not able to re-expand after drainage of an effusion if it is encased by tumour on the visceral pleural surface (*trapped lung*).

Chest pain is either pleuritic, or more deep-seated and 'gnawing' in nature as a consequence of chest wall and intercostal nerve invasion.

Examination

On examination, the physical signs are those of a pleural effusion.

EMPYEMA

An empyema is a collection of pus in the pleural space (Fig. 2.5).

An empyema develops from a parapneumonic effusion complicating a pneumonia. Only a small proportion of these effusions go on to become empyemas.

An iatrogenic empyema can complicate chest surgery or chest drain insertion. Untreated, serious complications can develop (Revision panel 2.6).

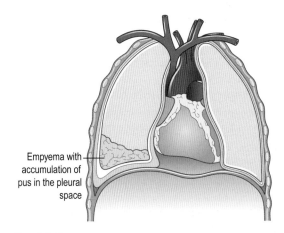

Empyema with accumulation of pus in the pleural space

Fig. 2.5 Empyema.

> ### Revision panel 2.6
> ## Complications of an empyema
> Bronchopleural fistula (invasion into the bronchial tree)
> Empyema necessitatis (invasion through the chest wall with spontaneous external drainage)
> Hemithorax contraction secondary to chronic pleural fibrosis
> Osteomyelitis (Fig. 2.6)
> Death

Fig. 2.6 Sternal osteomyelitis in an intravenous drug user following a traumatic sternal fracture.

There are three stages in the development of an empyema:

1. *Exudative.* A simple pleural effusion becomes complicated by infection.
2. *Fibrinopurulent.* A macroscopically purulent effusion develops with fibrin deposition, which may cause the effusion to become loculated.
3. *Organizing/chronic.* The pus is viscous and both the visceral and parietal pleurae become thickened, encasing the lung.

History

Age An empyema complicating a pneumonia can occur at any age.

Symptoms There is often a history of a respiratory tract infection, or symptoms of general malaise, over the previous few weeks or months.

Patients may be *breathless* caused by lung compression by the pleural pus, restriction of normal chest wall and lung excursion by scar tissue over the parietal and visceral pleura, or lung consolidation.

Vague ipsilateral *chest discomfort* or pleuritic chest pain is sometimes a dominant feature.

Fever is common, and the patient may experience sweats and rigors.

A *cough* with purulent sputum may still persist from the original pneumonia.

Examination

General appearance Although some patients look relatively well, others show signs of systemic sepsis (hypotension, tachycardia and respiratory distress).

A swinging fever, typical of a collection of pus, is often seen, and the patient may appear flushed and sweaty.

Inspection Chest movement may be reduced on the affected side. The trachea is only deviated if there is associated lung collapse (deviated to the ipsilateral side) or a massive effusion (deviated to the contralateral side).

Palpation Vocal resonance is reduced over an empyema, and there may be reduced chest wall excursion.

Percussion A dull or stony dull percussion note is characteristic of an effusion or empyema.

Auscultation Air entry is usually reduced or absent over the empyema, as is vocal resonance and whispering pectoriloquy.

PULMONARY EMBOLISM

Pulmonary embolism is usually a complication of venous thromboembolic disease (see Chapter 10) (Revision panel 2.7). Less frequently, air, fat and amniotic fluid embolize to the lungs. Reduced pulmonary blood flow, local inflammation and right heart strain are responsible for the ensuing signs and symptoms.

History

Age Although the incidence increases with age, pulmonary emboli can occur at any age.

Symptoms Many pulmonary emboli are symptomless, while some present as sudden death.

The most common clinical presentation is with a sudden onset of breathlessness, often accompanied by pleuritic chest pain. The pain may heighten

---

> ### Revision panel 2.7
> #### Risk factors for deep vein thrombosis/pulmonary embolus
> - Immobility
> - Surgery
> - Pregnancy
> - Obesity
> - Cancer
> - Increasing age
> - Genetic thrombophilias (e.g. protein C deficiency, protein S deficiency, antithrombin III deficiency, antiphospholipid syndrome)
> - Acquired prothrombotic disorders (e.g. nephrotic syndrome)

---

the sensation of breathlessness by preventing deep inspiration. Haemoptysis occasionally occurs.

Some patients present with a swollen painful leg secondary to an underlying deep venous thrombosis.

Examination

Inspection Patients who have had a massive pulmonary embolism may be centrally and peripherally cyanosed (see Chapter 1), with tachypnoea and signs of cardiovascular collapse (tachycardia, hypotension, cool peripheries).

A raised jugular venous pressure (JVP) is indicative of right heart strain.

Even in severe cases, examination of the chest is often normal except for the presence of tachypnoea.

Auscultation A pleural rub may appear later in the disease process. Right ventricular strain can produce a loud second heart sound as a result of loud pulmonary valve closure. Fixed splitting of the second heart sound may develop.

LUNG CANCER

Lung cancer is the most common cause of cancer death in the world. Smoking is the main risk factor, and around one in 10 smokers develop lung cancer. Around 40 000 new patients are diagnosed each year in the UK, of whom less than 10 per cent survive 5 years.

There are two main histological types: small cell, and non-small cell.

- *Non-small cell* tumours include adenocarcinomas, squamous cell carcinomas and large cell carcinomas.
- *Small cell* tumours are less common and are part of a spectrum of neuroendocrine lung malignancies that includes carcinoid tumours and large cell neuroendocrine carcinomas.

Common sites of distant spread include the mediastinal lymph nodes, the liver, the adrenal glands, the bones and the brain. Metastases are more common in small cell carcinoma than in other types.

History

Age The incidence of lung cancer increases with age and is uncommon before the age of 50 years.

Symptoms Around one-fifth of patients are symptomless when diagnosed, their lung cancer being picked up incidentally on a routine chest X-ray. These patients are likely to have operable disease, but those with symptoms tend to have more advanced disease.

Patients may also present acutely with chest sepsis, thromboembolic disease, hypercalcaemia or other symptoms of metastatic disease.

Shortness of breath may be caused by:

- pneumonia, lobar collapse or lung collapse distal to an obstructing bronchial tumour;
- partial obstruction of the major airways (trachea or main bronchi) by endobronchial tumour, causing impaired airflow;
- extrinsic compression of the major airways by mediastinal invasion or mediastinal lymphadenopathy;
- invasion and occlusion of a pulmonary artery;
- pulmonary emboli;
- pleural effusion secondary to metastatic spread of disease;
- pericardial effusion secondary to either metastatic spread or direct invasion of the pericardium;
- invasion of the phrenic nerve with diaphragmatic palsy;
- underlying COPD or emphysema;
- anaemia.

Cough is a common symptom. It may have an insidious onset and be persistent and non-productive in nature. Coughs are caused by local irritation of the airways or recurrent chest infections secondary to bronchial obstruction.

Haemoptysis may occur but is usually of small volume.

Chest pain can occur in more peripheral tumours. Pleuritic pain may be a consequence of repeated chest infections and pleural inflammation. Invasion of the chest wall produces a localized deep, gnawing pain. Subsequent involvement of the intercostal nerve causes pain referred anteriorly to the affected dermatome.

Non-specific symptoms such as loss of appetite, weight loss, malaise, fatigue and low-grade fevers are common. Significant weight loss is a poor prognostic sign.

Other symptoms caused by local spread include:

- stridor from involvement of the major airways by either endobronchial tumour or extrinsic compression;
- facial swelling as a result of superior vena cava obstruction (SVCO) secondary to mediastinal lymphadenopathy or invasive right hilar tumours;
- dysphagia from direct invasion or extrinsic compression of the oesophagus;
- hoarseness from invasion of the recurrent laryngeal nerve (usually the left nerve because of its origin in the aorto-pulmonary window and long course in the chest);
- arm pain (brachial plexus invasion in a Pancoast tumour, see below);
- palpitations from pericardial involvement.

Symptoms from distant spread are present in 30–40 per cent of patients at diagnosis. These include:

- bone metastases, causing bone pain and pathological fractures;
- brain metastases, resulting in space-occupying symptoms such as headache and nausea, and central nervous system signs;
- liver metastases with abdominal pain and jaundice (see Chapter15)
- paraneoplastic syndromes (Revision panel 2.8).

Risk factors Ninety per cent of patients with lung cancer will be current or ex-smokers. A smoking history should be expressed in pack years – one packet of 20 cigarettes a day for 1 year equates to a pack year (7300 cigarettes!).

Revision panel 2.8

Paraneoplastic syndromes associated with lung cancer

Endocrine/metabolic

Water retention with hyponatraemia (syndrome of inappropriate antidiuretic hormone secretion)

Hypercalcaemia (parathormone-like hormone)

Cushing's syndrome (adrenocorticotrophic hormone)

Gynaecomastia

Neurological

Peripheral neuropathy

Polymyositis

Eaton–Lambert syndrome

Skeletal

Finger clubbing

Hypertrophic pulmonary osteoarthropathy

Cutaneous

Hyperkeratosis

Hyperpigmentation

Dermatomyositis

Acanthosis nigricans

Fig. 2.7 Acute superior vena cava obstruction secondary to locally advanced non-small cell lung cancer. The upper half of the torso is erythematous with engorged veins and venous flaring.

A previously cured lung cancer, exposure to asbestos and exposure to radon gas are other risk factors for lung cancer.

Examination

General appearance Cachexia may be the result of metastatic lung cancer or pre-existing emphysema.

Jaundice suggests liver metastases, while anaemia may be the result of significant or prolonged haemoptysis or the consequence of chronic disease.

Finger clubbing is a paraneoplastic syndrome (see Chapter 1).

Examination of the neck may reveal metastatic cervical lymphadenopathy (see Chapter 12).

Distended neck veins are seen in both SVCO and pericardial effusion. The face and chest wall may also be engorged, swollen and plethoric in SVCO (Fig. 2.7).

Horner's syndrome is the result of invasion of the stellate sympathetic ganglion, normally by a Pancoast tumour (see Chapter 1).

Direct spread into the pericardium can produce arrhythmias or signs of cardiac tamponade (see below).

Examination of the respiratory system is often normal, but there may be signs of pneumonia, pleural effusion, lobar collapse, lung collapse or airway compression.

Inspection Stridor (see below) may be audible from the end of the bed, and is the result of critical airway narrowing. It is often associated with an increased respiratory effort.

Unilateral reduced chest movement can be caused by the collapse of a lobe or a lung secondary to bronchial obstruction.

Palpation The trachea is deviated to the side of any lobar or lung collapse. By contrast, reduced chest movement with tracheal deviation to the contralateral side is seen with massive pleural effusions.

Percussion This is dull over a collapsed lung or a pleural effusion.

Auscultation Stridor or a wheeze may be heard over an area of major airway compression or partial obstruction.

Air entry is reduced at the lung base in lobar collapse and throughout the whole lung in lung collapse.

Coarse upper airways noises may be heard throughout if there are problems clearing secretions past an obstruction.

HEART FAILURE

Heart failure is the final end result of all diseases of the heart. Over the age of 65 years, around 1 in 10 people will have heart failure. The causes are shown in Revision panel 2.9.

History

Shortness of breath/dyspnoea is the most common symptom and is the result of pulmonary oedema. It is not a symptom specific for heart failure, but when accompanied by orthopnoea, and in particular PND, heart failure is the likely diagnosis. Its severity is graded according to the NYHA Functional Classification (see Revision panel 2.3).

Nocturnal cough can also occur as part of the same process, and pulmonary oedema may also manifest itself as a *wheeze*.

Reduced exercise tolerance with lethargy and fatigue is due to exertional dyspnoea, muscle wasting and loss of sleep from PND.

Ankle swelling is another common but non-specific symptom, and is a result of right heart failure (itself usually a consequence of left heart failure).

Previous history

Previous ischaemic heart disease, hypertension and valvular heart disease are common.

Examination

General appearance Cachexia and muscle wasting occur in severe heart failure, but in less severe forms there may be few physical signs.

Examination of the pulse may reveal tachycardia (as a result of sympathetic overdrive) or *pulsus alternans* (the poor prognostic sign of alternating weak and strong beats sometimes seen in left ventricular failure). Arrhythmias are also common, especially atrial fibrillation.

Distended neck veins (elevated JVP) result from elevated right heart pressures (Fig. 2.8).

Oedema of the ankles and feet is a common but non-specific sign – immobility is a more common cause of ankle swelling. In gross heart failure, tender hepatomegaly and ascites may be present.

Revision panel 2.9

Causes of heart failure

Ischaemic heart disease
Myocardial infarction
Ongoing myocardial ischaemia ('hibernating myocardium')

Hypertension
Valvular heart disease
Mitral valve disease
Aortic valve disease

Congenital heart disease
Atrial septal defect
Ventricular septal defect

Cardiomyopathy
Cardiac arrhythmias
Alcohol and drugs
Alcohol
Beta-blockers, calcium antagonists

Pericardial disease
Constrictive pericarditis
Pericardial effusion

Primary right heart failure
Cor pulmonale
Pulmonary embolism
Primary pulmonary hypertension
Tricuspid valve regurgitation

Fig. 2.8 Distended neck veins in a patient with heart failure.

Palpation A displaced apex beat indicates an enlarged heart, while right ventricular heave is a sign of right heart failure.

Auscultation Fine inspiratory crackles heard at the lung bases indicate the presence of pulmonary oedema.

A third heart sound or 'gallop rhythm' is a classical sign but may be difficult to appreciate.

A murmur should be heard if the heart failure is secondary to valvular heart disease.

VALVULAR DISEASE

Mitral regurgitation

Mitral regurgitation is the most common heart valve disorder. It is usually a consequence of myxomatous degeneration, or 'floppy' valve prolapse. In the past, rheumatic heart disease was a common cause, usually associated with a degree of mitral stenosis.

Functional mitral regurgitation can occur as a result of left ventricular failure in ischaemic heart disease. It can also occur after an infarction of a papillary muscle following a myocardial infarction, or from valvular destruction in infective endocarditis.

Mitral regurgitation leads to volume overload (and increased preload) of the left heart because a significant proportion of the potential cardiac output is ejected back into the left atrium during systole, subjecting the lungs to persistently high pressure.

History

Initially, the heart compensates as a consequence of left atrial enlargement and left ventricular hypertrophy. Symptoms are often mild or non-existent. As the regurgitation becomes more severe, the heart decompensates, and breathlessness on exertion, fatigue and other symptoms of heart failure/pulmonary oedema develop.

Palpitations are very common, and usually the result of atrial fibrillation.

Examination

General features The irregularly irregular pulse of atrial fibrillation is common, and a tachycardia may be present in those patients with decompensated heart failure. With more severe regurgitation, other signs of heart failure such as ankle oedema and a raised JVP are likely.

Palpation The apex beat may be displaced to the left and become hyperdynamic.

Auscultation A pansystolic murmur loudest at the apex indicates mitral regurgitation. The murmur can radiate to the axilla or lower left back. Its loudness is not necessarily related to the severity of the regurgitation. A third heart sound is also sometimes heard.

Mitral stenosis

Rheumatic fever and heart disease following a throat infection with a beta-haemolytic *Streptococcus* is responsible for almost all cases of mitral stenosis. The bacterial antigens cross-react with various tissues including the heart valves, joints and basal ganglia (Sydenham's chorea). The commissures become fused, the leaflets thickened and the chordae shortened.

In countries where rheumatic fever is endemic (those with overcrowding and poor living conditions), mitral stenosis is the most common heart valve abnormality.

Narrowing of the mitral valve orifice leads to an increased pressure gradient across the valve during diastole. As the stenosis becomes more severe with time, the obstruction to the forward flow of blood becomes greater, resulting in increased left atrial pressures, atrial dilatation complicated by thrombosis, atrial fibrillation and pulmonary oedema. Right heart failure will also develop.

History

Initial symptoms are experienced 15–20 years after the first episode of rheumatic fever.

Breathlessness is the most common symptom, and is often worse on lying flat.

Fatigue and other symptoms of heart failure develop as the stenosis becomes more severe. Associated heart failure can cause haemoptysis.

Palpitations are commonly the result of atrial fibrillation, the risk increasing with the degree of stenosis.

Thromboembolic disease presents most commonly as a stroke secondary to cerebral emboli. Other sites for emboli are the legs and mesenteric vessels.

Examination

Appearance The term 'mitral facies' refers to the red cheeks but otherwise pallid complexion of those

CHAPTER 2 | THE HEART, LUNGS AND PLEURA

with severe mitral stenosis. It is not a specific sign and is seen in some normal individuals.

Cachexia is not uncommon (see Chapter 1) and progresses with the severity of the stenosis, as do the other signs of heart failure.

Atrial fibrillation is common, particularly in the later stages of the disease.

Palpation The increased shock of closure of the mitral valve may be appreciated as a 'tapping' apex beat. Sometimes the murmur of mitral stenosis can be felt as a thrill, which may be described as feeling like the back of a purring cat. A left parasternal or right ventricular heave indicates pulmonary hypertension and right heart failure.

Auscultation An opening snap is heard immediately after the second heart sound, followed by a low-pitched mid-diastolic murmur. These added sounds are heard best with the patient turned towards their left side.

Aortic regurgitation

Aortic regurgitation can often coexist with aortic stenosis, as any pathological process that restricts valve opening can also impair valve closure. Other causes of regurgitation include rheumatic fever, a congenitally bicuspid aortic valve, infective endocarditis, aortic dissection and syphilis. Dilatation of the aortic root and ascending aorta as a result of Marfan's syndrome or annulo-aortic ectasia is another cause.

The result is volume overload and increased preload of the left heart. A proportion of the cardiac output flows back into the left ventricle from the aorta during diastole. This leads to left ventricular hypertrophy and dilatation, and eventually to heart failure if left untreated.

History

Patients with acute aortic regurgitation secondary to infective endocarditis or aortic dissection can present with acute heart failure and cardiovascular collapse. Those with chronic aortic regurgitation may, however, be asymptomatic for a considerable period of time because the left ventricle adapts to the volume overload. As the heart begins to decompensate, symptoms of heart failure appear.

Examination

General appearance In the later stages of the disease, signs of heart failure may be obvious.

A number of specific signs can be attributed to the low diastolic blood pressure and wide pulse pressure found in aortic regurgitation:

- Water hammer pulse – accentuation of the radial pulse when lifting the arm.
- Quincke's sign – capillary pulsation in the nail beds.
- De Musset's sign – head nodding in time with the heart beat.
- Pulsatile liver – more often associated with tricuspid incompetence.

Palpation The apex beat is hyperdynamic and may be displaced laterally in later stages of the disease.

Auscultation An early diastolic murmur is almost always heard, loudest at the lower left sternal edge. It is sometimes easier to hear when the patient leans forward and pauses at the end of expiration. As the left ventricle decompensates with time, a third heart sound or gallop rhythm develops.

A regurgitant jet of blood can interfere with the opening of the mitral valve and produce a mid-diastolic murmur at the left apex similar to that of mitral stenosis. This is called the *Austin Flint murmur*.

Aortic stenosis

The most common cause of aortic stenosis is senile aortic calcification, followed by secondary calcification of a congenitally bicuspid aortic valve.

Rheumatic heart disease accounts for most of the remaining cases.

Narrowing of the aortic valve orifice leads to an increased pressure gradient across the valve during systole. Obstruction to the forward flow of blood from the left ventricle through the aortic valve and into the aorta leads to pressure overload (and increased afterload) that is compensated for by left ventricular hypertrophy. As the aortic stenosis becomes more severe with time, the left ventricular pressure increases further and ventricular dilatation develops, which subsequently causes the heart to fail.

History

Age Senile calcification is uncommon before the age of 65 years. With a bicuspid aortic valve, calcification and stenosis occurs in middle age.

The triad of symptoms Most patients with mild to moderate aortic stenosis are asymptomatic. As the stenosis becomes more severe, one or more of angina, breathlessness and syncope follow (Stokes-Adams attacks).

The stage at which the symptoms appear is a good prognostic indicator. The onset of angina is associated with a median survival of 5 years, syncope with 3 years, and breathlessness and other symptoms of heart failure with only 2 years.

Examination

Pulse The pulse is typically slow-rising or low in volume.

Palpation In severe stenosis with preserved ventricular function, a thrill may be felt in the second right intercostal space, at the sternal notch or over the carotid arteries.

Auscultation The murmur of aortic stenosis is an ejection systolic murmur heard loudest in the second right intercostal space. It can radiate to the neck and be confused with a carotid bruit. As the heart begins to fail, the murmur becomes softer.

Tricuspid regurgitation

This rarely develops in isolation, and the valve usually becomes incompetent as a consequence of high right-sided pressures and subsequent right ventricular dilatation. The most common cause is left heart failure. Another cause of such functional regurgitation is cor pulmonale. Infective endocarditis in intravenous drug users can result in destruction of the valve, causing regurgitation.

Examination

Inspection The JVP is raised, with large visible V waves occurring in systole. Peripheral oedema is often present.

Palpation A large pulsatile liver may be palpable in the right hypochondrium. Ascites may also be present.

Auscultation A pansystolic murmur can sometimes be heard, loudest at the lower left sternal edge on inspiration.

Pulmonary valve disease

This is rare. Pulmonary stenosis is congenital and can occur at the level of the pulmonary valve, below the valve (right ventricular outflow tract) or above the valve (pulmonary artery). It most commonly occurs in isolation, but is associated with other conditions such as tetralogy of Fallot.

In severe pulmonary stenosis, right atrial pressures rise and can force open the foramen ovale, causing a right to left shunt of deoxygenated blood and central cyanosis. In less severe cases, right heart failure can develop over time, producing the signs of elevated JVP, peripheral oedema and hepatomegaly.

Pulmonary regurgitation is usually acquired and may be the result of pulmonary hypertension (e.g. cor pulmonale), infective endocarditis, rheumatic fever, carcinoid syndrome or trauma (usually iatrogenic following surgery for pulmonary stenosis or tetralogy of Fallot). The symptoms that predominate are those of the underlying cause. Right ventricular hypertrophy produces a right ventricular heave on examination. The subsequent development of right heart failure produces the signs described above.

INFECTIVE ENDOCARDITIS

This is an infection of the endocardium that results in vegetations on the heart valves from a repeated cycle of bacterial infection and platelet and thrombus deposition.

In intravenous drug abusers, the tricuspid valve, as the first valve the infected material meets, is most commonly affected. In other cases, there is often pre-existing congenital or acquired valve pathology, and the left-sided valves (aortic and mitral) are usually affected.

Any bacteraemic episode can potentially cause endocarditis, Gram-positive cocci predominating. Causes include dental surgery or poor dental hygiene, any other surgery, and long-term central venous lines.

History

Age The elderly are most at risk.

Symptoms *Fever* is the principal symptom, with night sweats, rigors, lethargy, muscle aches and general malaise, easily confused with influenza. Once a heart valve becomes regurgitant as a consequence of local tissue destruction, the symptoms of heart failure become apparent.

Neurological symptoms result from septic emboli to the brain.

Risk factors include previous heart valve disease, a history of rheumatic fever, the insertion of prosthetic valves, congenital heart disease and intravenous drug abuse.

CHAPTER 2 | THE HEART, LUNGS AND PLEURA

Pyrexia of unknown origin Endocarditis should be suspected in any immunocompromised patient with a persistent fever.

Examination

General examination A fever is invariably present. Nowadays, the classic vascular phenomena secondary to septic emboli or an immune complex-mediated vasculitis are only occasionally seen. These include splinter haemorrhages (see Fig. 1.19), Janeway lesions (erythmatous non-tender lesions on the soles or palms), Osler's nodes (painful nodules on the finger pulps or digits) and Roth's spots (retinal haemorrhages with pale centres).

Septic emboli to the brain are not uncommon, and neurological signs will be present in 15 per cent of patients.

Chest A new or changing murmur, most commonly of aortic regurgitation, is heard in one-third of patients. Signs of heart failure such as a gallop rhythm or the bi-basal inspiratory crackles of pulmonary oedema occur in those with valve incompetence.

CONGENITAL HEART DISEASE

There are many congenital cardiac anomalies. They can be divided into septal defects, obstructive defects and cyanotic defects. The most common are:

- *Septal defect:*
  - Atrial septal defect (ASD)
  - Ventricular septal defect (VSD)
- *Obstructive defects:*
  - Aortic stenosis (see above)
  - Pulmonary stenosis (see above)
  - Coarctation of the aorta
- *Cyanotic defects:*
  - Tetralogy of Fallot
  - Transposition of the great vessels.

Other conditions affect the great vessels but are commonly classified with the congenital heart defects, including patent ductus arteriosus.

Patent ductus arteriosus

This common congenital cardiac defect (5–10 per cent of all cases) results from failure of the ductus arteriosus to close at birth (Fig. 2.9). When the shunt

Fig. 2.9 Patent ductus arteriosus. AO aorta; LA left atrium; LV left ventricle; PA pulmonary artery; RA right atrium; RV right ventricle.

is large, oxygenated blood flows from the systemic circulation into the pulmonary circulation, raising the pulmonary arterial and right heart pressures, and causing engorgement of the pulmonary vasculature. The left ventricle is subject to volume overload, and will fail with time if left untreated.

Many patients with small shunts have few symptoms and signs throughout life. *Symptoms* include dyspnoea and fatigue on exertion with failure to grow.

On examination, the pulses are bounding with cyanosis of the lower body. A continuous 'machinery' murmur is heard best in the left second intercostal space. Signs of heart failure eventually develop, occurring more quickly with larger shunts.

Atrial septal defect

The atria are connected through the foramen ovale before birth to allow oxygenated blood arriving in the right atrium from the placenta to bypass the non-functional fetal lungs and enter the systemic left heart circulation. When the lungs expand at birth, pulmonary vascular resistance drops, and the right atrial pressure falls below that of the left atrium. The flap valve (septum primum) in the foramen ovale closes and seals to the septum secundum (Fig 2.10). Failure of this process results in a patent foramen ovale. An ostium secundum (ASD) forms if this is associated with abnormal development of the septum secundum.

Fig. 2.10 Atrial septal defect.

Three patterns of ASD are recognized: ostium secundum (as above, accounting for 80 per cent of ASDs), and two less common but more complex defects (ostium primum and sinus venosus defects).

The compliant right ventricle allows a large left to right shunt, eventually causing the right heart size to increase and the pulmonary pressure to rise. In some cases, the pulmonary arterial pressure may rise sufficiently to reverse the shunt. This rare occurrence is known as *Eisenmenger's syndrome*.

Symptoms are often absent for many years, but some children may suffer from recurrent chest infections, fatigue and shortness of breath on exertion.

Decompensation usually occurs between 30 and 50 years of age, and is indicated by decreased exercise tolerance, fatigue, dyspnoea, palpitations secondary to atrial arrhythmias and syncopal attacks.

Some patients present in adulthood with paradoxical emboli. Thrombi from the lower limb veins pass through the defect into the systemic circulation and may cause strokes.

On examination atrial fibrillation or flutter is common.

Right ventricular dilatation and hypertrophy may be detected as a right heart 'heave'.

There is a fixed wide split of the second heart sound, which does not alter with respiration. An ejection systolic murmur is produced by increased flow across the pulmonary valve. Flow across the ASD cannot be heard.

Cyanosis and finger clubbing indicate the onset of Eisenmenger's syndrome.

Ventricular septal defect

Many congenital VSDs close spontaneously in early life. In children with persistent and large defects, blood flows into the right ventricle from the higher pressure left ventricle, causing pulmonary hypertension (Fig 2.11). There is an increased incidence of VSD in children with Down's syndrome and other congenital conditions.

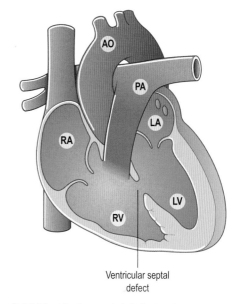

Fig. 2.11 Ventricular septal defect.

VSD may also be acquired in adulthood as a complication of myocardial infarction (see below).

Symptoms are usually minimal at first, but dyspnoea, recurrent chest infections, poor feeding and failure to thrive develop in children with large defects causing cardiac failure.

On examination, there is often evidence of an enlarged and displaced apex beat with a right heart heave and a thrill.

There is fixed splitting of the second heart sound, and a loud pansystolic murmur heard best at the left sternal edge.

Cyanosis indicates Eisenmenger's syndrome (see above).

Coarctation of the aorta

Coarctation means 'narrowing' and refers to obstruction of blood flow in the aorta, usually just distal to the origin of the left subclavian artery around the level of the ductus arteriosus. The defect varies in severity and length from a long-segment narrow stenosis to a discrete shelf. To supply blood to the lower body, large collaterals form between the branches of the subclavian arteries and the intercostals, and upper limb hypertension develops.

Males are affected twice as commonly as females. Associations include Turner's syndrome and left-sided congenital cardiac defects.

Symptoms may be absent in mild cases, and only present in later life with hypertension and its complications. Neonates with severe coarctations may present with cardiovascular collapse as the ductus closes. In between these two extremes, symptoms include dyspnoea, poor feeding and failure to thrive.

Increasing dyspnoea, faintness, chest pain and fatigue indicate the onset of heart failure. Headaches and nosebleeds may be caused by the associated hypertension, and impaired circulation to the lower limbs may cause intermittent claudication.

On examination, there are weak femoral and distal pulses that contrast with bounding 'hypertensive' pulses in the upper limbs. An associated discrepancy in the blood pressure of 20 mmHg or more (the pressure being higher in the brachial vessels) is diagnostic. Palpation of the peripheral pulses will reveal a radial-femoral delay.

An abnormal pulsation or thrill may be felt in the suprasternal notch. An ejection systolic murmur situated over the coarctation, to the left of the spine posteriorly, is often heard.

Tetralogy of Fallot

The four components are:

- a VSD;
- the aorta over-riding the defect (straddling the VSD), causing it to receive deoxygenated blood from the right ventricle;
- obstruction of the right ventricular outflow tract/pulmonary valve;
- an abnormally thick right ventricular wall (Fig. 2.12).

A proportion of the deoxygenated blood in the right ventricle passes through the VSD into the left ventricle and aorta, producing varying degrees of cyanosis. When the child becomes upset, the right ventricular outflow tract muscle can contract, exacerbating the obstruction and causing more right to left shunting of deoxygenated blood. The resulting cyanotic episodes are known as 'blue spells' or 'tet spells'.

(a) Normal heart.

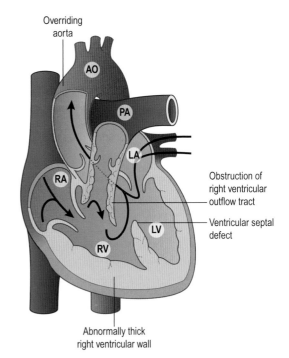

(b) Tetralogy of Fallot

Fig. 2.12 TETRALOGY OF FALLOT

History

Symptoms The child may be 'blue' or cyanotic at birth, or become blue when active, feeding or upset. In older children, a characteristic squatting posture may relieve the hypoxaemia caused by these spells by kinking the femoral arteries, raising the systemic resistance, reducing the right to left shunt and forcing more blood through the lungs.

On examination, central cyanosis suggests the diagnosis. Finger clubbing develops early. Right ventricular heave is often present.

There is a systolic murmur from the pulmonary stenosis heard best at the left sternal edge and associated with a palpable thrill. It may disappear during a cyanotic spell.

Transposition of the great vessels

In this rare condition, the aorta arises from the right ventricle, and the pulmonary artery from the left ventricle. Survival after birth is dependent on arterial and venous blood mixing through various septal defects and a patent ductus arteriosus. The condition is incompatible with life without surgical intervention.

Cyanosis is usually present at birth, and a number of murmurs indicate the existence of the shunts described above.

LEFT ATRIAL MYXOMA

This rare benign tumour can present in three distinct ways:

- As the tumour enlarges, it can obstruct blood flow, mimicking mitral stenosis, causing dyspnoea, orthopnoea and PND. There may be a murmur that varies with posture.
- A distal embolus or stroke may occur. All recovered embolic material should always be sent for histological examination.
- There may be non-specific symptoms of fever and malaise, with raised inflammatory markers.

COUGH

A cough is a forced expulsion of air from the lungs, initially against a closed glottis, accompanied by a characteristic sound. It may be a voluntary manoeuvre or an involuntary reflex. Its purpose is protective, and it serves to move and clear secretions, foreign bodies or other irritants from the airways. An occasional cough is, of course, a normal and necessary part of everyday life, but a persistent or troublesome cough may be the first symptom of underlying disease.

By far the most common cause of an acute cough is a viral upper respiratory tract infection. A chronic cough is most commonly caused by postnasal drip, asthma, eosinophilic bronchitis or gastro-oesophageal reflux disease. Other causes are listed in Revision panel 2.10.

Revision panel 2.10

The causes of cough

Infective
Viral upper respiratory tract infections
Bacterial infection (acute bronchitis)
Pneumonia
Tuberculosis
Aspergillosis
Bronchiectasis
Lung abscess

Airways
Asthma
Eosinophilic bronchitis
Chronic obstructive pulmonary disease
Inhaled foreign body
Allergy
Endobronchial tumours (e.g. lung cancer, carcinoid tumour, metastatic disease)

Other lung disease
Lung cancer
Interstitial lung disease
Sarcoidosis
Cystic fibrosis

Heart
Pulmonary oedema

Drugs
Angiotensin-converting enzyme inhibitors

Environment
Smoking (chronic bronchitis)
Pollution

Other
Postnasal drip (secondary to rhinitis or sinusitis)
Gastro-oesophageal reflux
Oesophageal dysmotility
Mediastinal masses
Psychogenic

CHAPTER 2 | THE HEART, LUNGS AND PLEURA

Characteristics of a cough

History

Duration A cough lasting less than 3 weeks is termed acute, while one lasting more than 8 weeks is termed chronic. An acute cough will in all likelihood be benign in nature, and is usually caused by a viral upper respiratory tract infection. Remember that a very sudden onset cough may be the result of an inhaled foreign body.

A chronic cough is also likely to be benign, but a careful history and examination may reveal a more sinister underlying disease process.

Sputum production Most coughs are dry or non-productive. The production of significant amounts of sputum suggests pathology of pulmonary origin.

Sputum is mucus from the lower airways. Its colour or consistency may provide clues to the underlying disease:

- Mucoid sputum is clear or white and seen commonly in smokers with chronic bronchitis.
- Purulent sputum is usually the result of underlying infection. Pus within the sputum results in a thick yellow or green appearance. It may be present acutely (upper respiratory tract infection, pneumonia, lung abscess) or in a chronic infection (chronic bronchitis, bronchiectasis).
- Rust-coloured sputum is typical of pneumococcal pneumonia.
- Blood-streaked sputum, or haemoptysis, occurs in acute inflammation (bronchitis, pneumonia) or lung cancer.
- Large-volume haemoptysis is much less common, and tends to occur in chronic inflammatory conditions (bronchiectasis, aspergillosis, tuberculosis).
- White and frothy sputum is seen in acute pulmonary oedema. Chronic and copious amounts of frothy sputum (*bronchorrhoea*) may be seen with lepidic-predominant adenocarcinoma of the lung (previously known as bronchoalveolar cell carcinoma).
- Pink and frothy sputum is also typical of pulmonary oedema. The pink colour is caused by red blood cells present in the alveoli.

Diurnal variation

Most patients cough less at night as the cough reflex is to some degree suppressed. The cough in asthma and chest infection does not lessen overnight and may wake the patient. Some conditions become worse on lying flat (e.g. pulmonary oedema, gastro-oesophageal reflux) and may manifest themselves as a nocturnal cough.

Association with eating, drinking or talking

A cough associated with eating, or one that occurs in the immediate postprandial period, may be the result of gastro-oesophageal dysmotility (see Chapter 15).

Associated symptoms

Although an acute cough is usually benign and self-limiting, certain additional symptoms suggest more serious pathology:

- Haemoptysis of small volume may be a symptom of lung cancer or an inflammatory or infective process.
- Shortness of breath occurring acutely with a cough is often caused by acute bronchitis, but asthma, an inhaled foreign body or anaphylaxis must be excluded.
- Fever and cough of acute onset may indicate pneumonia.
- Acute-onset pleuritic chest pain with a cough may result from underlying pneumonia. A more gradual onset of symptoms may also represent an infective process, but lung cancer must be considered in the differential diagnosis. Mediastinal masses may also cause these symptoms but are much less common.
- Weight loss can be dramatic, and is most commonly seen with lung cancers and chest sepsis.

Specific sounding coughs

- A barking cough is characteristic of *croup*.
- Pertussis, or whooping cough, is so-named because of the high-pitched 'whoop' sound made by an affected child when inhaling air immediately after coughing.
- A bovine cough, weak and non-expulsive, is associated with hoarseness from recurrent laryngeal nerve palsy, often from a lung cancer.

Complications of acute and chronic cough

Vomiting and syncope may be seen following bouts of severe coughing.

In parous females, a cough can induce stress incontinence.

Rib fractures are uncommon but can occur following episodes of severe coughing. An abdominal hernia, on the other hand, is found commonly in patients with a chronic cough.

INHALED FOREIGN BODY

The inhalation of objects is more common in young children. Because of the small size of the airways, there is a greater chance of complete obstruction.

Adults also inhale foreign bodies, commonly teeth and crowns (often while undergoing a dental examination), food (especially peas and peanuts), coins, pins and tacks.

Most inhaled objects lodge in the right main bronchus, bronchus intermedius or right lower lobe segmental bronchi, because of the shape of the bronchial tree.

History

In adults, the most common symptoms are cough, wheeze or stridor, and breathlessness of acute onset, but many cases are asymptomatic. There is usually a clear history of an inhalation event. If a patient presents late, they may be unaware or have forgotten that they had inhaled anything, and the symptoms and signs of pneumonia predominate.

Examination

Physical examination is often unremarkable, but tachypnoea may be evident. Proximal obstruction of a lung will cause collapse of the lung with tracheal deviation to that side, with possible reduced air entry and a localized wheeze.

PNEUMONIA

Pneumonia is inflammation and consolidation of the lung, normally caused by infection. Most cases are bacterial or viral, but fungi and parasites may be responsible in immunocompromised individuals.

Non-infectious idiopathic pneumonias such as non-specific interstitial pneumonia, usual interstitial pneumonia and organizing pneumonia are better classified as interstitial lung diseases, and have different symptoms and signs.

In bacterial pneumonia, *Streptococcus pneumoniae* (the pneumococcus) is the most commonly isolated pathogen.

Pneumonia is a significant cause of death in the very young and the very old, in patients with chronic illness and in patients admitted to hospital. It is also a significant cause of postoperative death.

History

Age All ages are affected, but those older than 65 years are most at risk.

Symptoms Onset may be rapid, with significant symptoms developing in less than 24 hours.

Cough is most common and may produce purulent sputum. In pneumococcus infection, this classically has a rusty colour.

Haemoptysis is occasionally seen.

Non-specific symptoms Malaise and fatigue are present in most cases. Fever may be associated with sweats and rigors. Joint and muscle aches are frequent.

Shortness of breath is reported by two-thirds of patients, often exacerbated by pleuritic chest pain. Severe, sharp pain on inspiration can prevent adequate ventilation and lead to respiratory failure.

Hiccough is an occasional symptom.

Previous history

Smoking is the biggest risk factor in those who were previously fit and well.

Specific conditions that increase the risk of pneumonia include a history of COPD, other chronic illness, alcohol dependency, immunocompromise, and gastro-oesophageal reflux disease. Malnutrition and immobility are other factors.

In some patients, an episode of pneumonia may be the first presentation of lung cancer. There is, however, often a history of non-specific symptoms such as weight loss and fatigue.

Examination

General appearance Some individuals look relatively well. Others are very ill, with cardiovascular

CHAPTER 2 | THE HEART, LUNGS AND PLEURA

compromise (tachycardia, hypotension) and signs of respiratory distress (tachypnoea, central cyanosis). In the elderly, confusion may be predominant.

Inspection Tachypnoea is common in unwell patients. Reduced chest movement on the affected side is sometimes seen.

Palpation The trachea is normally central, but collapse of a lobe or lung results in deviation towards the affected side.

Increased tactile vocal fremitus results from a better conduction of sound through consolidated lung. This will be absent if there is an associated pleural effusion.

Percussion The percussion note will be dull over the affected area.

Auscultation Air entry may be reduced or *bronchial breathing* heard over the area of consolidated lung, particularly at the bases. Coarse inspiratory crackles are common.

Increased vocal resonance (the auscultatory equivalent of tactile vocal fremitus) with reduced air entry differentiates lung consolidation from a pleural effusion. *Whispering pectoriloquy* (increased quality and loudness of whispered words) is also the result of increased transmission of sound through consolidated lung.

A *pleural rub* is occasionally heard and occurs as inflamed pleural surfaces move against each other during both inspiration and expiration. The sound may be likened to creaking leather or treading on fresh snow.

LUNG ABSCESS

This is a localized collection of pus contained within a cavity formed by the disintegration of the surrounding lung parenchyma. Multiple abscesses may be present in the immunocompromised patient.

A primary lung abscess is either caused by aspiration or a complication of pneumonia.

Secondary lung abscesses occur as a result of another pathology such as metastatic septic emboli, an obstructing bronchial carcinoma or an infected bulla.

Anaerobic organisms (particularly *Bacteroides*) are commonly isolated from the pus, having gained access from aspiration or periodontal disease. Aerobic bacteria such as *Streptococcus pneumoniae* and *Staphylococcus aureus* are becoming more common.

History

Age Lung abscesses occur more commonly in the elderly as they are more likely to develop pneumonia or suffer from dysphagia and aspiration, and to have poor oral health.

Onset The onset may be gradual in anaerobic infections but can be quite rapid with aerobic bacteria.

Symptoms Cough and fever are the most common symptoms. Later in the disease process, as the abscess drains spontaneously into the bronchial tree, the cough produces pus. In anaerobic infections, this purulent sputum tastes and smells foul.

Haemoptysis occurs in one-third of patients.

Night sweats and rigors may accompany the fever.

General symptoms include malaise, fatigue and weight loss.

Shortness of breath is sometimes a feature and may be exacerbated by pleuritic chest pain.

Previous history

Aspiration is a cause of primary lung abscess, and risk factors such as alcohol abuse, recent dental work and bulbar palsy may be present.

A lung abscess should be considered in any patient who has failed to respond to the treatment of pneumonia (although empyema is more likely).

Examination

General appearance Cachexia and fever are usually present. The fever is often swinging and associated with a tachycardia.

Finger clubbing is seen in one-third of patients.

Some patients, particularly those with aerobic infections, can be very unwell with high fever, signs of respiratory failure, and cardiovascular compromise, with tachycardia and hypotension.

The chest signs are usually the same as in pneumonia and lung consolidation. A dull percussion note with reduced air entry and reduced vocal resonance will be present when a pleural effusion or empyema has complicated the lung abscess.

BRONCHIECTASIS

Bronchiectasis is a chronic condition characterized by abnormal and permanent dilatation of the subsegmental bronchi. Its pathogenesis requires infection, and either impairment of bronchial drainage, airway obstruction or impaired immunity (Fig. 2.13).

Fig. 2.13 Bronchiectasis (dilated bronchi).

History

Age More common over the age of 60 years. Congenital bronchiectasis, often the result of cystic fibrosis, presents in childhood.

Symptoms Cough is the dominant symptom. While this may be unproductive, the majority of patients produce large volumes of purulent sputum of a thick yellow or green consistency. The daily volumes of sputum can be impressively large and prove embarrassing.

Repeated respiratory tract infections cause shortness of breath, wheezing and pleuritic chest pain.

Halitosis is noticed by patients or those around them, and may indicate an exacerbation.

Haemoptysis is common, on occasion massive.

Previous history

Congenital causes of bronchiectasis include:

- cystic fibrosis;
- hypogammaglobulinaemia;
- alpha-1 antitrypsin deficiency;
- Kartagener's syndrome (failure of ciliary motility).

While bacterial infection is the most common cause of acquired bronchiectasis, other associations include acquired immune deficiency syndrome (AIDS) and tuberculosis, ulcerative colitis, rheumatoid arthritis, and male infertility as part of Kartagener's syndrome.

Examination

General appearance Cachexia and evidence of weight loss may be present. Finger clubbing is seen only in patients with severe disease, but nasal polyps and chronic sinusitis are common.

Auscultation All manner of added sounds, including crackles, wheezes and squeaks can be heard throughout all lung fields. These sounds are more pronounced during exacerbations.

CHEST PAIN

Pain in the chest is a common presenting symptom. It may arise from almost any structure within the thorax, including the heart, pericardium, lungs, pleura, chest wall, oesophagus, mediastinum or thoracic spine. Some causes are benign and self-limiting, while others are immediately life threatening. The causes are listed in Revision panel 2.11.

Characteristics of chest pain

Site

Central, retrosternal or midline chest pain normally arises from structures in the midline such as the heart, pericardium and oesophagus. Similarly, mediastinal masses are likely to cause central chest pain or discomfort.

It is unusual for lateral structures such as the lung, pleura or lateral chest wall to cause midline pain. Pain tends to be localized to the site and side of origin.

Radiation

Pain felt away from the site of the cause may either be *referred*, or due to *extension of the underlying disease*. There are times when referred pain is the only feature, making diagnosis difficult.

History

Referred pain

Myocardial ischaemia classically causes central chest pain. Common sites of radiation include the arms (especially the left), neck, jaw, epigastrium and back.

Aortic pathology such as a dissection may present with symptoms identical to myocardial ischaemia, or with back pain between the shoulder blades. Oesophageal pain, such as in reflux disease

---

Revision panel 2.11

The causes of chest pain

Heart
Chronic stable angina
Acute coronary syndromes
Aortic dissection
Aortic stenosis

Pericardium
Pericarditis
Pericardial cyst

Mediastinum
Mediastinitis
Oesophagitis
Oesophageal tumour
Oesophageal motility disorders
Ruptured oesophagus
Other mediastinal masses (e.g. thymoma, lymphadenopathy, germ cell tumour, neurogenic tumour, foregut cysts)

Spontaneous pneumomediastinum (Hamman's syndrome)

Pleura
Pneumonia
Pulmonary embolus
Pneumothorax
Pleural effusion
Empyema
Tumour (e.g. invasive lung cancer, mesothelioma, metastatic disease)

Chest wall and spine
Trauma (e.g. rib fractures)
Tumour (e.g. invasive lung cancer, secondary bony deposits, mesothelioma, primary chest wall sarcomas)
Costochondritis
Tietze's syndrome (see Chapter 13)

---

or oesophageal spasm, may also be very similar to cardiac pain in terms of site and radiation.

Lung cancers invading the chest wall, chest wall tumours, neurogenic tumours arising in the paravertebral region and pleural disease may produce pain localized to the site of origin. Often, however, intercostal nerve involvement causes neurogenic pain felt in the dermatome of the affected nerve. If this is only felt anteriorly, it mimics conditions causing midline chest or abdominal pain.

Extension of the underlying disease process

As an aortic dissection extends from the ascending aorta to the descending aorta, pain may migrate from the retrosternal area to the back. Mediastinal tumours are often asymptomatic, but may cause central chest pain. Spread into the pleural cavity may produce more lateral symptoms. Pneumothorax is often associated with sharp pleuritic chest pain on the side of the disease. Extension of air into the mediastinum can result in central chest pain.

Character

Pain may be described in multiple different ways by the patient: 'sharp', 'stabbing', 'dull', 'crushing', 'tight', 'gnawing', 'aching', 'tearing'.

The central aspect of cardiac pain is often described as 'crushing', 'heavy', 'tight', 'like a band around my chest' or 'like a weight on my chest'. Interestingly, referred cardiac pain often has a different quality.

Oesophageal pain can mimic cardiac pain in character as well as site, as can pain from other mediastinal pathology.

Aortic dissection may produce a 'tearing' sensation, often felt between the shoulder blades.

Pleural pain is sharp or stabbing in nature, and any pleural or chest wall pathology can cause it. It results from inflammation of the pleural surfaces, and the pain is felt as they move against one another, typically on deep breathing, coughing, laughing or sneezing. Chest wall invasion by tumour does not always produce pleuritic pain. It tends to be dull, gnawing or aching.

Severity

Severity of pain is subjective, varying considerably from person to person and on the situation. A chest injury sustained on the rugby pitch will be tolerated better than a similar injury in the home.

Some chest pathologies such as myocardial infarction, aortic dissection, oesophageal rupture and multiple rib fractures typically cause severe pain. Bizarrely, however, some patients experience little or no pain. This is more likely in the elderly, and in those with autonomic neuropathy due to diabetes.

Onset and duration

Subjective reporting of pain duration is unreliable. Pain of a few seconds duration is unlikely to be significant (e.g. precordial catch syndrome).

The pain of chronic stable angina will have come on and resolved in a period of minutes, whereas pain from a myocardial infarction may last for hours.

Acute diseases causing pleural pain, such as pneumothorax, usually produce pain with an acute onset, which may be persistent.

Tumours of the mediastinum and chest wall are often asymptomatic, but there may be pain with an insidious onset that persists.

Frequency and periodicity

There is no chest equivalent to the colicky pain of intestinal origin. The pain tends to be constant, the exception being pleuritic chest pain related to breathing.

Precipitating and aggravating factors

The symptoms of chronic stable angina are usually brought on by exercise. As the coronary artery disease progresses and blood flow to the heart reduces, symptoms appear with less and less exertion, even on brushing the teeth. Other precipitating factors include emotional stress, cold weather and eating.

Pleuritic pain is classically worse on inspiration. Sometimes it may only be felt on deep inspiration, while at others times pain may be experienced even during shallow respiration. Other aggravating factors include any chest movement, including coughing, laughing and sneezing.

Pericarditis causes a sharp central pain, typically aggravated by lying flat and relieved by sitting up or leaning forward. Like pleuritic pain, it is worse on inspiration.

Oesophageal pain is often identical to cardiac pain, and telling the two apart can be difficult. Precipitation by eating or aggravation by posture is more likely with oesophageal pain, while exercise is associated with cardiac pain.

Musculoskeletal chest wall pain, in common with pleuritic pain, is aggravated by any form of chest movement, including inspiration. Local pressure may precipitate or exacerbate the pain. Pressing on the sternum causes pain over the sites of rib fractures.

Relieving factors

Sometimes an action or event coincides with the spontaneous resolution of pain, and the patient wrongly attributes this as a relieving factor. There are, however, true relieving factors classically associated with different causes of chest pain.

The central chest pain of stable chronic angina typically passes off after a few minutes of rest or use of sublingual nitrates. Failure to resolve with rest or nitrates suggests a different diagnosis, such as acute coronary syndrome or non-cardiac pain.

Oesophageal pain is often similar to cardiac pain, and confusingly may also be relieved by nitrates. Relief of symptoms with antacids suggests an oesophageal cause.

Partial relief of musculoskeletal and pleuritic pains may be achieved by keeping as still or as rigid as possible.

Associated symptoms and signs

Pain is often associated with features that are the result of sympathetic over-stimulation, such as tachycardia and hypertension. Nausea and sweating are frequently associated with the severe pain of acute coronary syndrome.

Regurgitation of gastric acid in association with central chest pain is not seen with cardiac ischaemia and is typical of gastro-oesophageal reflux disease. Breathlessness, however, is commonly seen with cardiac ischaemia but not with oesophageal disease.

CHRONIC STABLE ANGINA

Angina, or angina pectoris, is the symptom of chest pain or discomfort experienced during transient cardiac ischaemia. The most common cause is atherosclerosis of the coronary arteries. As a consequence, coronary artery blood flow is reduced, and pain develops when the heart is asked to work harder during exercise. Other conditions that reduce coronary artery blood flow include neointimal hyperplasia within a coronary stent, neointimal hyperplasia in areas of previous coronary angioplasty and coronary artery spasm (known as variant or Prinzmetal's angina). Angina is also a late and worrying symptom in aortic valve stenosis (see above).

CHAPTER 2 | THE HEART, LUNGS AND PLEURA

History

Age and sex The likelihood of angina increases with age. In the UK, it is rare before the age of 45 years and unusual before 55 years. The incidence of angina then increases steeply with each decade of life, being 1.7 times more common in males than females. Over the age of 75 years, 16 per cent of males and 11 per cent of females experience angina as a symptom of ischaemic heart disease.

Symptoms The main symptom is central retrosternal chest pain or discomfort brought on by effort or exercise. Other precipitating factors include stress, cold weather and heavy meals. The pain is variously described as 'tight', 'like a band', 'constrictive' or 'heavy'. Radiation to the jaw or neck may produce a 'choking' sensation. Other sites of radiation include the arms (principally the left arm) and the back. The pain abates after a few minutes of rest or the use of sublingual nitrates.

The severity of angina pain is not necessarily related to the degree of ischaemia. Indeed, myocardial ischaemia may be silent, particularly in patients with autonomic neuropathy (such as diabetics).

The thresholds for the precipitation of angina symptoms are summarised by the Canadian Cardiovascular Society angina classification (Revision panel 2.12). Patients in classes 3 and 4 have a worse prognosis than those in classes 1 and 2.

Angina can be aggravated by anaemia, hyperthyroidism and obesity.

Revision panel 2.12

Canadian Cardiovascular Society angina classification

1. Angina with strenuous, rapid or prolonged exertion, not ordinary physical activity.
2. Slight limitation of activity. Angina occurs when walking uphill or climbing stairs rapidly.
3. Marked limitation of activity. Symptoms occur with everyday activities such as walking one or two blocks on the level or climbing one flight of stairs at a normal pace.
4. Severe limitation. Inability to carry out any physical activity without angina or angina at rest.

Patients with ischaemic heart disease and angina often experience breathlessness and autonomic symptoms such as nausea with their pain.

Pain caused by oesophageal pathologies such as oesophageal motility disorders and reflux disease is the most important differential diagnosis (see above).

Risk factors include smoking, a family history of ischaemic heart disease, obesity, advancing age and a sedentary lifestyle. Their presence makes myocardial ischaemia a more likely diagnosis.

Previous history

Hypertension, diabetes and hypercholesterolaemia are additional risk factors. Patients with renal failure are also at significant risk. A history of peripheral vascular or cerebrovascular disease is more likely in patients with ischaemic heart disease.

Examination

General appearance There are frequently no abnormal physical signs in patients with chronic stable angina. Nicotine staining of the fingers may be seen in smokers. Xanthelasmata, or cholesterol deposits in the skin of the eyelids, are a sign of hypercholesterolaemia (see Chapter 1). Similarly, a corneal arcus may also indicate hypercholesterolaemia in young patients, but in older people is a relatively non-specific sign.

Blood pressure should be checked, as hypertension is a major risk factor.

The pulse will normally be regular, but cardiac ischaemia is a known cause of atrial fibrillation, in which case the pulse will be irregularly irregular. Signs of heart failure, such as raised JVP and ankle oedema should also be sought.

Chest examination This is usually normal. If there is an element of heart failure, fine inspiratory crackles may be heard at both lung bases. Mitral regurgitation as a result of cardiac ischaemia may result in a pansystolic heart murmur.

ACUTE CORONARY SYNDROMES

The acute coronary syndromes occur following occlusion of a coronary artery, usually by thrombus formation over the site of a ruptured atherosclerotic plaque within the wall of the coronary artery. They are almost always accompanied by central chest pain. There are three patterns:

1. Unstable angina
2. ST elevation myocardial infarction (STEMI)
3. Non-ST elevation myocardial infarction (NSTEMI)

A *STEMI* is characterized by electrocardiogram (ECG) changes typical of myocardial infarction (ST elevation or new left bundle branch block) with evidence of myocardial damage (raised serum cardiac markers such as troponin I or T).

An *NSTEMI* does not produce typical ECG changes, but there is biochemical evidence of myocardial damage.

Unstable angina typically has neither ST elevation on ECG nor positive serum cardiac markers.

Symptoms are often identical for all three syndromes.

History

The age, risk factors and previous history are the same for the acute coronary syndromes as for chronic stable angina. It is the onset, severity and resolution of symptoms that differentiate the two. While many patients presenting with an acute coronary syndrome have a history of chronic stable angina, it is often the first presentation of ischaemic heart disease.

Symptoms The predominant symptom is central, retrosternal chest pain, often with radiation to the neck, jaw, arms or back.

In those with a previous history of chronic stable angina, the pain is often described as being more severe or oppressive in nature. Whereas stable angina is brought on by effort and is relieved after a few minutes by rest or sublingual nitrates, the acute coronary syndromes have an unpredictable onset or occur at rest. Furthermore, rest and nitrates have little effect. Pain may persist for many minutes or indeed hours.

Patients often have a sense of impending doom or death. Sympathetic symptoms such as nausea, vomiting and sweating are a more dominant feature than in stable angina, particularly for inferior STEMIs.

Acute left ventricular failure is a complication of an acute coronary syndrome, and sudden onset breathlessness and orthopnoea may be a presenting feature. Rhythm disturbances such as atrial fibrillation, atrial flutter, ventricular ectopics, heart block and ventricular tachycardia are also common, causing palpitations, light-headedness or syncope. Ventricular fibrillation leading to sudden death is not uncommonly the first presentation of ischaemic heart disease.

Examination

General appearance As with stable angina, the stigmata of smoking or hypercholesterolaemia may be evident.

The patient often looks unwell, with autonomic signs such as sweating, pallor and vomiting as a consequence of the pain.

Tachycardia A weak and rapid pulse indicates cardiogenic shock that can complicate some acute coronary syndromes, particularly STEMIs. Arrythmias may also be detected. *Blood pressure* may be elevated as a result of either long-standing hypertension or the acute pain. Low blood pressure with cool peripheries, peripheral cyanosis, sweating and pallor indicates cardiogenic shock, and there may be other signs of heart failure such as a raised JVP.

Chest In the presence of heart failure, fine inspiratory crackles are heard at the lung bases.

Auscultation of the heart is usually normal unless there is concomitant valvular heart disease.

Complications of myocardial infarction may produce additional signs:

- A gallop rhythm indicates left ventricular failure.
- Ischaemic rupture of the chordae tendineae will result in acute mitral regurgitation and a pansystolic murmur.
- Postinfarct VSD causes a harsh systolic murmur, loudest at the lower left sternal edge.
- Some patients who survive a large full-thickness infarct may develop a left ventricular aneurysm. This may lead to heart failure, and arrhythmias.

AORTIC DISSECTION

A dissection forms as blood enters the muscular layer of the wall of the aorta via a tear at a weak spot in the intimal lining. Two-thirds of cases originate in the ascending aorta, with the remainder in the arch or proximal descending aorta. While this false lumen may remain localized, the pressure of the blood can force it to extend (*dissect*) proximally towards the heart or distally towards the aortic iliac bifurcation. The process can then occlude branches of the aorta (the coronary, carotid or coeliac arteries), or the thinned outer layer of the aorta can rupture, usually fatally (Fig. 2.14).

Fig. 2.14 Aortic dissection.

The Stanford classification divides aortic dissections into two groups:

- Type A dissections involve the ascending aorta and require immediate surgery.
- Type B dissections do not involve the ascending aorta and can be managed without surgery initially, although endovascular stenting or surgery may be required later to treat complications.

History

Age Most patients (90 per cent) are over 60 years old, and dissection is twice as likely in males. Many patients die before reaching hospital.

Symptoms Pain is the principal symptom and is related to the site of the dissection. Central chest pain, not dissimilar to angina, is experienced in dissections involving the ascending aorta. The onset is usually sudden, and it is sometimes described as tearing in nature.

Back, or intrascapular, pain is a feature of dissections involving the descending aorta. Pain that began centrally radiating to the back is ominous, indicating possible extension of the dissection.

Sharp, central, pleuritic-type pain may indicate involvement of the pericardial sac and the impending development of cardiac tamponade.

Involvement of the heart or aortic branches can result in end-organ damage and further symptoms.

One-third of type A dissections involve the aortic valve, causing aortic regurgitation and symptoms of heart failure.

Involvement of the coronary arteries may produce additional symptoms of myocardial ischaemia, although these are difficult to separate from the symptoms of the dissection itself.

Neurological symptoms and stroke occur with occlusion of the aortic arch branches.

Extension distally may produce abdominal pain (coeliac and mesenteric vessels) or symptoms of lower limb ischaemia.

Risk factors Hypertension is the most common risk factor.

Other predisposing conditions include connective tissue disorders such as Ehlers–Danlos syndrome (Fig. 2.15) and Marfan's syndrome (see Chapter 1), and bicuspid aortic valve.

Hypervolaemic states such as pregnancy in conjunction with connective tissue abnormalities may initiate dissection.

Fig. 2.15 Hyperflexibility of the fingers in Ehlers–Danlos syndrome. This condition is a risk factor for aortic dissection.

Previous history

Recent cardiac surgery, particularly on the aortic valve, can predispose to dissection.

Examination

General appearance The surviving patients may have obvious stigmata of underlying connective tissue disorders, or signs of stroke or limb ischaemia. Paraplegia, if present, is a result of spinal artery occlusion.

Blood pressure is variable. Pain or long-standing hypertension may result in high blood pressure, but loss of blood, cardiac failure or cardiac tamponade is associated with hypotension.

Hypotension is more common in type A dissections and is a poor prognostic sign. Aortic regurgitation results in a low diastolic pressure with a wide pulse pressure.

If the blood pressure is measured in an ischaemic upper limb, there will be apparent hypotension. Check the peripheral pulses first.

Auscultation Auscultation of the heart reveals an early diastolic murmur if the dissection has caused aortic regurgitation. Muffled heart sounds suggest cardiac tamponade.

Pleural fluid collections can develop from either rupture of the aorta or an inflammatory reaction to the dissection process. The left chest is usually involved, with signs of a pleural effusion (see above). If severe aortic regurgitation has complicated the dissection there will be signs of pulmonary oedema (fine bi-basal crackles).

MEDIASTINAL MASSES AND TUMOURS

Masses arising in the mediastinum are inaccessible to clinical examination. Modes of presentation are:

- no symptoms, with an incidental finding on imaging studies such as a chest X-ray or CT scan;
- chest pain, normally central; paravertebral masses may produce pain in the affected dermatome;
- shortness of breath as a consequence of airway compression or invasion by large mediastinal masses or lymphadenopathy;
- cough;
- dysphagia from compression of the oesophagus;
- fever or night sweats in mediastinal lymphadenopathy caused by lymphoma or tuberculosis;
- general malaise;
- muscle weakness secondary to myasthenia gravis associated with a thymoma.

Up to one-half of all mediastinal masses are asymptomatic. The presence of symptoms or signs is more likely to represent a sinister pathology.

Anatomically, the mediastinum is divided into the superior, anterior, middle and posterior compartments. A more useful surgical description of the mediastinum divides it into three compartments: anterior (containing the thymus gland, fat and lymph nodes), visceral (containing the trachea and main stem bronchi, lymph nodes, heart, pericardium, great vessels, oesophagus and thoracic duct) and paravertebral (containing the sympathetic chain and thoracic spinal ganglia).

The cause and sites of mediastinal masses are listed in Revision panel 2.13.

Revision panel 2.13
Sites and causes of mediastinal masses

Anterior compartment

Thymoma or thymic hyperplasia

Thyroid (retrosternal goitre)

Germ cell tumours

Lymphadenopathy

Visceral compartment

Tracheal and bronchial tumours (e.g. lung cancer, benign tracheobronchial tumours)

Lymphadenopathy

Foregut cysts (bronchogenic, oesophageal)

Pericardial cysts

Cardiac tumours

Aortic aneurysm

Oesophageal tumours

Hiatus hernia

Paravertebral compartment

Neurogenic tumours (e.g. neurofibroma, schwannoma, ganglioneuroma, phaeochromocytoma)

Lymphadenopathy

OTHER SYMPTOMS/SIGNS

STRIDOR

Stridor is the harsh, high-pitched or wheezing sound of breathing associated with a partially obstructed airway. Turbulent and restricted airflow occurs secondary to either intrinsic obstruction or extrinsic compression of the airway, anywhere between the larynx and the main bronchi. The onset of stridor is always an emergency and must be investigated promptly.

Stridor is loudest in inspiration and is accentuated by coughing. It is often, although not always, associated with shortness of breath. A sudden onset is typical of an inhaled foreign body, while a gradual onset may be from endobronchial malignancy or extrinsic compression by tumour masses (Revision panel 2.14).

Revision panel 2.14

Causes of stridor

Laryngeal disease

Infection (croup, epiglottitis, retropharyngeal abscess)

Tumour (laryngeal papillomatosis, laryngeal cancer)

Oedema (instrumentation of airway, anaphylaxis)

Endobronchial disease

Lung cancer

Primary tracheal tumours

Metastatic cancer (e.g. renal cell)

Locally invasive cancer (e.g. lung, oesophagus, thyroid)

Inhaled foreign body

Benign stenosis (e.g. secondary to prolonged intubation or tracheostomy)

Extrinsic compression

Mediastinal lymphadenopathy (e.g. metastatic lung cancer, lymphoma)

Mediastinal tumours (thymoma, germ cell tumour)

Thyroid swelling

Thoracic aortic aneurysm

Vascular anomalies (e.g. vascular ring secondary to a double aortic arch)

Other

Tracheomalacia

HAEMOPTYSIS

Haemoptysis is the clearing of blood or blood-stained sputum from the lungs by coughing. It is sometimes difficult to differentiate from bleeding from the nasopharynx, or the oesophagus and stomach.

Massive haemoptysis means that enough blood has been lost into the bronchial tree to threaten life, usually more than half a litre in 24 hours. The threat is from asphyxiation (drowning) rather than exsanguination.

The causes of simple haemoptysis are the same as those for massive haemoptysis (Revision panel 2.15). While small-volume haemoptysis in a smoker may be a symptom of lung cancer, massive haemoptysis is more commonly caused by an inflammatory process.

Revision panel 2.15

The causes of haemoptysis

Inflammation and infection (including tuberculosis and *Aspergillus*)

Bronchiectasis

Lung cancer and other tumours of the tracheo-bronchial tree

Trauma (e.g. pulmonary artery catheter, penetrating trauma)

Pulmonary embolus

Pulmonary arterio-venous malformations

Mitral stenosis

DISTENDED NECK VEINS

Distention of the neck veins is most commonly due to raised JVP secondary to heart failure. Consequently, there are normally other signs of right heart failure including ankle swelling. However, any pathology that interferes with drainage of the blood from the head and neck into the heart via the brachiocephalic veins and superior vena cava can cause distension of the neck veins (Revision panel 2.16).

Pericardial effusion

A pericardial effusion is a collection of fluid in the non-distensible pericardial sac that encloses the heart. If the pressure is sufficient to impair cardiac function, cardiac tamponade (literally 'packing') ensues. The cause may be benign (usually

Revision panel 2.16

Causes of distended neck veins

Cardiac disease
Left and right heart failure
Cor pulmonale
Pulmonary embolism
Primary pulmonary hypertension
Tricuspid valve regurgitation

Pleural disease
Tension pneumothorax
Massive pleural effusion
Massive haemothorax

Pericardial disease
Constrictive pericarditis
Pericardial effusion
Cardiac tamponade

Superior vena cava obstruction

Revision panel 2.17

Causes of a pericardial effusion

Pericarditis
Idiopathic
Viral
Bacterial (including tuberculosis)
Post myocardial infarction (Dressler's syndrome)
Collagen disease (e.g. systemic lupus erythematosus)
Uraemia of renal failure

Malignant
Metastatic spread (lung cancer and other cancers such as breast)
Direct spread (lung cancer)

Trauma
Postcardiac surgery

Other
Hypothyroidism

inflammatory) or malignant (invariably metastatic) (Revision panel 2.17).

History

Symptoms Small pericardial effusions are usually symptomless. As the effusion becomes more significant, there may be central chest discomfort. Breathlessness, light-headedness and syncope are symptoms of impending cardiac tamponade.

If pericarditis is the cause, there is pleuritic central chest pain, worse on inspiration and lying flat, but eased by bending forwards.

Previous history

A myocardial infarction within the previous 2–6 weeks suggests Dressler's syndrome (pericardial effusion, fever and pleuritic pain). Postcardiotomy syndrome after cardiac surgery is similar, and probably has the same autoimmune cause.

Examination

General examination In the presence of a pericardial effusion, the stroke volume of the heart cannot be increased. The only way to increase the cardiac output is to increase the rate, so there is tachycardia. Tamponade with hypotension and shock will eventually follow (see below).

The JVP is usually raised, shown by distended neck veins. There may be a paradoxical rise in the JVP in inspiration, known as Kussmauls's sign (not to be confused with Kussmaul's breathing in acidosis). Other signs of right heart failure, such as ankle swelling, may also be present.

Auscultation of the heart in acute pericarditis may reveal a pericardial friction rub, best heard at the lower left sternal edge with the patient leaning forwards. With significant effusions, the heart sounds are muffled or distant.

Cardiac tamponade

Cardiac tamponade is the end-stage of a pericardial effusion or haemo-pericardium. Fluid under pressure in the constricted space around the heart impairs normal cardiac function, mainly by preventing adequate filling of the heart in diastole. Preload is therefore reduced, which in turn reduces stroke volume. Tachycardia develops to maintain cardiac output. Eventually, the heart can no longer compensate, and shock ensues.

As little as 100 mL of fluid in the pericardial sac is enough to cause tamponade. It is seen most commonly after trauma and cardiac surgery.

CHAPTER 2 | THE HEART, LUNGS AND PLEURA

History

Patients feel generally unwell and complain of breathlessness, fatigue, light-headedness and fainting.

Examination

The classical triad of signs in cardiac tamponade is known as *Beck's triad*. This consists of:

- hypotension (reduced stroke volume and cardiac output);
- distended neck veins (impaired diastolic filling of the heart);
- muffled heart sounds (the presence of pericardial fluid).

Other signs include tachypnoea, tachycardia, pulsus paradoxus (an exaggerated drop in blood pressure during inspiration), and a reduced level of consciousness.

Superior vena cava obstruction

The superior vena cava is a short segment of the venous system connecting the junction of the left and right brachiocephalic veins with the right atrium. It drains blood from the arms, head, neck and upper thorax. It is a thin-walled, low-pressure conduit and is susceptible to external compression and obstruction by mediastinal pathology.

The most common cause of SVCO is lung cancer, either invasive right-sided tumours or metastatic mediastinal lymph nodes. Other causes are shown in Revision panel 2.18.

History

Age Except for mediastinal tumours, the other causes of SVCO occur in older age groups.

Symptoms Breathlessness usually of gradual onset is the most common symptom. At the same time, the neck and face swell, most pronounced in the morning. This improves during the day because standing aids venous drainage of the head.

Examination

There is obvious swelling and venous congestion, with flaring of the arms, neck, face and anterior chest wall.

In chronic SVCO, veins over the anterior chest wall may become very prominent, as venous blood finds alternative routes to the right atrium (Fig. 2.16).

Revision panel 2.18
Causes of superior vena cava obstruction

Benign

Fibrosing mediastinitis

Great vessel arterial aneurysm

Retrosternal goitre

Malignant

Lung cancer

Mediastinal lymphadenopathy (e.g. lymphoma, metastatic disease)

Mediastinal masses (e.g. thymoma, germ cell tumours)

Iatrogenic

Internal jugular and subclavian central venous lines

Transvenous pacing systems

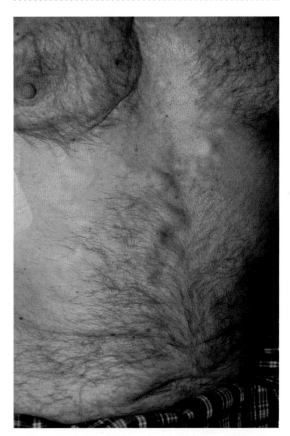

Fig. 2.16 Chronic superior vena cava obstruction secondary to trauma. There are enlarged and tortuous superficial veins over the anterior chest wall.

CHEST AND CARDIAC TRAUMA

Chest trauma has been covered fully in Chapter 5.

Aortic rupture

This serious injury occurs in severe high-speed deceleration accidents such as car crashes. The site of rupture is just beyond the left subclavian artery at the level of the ligamentum arteriosum.

In patients who survive the initial incident, the adventitia remains intact, temporarily containing the bleeding. The diagnosis is suspected from finding weak femoral pulses or unequal blood pressures in the two arms. Investigation usually reveals a wide mediastinum.

Blunt cardiac injury

The heart is compressed between the sternum and the vertebral column.

If the heart ruptures, the patient dies immediately, but myocardial contusions can occur. These behave like myocardial infarcts (see above).

Very occasionally, heart valves rupture. Presentation is with symptoms of acute regurgitation.

Penetrating cardiac injury

An appropriately sited entry wound (normally medial to the nipple) and evidence of tamponade or hypovolaemia suggest the diagnosis.

CHEST WALL ABNORMALITIES

The chest wall may have an abnormal shape, which is either congenital or acquired later in life (Revision panel 2.19).

Pectus deformities are common, and occur in more than 1 in every 1000 children. Trauma (including iatrogenic) is probably the most common cause of acquired chest wall deformity.

Primary chest wall tumours (chondromas and sarcomas) are rare (Fig. 2.17).

Lung hernias usually occur following a thoracic or cardiac operation (Fig. 2.18), but can occur spontaneously following a bout of severe coughing.

Revision panel 2.19

The causes of chest wall deformity

Congenital

Pectus excavatum

Pectus carinatum

Poland syndrome

Acquired

Trauma (e.g. rib fractures, sternal fracture)

Iatrogenic (e.g. thoracoplasty)

Lung hernia

Thoracic aortic aneurysm

Benign tumours (e.g. chondroma)

Malignant tumour (e.g. metastasis, primary sarcoma)

Syphilitic ascending thoracic aortic aneurysms eroding the anterior chest wall are nowadays exceptionally rare.

Fig. 2.17 Chest wall osteosarcoma arising from the left fourth rib laterally just below the axilla.

CHAPTER 2 | THE HEART, LUNGS AND PLEURA

Fig. 2.18 Lung hernia. This occurred following placement of a chest drain in a patient with bullous emphysema.

Pectus deformities

Pectus excavatum is a depression of the anterior chest wall, and is sometimes known as funnel chest (Fig. 2.19).

Fig. 2.19 Symmetrical pectus excavatum deformity.

Pectus carinatum is the opposite, with protrusion of the anterior chest wall (Fig. 2.20). It is sometimes called pigeon chest.

The cause is thought to be abnormal growth patterns of the costal cartilages. Excavatum and carinatum deformities can coexist.

History

Age Pectus deformities often become apparent during adolescent growth spurts.

Symptoms The major symptom, and the reason why surgical correction is offered, is sensitivity about the shape of the chest causing lack of confidence, depression and an inability to interact with peers.

Fig. 2.20 Pectus carinatum deformity, more marked on the right.

Vague chest pains, fatigue and shortness of breath on exertion are sometimes reported.

Previous history

Scoliosis (see Chapter 9) is associated with both deformities. Pectus excavatum is often present in Marfan's syndrome (see Chapter 1).

Examination

General appearance In addition to an assessment of the pectus deformity, look for costal flaring and scoliosis.

Auscultation Auscultation of the heart in Marfan's syndrome may reveal a murmur of either mitral or aortic regurgitation.

FINGER CLUBBING

The pathological process leading to finger clubbing is poorly understood. Nevertheless, it is a common sign in chest disease and is most frequently seen as a paraneoplastic syndrome, in chronic chest sepsis or in chronic cyanotic conditions. Lung cancer is the most common pulmonary cause, and congenital cyanotic heart disease – in which a right to left shunt exists – is the most common cardiac cause. Other causes are listed in Revision panel 2.20.

Finger clubbing is characterized by:

- a fluctuant nail bed;
- loss of the nail bed angle;
- increased curvature of the nail;
- swelling and thickening of entire finger pulp, producing the classic drumstick appearance.

ANKLE SWELLING

Ankle swelling as a result of right heart dysfunction and peripheral oedema is a classical sign in patients with heart failure. It is more commonly associated with immobility, and is most marked in low-protein states (for example, in postoperative patients who are recovering from complications).

Peripheral oedema is characterized by ankle swelling that pits on sustained pressure with an examining thumb, 'pitting oedema' (Fig. 2.21). The causes are listed in Revision panel 2.21.

Fig. 2.21 Gross pitting ankle oedema in a patient with heart failure. There is a thumb indentation on the right shin.

CYANOSIS

Cyanosis is the blue discolouration of the skin or mucous membranes seen when there are high levels of deoxygenated haemoglobin in the blood.

Central cyanosis is a sign of arterial hypoxia, and is noticed when the arterial oxygen saturation falls below 85 per cent. The lips or tongue take on a bluish tinge, and it can be present in any condition causing severe hypoxaemia.

Peripheral cyanosis refers to a blue discolouration of the fingers and toes. It is also seen in hypoxia, but is additionally observed as a result of poor tissue perfusion. Examples include low cardiac output states such as shock or severe heart failure, and local vasoconstrictive states such as Raynaud's phenomenon.

HORNER'S SYNDROME

The most common thoracic cause of Horner's syndrome is lung cancer. Tumours at the apex of the upper lobes can invade the surrounding structures, including the brachial plexus, subclavian vessels, chest wall and vertebral bodies. These Pancoast tumours may also invade the stellate ganglion of the sympathetic chain, causing an ipsilateral Horner's syndrome (Fig. 2.22).

Interruption of the sympathetic nervous supply to the face produces:

- ptosis (a droopy eyelid);
- miosis (a constricted pupil);
- anhidrosis (a dry cheek due to a lack of sweating);

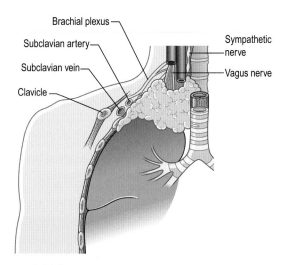

Fig. 2.22 Pancoast tumour.

- enophthalmos (a sunken eyeball).

Other causes within the chest include high paravertebral mediastinal tumours (normally neurogenic in origin), trauma, and intercostal chest tube drains.

3

The brain, central nervous system and peripheral nerves

In the nervous system, it is usually possible to localize the likely pathology by clinical assessment alone, because the different functions are located in different sites connected by well-defined anatomical pathways. Advances in neurological imaging have not reduced the importance of taking a full history and carrying out a thorough examination.

HISTORY

Establish the patient's age, whether they are right or left handed and their occupation, and try to assess their mental status. The ability to give a history may be impaired by neurological disease, and help will be needed from family members, paramedics or other witnesses to the event (see Chapter 5).

For a child, include details of the birth, early milestones and school progress.

The nervous system is bilaterally symmetrical, and establishing the correct side is vital, so write out 'right' or 'left' in full. It is also important to understand the impact of the condition on the patient's day-to-day activities.

Start with open questions, but then supplement the information with direct questions such as 'What do you mean by weakness?'

At the end of the history, it is worth going through a summary with the patient because they will often remember further details of their condition.

NEUROLOGICAL SYMPTOMS ARISING FROM CRANIAL CONDITIONS

Common neurological symptoms include:

- Headache.
- Fits.
- Visual disturbance.
- Weakness.
- Deafness.
- Loss of balance.

Intracranial conditions presenting with severe headache

Headache is a common complaint at all ages, but severe headaches in a sick patient must not be ignored (see Revision panel 3.1).

Subarachnoid haemorrhage usually presents as the worst headache the patient has ever experienced, as if they have been struck over the head with a hammer. This pattern of headache must not be missed as there is major risk of further bleeds. Misdiagnosis as 'sinusitis' or 'atypical migraine' is common even though the patient has described the headache as:

- 'like no other, worst at the beginning';
- 'as though I have been hit over the head';
- 'definitely the worst headache of my life'.

Pituitary apoplexy also presents with sudden-onset severe headache and may involve loss of vision and disturbed eye movements. It may be caused by a spontaneous bleed into an existing pituitary macroadenoma, and may be taking anticoagulants.

Acute hydrocephalus can arise as a result of a blocked ventriculo-peritoneal shunt or rarely from a colloid cyst of the third ventricle blocking the foramina of Munro, causing acute obstruction. Early diagnosis is vital to avoid rapid deterioration and death.

Headaches associated with nausea and giddiness are common after a head injury and may not settle for days or weeks. However, increasing headache after a head injury in the elderly or a patient on anticoagulants suggests a chronic subdural collection.

Raised intracranial pressure from any cause (tumour, haematoma, abscess or hydrocephalus) typically causes severe, progressive headaches that are worse in the morning and are often accompanied by vomiting. When a person is asleep in the recumbent position, there is a relative rise in pCO_2 and a degree of vasodilatation. This relative expansion of the vascular space, with the loss of compliance as a result of the space-occupying lesion, leads to an exponential rise in pressure, manifest as an intense headache that can wake the patient. Vomiting and hyperventilation follow the onset of the headache, which can in turn ease the headache, only for it to return the next day. Such headaches always require urgent referral.

Headache with a fever, photophobia and neck stiffness is characteristic of meningitis, and can progress to a subdural empyema.

A 'cough headache' experienced 'intensely at the back of the head' is a presenting feature of a type 1 Chiari malformation which is associated with herniation of the cerebellar tonsils through the foramen magnum.

There are therefore a number of important questions to be explored with any patient with a headache:

- Severity.
- Character.
- Duration.
- Speed of onset.
- Are you unwell?
- What provokes the headache?
- What makes it better?

- Is it different from previous headaches?
- Is there any aura or accompanying visual symptoms or nausea?

Never forget that the headache may be the result of a brain haemorrhage, although most headaches are the result of migraines or tension.

Revision panel 3.1
Causes of acute headache

Infection

Meningitis

Encephalitis

Ventriculo-peritoneal shunt infection and blockage

Subdural empyema

Brain abscess

Vascular

Arteriovenous malformation

Subarachnoid haemorrhage

Intracerebral haemorrhage

Carotid dissection

Pituitary apoplexy

Sagittal sinus thrombosis

Increased intracranial pressure

Hydrocephalus

Tumours

Local causes

Temporal arteritis

From the eye (acute angle-closure glaucoma)

Sinusitis

Intracranial conditions presenting with 'fits'

A 'fit' will always provoke major concerns for the patient and their family.

The diagnosis of 'epilepsy' is usually straightforward, but exclude:

- a blackout from a cardiac event;
- a simple faint (vasovagal attack).

It is important to establish whether the fit was focal and stayed focal, or whether it became generalized. Did the 'twitching' start in the face or arm?

Was there any weakness after the attack (postictal weakness, Todd's paresis)?

Family and friends may describe:

- a brief blank look and 'lip-smacking' in a petit mal attack;
- major body movements in a generalized tonic/clonic grand mal attack.

Many patients bite their tongue and are incontinent during a generalized fit.

In an acutely unwell patient the following conditions must be considered:

- Infection.
- Stroke.
- Head injury.
- Cerebral haemorrhage.
- Supratentorial brain tumour.
- Metabolic disorder.

Partial or generalized epilepsy is a frequent symptom of frontal and temporal lobe tumours.

Seizures beginning after adolescence should always raise the suspicion of an underlying brain tumour.

When recording the history of a 'fit', ask what the patient experienced, as well as what was observed by family or friends. Ask about the onset of the fit:

- Were there any warning symptoms?
- Were there any abnormal tastes or smells?
- Were there any 'butterflies' in the stomach?

These may indicate an origin in the temporal lobe.

Subsequent attacks often follow a particular pattern, and can be triggered by lack of sleep, alcohol and stress.

Note A brain abscess carries the highest risk of long-term fits.

Intracranial conditions presenting with disturbance of vision (visual loss and double vision)

Failing vision

The cause is ocular (cataract, macular degeneration and glaucoma) more often than neurological.

Key points in the history

Is the visual loss monocular or binocular? Monocular visual loss arises in one eye or optic nerve. Binocular visual loss, such as a homonymous hemianopia, is related to the visual pathways posterior to the optic chiasm.

A vascular cause such as amaurosis fugax (fleeting blindness) should be suspected from the history (see Chapter 10). Smoking, diabetes and hypertension are associated factors.

Coexisting headache or retro-orbital pain raises the possibility of retro-orbital neuritis, a carotid dissection or an expanding aneurysm.

Other important elements in the history are the speed and degree of visual loss, whether it is painful and the exact pattern of the defect.

Neurosurgical causes for visual loss

Tumours in the suprasellar region compressing the optic nerves and chiasm. Meningiomas and pituitary tumours present with gradual painless visual loss. Compression of the optic nerves and chiasm leads to a reduction in the peripheral visual fields, sometimes unnoticed for years. The patient will eventually present with visual failure when the tumour is much larger and the central visual fields are lost, limiting reading and writing.

Pituitary apoplexy with headache is associated with rapid loss of vision in one or both eyes, often with temporal visual field loss, and is caused by haemorrhage in a pre-existing pituitary tumour.

Raised intracranial pressure can lead to transient loss of vision with postural change (obscuration). It is often described as a brief blackout, like a curtain coming down, and lasting only seconds. Look for papilloedema.

Temporal arteritis. In the elderly, transient visual loss can be caused by temporal arteritis, which, without treatment, can lead to irreversible blindness. There may be tenderness and prominence of the temporal artery and 'claudication' on chewing.

CHAPTER 3 | THE BRAIN, CENTRAL NERVOUS SYSTEM AND PERIPHERAL NERVES

Double vision

(Diplopia)

To identify which group of muscles are involved ask whether the double vision is:

- worse looking up or down;
- worse looking left or right;
- better with the head tilted.

If the double vision is worst in one particular direction, horizontal, vertical or diagonal, this will indicate which muscle and hence which nerve is involved. For example, if the left lateral rectus is weak, double vision will be maximal looking to the left.

A painful IIIrd nerve palsy with ptosis, a dilated pupil and an inability to move the eye in any direction but outwards is a classical presentation of an expanding aneurysm behind the eye (Fig. 3.1).

Fig. 3.1 IIIrd cranial nerve palsy.

A pupil-sparing IIIrd nerve palsy is often attributed to diabetes and an ischaemic neuropathy.

When a tumour or aneurysm involves the cavernous sinus there is a characteristic combination of IIIrd, IVth and VIth cranial nerve palsies, often with proptosis. If the branches of the trigeminal nerve are also involved, there is altered sensation over the cheek or the forehead

Painless diplopia secondary to an isolated IVth or VIth cranial nerve palsy is often unexplained.

When the eyes obviously point in different directions and there is no complaint of double vision, there must be a long-standing squint, or an accompanying loss of vision in one eye with the squint (**amblyopia**).

Intracranial conditions presenting with weakness (focal neurological deficit)

Focal neurological deficits such as weakness of the arm or leg allow the site of the pathology to be localized whatever its cause (Table 3.1).

The motor homunculus is a cortical representation of control of movements (Fig. 3.2). It is important to distinguish *cortical* from *spinal* motor paresis. A parasagittal meningioma compressing the medial aspect of the motor strip in the posterior frontal region can give rise to a stiff spastic leg.

Table 3.1   Localization of pathology within the brain

Site of focal lesion	Symptom
Frontal lobe	Dementia and personality change with hemiparesis
Temporal lobe	Auditory or olfactory hallucinations, memory impairment, visual field defect and with dominant lobe, dysphasia
Parietal lobe	Hemiparesis with sensory neglect and visual field defect
Occipital lobe	Contralateral visual field defect
Posterior fossa	Cranial nerve palsies and ipsilateral ataxia

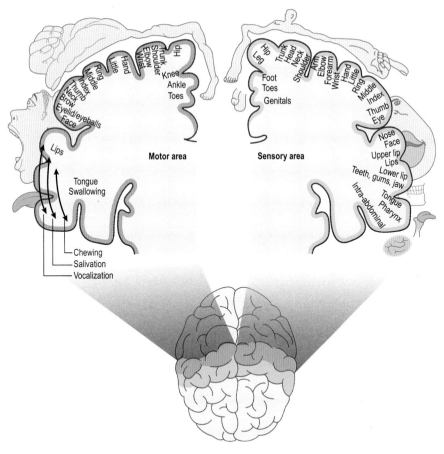

Fig. 3.2 Motor and sensory homunculus.

Intracranial conditions presenting with deafness and loss of balance

Deafness is common and has many causes.

Ask directly about:

- Speed of onset.
- Degree of hearing loss.
- Unsteadiness.
- Facial numbness.
- Change of voice.
- Difficulty swallowing.

Unilateral progressive deafness may indicate the early stages of an infratentorial tumour such as a vestibular schwannoma or a meningioma.

As these tumours enlarge, they distort the brainstem, which produces multiple cranial nerve palsies, seen with any space-occupying lesion in the cerebellopontine angle.

Early symptoms with small tumours include:

- unilateral hearing loss;
- high-pitched tinnitus;
- unsteadiness.

Examination reveals a sensorineural hearing loss. In contrast, a conductive deafness may be caused by chronic otitis media.

Symptoms of a vestibular schwannoma correlate closely with tumour size. Large tumours can cause facial pain or numbness from trigeminal nerve compression, as well as unsteadiness from brainstem distortion.

Bilateral symptoms are rare and suggest type 2 neurofibromatosis.

Very large tumours cause brainstem signs with ataxia, double vision and eventually hydrocephalus. Lower cranial nerve involvement produces hoarseness and difficulty in swallowing.

CHAPTER 3 | THE BRAIN, CENTRAL NERVOUS SYSTEM AND PERIPHERAL NERVES

NEUROLOGICAL SYMPTOMS ARISING FROM SPINAL CONDITIONS

These are discussed in Chapter 9.

Chronic spinal cord compression

Cervical myelopathy causes abnormalities of gait and weakness or stiffness of the legs. It can also present with a loss of manual dexterity, difficulty in writing and abnormal sensations, which patients describe as numb, clumsy hands.

Signs of spasticity are often present, but loss of sphincter control and urinary incontinence are unusual.

Acute spinal cord compression

The clinical features of acute cord compression are:

- progressive paraparesis;
- a 'sensory level' (the sensory segmental level of the spinal cord below which sensation to a pin or light touch is impaired);
- often disturbance of sphincter control;
- back pain, usually intense.

Speed of onset

An acute onset is typically associated with transverse myelitis or a bleed from a spinal arteriovenous malformation. Infection and malignant tumours present with a steady deterioration over some weeks.

A slow painless progression over months suggests a benign intradural tumour such as a meningioma or schwannoma.

Evidence of cutaneous neurofibromatosis (see Chapter 4) increases the likelihood of a spinal tumour. Long-standing plexiform neurofibromas are known to undergo late malignant transformation.

NEUROLOGICAL EXAMINATION

You need to become confident with the ophthalmoscope, red pin and reflex hammer.

Observe the patient as they enter, noting their general appearance, mood and mobility, and how they sit and stand, undress and dress. A number of neurological conditions can be diagnosed at this point.

Acromegaly (see Chapter 1) is caused by the stimulation of growth after normal growth has ceased. The patient has a large face and large hands, with overgrowth of the soft tissues of the face, nose, lips and tongue, and of the frontal sinuses and jaw (see Fig. 1.9).

The **neurocutaneous syndromes** (see Chapter 4) are readily diagnosed on sight:

- Type 1 neurofibromatosis (café-au-lait patches, subcutaneous nodules, plexiform neuromas with a risk of sarcomatous change).
- Sturge–Weber syndrome (epilepsy and a port wine stain on the forehead).
- Tuberous sclerosis (adenoma sebaceum on the cheeks and nose, subungal fibromas).

HEAD AND SPINE

Measure the circumference of a large or abnormally shaped head with a tape measure. Over 60 cm is abnormal. Larger heads can indicate:

- chronic hydrocephalus (see Chapter 1);
- acromegaly (see Chapter 1);
- Paget's disease in the elderly (Fig. 3.3)

Fig. 3.3 Paget's disease. Large head circumference.

Often standard headwear, caps and hats will not fit (see Chapter 6).

Scalp swellings are inspected and palpated. Determine whether they are mobile in relation to the skull, such as a dermoid of the scalp (see Chapter 4), or are fixed to the skull and hard, such as an osteoma of the skull (see Chapter 6). Very rarely, a hard bony lump indicates an underlying meningioma.

In the elderly, feel the temporal arteries looking for tenderness and thickening. In a patient with the headache of temporal arteritis, the abnormal arteries stand out.

If there is proptosis, listen with your stethoscope over the closed eye, the cheek and the mastoid area. If there is a carotico-cavernous fistula or a cerebral arteriovenous malformation, there will be bruit, a whooshing noise.

Inspect the spine for any midline cutaneous abnormalities such as an angioma, dimple or hairy patch that may be a cutaneous manifestation of underlying spinal dysraphism (see Chapter 9).

Examine the spine with the patient standing. Note any deformity or swelling. Look for kyphosis and scoliosis. Assess the full range of movement, with the patient bending forwards and backwards, with lateral flexion and with rotation to either side. Note any fatty swelling such as a lipoma over the lower spine, also in keeping with dysraphism. Palpate for tenderness and paravertebral spasm.

The neurological examination starts with the higher functions and then works systematically down from the head to the arms and legs.

Explain what you are doing and why. The examination finishes as you watch the patient leave the consulting room.

PRACTICAL NEUROLOGICAL EXAMINATION

Testing of higher cortical function

Assess the patient's orientation in time and place. Ask their views of current events, perhaps sport results or newspaper headlines. Routine tests of memory and intellectual function are undertaken if there are doubts about short-term memory.

A useful test is to ask the patient to memorize three objects immediately, and recall them immediately after 5 minutes. An alternative is to ask them to carry out a serial subtraction of seven from 100.

Any speech or language disorder should become evident during the history-taking.

Do not use the term 'confused'. It is better to state whether the patient is fully orientated or disorientated, and whether they are able to express themselves or not, that is, they are dysphasic. Dysphasia can make patients appear muddled because of difficulty in expressing themselves.

Other tests of language include reading and the ability to execute spoken commands and name objects.

Visuospatial difficulties can be assessed by asking the patient to copy a figure or draw a clock face with hands.

Examination of the cranial nerves

Examine the cranial nerves systematically to ensure that all 12 nerves are tested on every occasion.

I Olfactory

The sense of smell can be tested formally with bottles containing cloves or cinnamon. If not available, you can use orange peel or soap! The nose is supplied by the Ist (smell only) and Vth cranial nerves.

An anosmic patient can still sense noxious agents such as ammonia through the trigeminal nerve, but can taste only salt, sweet, sour and bitter, not enough to savour food or wine. *They cannot smell smoke if there is a fire.*

Neurological loss of smell results from head injury or a large anterior skull base tumour such as a bifrontal meningioma presenting with dementia and anosmia.

Nasal causes of anosmia such as sinusitis and polyps are more common.

II Optic

Fundoscopic examination is key.

Look for swelling of the optic disc (**papilloedema**) in any patient with suspected raised intracranial pressure (Fig. 3.4). The optic disc is normally pale pink or yellow with crisp margins. An early sign of papilloedema is the loss of venous pulsation. If there is any doubt, standing the patient up increases the pulsation. Blurring of the optic disc is characteristic, particularly on the temporal side, and retinal haemorrhages are common.

The visual acuity is often normal, with a concentric restriction of the visual fields, and enlargement of the blind spot (see below). Note that papilloedema may not occur in elderly patients who have raised intracranial pressure.

Optic atrophy (pallor of the optic disc) secondary to chronic compression is found in patients with expanding lesions in the suprasellar region, pituitary tumours, meningioma and aneurysms (Fig 3.5).

Fig. 3.4 Papilloedema.

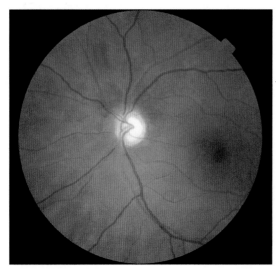

Fig. 3.5 Optic atrophy.

Confidence using the ophthalmoscope requires practice at every opportunity. The pupil gets smaller with age, so learn to use the instrument on younger patients or colleagues. A darkened room helps.

Visual acuity is a test of how well patients see using their central visual field.

Distant vision is tested with a well-illuminated Snellen chart, at a distance of 6 m. Details can be found in ophthalmology texts.

Asking the patient to read newspaper headlines is a crude alternative.

Impaired vision can be graded as the ability to count fingers, detect hand movements and tell light from dark.

Near vision is tested with reading cards with varying sizes of print.

Visual fields can be tested rapidly and reliably at the bedside.

Sit directly in front of the patient. Ask them to close one eye and look straight at you with the other. Keeping your hand midway between you and the patient, move your hand holding a red pin beyond your own visual field. Then gradually move the pin towards the midline until you can see it

If you and the patient see the red colour at the same time, the visual field is normal.

Any abnormality can be investigated further by testing each quadrant.

The visual pathways are important in localizing cerebral lesions because they travel from the temporal lobe through the parietal lobe to the occipital cortex. The pattern of visual field loss enables the lesion to be localized (Fig. 3.6).

A lesion of the optic radiation leads to an homonymous hemianopia or quadrantanopia (Fig 3.6).

Lesions of the optic nerve lead to monocular visual loss, and those of the optic chiasm to bitemporal hemianopia (Fig 3.6).

Lesions of the optic tract, optic radiation or geniculostriate tract cause varying degrees of homonymous hemianopia (Fig 3.6).

Lesions of the striate cortex, particularly if vascular, can be associated with sparing of macular vision. Some fibres course inferiorly around the occipital horn of the lateral ventricle (Meyer's loop), and lesions here cause a homonymous upper quadrantanopia (Fig 3.6).

Lesions affecting the upper, more direct fibres of the tract cause a homonymous lower quadrantanopia (Fig 3.6).

The **pupils** are inspected for size, shape and reaction to light. Horner's syndrome (see Chapter 1) and Holmes Adie syndrome will be obvious.

Eye movements

There are six muscles attached to each eye. To test the eye movements, ask the patient to keep their head still and follow your finger, and to tell you if they see double at any stage.

Draw a large H to test lateral and vertical movements.

The medial and lateral rectus are involved in horizontal movement.

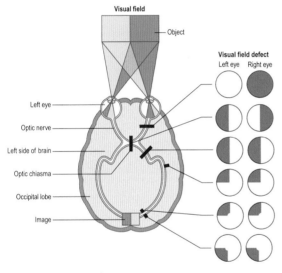

Fig. 3.6 Visual pathways.

The inferior and superior rectus are involved in vertical movements.

Torsional movements are controlled by the inferior and superior obliques.

III Oculomotor nerve

This supplies four of the six extrinsic eye muscles, as well as the levator palpebrae superioris and the muscle of accommodation. When it fails to function, the eye turns downwards and outwards, the upper lid droops (ptosis) and the pupil becomes fixed (not responding to light or accommodation) (Fig 3.7).

Sometimes individual muscles supplied by the third nerve can be paralysed.

To test the superior rectus muscle, ask the patient to 'look up'.

To test the inferior rectus ask the patient to 'look down'.

Oculomotor function is examined by looking for ptosis, the size of the pupils, and their reactivity to light and accommodation.

Remember that the IVth and VIth cranial nerves also have a role in eye movements. Attention should be paid to the direction in which maximal diplopia is noted by the patient, because this indicates the most likely weak muscle and responsible cranial nerve.

IV Trochlear nerve

This supplies the superior oblique muscle, which turns the eye downwards and outwards. If the nerve is damaged, the eye will look inwards (Fig. 3.8)

Fig. 3.7 Third nerve palsy. Ptosis and difficulty looking up and down.

Fig. 3.8 Damage of the right IVth cranial nerve.

and the patient will experience diplopia below the horizontal plane, for example when walking downstairs.

V Trigeminal nerve

This has three main divisions and is sensory to the face and up to the crown of the head (vertex). Test sensation close to the midline and compare the two sides. Note that the angle of the jaw is supplied by the great auricular nerve from the C2 and C3 roots. The cutaneous distribution of the ophthalmic, maxillary and mandibular divisions are shown in Fig. 3.9.

The corneal reflex has the Vth nerve as its afferent pathway and the VIIth nerve as its efferent. It therefore assesses the facial nerve as well as the trigeminal nerve. It is tested by touching the 'cornea of the eye' with a twisted pointed roll of tissue paper or cotton wool. This normally elicits a blink. The reflex/blink is lost if the ophthalmic division is damaged.

The trigeminal nerve also supplies the muscles of mastication. Motor fibres of the trigeminal nerve run in its mandibular division to the masseter, temporalis and medial and lateral pterygoid muscles.

Ask the patient to clench the teeth, and feel the contraction of the temporalis and masseter

Do not test power by trying to close an open jaw. This may cause dislocation.

If there is Vth nerve damage, the jaw deviates towards the side of the lesion, pushed across by the unopposed pterygoid muscles.

VI Abducens nerve

This nerve supplies the lateral rectus muscle, which turns the eye outwards. If it is damaged, the eye does not move when the patient tries to look sideways and there is diplopia, maximal when looking towards the side of the lesion (Fig 3.10).

A VIth nerve palsy can occur with any rise in intracranial pressure, so it is not a useful localizing sign.

VII Facial nerve

This is the motor nerve to the muscles of facial expression.

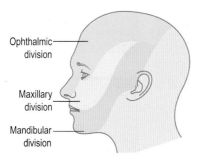

Fig. 3.9 Trigeminal nerve sensory distribution.

Fig. 3.10 Bilateral VIth cranial nerve palsies.

To test the facial nerve:

- Ask the patient to look up – the forehead should wrinkle (Fig. 3.11a).
- Ask them to close their eyes tightly. Any weakness is obvious (Fig. 3.11b).

With a facial nerve lesion, the ability to blink is lost and the eyelids do not cover the eye fully.

When the patient is asked to show you their teeth, the mouth becomes asymmetrical.

The patient cannot whistle.

Any damage to the tract of the nerve distal to the nucleus (lower motor neuron) causes paralysis of the whole of one side of the face (see Fig. 1.12).

If there is an upper motor neuron lesion, there is bilateral representation and function of the forehead is persevered.

Facial movements should also be observed with the patient talking and smiling, as a mild upper motor neuron weakness may be missed at rest.

The most important sensory function of the facial nerve is taste to the anterior two-thirds of the tongue via the chorda tympani. Taste may be tested using sweet, sour, salt and bitter substances.

VIII Auditory nerve

This nerve has two distinct components, both passing through the internal auditory meatus:

- The *cochlear* (auditory) division is responsible for hearing and transmits sound from hair cells in the organ of Corti within the inner ear.
- The *vestibular* division is responsible for balance and transmits information from the semicircular canals.

This nerve may be damaged by fractures of the base of the skull or compressed by acoustic neuromas.

Hearing can be tested simply by whispering in one ear while the opposite ear is closed by pressure on the tragus. The patient is asked to repeat what they can hear.

Hearing loss is either *conductive*, when the sound does not reach the cochlea, or *sensorineural*, where there is dysfunction of the cochlea, the auditory nerve or the brain itself. First look with an auroscope

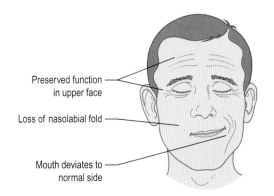

Preserved function in upper face

Loss of nasolabial fold

Mouth deviates to normal side

(a) Wrinkling of the forehead, UMN.

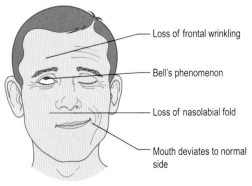

Loss of frontal wrinkling

Bell's phenomenon

Loss of nasolabial fold

Mouth deviates to normal side

(b) Weakness of eye closing, LMN.

Fig. 3.11 FACIAL NERVE PALSY

to ensure there is no obstruction in the outer or middle ear causing conductive deafness.

Rinne's and Weber's tests distinguish sensorineural hearing loss from conductive hearing loss.

- *Rinne's test.* Hold a vibrating tuning fork next to the external auditory meatus until the patient indicates that the sound can no longer be heard. The base of the tuning fork is then placed on the mastoid process. If the sound can still be heard, the patient has a conductive deafness (*negative* Rinne's test).
- *Weber's test.* Place the tuning fork on the centre of the forehead. Normally, both ears hear the sound equally. If there is sensorineural deafness, the sound will be loudest in the normal ear. If there is conductive deafness, the sound will be loudest in the abnormal ear.

Nystagmus, a rapid, brief to and fro movement of the eyes, suggests impairment of the vestibular division of the auditory nerve. The patient may complain of giddiness, and the abnormal eye movements may be seen on extremes of gaze.

The Romberg and stepping tests are also useful in evaluating vestibular function (see below).

IX Glossopharyngeal nerve

This nerve is the sensory nerve of the posterior third of the tongue. It also supplies the taste receptors and sensory endings of the mucous membrane of the pharynx.

It can be assessed by testing the gag reflex.

X Vagus nerve

The vagus nerve carries motor function to the soft palate.

When patients are asked to open the mouth widely and say 'Aarrh', the soft palate should move upwards symmetrically. If one side of the palate is paralysed, the uvula will be pulled towards the functioning side.

Lesions of the glossopharyngeal nerve usually also involve the vagus nerve as they travel together through the jugular foramen, where they can be compressed by, for example, a glomus jugulare tumour.

The IXth and Xth nerves control the pharynx and larynx, and are tested together. The voice and the ability to cough and swallow are functions of the two nerves. Loss of function should be suspected if

the patient is hoarse or has a bovine cough. They are then at risk of aspiration and chest infection.

XI Spinal accessory nerve

This nerve arises from medulla and upper spinal cord. It is a pure motor nerve and supplies the trapezius and sternomastoid muscles.

The function of these muscles is tested by asking the patient to shrug the shoulders and to turn the head against resistance.

It is very rare to have a spontaneous XIth nerve palsy. The usual cause is damage during surgical dissection of the posterior triangle of the neck (Fig. 3.12).

Fig. 3.12 Spinal accessory nerve. Damaged by block dissection of neck on the left side.

XII Hypoglossal nerve

This is also a purely motor nerve and supplies the muscles of the tongue. When one hypoglossal nerve is paralysed, the tongue is wasted on that side, and the tongue deviates towards the weak side (Fig 3.13).

Fig. 3.13 Hypoglossal nerve. Damaged by right carotid endarterectomy.

Examining motor function

Start by inspecting and testing the tone of the resting muscles (Revision panel 3.2). *Wasting and reduced tone indicate a lower motor neuron lesion.* Muscle bulk can be assessed by comparing the maximum circumference of the calves or thighs (Fig. 3.14). There should be no more than 1 cm difference. With an upper motor neuron lesion, there is no wasting; increased spinal activity maintains the muscle bulk.

- Examine the upper limbs with the patient sitting (Fig. 3.15).
- Examine the lower limbs with the patient supine.
- Examine the range of spinal movements with the patient standing.

Ask the patient to stand on their toes, testing S1, and then on their heels, testing L4/5. Then ask them

> ### Revision panel 3.2
> #### Types of weakness and region affected
> Monoplegia: single limb
> Hemiplegia: one side of the body, arm and leg
> Paraplegia: both lower limbs
> Quadriplegia: all four limbs

to stand on each leg, and then hop on each leg, thus checking power and coordination.

Watch the patient walking.

Look out for proximal weakness, which may be indicated by difficulty with getting out of a chair.

Upper limb

Power is graded from 0 to 5.

Fine finger movement is tested by asking the patient to pretend to play the piano.

The fingers are spread wide, testing the intrinsic muscles of the hand supplied by T1 (Fig. 3.16).

The fingers are brought together and held straight, which tests the long extensors (C8) (Fig. 3.17) and curled to test the flexors (Fig. 3.18).

The fist is clenched and locked at the wrist. Resistance to movement assesses muscle power.

Test elbow flexion (C6) and extension (C7) (Fig. 3.19).

Fig. 3.14 Measuring to assess muscle bulk.

Fig. 3.15 Examining the upper limbs with the patient seated.

Fig. 3.16 Testing the power of the intrinsic muscles of the hand (T1).

Fig. 3.17 Testing the power of the long extensors of the hand (C7/8).

(a) Testing the power of extension of the elbow (C7).

Fig. 3.18 Testing the long flexors (C8).

(b) Testing the power of flexion of the elbow (C5/6).

Fig. 3.19 ELBOW FLEXION AND EXTENSION

Finally, test the power of shoulder abduction (C5) (Fig. 3.20).

Upper limb reflexes

These are supinator (C6) (Fig. 3.21) biceps (C6) (Fig. 3.22), triceps (C7) (Fig. 3.23) and deltoid (C5).

The tendon hammer is held lightly at the far end and swung smoothly onto the tendon covered by your finger or thumb. This allows you to see and feel the reflex, or its absence.

An 'inverted' or paradoxical reflex is a useful localizing sign, particularly in patients with multilevel cervical myelopathy. On testing, the biceps reflex (C6) is absent, but there is brisk finger flexion (C8) (Fig. 3.18). This indicates a lower motor neuron lesion at C6 level (absent reflex) and an upper motor neuron lesion at C8 (finger flexion brisk).

Fig. 3.20 Testing the power of shoulder abduction (C5).

Rapid screening tests

Ask the patient to hold their arms out straight. If one arm drifts down or the wrist pronates, there may be pyramidal weakness. A rising arm is a sign of a cortical sensory loss in the parietal region with loss of spatial awareness.

Oscillation of the arms indicates a cerebellar problem with lack of coordination.

Simple tests of coordination

Ask the patient to alternately touch their nose and the examiner's finger, and run a heel down their contralateral shin.

These should always be part of your examination.

Fig. 3.21 Supinator (C6) reflex.

Fig. 3.22 Biceps (C5/6) reflex.

Fig. 3.23 Triceps (C7) reflex.

Lower limb

With the patient supine, begin with straight leg raising, which should be to 80–90°. Look for muscle wasting, and then test power, tone and reflexes (Fig. 3.24).

Start distally at the ankles, with dorsiflexion (L4/5) and plantar flexion (S1/2) (Fig. 3.25).

Place the patient's heels together and test inversion (L4) (Fig. 3.26a) and eversion (L5) (Fig. 3.26b).

Fig. 3.24 Straight leg raising.

(a) Testing dorsiflexion of the ankle (L4/5).

(b) Testing plantar flexion of the ankle (S1/2).

Fig. 3.25 DORSIFLEXION AND PLANTAR FLEXION

CHAPTER 3 | THE BRAIN, CENTRAL NERVOUS SYSTEM AND PERIPHERAL NERVES

(a) Testing inversion of the ankle (L4).

(b) Testing eversion of the ankle (L5).

Fig. 3.26 INVERSION AND EVERSION OF THE ANKLE

(a) Hip flexion (L1, L2, L3).

(b) Hip extension (L5, S1).

(c) Knee extension (L3, L4).

Fig. 3.27 TESTING POWER OF MOVEMENTS OF THE KNEE AND HIP

Movements at the knee and hip are then examined (Fig. 3.27).

Test the patellar and ankle reflexes (Fig. 3.28). Gently draw a thumbnail or pointed end of patellar hammer along the outer edge of the sole (Fig. 3.28). If there is tonic dorsiflexion (upgoing) of the big toe accompanied by fanning of the other toes, this is a positive plantar reflex, called Babinski's sign.

Always check the peripheral pulses. Claudication may be vascular or neurological, and the presence or absence of pulses can be indicative (see Chapter 10).

Finally, ask the patient to lie prone so the back can be inspected, and test perineal sensation.

The patient may sometimes be unable to stand, as for example in acute lumbar disc prolapse with sciatica. However, it is possible to gain diagnostic information from the reflexes and restricted straight leg raising.

Examining sensory function

This is the most time-consuming and difficult part of the neurological examination. Test the whole body, with different methods.

(a) The knee reflex L3/L4.

(b) The ankle reflex S1.

(c) Testing the plantar response.

Fig. 3.28 TESTING LOWER LIMB REFLEXES

Some variations in sensation are actually normal. For example, the outer aspect of the thigh is less sensitive than the inner.

Start with a general survey of sensation to light touch and pinprick. Any obvious abnormality can then be looked at in more detail.

When mapping numbness, test the region with reduced sensation before the area with normal sensation. This makes it easier for the patient to recognize the difference.

The examination should include a testing of sensations subserved by:

- the lateral spinothalamic pathway – pain, temperature;
- the anterior spinothalamic tract – touch/deep pressure;
- the posterior column/medial lemniscal system – light touch, proprioception, vibration and position sense.

The sensory level is vital to establish in patients presenting with cord compression.

Perception of passive motion

Proprioception is first tested in the fingers and toes, as any abnormality here is more likely to be noticed by the patient. Then move proximally.

Vibration sense

Vibration sense is tested by placing a low-frequency tuning fork over a bony prominence. Explain that you want to see if the patient detects vibration and not just pressure. Vibration and position sense are usually lost together, vibration sense usually more obviously. With increasing age, vibration sense is commonly reduced in the feet.

Reflexes

These can be both seen and felt, as described above.

Increased reflexes may indicate *upper motor neurone* disease, but remember that reflexes are often brisk in the young or anxious patient.

CHAPTER 3 | THE BRAIN, CENTRAL NERVOUS SYSTEM AND PERIPHERAL NERVES

Decreased or absent reflexes are a sign of a *lower motor neuron* lesion and will often be accompanied by reduced tone and loss of muscle bulk (Revision panel 3.3).

Revision panel 3.3

Upper and lower motor neuron lesions

Upper motor neuron lesions

There is damage above the level of the anterior horn cell, anywhere from the spinal cord to the primary motor cortex. There is:

No muscle wasting
Increased tone – spasticity like a clasp knife due to hypersensitivity of the stretch reflex
Weakness in a typical pattern, termed 'pyramidal'
In the upper limbs – weak abductors and extensors
In the lower limbs – weak abductors and flexors
Increased reflexes causing slow involuntary contractions (clonus)
Up-going plantar response (extensor)

Lower motor neuron lesions

Damage below the level of the anterior horn cell resulting in:

Muscle wasting
Fasciculations – rapid twitches
Decreased tone
Flaccid weakness
Decreased tendon reflexes
Plantar response that is down-going or absent (flexor)

At the start of the examination explain (as always) what you are going to do, and make sure the patient is warm and relaxed.

Test the biceps, triceps, supinator, patellar, Achilles and plantar reflexes.

Gait and stance

This usually concludes the examination of the neurological system.

An abnormality of gait and stance may be the only neurological abnormality if there is a midline cerebellar lesion.

Asking the patient to walk heel to toe may unmask subtle problems with balance not seen with their normal gait.

A *spastic* gait is a stiff scraping walk often tripping over kerbs.

An *ataxic* gait can be due to cerebellar disease or to loss of the dorsal column pathways caused by vitamin B12 deficiency or syphilis (sensory ataxia). The patient will describe being unsteady in the dark and having difficulty walking across rough ground. They often have a loud slapping step and rely on visual clues.

A *Parkinson's* gait is short shuffling steps with difficulty starting and stopping. There may be resting tremor and a lack of facial expression.

Perform the *Romberg* test. Ask the patient to stand still with their heels together and eyes closed. If the patient loses balance, the test is positive. The usual cause is a sensory problem in the posterior columns.

SPECIFIC INTRACRANIAL CONDITIONS

HEAD INJURY

When taking a history and examining a patient with a head injury who is conscious and alert, it is important to decide whether the patient has suffered a superficial head injury or a brain injury.

Try to establish a clear history of the forces involved and the speed of the accident. Question any available witness, police or attending paramedics for further information.

Record the Glasgow Coma Scale score in all patients. This is an essential tool in the assessment and management of patients with a head injury. Establish the best score in eye opening, verbal response and motor examination (Table 3.2, Revision panel 3.4).

Assess the post-traumatic amnesic (PTA) period, which is a good guide to the severity of the injury. This is the time from the accident to the recovery of full orientation. Amnesia for a significant length of time indicates diffuse head injury. PTA of less than 1 hour is graded mild, 1–24 hours moderate, and more than 24 hours severe.

Examine the head looking for laceration and bruising, shaving the hair if necessary. An apparently innocent laceration may be a sign of penetrating injury.

Table 3.2 The Glasgow Coma Scale

	Patient response	Score
Eye opening	Spontaneous	4
	To speech	3
	To pain	2
	None	1
Best verbal response	Orientated	5
	Confused	4
	Inappropriate words	3
	Incomprehensible sounds	2
	None	1
Best motor response	Obeys commands	6
	Localizes to pain	5
	Normal flexion	4
	Abnormal flexion	3
	Extends to pain	2
	None	1

Look for blood or cerebrospinal fluid (CSF) leaking from the ear or nose. This indicates a skull base fracture, with a risk of meningitis (see below).

Look for bruising behind the ear over the mastoid process (Battle's sign). This reflects a fracture of the middle cranial fossa (see Fig. 5.9).

Bruising around the eyes (the racoon sign) indicates a fracture of the anterior skull base (see Fig. 5.7).

Decide whether this is a closed or an open head injury. Patients with compound depressed fractures may not have been knocked out and may be fully alert and orientated by the time they arrive at hospital. Examine the wound for foreign bodies. Feel around the laceration as a depressed fracture may not be directly under the wound.

Concussion

This means temporary loss of consciousness occurring from the time of impact.

It can be *moderate*, with complete recovery in less than 5 minutes, or *severe* if the patient is unconscious for more than 5 minutes.

The majority of patients do not deteriorate but still require neurological monitoring until the symptoms have resolved. They may also be under the influence of drugs or alcohol and have no reliable companion at home.

Postconcussive syndrome includes headache, mild impairment of memory, giddiness and alteration of mood. These symptoms usually regress spontaneously but can persist for weeks or months.

Head injury and reduced conscious level

You must decide if there are focal signs or whether it is a diffuse head injury.

A patient with focal neurological signs, such as a unilateral dilated pupil who is flexing to pain on one side and extending on the other with a deteriorating conscious level, is very likely to have an expanding intracranial haematoma such as an acute subdural haematoma.

In contrast, a patient who is involved in a high-speed accident who is deeply unconscious from the time of the accident with symmetrical pupils and no lateralizing signs is more likely to have suffered a diffuse head injury (diffuse axonal injury) without any intracerebral haematoma.

Diffuse axonal injury is the most severe form of diffuse brain injury and is the most common cause of prolonged post-traumatic coma that is not the result of a mass lesion or ischaemia

It is characterized by small haemorrhages from microscopic shearing injuries between the grey and white matter tracts, involving the corpus callosum, rostral mid brain and superior cerebellar peduncles.

Patients frequently show abnormal posturing and autonomic dysfunction in addition to their prolonged coma. The intracranial pressure is often normal.

The prognosis is generally poor, with a 50 per cent mortality.

Cerebral contusion is focal brain injury caused by the impact of the brain surface against the internal ridges of the skull. Cerebral contusions are common in the frontal and temporal poles, as a result of impact against the corrugations in the floor of the skull.

A characteristic pattern of cerebral contusion is the **coup and contrecoup** injury. The coup occurs at the point of impact and the contrecoup at the point diametrically opposite (Fig 3.29).

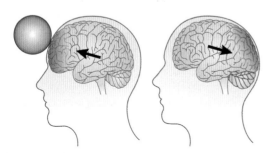

Fig. 3.29 Coup and contrecoup in cerebral contusion.

A contusion can cause fits, or may lead to an expanding haematoma producing late deterioration.

The neurological condition of patients with severe brain injury is notoriously fluctuant. Any deterioration in a patient's condition may require urgent intervention, so such patients must be monitored carefully and any change acted upon.

Many patients with head injuries are found unconscious at the scene of a high-speed accident, with focal neurological signs. Associated extracranial injuries are common, so that the primary brain injury is compounded by secondary damage from ischaemia and hypoxia. Swelling and bleeding from the surface of the hemisphere at the site of impact is also common. The blood clot can cover the whole hemisphere and cause major brain shift (see below) with elevated intracranial pressure (Fig. 3.30).

Revision panel 3.4

Severity of head injury

Severe head injury
Glasgow Coma Scale score 3–8

Moderate injury
Glasgow Coma Scale score 9–14

Minor head injury
Glasgow Coma Scale score 15

Brain shift and herniation

In brain herniation, a rise in intracranial pressure displaces the brain either downwards or across a fixed intracranial structure, leading to deepening coma.

Major herniations are common in severe head injuries. As the brain shifts, the brainstem is compressed against the contralateral tentorial edge. This results in an ipsilateral dilated pupil and a contralateral hemiplegia. Initial midbrain dysfunction progresses to involve the brainstem.

Brainstem signs are associated with deepening coma and imminent death. They include profound bradycardia, raised blood pressure and an irregular respiratory pattern.

Coning is an example of brain herniation. There is vertical displacement of the hindbrain. The cerebellar tonsils and lower brainstem become impacted in the foramen magnum, often producing irreversible brainstem ischaemia (Fig. 3.30).

Extradural haematoma

A fracture, commonly of the temporal bone, tears an adjacent meningeal vessel, and a haematoma develops in the extradural space (Fig. 3.31). This

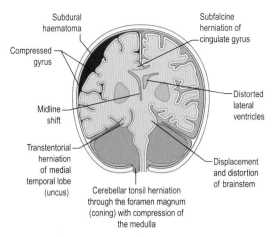

Fig. 3.30 Lateral and vertical brain shift due to expanding space occupying lesion (e.g. haematoma).

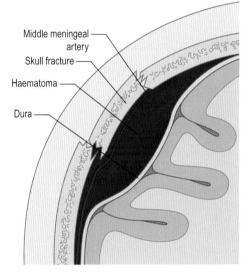

Fig. 3.31 Extradural haematoma formation after a skull fracture and torn middle meningeal artery.

increases the intracranial pressure (which is normally less than 20 mmHg). The brain itself is often initially undamaged. The rapidly expanding haematoma in the middle cranial fossa displaces the brain medially, causing the inner aspect of the temporal lobe (uncus) to be stretched over the free edge of the tentorium. This compresses the ipsilateral IIIrd cranial nerve and posterior cerebral artery, resulting in a dilated pupil on the side of the injury (Fig. 3.32), and then posterior cerebral ischaemia, which produces paralysis on the opposite side because of the crossed nerve tracts.

Symptoms Typically, a young person is struck forcibly on the side of the head, and there may be no loss of

(a) Fixed dilated pupil with decreased conscious level due to expanding space occupying lesion.

(b) Traumatic fixed dilated pupil.

Fig. 3.32 FIXED DILATED PUPIL

consciousness. There is headache from local bruising and the underlying fracture. There follows a progressive deterioration in the clinical condition, with increasing headache, vomiting and drowsiness progressing to coma. There is often no lucid interval but rather progression of signs and symptoms of raised pressure.
Signs There is bruising and swelling over the temporal area of the skull where the impact occurred. Deterioration to a contralateral hemiplegia and an ipsilateral dilated pupil can occur within hours and requires urgent surgery.

Penetrating brain injuries

Low-velocity injuries, such as those produced by a knife blade, cause local injury to the brain along the track but may not cause loss of consciousness or leave a permanent neurological deficit. The prognosis is good if no vital structures are torn.

High-velocity injuries, by a bullet, produce wide spread damage to the brain, from the missile itself and from the associated shock wave. Patients in coma have a very poor prognosis.

CSF fluid leak Fractures of the base of the skull may be associated with leakage of blood and CSF from the nose or ear. There may also be injury to the optic nerve, the pituitary gland, the hearing mechanisms and the facial nerve.

Persistent CSF rhinorrhoea carries the risk of meningitis and tension pneumocephalus.

Injuries of the brachial plexus

It is important to remember the possibility of a brachial plexus injury in any unconscious patient, especially when there are fractures of the shoulder girdle, proximal humerus or first rib. Complete plexus lesions can be caused by trauma to the cervical spine, gunshot wounds, stabbings, fractures of the clavicle, dislocations of the humerus and motorcycle accidents (in which the shoulder and neck are forcibly pulled apart, causing complete or partial disruption of the plexus).

The prognosis relates to the level of the damage. There are three main types of injury:

- *Root avulsion.* The nerve roots are avulsed from the spinal cord within the vertebral column. Spontaneous improvement is unlikely, and the injury is not amenable to surgical repair.
- *Rupture outside the vertebral column.* Spontaneous improvement is unlikely but the injury may benefit from surgical repair.
- *Nerve damage without rupture.* A neuropraxia or axonotmesis (see later in the chapter) with preservation of the nerve sheaths is likely to improve spontaneously.

In road traffic accidents, a low-velocity injury points to neuropraxia and axonotmesis, while a high-velocity impact is more likely to produce a complete disruption of the plexus.

The clinical picture depends on the level of injury (Fig. 3.33):

- In *root damage*, there will be paralysis of the scapular muscles and the diaphragm, and a Horner's syndrome.
- In *upper plexus damage*, sensation is lost over the C5 and C6 dermatomes. There is paralysis of the deltoid, the external rotators of the shoulder and the biceps, resulting in loss of shoulder abduction and inability to externally rotate the arm. Elbow flexion and forearm supination are weak. The *internally rotated* arm hangs against the trunk in the 'waiter's tip' position.

(a) Preservation of the deltoid (C5).

(b) All other muscles are wasted, and the hand is clawed.

Fig. 3.33 BRACHIAL PLEXUS INJURY FROM MOTORCYCLE ACCIDENT, RUPTURE OCCURRED OUTSIDE VERTEBRAL COLUMN

- Isolated *lower plexus damage* is rare. Sensation is lost over the inner ulnar aspect of the arm. The small *muscles of the hand* are paralysed, producing a claw hand.
- In *total plexus damage*, there is a numb flail upper limb with severe muscle wasting.

In a conscious patient, a careful examination of sensation and motor function will distinguish a brachial plexus injury from a radiculopathy (see Revision Panel 9.1). Pain and sensory changes are generally dominant in a plexus injury, and the sensory changes do not follow typical dermatomal patterns.

Chronic subdural hematoma

In the elderly, the subdural space is enlarged because of brain atrophy. Relatively minor head injuries such as striking the head against a door can tear a cortical bridging vein. The subsequent chronic subdural venous hematoma enlarges slowly, with episodes of rebleeding (Fig. 3.34).

Time of onset Clinical presentation is typically 6–8 weeks after a minor head injury.

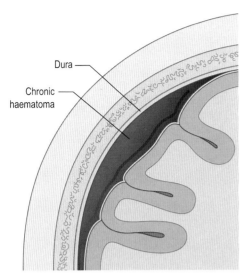

Fig. 3.34 Chronic subdural haematoma.

Risk factors The risk factors are advanced age and cerebral atrophy, coagulopathy, anticoagulants and alcohol abuse.

Symptoms These are of raised intracranial pressure, namely headache and drowsiness.

Signs The haematoma causes a mass effect, leading to – hemiparesis, dysphasia and tremors.

Differential diagnosis The clinical picture can easily be mistaken for a stroke, but the prognosis can be good, because there is no primary brain injury.

BRAIN TUMOURS

Presentation This depends on the location and speed of growth of the tumour. In general, a brain tumour can present with the signs of raised intracranial pressure, focal signs and/or fits. Progressively severe headaches and vomiting are typical symptoms. Drowsiness is an early sign of raised intracranial pressure. Hemiparesis and ataxia are examples of focal signs.

Family history The vast majority of primary brain tumours are sporadic. Of the small number that are familial, there is usually a hereditary disease known to be associated, such as tuberous sclerosis, neurofibromatosis, familial polyposis or Li–Fraumeni syndrome.

Symptoms The most common presentation is a progressive, usually motor neurological deficit, followed by headaches and then fits.

Brain tumours are classified by tumour location as supratentorial or infratentorial, and by tumour type.

Frontal brain tumours characteristically present with mental apathy, and personality change and dementia. Anosmia in such a patient would suggest a meningioma arising from the floor of the anterior cranial fossa.

Temporal tumours will often present with fits and speech disturbance if the dominant hemisphere is involved. On examination there may be a contralateral hemiparesis and a visual field defect.

Parietal tumours classically present with a contralateral weakness depending on which region of the motor strip is involved.

Patients with occipital tumours are often found to have a visual field defect.

Infratentorial tumours (cerebellum/brainstem) often present with loss of balance (ataxia) and disturbance of vision. Headache, when present, is often severe due to obstructive hydrocephalus.

The location of the headache is not normally related to the site of the tumour, although rarely downward displacement of the cerebellar tonsils can cause severe neck pain.

Brain tumours may be intrinsic, namely arising from the brain itself, or they may be extrinsic and arise from the surrounding structures (Revision panel 3.5).

Revision panel 3.5

Intrinsic and extrinsic brain tumours

Intrinsic tumours
Cerebral metastases
Glioblastoma multiforme
Astrocytoma
Oligodendroglioma
Ependymoma

Extrinsic tumours
Meningioma
Pituitary adenoma
Schwannoma

Intrinsic tumours

Gliomas, the most common type, are classified by cell type and histological grade. The incidence of high-grade glioma is increasing as the population grows older.

Grade 1 gliomas, such as the well-circumscribed pilocytic astrocytoma, occur in children and young adults and can involve both the cerebellum and the cerebral hemispheres. They generally carry a good prognosis.

Grades 2, 3 and 4 are infiltrating astrocytomas and usually involve the cerebral hemispheres and spare the cerebellum. The prognosis deteriorates with increasing grade. Grades 3 and 4 are clearly malignant tumours with a poor prognosis.

Older patients tend to have more aggressive higher grade tumours. The mean ages for these tumours are:

- grade 2 astrocytoma in adults – 34 years;
- anaplastic grade 3 astrocytoma – 41 years;
- grade 4 malignant glioblastoma multiforme – 63 years.

It is very unusual for a primary tumour of the central nervous system to spread outside the brain and spinal cord. Rarely, an aggressive primary tumour of the central nervous system such as a high-grade glioma will metastasize within the craniospinal axis (Revision panel 3.6).

Revision panel 3.6

Cerebral metastases

These are the most common intracranial tumours

Their incidence is increasing as more patients survive the primary treatment of carcinomas

Common primary tumours for blood-borne metastases are:

> Lung carcinoma
> Breast carcinoma
> Kidney carcinoma
> Gut carcinoma
> Melanoma

Extrinsic tumours

Pituitary tumours

These present with endocrine dysfunction caused by either overproduction of hormones or underproduction because of pressure from a tumour leading to failure of the rest of the gland (hypopituitarism).

Prolactinomas (lactotroph) secrete excessive prolactin, and a microprolactinoma is typically responsible for amenorrhoea and galactorrhoea in young females.

Somatotroph adenomas produce excessive growth hormone, causing acromegaly.

Pituitary tumours may also produce adrenocorticotropic hormone causing Cushing's disease (see Chapter 1), or thyroid-stimulating hormone leading to thyrotoxicosis (see Chapter 12).

Functioning tumours are seen more often in younger age groups, and are generally small benign adenomas.

Non-functioning tumours typically occur in the elderly. Symptoms do not appear until the tumour has reached a considerable size (macroadenoma). The tumour fills the pituitary fossa and grows upwards to compress the optic chiasm and optic nerves. The central crossing fibres are compressed, resulting in a bitemporal hemianopia (see Fig. 3.6).

There may be associated hypopituitarism, but the visual loss is usually the presenting feature.

Craniopharyngiomas

These arise in the suprasellar region, often from the pituitary stalk, so the endocrine dysfunction produced is diabetes insipidus, because of a loss of antidiuretic hormone. This causes polyuria and polydipsia.

Craniopharyngiomas occur more frequently in the young, causing short stature from a lack of growth hormone. The local mass effect causes headaches, and visual loss is usually asymmetrical.

Meningiomas

Meningiomas arise from meningothelial cells of the arachnoid layer, a membranous layer surrounding the brain and spinal cord. They occur primarily at the base of the skull, in the parasellar regions and over the cerebral convexities. They are usually solitary, except in neurofibromatosis type 2.

Ninety per cent of meningiomas are benign, but a few are atypical or frankly malignant. There are many histological varieties of benign meningioma, including syncytial, fibrous and transitional, but the distinction is usually of little clinical significance.

Meningiomas typically grow very slowly and can reach a considerable size without producing symptoms.

Symptoms and signs often present in the middle aged and elderly include progressive motor weakness, visual disturbance and infrequent headaches.

Asymptomatic meningiomas are often uncovered in the elderly after a stroke or head injury, and can usually simply be kept under periodic review.

Vestibular schwannomas (acoustic neuroma)

These are benign tumours of myelin-forming cells of the VIIIth cranial nerve. They cause unilateral deafness that may be preceded or accompanied by tinnitus.

In the early stages, there is nothing to find apart from deafness, but as the tumour gradually enlarges, there is displacement and distortion of the brainstem. The diagnosis should be considered in any patient with unilateral deafness.

BRAIN HAEMORRHAGE

Twenty per cent of strokes are caused by a cerebral haemorrhage, the rest being due to thrombosis and embolism.

Spontaneous intracranial haemorrhage

Causes of spontaneous intracranial haemorrhage vary with age (Revision panel 3.7). In the elderly, vascular disease associated with hypertension is common, but in younger patients coagulopathy is more likely.

Clues to the cause of an intracranial bleed may be gleaned from the site. For example, hypertensive haemorrhage tends to damage the basal ganglia, and a lobar haematoma is seen with amyloid angiopathy.

Subarachnoid haemorrhage from berry aneurysms:

Cerebral aneurysms occur at the branching points of the cerebral arteries around the circle of Willis, in the subarachnoid space (Fig. 3.35). They are commonly known as berry aneurysms because of their size and shape.

Revision panel 3.7

Risk factors for intracranial haemorrhage

General

These are similar to those for ischaemic stroke:

  Increasing age
  Male gender
  Hypertension
  Smoking
  Diabetes
  Alcohol abuse

Underlying vascular conditions

Arteriovenous malformation

Aneurysm

Cavernoma

Amyloid angiopathy

Cerebral venous thrombosis

Abnormal haemostasis

Anticoagulant drugs

Antiplatelet drugs

Coagulation disorders

Thrombolytic drugs

Other causes

Drug abuse (cocaine)

Moyamoya syndrome

Haemorrhage into a primary or secondary brain tumour

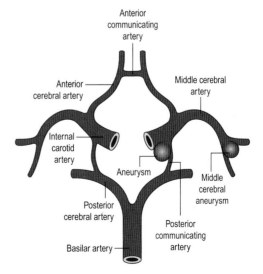

Fig. 3.35 Circle of Willis with sites of aneurysm formation. These may rupture and cause subarachnoid haemorrhage.

Incidence As many as 1 per cent of adults in the UK are affected.

Age They are increasingly common with age.

Sex Berry aneurysms are twice as common in females.

Risk factors Hypertension, and smoking. In countries with a high prevalence such as Finland, the condition may be familial.

Symptoms There are usually no symptoms from an unruptured aneurysm, although large lesions can compress surrounding brainstem structures and can, for example, interfere with vision. Patients may experience a less severe, sentinel headache a few days before a major rupture.

The patient may make a full recovery from a small bleed.

Where there is no neurological deficit, the decision to investigate this group of patients is then based on the history alone.

Signs The patient with a typical subarachnoid is drowsy and disorientated with neck stiffness. The site of the ruptured aneurysm will dictate the presence of any focal signs. Vasospasm can occur in the weeks after the initial bleed leading to cerebral ischaemia with further neurological deficit.

Cerebral arteriovenous malformation

Incidence They are only one-tenth as common as cerebral aneurysms.

Pathology The malformations are congenital, usually solitary lesions. There is shunting of blood from arteries to veins.

Symptoms and signs Some patients describe a pulsatile noise in the head, but the usual presentation is with an intracerebral haemorrhage that may be intraparenchymal, intraventricular or subarachnoid. This haemorrhage may produce severe headache, fits and/or a stroke.

Cavernoma

This lesion is a cavernous haemangioma of the brain, spinal cord or cauda equina, and consists of vascular channels under low pressure. It is often small and looks like a blackberry. One-quarter are multiple.

Aetiology Cavernomas are often familial. Multiple sporadic lesions may result from trauma or radiation.

Symptoms The cavernoma may enlarge and present as a space-occupying lesion. Once a lesion bleeds there is a small risk of further local small bleeds. Fitts may also be a symptom of repeated haemorrhage.

Signs When the cavernoma is in the posterior fossa or the spinal cord, there may be a progressive neurological deficit due to repeated local bleeds.

INFECTIONS OF THE BRAIN

Cerebral abscess

A brain abscess may be the result of a local spread of infection from the frontal sinuses, mastoids or teeth, or less commonly via the bloodstream from the heart or lungs.

Presentation The classical triad is fever, headache and focal neurological signs.

Fever is often absent or low grade.

Headache is often accompanied by drowsiness because there is raised intracranial pressure.

The *focal signs* depend on the site of the abscess:

- Fits suggest a frontal or temporal lobe abscess.
- A temporal lobe abscess arising from a chronic middle ear infection can present with a contralateral hemiparesis and a visual field defect.
- Nystagmus and ataxia suggest a cerebellar abscess arising from the middle ear.

Subdural empyema

Infection from the sinuses or skull bones may be confined to the subdural space. It may cause thrombosis of the cortical veins leading to infarction and swelling of the brain.

Symptoms Because of the confined space, the headache is severe and rapidly progressive.

Signs The patient is unwell with a high fever and neck stiffness from meningeal irritation.

There is often tenderness over the infected sinus.

Eventually, the patient, who is often young, develops fits, a decreasing conscious level and hemiparesis.

Traumatic cerebrospinal fluid leak and meningitis

A skull base fracture involving the anterior or middle fossa may lead to a CSF leak. The fluid may initially be bloodstained but becomes clear. This is a compound fracture, and meningitis can follow.

The bacteria responsible depend on the site: pneumococcus from the nose, and multiple organisms such as *Staphylococcus*, *Pseudomonas* and coliforms from the ears.

Air may pass into the cranium under pressure if a patient with CSF rhinorrhoea blows their nose, causing a *tension pneumocephalus* and collapse.

HYDROCEPHALUS

This is excessive accumulation of CSF caused by a disturbance of its formation, flow or absorption.

The volume of CSF in an adult is 120–150 mL, and the normal production of CSF is 450 mL/24 hours. Therefore the CSF is recycled three times every day.

Types of hydrocephalus

- *Communicating hydrocephalus* occurs when there is impaired CSF reabsorption by the arachnoid granulations and leads to increased CSF pressure and ventricular enlargement. It is generally safe to undertake lumbar puncture in this group of patients, but not in patients with an obstructive hydrocephalus.
- *Non-communicating or obstructive hydrocephalus* occurs when the CSF outflow tracts are obstructed, such as at the exit foramina (Magendie and Luschka) of the fourth ventricle (see Fig. 1.15).
- *Hydrocephalus ex vacuo* occurs when compensatory ventricular enlargement develops secondary to brain atrophy.

- *Arrested hydrocephalus* usually occurs as a result of an incomplete obstruction in a communicating hydrocephalus where CSF production is balanced by absorption. The intracranial pressure is normal, despite the ventricles remaining dilated. The head circumference may be increased if the hydrocephalus is congenital and presenting in infancy. These patients can decompensate after a head injury later in life.
- *Normal-pressure hydrocephalus* is a condition in which the ventricles remain enlarged after a previous period of raised pressure.

Acute hydrocephalus

The causes of acute hydrocephalus are shown in Revision panel 3.8.

Revision panel 3.8

Causes of hydrocephalus

Acute

Posterior fossa tumours

Cerebellar haemorrhage or infarction

Colloid cyst of the third ventricle

Ependymoma of the fourth ventricle

Subarachnoid haemorrhage

Trauma

Acute meningitis

Chronic

Slow-growing posterior fossa tumours

Subarachnoid haemorrhage

Chronic meningitis

No demonstrable cause (30% of cases)

History

There is headache and vomiting because of the raised intracranial pressure. There may be diplopia caused by a VIth nerve palsy.

Occasionally, there is rapid loss of consciousness and death. For example, acute hydrocephalus with a colloid cyst blocking the foramina of Monro.

Examination

On examination, there may be an impaired conscious level and an inability to look upwards (Parinaud's syndrome, a result of compression of the upper brainstem). Papilloedema may be present.

Chronic hydrocephalus

Presentation is usually in the elderly with a decline in intellect and memory, an ataxic gait and urinary incontinence.

PERIPHERAL NERVE INJURY

There are three grades of peripheral nerve injury.

Neurapraxia

Axonal continuity is maintained, and nerve conduction is preserved both proximal and distally but not across the injured segment. This type of injury is usually reversible, and a full recovery may occur within days to weeks.

It results from:

- direct mechanical compression;
- ischaemia secondary to vascular compromise;
- metabolic derangements;
- diseases or toxins causing demyelination.

In the last two categories, conduction is restored once either the metabolic derangement has been corrected or remyelination occurs.

Axonotmesis

This is a more severe grade of nerve injury in which there is interruption of the axons with preservation of the surrounding myelin and connective tissue sheath. It is followed by degeneration of the axon and myelin distal to the site of injury, occurs over several days and is called *Wallerian degeneration.*

Electrical stimulation of the disconnected distal nerve stump does not produce nerve conduction or muscle contraction. Recovery can occur from axonal regeneration through the preserved Schwann cells and their basal lamina. The Schwann cells proliferate and form longitudinal conduits through which the axons regenerate.

This type of injury usually recovers, but over a period of months. The timing and degree of recovery depend on the extent of the retrograde axonal loss. Peripheral nerve fibres usually regenerate at approximately a millimetre per day or an inch per month. More proximal injuries take longer to recover.

Neurotmesis

In the most severe grade of peripheral nerve injury, there is disruption of the axon, myelin and connective tissue components of the nerve. Therefore recovery through regeneration is impossible.

Division may be obvious, but sometimes the continuity of the nerve appears intact although intraneural fibrosis has blocked axonal regeneration. Continuity of the nerve can only be re-established by surgery to remove scar tissue and restore alignment.

It is often difficult to diagnose the grade of nerve injury by clinical examination at the time of injury. In general, movement recovers before sensation.

Examination

First grade the strength of the individual muscles or muscle groups. Then perform a sensory examination, testing for light touch, pinprick, two-point discrimination, vibration and proprioception. Look carefully at the autonomous zones of a nerve where there is minimal overlap from adjacent nerves.

Map out the distribution of the sensory loss to determine whether it corresponds to a dermatome or a single nerve (Fig. 3.36).

Tinel's sign is paraesthesia distal to the injury, described by the patient as tingling, that is elicited by tapping over the nerve. It indicates a partial lesion or the beginning of regeneration of the nerve, and can be used to map nerve regeneration. The presence of this sign does not, however, guarantee motor recovery.

A return of sweating signifies sympathetic nerve fibre regeneration.

Reflex changes are sensitive indicators of nerve damage.

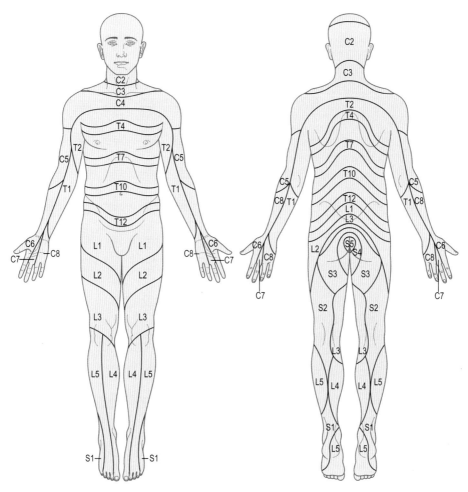

Fig. 3.36 Upper and lower limb dermatomes.

Nerves of the upper limb

Median nerve

The nerve can be damaged by:

- penetrating injuries of the arm and forearm;
- lacerations at the wrist;
- wrist dislocation;
- carpal tunnel compression.

Sensory loss The median nerve is sensory to the palmar aspect of the thumb, index and middle fingers, and the dorsal aspect of the distal phalanx and half of the middle phalanx of the same fingers. It also supplies sensation to the radial side of the palm.

Motor malfunction If the injury is at wrist level, there is:

- wasting of the muscles of the thenar eminence;
- loss of abduction and opposition of the thumb (Fig. 3.37).

If the injury is above the antecubital fossa (elbow level), there is:

- wasting of the muscles of the forearm and thenar eminence;
- loss of flexion of the thumb and index finger;
- holding of the hand in the 'benediction' position, with the ulnar fingers flexed and the index finger straight.

(a) Bilateral median nerve compression with wasting of the thenar eminences.

(b) Ulnar nerve lesion.

Fig. 3.37 LOSS OF ABDUCTION AND OPPOSITION OF THE THUMB

Ulnar nerve

This nerve can be damaged by:

- compression or injury at the elbow;
- penetrating injuries of the arm or forearm;
- fractures of the medial epicondyle;
- lacerations at the wrist;
- long-standing marked cubitus valgus.

Sensory loss The ulnar nerve is sensory to the anterior and posterior surfaces of the little finger, and the ulnar side of the ring finger. It also provides sensation to the skin over the front and back of the hypothenar eminence.

Motor malfunction If the injury is at wrist level there is:

- wasting of the hypothenar eminence and between the metacarpals;
- loss of flexion of the little and ring fingers;

- a 'claw' hand, in which the ring and little fingers are hyperextended at the metacarpo-phalangeal joints and flexed at the interphalangeal joints (Fig 3.38);
- an absence of both abduction and adduction of the fingers, with a positive Froment's sign (inability to hold a sheet of paper between thumb and index finger) (Fig 3.39).

If the injury is at elbow level, there is:

- wasting of the intrinsic muscles of the hand and hypothenar eminence;
- a claw hand without the flexion of the terminal interphalangeal joints because of paralysis of half the deep flexors of the fingers;
- a positive Froment's sign.

If the injury is well above the elbow, there is:

- wasting of the intrinsic muscles of the hand and hypothenar eminence;
- loss of flexion of the little and ring fingers;

Fig. 3.38 Claw hand in syringomyelia.

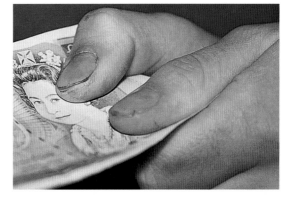

Fig. 3.39 Froment's sign.

- a 'claw' hand in which the ring and little fingers are hyperextended at the metacarpophalangeal joints without flexion of the interphalangeal joints;
- absence of both abduction and adduction of the fingers, with a positive Froment's sign;
- a paralysed flexor carpi ulnaris.

Radial nerve

This nerve can be damaged by:

- fractures of the humeral shaft;
- prolonged pressure from a crutch in the axilla;
- penetrating injuries of the back of the arm or forearm.

Sensory loss The radial nerve supplies sensation to a small area on the lateral aspect of the first metacarpal and the back of the first web space and thumb.

Motor malfunction If the nerve is injured in the axilla:

- there will be dropping of the wrist with inability to extend (Fig 3.40);
- the triceps will be paralysed, so the elbow will not extend.

If the nerve is injured as it wraps round the humerus in its middle third:

- the brachioradialis, an elbow flexor, is spared;
- there is still a wrist drop and loss of triceps action.

If the injury is to the posterior interosseous nerve:

- the hand deviates radially during wrist extension;
- there is an inability to maintain opposed finger extension.

Quick screen of the motor function of the nerves of the upper limb

Three simple tests will give you an idea of which nerve is injured:

- Median nerve: abduction of thumb (Fig. 3.41a).
- Ulnar nerve: abduction of little finger (Fig. 3.41b).
- Radial nerve: extension of the wrist (Fig. 3.41c).

(a) Median nerve – abduction of the thumb.

(b) Ulnar nerve – abduction of the little finger.

(c) Radial nerve – extension of the wrist.

Fig. 3.41 QUICK SCREEN OF MOTOR FUNCTION IN THE UPPER LIMB

Fig. 3.40 Wrist drop of right hand, caused by radial/posterior intraosseous nerve damage.

CHAPTER 3 | THE BRAIN, CENTRAL NERVOUS SYSTEM AND PERIPHERAL NERVES

Quick screen of sensory loss of the upper limb

Axillary nerve

This nerve can be damaged by:

- shoulder dislocation or fracture;
- penetrating axillary injuries.

Sensory loss The loss covers a small area over the deltoid equivalent to the C5 dermatome.

Motor malfunction The deltoid muscle is paralysed, so shoulder abduction is lost.

Nerves of the lower limb

Femoral nerve

This is commonly damaged by knife or bullet injuries to the femoral triangle.

Iatrogenic injuries also occur.

The sensory loss is over the anterior and medial surfaces of the thigh.

The quadriceps muscles are paralysed, causing weakness of knee extension.

The patellar tendon reflex is lost.

Sciatic nerve

This nerve can be damaged by:

- usually knife and gunshot wounds (e.g. knee-capping);
- gluteal injections, hip replacement surgery and repair of acetabular fractures;
- compound fracture dislocation of the hip.

Sensory loss is variable, depending on the level of nerve damage.

Motor malfunction The muscles of the lower leg are paralysed and later become wasted. The limb is 'flail'.

The ankle jerk is lost.

Common peroneal nerve

This nerve is easily damaged as it winds around the neck of the fibula.

This nerve can be damaged by:

- local trauma;
- external pressure from a splint or plaster;

- iatrogenic damage during surgery on the limb, usually caused by poor positioning.

Sensory loss Sensation is lost over the outer side of the leg foot and sole.

Motor malfunction There is foot drop with weakness of eversion and dorsiflexion of the ankle.

Quick screen of the motor function of the nerves of the lower limb

Test plantar flexion (Fig. 3.42a) and dorsiflexion (Fig. 3.42b).

(a) The patient standing on their toes to test plantar flexion S1, S2.

(b) The patient standing on their heels to test dorsiflexion L4/5 and exclude any footdrop.

Fig. 3.42 QUICK SCREEN OF MOTOR FUNCTION IN THE LOWER LIMB

The skin and subcutaneous tissues

ANATOMY AND FUNCTION

The skin is a complex organ that provides protection from ultraviolet light and microbiological invasion. It has an important sensory role, containing mechanoreceptors, thermoreceptors and nocioreceptors (for pain sensation). It also controls body temperature, is important in maintaining fluid balance and provides immunological surveillance.

The skin consists of two layers: the epidermis, derived from ectoderm, and the dermis, derived from the mesoderm.

The epidermis

The epidermis is a stratified squamous epithelium composed of five layers:

- the *stratum germinativum* – containing basal cells;
- the *stratum spinosum* – containing prickle cells;
- the *stratum granulosum* – containing granular cells;
- the *stratum lucidum* – a clear layer present only in the palms of the hands and soles of the feet;
- the *stratum corneum* – containing keratinized cells.

The thick cells of the **stratum corneum** protect against trauma and bacterial invasion, and also insulate against fluid loss.

Melanoblasts, derived from the neural ectoderm of the anterior horn cells, migrate into the basal layers of the epidermis. They produce the pigment melanin in response to a number of stimuli, and transfer this to the nearby keratinocytes through their dendritic processes.

Langerhans cells are also present in the epidermis, and are part of the monocyte–macrophage system, which processes antigens.

Merkel cells are mechanoreceptors present in the epidermis.

Hair and nails are derived from modified keratin by invagination of the epidermis.

The dermis

The dermis is made up of collagen bundles and various proteoglycans that form a supporting framework for the blood vessels, lymphatics, nerves, sebaceous glands, sweat glands and hair follicles. The dermis also contains **histiocytes** and **mast cells**, which can act as antigen-presenting cells and are part of the reticulo-endothelial system.

The dermis is subdivided into the papillary dermis and the deeper reticular dermis, which sits on the deep fascia.

DIAGNOSIS OF SKIN CONDITIONS

There are many skin problems that require surgical treatment and form an important part of general surgical practice. This chapter concentrates on the common skin problems that are likely to be seen in a surgical clinic. The important features that should be elicited in the history and examination are summarised in Revision panel 4.1.

It is difficult to draw up a set of simple diagnostic pathways suitable for all skin lesions because they have such varied features. For example, a basal cell carcinoma can be a raised nodule, a flat plaque or an ulcer, and can be skin coloured, pearly white, brown or pink. It is therefore better to learn the physical features of each skin lesion, and the best way to do this is by examining as many patients with 'skin conditions' as you can. The diagnosis relies heavily

Revision panel 4.1

Features of the history and examination of a lump or skin lesion that must be elicited

History

Age

Sex, ethnic group, occupation

First local symptom

Other symptoms

Duration of symptoms

Development of symptoms

Persistence of symptoms

Multiple or single lesions

Systemic symptoms (direct questions)

Possible cause

Family history

Social history

Local examination

Site

Shape

Size

Colour

Temperature

Tenderness

Surface

Edge

Ulcer (edge, base, depth, discharge, surrounding tissues)

Composition/contents:

   Consistency
   Fluctuation
   Resonance
   Fluid thrill
   Translucency
   Pulsatility
   Compressibility
   Bruit

Reducibility

Relations to surrounding structures

Lymph drainage

State of local tissues (arteries, nerves, bones and joints)

General examination

on careful inspection and pattern recognition. Tactile and auditory skills are less important.

Always examine every skin blemish carefully before making a diagnosis, however familiar the condition.

Skin lesions have two basic distinguishing features: **their colour** and **their relationship to, and effect on, the overlying epidermis**. The overlying epidermis is likely to be raised and look abnormal if abnormal tissue is present in the superficial part of the dermis. An ulcer will develop if a localized area of the epidermis is destroyed. Alternatively, the overlying epidermis may be stretched but remains normal if there is an abnormality deep in the dermis. The terms used to describe the clinical appearances of different skin conditions are summarised in Revision panel 4.2.

Revision panel 4.2

Terms used to describe skin pathology

Macule – a localized change in colour of the skin that is not elevated (or palpable) or freckled

Papule – a small, solid elevation, flat-topped, conical, round, polyhedral, follicular (hairy), smooth or scaly

Vesicle – a small collection of fluid between the dermis and epidermis (a blister)

Bulla – a collection of fluid larger than a vesicle, under the epidermis

Wheal – a transient elevation of the skin caused by oedema

Cyst – a tumour that contains fluid

Naevus – a lesion present from birth, composed of mature structures normally found in the skin but present in excess, or in an abnormal disposition. The term 'naevus' is also used to describe lesions composed of naevus cells, as in melanocytic or pigmented naevi

Papilloma – a benign overgrowth of epithelial tissue

Tumour – literally, a swelling; commonly but inaccurately used to mean a malignant swelling

Hamartoma – an overgrowth of one or more cell types that are normal constituents of the organ in which they arise; the most common examples are haemangiomas, lymphangiomas and neurofibromas

Ulcer – an area of 'dissolution' of an epithelial surface

It is possible, therefore, to subdivide all skin lesions into three categories:

- those with an intact but abnormal epidermis;
- those in which an area of the overlying epidermis is destroyed (ulcers);
- those covered with a normal epidermis.

In the last of these, the bulk of the pathology is likely to be in the subcutaneous tissues, and even though it may be derived from a skin structure (e.g. a sebaceous gland), it is usually classified as a subcutaneous lesion.

The colour of a skin lesion may be helpful in making a diagnosis. Skin lesions may be black, brown, yellow, red or normal skin colour.

The following classification, based on the condition of the overlying epidermis and its colour, gives some idea of the multitude of lesions that you must learn to recognize.

Epidermis intact but abnormal (Fig. 4.1)

- Black:
  - ○ Gangrenous skin.
  - ○ Early pyoderma gangrenosum.
  - ○ Early anthrax pustule.
- Brown:
  - ○ Freckles.
  - ○ Seborrhoeic keratosis.
  - ○ Moles of all varieties.
  - ○ Malignant melanoma.
  - ○ Pigmented basal or squamous cell carcinoma.
  - ○ Café-au-lait patch.

- ○ Pigmentation following a bruise, thrombophlebitis or venous hypertension (the epidermis may be normal in these conditions).
- Greyish-brown:
  - ○ Wart.
  - ○ Seborrhoeic keratosis.
  - ○ Keratoacanthoma.
- Yellow–white:
  - ○ Xanthoma.
  - ○ Lymphangioma.
  - ○ Pustules of furunculosis and hidradenitis, subcutaneous calcinosis.
- Red–blue:
  - ○ Strawberry naevus.
  - ○ Port wine stain.
  - ○ Spider naevus.
  - ○ Campbell de Morgan spot.
  - ○ Telangiectases.
  - ○ Pyogenic granuloma.
- Skin colour:
  - ○ Papilloma.
  - ○ Early basal and squamous cell carcinoma.
  - ○ Keloid scar.
  - ○ Keratoacanthoma.

Destruction of the overlying epidermis: ulceration (Fig. 4.2)

- *Sloping edge*: a venous, ischaemic, trophic or neuropathic ulcer.
- *Punched-out edge*: an ischaemic, trophic or syphilitic ulcer.
- *Undermined edge*: chronic infection (tuberculosis, carbuncle), pressure sore.
- *Rolled or everted edge*: malignant ulceration.

Fig. 4.1 Epidermis intact but abnormal.

Fig. 4.2 Destruction of the overlying epidermis – ulceration.

CHAPTER 4 | THE SKIN AND SUBCUTANEOUS TISSUES

Overlying epidermis normal (Fig. 4.3)

Although these lesions may have arisen from a skin structure, their mass is beneath the skin and does not affect its structure. They are usually classified as subcutaneous conditions.

Fig. 4.3 Overlying epidermis normal.

Individual skin disorders

Throughout this book, each disease is described using the standard plan of history-taking and examination presented in Chapter 1. These headings appear regularly because repetition is the secret of learning. Revise the plan of history-taking and clinical examination set out in Revision panel 4.1.

CONGENITAL SKIN DISORDERS

These may be genetic or non-genetic. The latter are more common and mostly hamartomas, i.e. tumour-like malformations in which there is an overgrowth of normal tissues arranged in an irregular fashion. The common congenital skin disorders are summarised in Revision panel 4.3.

GENETIC SKIN DISORDERS

Rare genetic skin disorders such as **ichthyosis** (a disorder of keratin formation that looks like lizard scales) or **epidermolysis bullosa** (in which the skin develops massive blisters after friction or minor trauma) are only likely to be encountered in a specialist dermatology clinic, whereas inherited neurofibromatosis is much more commonly seen in a surgical clinic.

Von Recklinghausen's disease

(Multiple neurofibromatosis)

This is an autosomal dominant condition in which multiple neurofibromas are present at birth and increase in number. Patients may have just a few tumours or multiple tumours over the whole body surface. The tumours are benign, and contain a mixture of neural (ectodermal) and fibrous (mesodermal) tissue. The condition is associated with a number of related abnormalities, such as:

- fibroepithelial skin tags (Fig. 4.4);
- patches of light brown discolouration of the skin (café-au-lait patches) (Fig. 4.5);
- neuromas on major nerves, especially the acoustic nerve (acoustic neuroma) and the sensory roots of the spinal nerves (dumb-bell neuroma);
- malignant change to a neurofibrosarcoma (seen in 5 per cent of neuromas);
- phaeochromocytoma of the adrenal gland, which commonly coexists.

History

Most neurofibromas are present at birth, but they increase in size and number during life. As the disease is inherited through a dominant gene, one of the patient's parents and half of their brothers and sisters will be affected.

Fig. 4.4 Multiple neurofibromatosis.

Fig. 4.5 A café-au-lait patch on the forearm.

Examination

The patient is covered with nodules of all sizes (see Fig. 4.4). Some are in the skin, some are tethered to it, and some become pedunculated. The nodules vary

in consistency from soft to firm, but each is distinct. They are often a darker pink than the surrounding skin. Careful inspection of the skin nearly always reveals irregular patches of pale brown pigmentation. The pigment is melanin, and the patches are known as **café-au-lait patches** (see Fig. 4.5). These are a diagnostic feature of von Recklinghausen's disease.

The blood pressure should be measured, as a **coexisting phaeochromocytoma** may cause hypertension. Neurological abnormalities are also common. It is important to test hearing and to examine the spinal nerves, to exclude the presence of major nerve malfunction caused by **neuromas on the acoustic and spinal nerves** (see Chapter 3).

NON-GENETIC CONGENITAL SKIN DISORDERS

Almost all of the following conditions are hamartomas.

Benign papilloma

A benign papilloma of the skin is a simple overgrowth of all layers of the skin, with a vascular core (Fig. 4.6). This is a hamartoma, and should be called a 'skin tag'.

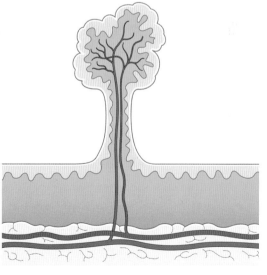

Fig. 4.6 A papilloma is an overgrowth of all layers of the skin with a central vascular core.

CHAPTER 4 | THE SKIN AND SUBCUTANEOUS TISSUES

History

Age They can appear at any age, and a few are congenital.

Symptoms The most common complaint is that the pedunculated swelling catches on clothes or rubs against another part of the body. It can become red and swollen and ulcerate, or even infarct if it is injured. The skin that forms a papilloma contains sweat glands, hair follicles and sebaceous glands. All of these structures can become infected and make the papilloma swollen and tender. The swelling can look like a carcinoma if the granulation tissue that forms in response to the infection becomes exuberant.

Examination

Site Papillomas occur anywhere on the skin.
Shape and size They vary from a smooth, raised plaque to a papilliferous, pedunculated polyp (Fig. 4.7). Their size is equally variable.
Colour They are the colour of normal skin.
Composition Papillomas are soft and not compressible.
Lymph glands These are not be enlarged.
Local tissues These are normal.

(a) A smooth papilloma with a narrow pedicle.

(b) A sessile polyp with excess epithelium covering the clefts and corrugations.

Fig. 4.7 PAPILLOMAS

Congenital dermoid cyst

This cyst lies beneath the skin and is lined by 'skin'. The two ways in which a piece of skin can become trapped deep to the normal skin are:

- as an accident during antenatal development;
- following an injury, which implants some skin into the subcutaneous tissue.

Dermoid cysts are therefore either congenital or acquired.

History

Duration They may be present at birth, but usually become obvious a few years later when they begin to distend. They are rarely multiple.
Symptoms Most congenital dermoid cysts occur in the head and neck, and parents are therefore concerned about their 'unsightliness' as well as the diagnosis. They rarely become very large or infected.

Examination

Site Congenital dermoid cysts develop where the skin dermatomes fuse. They therefore occur in the **midline of the trunk**, and are particularly common in the neck and face, along the lines of fusion of the ophthalmic and maxillary facial processes, especially at the **inner and outer ends of the upper eyebrow** (Fig. 4.8).
Shape and size They are usually ovoid or spherical and 1–2 cm in diameter.
Surface Their surface is smooth.
Composition Cysts on the face often feel soft, not tense and hard. They fluctuate, but only transilluminate if

Fig. 4.8 A right external angular dermoid cyst, so called because it lies beneath the outer end of the eyebrow over the external angular protuberance of the skull. This is a congenital dermoid cyst.

they contain clear fluid, instead of the usual thick, opaque mixture of sebum, sweat and desquamated epithelial cells. They are not pulsatile, compressible or reducible.

Relations Dermoid cysts lie deep to the skin, in the subcutaneous tissue. Unlike sebaceous cysts, they are not attached to the skin.

HAEMANGIOMAS/LYMPHANGIOMAS

These are vascular hamartomas in which the blood and lymphatic vessels are irregularly arranged. They have many forms, such as **strawberry naevus, port wine stain, spider naevus, vin rosé patch** and **Campbell de Morgan spot**. Virtually all are various shades of pink or red, but each one has distinctive features. The majority blanch on pressure.

Strawberry naevus

The name is an accurate description because this bright red 'tumour', which sticks out from the surface of the skin, looks just like a strawberry. The term 'naevus' is correct because strawberry naevi are present at birth. They are congenital intradermal haemangiomas (Fig. 4.9).

History

Age Strawberry naevi are present at birth.
Sex They are equally distributed.
Duration They often regress spontaneously, a few months or years after birth.

Symptoms The child is almost always brought to the clinic because the red lump is disfiguring or a nuisance. Naevi that are rubbed or knocked may ulcerate and bleed. When they are on the buttocks, they can get wet and infected. More than one strawberry naevus may be present.

Examination

Site They can occur on any part of the body, but are most common on the head and neck.
Shape and size They protrude from the skin surface. Small naevi are sessile hemispheres, but as they grow they can become pedunculated.

They are usually 1–2 cm in diameter, but they can become quite large (5–10 cm).

Surface Their surface is irregular, but covered with a smooth, pitted epithelium. There may be small areas of ulceration covered with scabs.
Colour They are either bright or dark red (Fig. 4.10).
Consistency A strawberry naevus is soft and compressible, but not pulsatile. Gentle sustained pressure squeezes most of the blood out of the 'tumour', leaving it collapsed, crinkled and colourless. The rate of refilling depends upon the number of feeding vessels.
Relations Strawberry naevi are confined to the skin, and are freely mobile over the deep tissues.
Lymph drainage The regional lymph glands should not be enlarged.
Surrounding tissues The blood supply of the surrounding skin is normal. They are not associated with any other congenital vascular anomalies.

Fig. 4.9 Diagram showing that a strawberry naevus is an intradermal and subdermal collection of dilated blood vessels.

Fig. 4.10 A close-up view of a strawberry naevus on the forehead, showing the smooth epithelial covering and little pits, which, with the red colour, make the lesion look like a strawberry.

CHAPTER 4 | THE SKIN AND SUBCUTANEOUS TISSUES

Port wine stain

This is an extensive intradermal haemangioma, which is mostly made up of small venules and capillaries (Fig. 4.11). It gives the skin, a deep purple–red colour; hence its name.

Fig. 4.11 A port wine stain is a collection of dilated venules and capillaries just below the epidermis.

Fig. 4.12 An extensive port wine stain of the lower face and neck.

History

Age They are present at birth, and subsequently do not change in size relative to the size of the rest of the body, although their colour may alter.

Symptoms The distress these stains cause the patient's parents and the subsequent disfigurement noticed by the patient are entirely related to their colour and position. They are often very noticeable as they commonly occur on the face. Occasionally, small vessels within the stain become prominent and bleed.

The port wine stain may be part of a more extensive vascular deformity.

Examination

Site Port wine stains are common on the face, and at the junctions between the limbs and the trunk, i.e. the shoulders, neck and buttocks.

They sometimes seem to be confined to a single dermatome, especially when they are part of a generalized vascular deformity, but they are never associated with any neurological abnormalities.

Shape and size Both are very variable.
Surface This is usually smooth, but the vessels can be prominent, and many bleed.
Colour Their distinctive feature is their deep purple–red colour (Fig. 4.12). There may be paler areas at the edge of the patch. The colour can be diminished by local pressure, but pressure rarely returns the skin to its normal colour because all the blood vessels within the patch are abnormal.
Surrounding tissues There may be some dilated subcutaneous veins beneath and around the lesion.

Venous angioma

Venous angiomas are usually situated in the deeper levels of the subcutaneous tissues and can extend into the muscles or joints (see Chapter 10). There are often some irregularly arranged distended veins in the skin over the surface of the subcutaneous soft mass that empty with pressure.

It is always wise to listen over the swelling for a bruit (see below).

Spider naevus

This consists of a solitary dilated skin arteriole feeding a number of small branches that leave it in a radial manner (Fig. 4.13). It is an acquired condition, and may be associated with a generalized disease such as cirrhosis.

History

Spider naevi are rarely noticed by the patient unless they are in a prominent position on the face. They cause no symptoms. They are usually multiple, and tend to increase in number over the years. It is important to enquire about the patient's consumption of alcohol because they are known to be associated with chronic liver disease.

Fig. 4.13 A spider naevus is a solitary dilated arteriole with visible radiating branches.

Fig. 4.14 A spider naevus.

Examination

Site Spider naevi appear on the upper half of the trunk, the face and the arms. This is the area of drainage of the superior vena cava, but it is not clear how this could affect their distribution.

Shape and size They look like little red spiders (Fig. 4.14). The central arteriole is 0.5–1.0 mm in diameter, and the radiating vessels usually spread for a varying distance of 1–2 mm.

Colour The central arteriole is bright red, and the vessels radiating from it are of a similar colour.

Compressibility Spider naevi are not tender, and fade completely when compressed with the finger or, preferably, a glass slide. Compression of the central arteriole with the head of a pin makes the radiating 'legs' fade. They refill as soon as the pressure is released.

Local tissues The local circulation is normal.

General examination They are known to be associated with **liver cirrhosis**, and other stigmata of liver disease may be present (see Chapter 15). They are also associated with tumours destroying the liver, and with oestrogen-producing tumours.

Vin rosé patch

This is a congenital intradermal vascular abnormality in which mild dilatation of the vessels in the subpapillary dermal plexus gives the skin a pale pink colour. It is often associated with other vascular abnormalities such as extensive haemangiomas, giant limbs caused by arteriovenous fistulas and lymphoedema (see Chapter 10).

A vin rosé patch can occur anywhere and causes no symptoms. It is not dark enough to be disfiguring,

and the patient has often accepted its presence as a minor birthmark and forgotten about it.

Campbell de Morgan spot

This is a bright red, clearly-defined spot caused by a collection of dilated capillaries fed by a single or small cluster of arterioles. The cause of these spots is unknown, and they are not associated with any other disease.

History

Age They increase in number with age, being uncommon before the age of 45 years.

Duration They appear suddenly, usually one at a time, but sometimes a cluster of spots will appear in one area of the skin.

Symptoms They are not painful or tender, and are rarely disfiguring.

Examination

Site They appear on both aspects of the trunk, more commonly on the chest. They occasionally arise on the limbs and rarely on the face.

Shape and size They are circular and have a sharp edge, which is sometimes slightly raised. They are usually 1–3 mm in diameter.

Colour They have a uniform deep red or purple colour that makes them look like drops of dark red paint or sealing wax just under the epidermis (Fig. 4.15).

Compressibility Although they comprise a collection of dilated capillaries, they do not always empty when compressed, although they always fade slightly.

CHAPTER 4 | THE SKIN AND SUBCUTANEOUS TISSUES

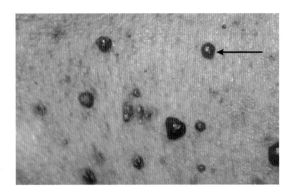

Fig. 4.15 A Campbell de Morgan spot.

Lymphangioma circumscriptum

This is a circumscribed cluster of many small dilated lymph sacs in the skin and subcutaneous tissues that do *not* connect with the normal lymph system. These blind sacs may be clusters of lymph sacs that failed to join into the lymph system during its development. Large, translucent lymph cysts confined to the subcutaneous tissues are called **cystic hygromas** (see Chapter 12).

History

Sex They are present at birth, but may not be noticed until the skin vesicles appear a few years later. They are equally common in males and females.

Symptoms They are usually noticed by the child's parents, who consult the doctor because they are concerned about the disfigurement. The vesicles sometimes leak clear fluid, and when very prominent, the vesicles can be rubbed by clothes and may get infected and painful.

Development As the years pass, the subcutaneous cysts enlarge and become prominent, and the number and extent of the skin vesicles increases.

Examination

Site They are found at the junction of the limbs with the trunk, i.e. around the shoulder, axilla, buttock and groin.

Shape and size They may present as a single or multiple lumps. A large area of skin may be involved – the whole of the buttock or shoulder may be abnormal – and most lymphangiomas cover an area 5–20 cm across by the time that they present.

Surface Their surface is smooth, but their edge is often ill defined and indistinct.

Colour The skin vesicles contain clear fluid, which looks watery or yellow. Blood in the vesicles turns them red–brown or even black (Fig. 4.16).

Overlying skin The subcutaneous cysts make the abnormal area bulge slightly, but the edges of this swelling are indistinct. The skin contains vesicles of varying sizes and colour, ranging from 0.5 to 3 or 4 mm in diameter (Fig. 4.16).

Composition The whole swelling is soft and spongy, although as it is usually composed of multiple cysts, it does not fluctuate. Occasionally, it may contain one or two large cysts, which may fluctuate. The mass is not compressible. The dark red or brown vesicles do not fade with pressure.

Lymph drainage The local lymph glands are not enlarged unless the lesion has become infected.

(a) Many of the vesicles are red, black or brown because they contain old blood.

(b) This malformation involves the whole of the side of the chest just below the axilla.

Fig. 4.16 LYMPHANGIOMATA CIRCUMSCRIPTUM

Arteriovenous fistulas

These may cause a swelling in the skin or subcutaneous tissues, which may have a vascular appearance. The veins are also often distended, but careful inspection may reveal pulsation, which is confined by palpation. Arteriovenous fistulas are not compressible, but should have a loud machinery murmur situated over them providing that they have a high flow (see Chapter 10).

ACQUIRED DERMATOLOGICAL CONDITIONS

CONDITIONS OF THE SKIN CAUSED BY TRAUMA

Keloid and hypertrophic scars

An incised wound heals in four phases:

- Phase one encompasses **haemostasis**, in which the gap in the tissue is filled by blood and fibrin.
- This is then followed by the **inflammation phase**, where there is an influx of mononuclear cells (monocytes and macrophages) into the wound.
- The **proliferation phase** involves the production of fibrous tissue/collagen in the wound.
- Reorganization then follows in the **remodelling phase** to give the wound its maximum strength.

This process, which is called healing by **primary intention**, is remarkably well controlled. Most surgical scars in the skin are thin lines containing the minimum amount of scar tissue. Sometimes, however, the fibrous tissue response is excessive, and the result is a **hypertrophic or keloid scar**.

In a **hypertrophic scar**, excessive amounts of fibrous tissue form, but this is confined to the scar; i.e. it is between the incised skin edges (Figs 4.17 and 4.18). Hypertrophic scars are quite common, particularly if there has been some additional stimulus to fibrous tissue formation during healing, such as infection or excessive tension, both of which are

Normal scar

Hypertrophic scar

Keloid scar

Fig. 4.17 Normal, hypertrophic and keloid scars.

common complications of scars crossing skin creases. Hypertrophic scars only enlarge for 2–3 months.

In a **keloid scar**, the hypertrophy and overgrowth of the fibrous tissue extend beyond the original wound into normal tissues (Fig. 4.19). This means that the scar has some of the characteristics of a locally invasive malignant neoplasm.

The tendency to produce keloid scars is a congenital trait, common in black individuals. Some tribes exploit the trait for the production of decorative scars on the face and trunk.

Keloid scars continue to enlarge for 6–12 months after the initial injury. They are almost certainly the result of a local release of *fibroblast growth factors*, which are unsuppressed.

As a keloid scar grows, it can become very unsightly, it is often tender to the touch, and it may itch. Although the disfigurement produced

THE SKIN AND SUBCUTANEOUS TISSUES

CHAPTER 4 |

Fig. 4.18 A hypertrophic scar on the medial side of the thigh.

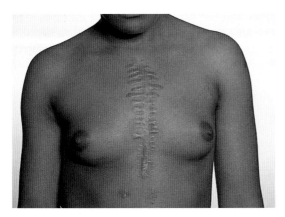

Fig. 4.19 A keloid scar after a median sternotomy.

by a hypertrophic scar may be as great as that of a keloid scar, it is important to try to distinguish the two abnormalities because hypertrophic scars do not recur after they have been excised if the causative factors are eliminated, whereas keloid scars will recur unless special measures are taken.

Acquired implantation dermoid cysts

History

These cysts develop when a piece of skin survives after being forcibly implanted into the subcutaneous tissues by an injury – often a small, deep cut or stab. The patient may not remember the initial injury.

Symptoms Implantation dermoid cysts are usually small and tense. They may be painful and tender because they usually occur in areas subject to repeated trauma. Cysts on the fingers may interfere with grip and touch.

Examination

Site Implantation dermoid cysts are commonly found where injuries are likely to occur, such as the fingers. Surprisingly, surgical incisions rarely cause these cysts.

Shape and size The cysts are spherical, smooth and small, about 0.5–1.0 cm in diameter (Fig. 4.20).

Composition Implantation dermoid cysts feel hard and tense, sometimes stony hard. Their small size makes the detection of their cystic nature – fluctuation – almost impossible. The deduction that they are cystic usually depends solely on their shape. They may occasionally transilluminate.

Relations A scar is usually present in the overlying skin. The cyst may be tethered to the deep aspect of the scar or even lie within it. The deeper structures should be normal, and the cyst is freely mobile over them unless they were involved in the initial injury.

Lymph drainage The regional lymph glands should be normal.

Fig. 4.20 An implantation dermoid cyst that appeared following a small stab wound.

Differential diagnosis A **sebaceous cyst** (see below) is often confused with an implantation dermoid. The history of an old injury and the presence of a scar are the most significant diagnostic features.

Pyogenic granuloma

Small capillary loops develop in a healing wound to knit it together and provide sustenance and support for the covering epithelium. In the base of a healing ulcer, these capillary loops form a layer of bright red tissue known as **granulation tissue**.

When the capillary loops grow too vigorously, they may form a protruding mass of tissue that becomes covered with epithelium and is called a pyogenic granuloma. *It is probably neither pyogenic nor granulomatous.* Its surface is often ulcerated and infected. The infection is a secondary event and probably not the initiating stimulus.

History

Age They are uncommon in children.
Symptoms There may be a history of a minor injury, usually a cut or scratch, but the patient often cannot remember the initial injury. They sometimes occur in response to a chronic infection such as a paronychia.

The patient complains of a rapidly growing skin lump, which bleeds easily and discharges serous or purulent fluid. The lump usually grows rapidly (it may double in size in a few days), and as a consequence many patients think it is a tumour. The bleeding, weeping and pain stop when it is completely covered with epithelium.

Examination

Site Pyogenic granulomas are commonly found where injuries are most likely to occur, such as the hands and face.
Shape and size They begin as a hemispherical nodule that grows upwards and outwards (Fig. 4.21). The lump is rarely more than 1 cm across because its blood supply becomes inadequate. Growth from a few millimetres to full size can occur in a few days.
Surface Before the surface is epithelialized, it has a covering of dried blood or plasma, and bleeds easily.
Colour At first, they are the bright red colour of healthy granulation tissue (Fig. 4.21), but as they get bigger and less vascular, they fade to a pale pink.

Fig. 4.21 A pyogenic granuloma on the skin of the chest.

When they become covered with epithelium, they turn pink or white.
Tenderness and composition They are sometimes slightly tender, and they feel soft.
Relations They are confined to the skin.
Complications They bleed easily when knocked, and can break off at their base. The granuloma may reform in the next few days, or the base can re-epithelialize.
Natural history Once the granulations have become completely covered with epithelium, the nodule begins to shrink, but it rarely completely disappears.
Differential diagnosis The important conditions to exclude are:

- **Squamous carcinoma.**
- **Non-pigmented melanoma.**
- **Kaposi's sarcoma.**

A history of trauma and the very rapid growth are the particular features of a pyogenic granuloma, but an excisional biopsy is often needed to confirm the diagnosis.

Fat necrosis

Dead fat becomes hard and fibrous. The skin then becomes tethered or fixed to it, and indrawn.

In the breast, which is an organ that is frequently knocked and bruised, fat necrosis may be mistaken for a carcinoma (see Chapter 13). The buttock is also a common site of fat necrosis, particularly in patients who have frequent subcutaneous injections, such as those with diabetes (Fig. 4.22).

CHAPTER 4 | THE SKIN AND SUBCUTANEOUS TISSUES

Fig. 4.22 Fat necrosis of the buttock fat caused by repeated injections of insulin. Note the tethering, indrawing and pigmentation of the skin. Beneath these areas were hard lumps of necrotic fat.

Common ulcers of the skin

An ulcer is a 'dissolution' of the continuity of an epithelial surface. Ulcers follow traumatic removal, or death and desquamation by disease, of the whole or part of an epithelium, and most occur in the lower limb (see Chapter 1).

Ulcers are discussed here because trauma is often the final cause of the skin breakdown, although there are many underlying causes that make the skin susceptible to injury and impede subsequent healing. The common causes are listed in Revision panel 4.4.

Revision panel 4.4
Causes of ulceration of the skin of the lower limb

Venous – 60% (one-half varicose and one-half post-thrombotic)

Ischaemic – 20% (one-quarter have an associated venous cause)

Collagen disease – 5% (rheumatoid and systemic lupus erythematosus)

Neuropathic – 2%

Traumatic – 1%

Neoplastic – 1%

Many rare causes – 5%

Unknown – 10%

Venous ulcers

Venous ulcers are found in the lower medial third of the lower limb. Their site is a diagnostic feature. They are described in detail in Chapter 10.

Ischaemic ulcers

Arterial insufficiency is usually manifest at the ends of the limbs. It is rare to see ulcers caused by arterial disease at the base of the limbs or on the trunk. Ischaemic ulcers are described in detail in Chapter 10.

Trophic ulcers

A trophic ulcer is an ulcer that has developed as the result of the patient's insensitivity to repeated trauma. These ulcers are commonly associated with those forms of neurological disease which cause loss of the appreciation of pain and light touch in weight-bearing areas (see Chapters 3 and 10).

Neoplastic ulcers

The ulcers caused by basal and squamous cell carcinomas are described in detail later in this chapter (see page 152).

When metastases from distant or underlying cancers appear in the skin, they may ulcerate and have features similar to those of a primary carcinomatous ulcer – an everted edge and a proliferating base.

Burns

The skin can be burnt by heat, irradiation, electrical or chemical noxious stimuli. A 'heat' burn is usually caused by direct flames, an explosion, contact with a hot object, steam or hot fluid. Burns caused by steam or hot water are called '**scalds**'. All burns cause local inflammation, and systemic effects occur if more than 20 per cent of the total body surface area is burnt.

Prophylaxis The fitting of household fire alarms and sprinkler systems and the increasing use of non-flammable fabrics and fittings are all designed to try to reduce the incidence of household and workplace burns. Poor electrical wiring and gas leaks are potentially avoidable, but continue to be a common cause of major burn injuries. Children and the elderly are particularly at risk: the young fail to recognize the hazard, and the elderly are often unable to avoid it as a consequence of immobility and frailty. Education and safeguards are the best form of defence in these age groups.

First-aid Wherever possible, burnt parts should be placed under cold running water. This is easy after a scald of the hand but impractical if the whole body has been burnt.

Assessment and resuscitation As in a major injury (see Chapter 5), these two must proceed simultaneously. Intravenous access and fluid replacement are essential in any patient who has a sizeable burn, and cannulae should be placed in large veins in an area of unburnt skin.

The size and depth of the burn must be carefully assessed.

The **burn size** is measured as a percentage of total body area using the 'Rule of nines' (Fig. 4.23). For a child, this must be modified – the head and neck being scored as 18 per cent, and the lower limbs downgraded from 18 per cent to 14 per cent.

The **burn depth** can be subdivided into superficial, superficial dermal, mid-dermal, deep dermal and full thickness (Fig. 4.24).

Superficial burns are usually blistered and very painful, while **full-thickness burns** are often pale or white, with absent sensation.

A number of formulae exist for calculating the patient's early fluid requirement based on the extent and depth of the burn, the weight of the patient and the time the burn was sustained. These are described in detail in *Investigation and Management*, Chapter 5. It must be stressed that early and adequate fluid replacement is the most important initial treatment.

Clinical features

Pain This is the main symptom, especially in patients with superficial burns.

Skin sensation Sensation must be carefully tested whenever a full-thickness burn is suspected, and re-tested 24 hours later, when the lack of sensation may be easier to determine.

The airway It is important to assess the face, mouth and airways, as an inhalation injury of their lining commonly complicates extensive burns. Burns around the mouth, nose and lips are highly indicative of an inhalation injury. The buccal mucous membrane and tongue must be inspected for mucosal burns. An urgent anaesthetic review is essential if airway burns are suspected.

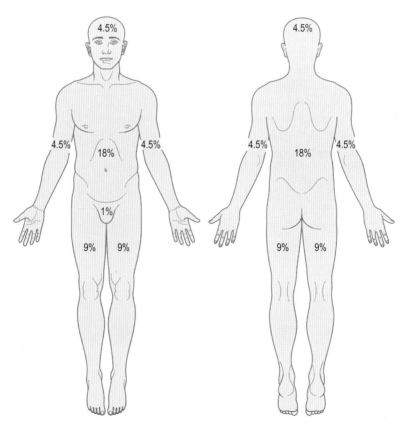

Fig. 4.23 The 'Rule of nines' method for calculating the proportion of the body surface that has been burnt.

CHAPTER 4 | THE SKIN AND SUBCUTANEOUS TISSUES

(a) A superficial burn: hyperaemia, blistering and pain.

Fig. 4.24 BURNS

(b) A mixture of partial-thickness and full-thickness burns.

(c) A partial-thickness burn: loss of epithelium, some superficial capillary bleeding and a few pale patches that may turn out to be deeper burns.

(d) An extensive scald, probably mostly a partial-thickness burn.

Breathing **The airway and breathing must be carefully monitored.** Special attention must be paid to any circumferential burns of the neck or chest, as these may constrict breathing. The occurrence of stridor or a difficulty with breathing is an indication for intratracheal intubation and ventilation, especially if the patient is unconscious.

Circulation The state of the circulation must be repeatedly assessed, as burns are associated with massive losses of fluids, electrolytes and protein from their surface, and red cell damage or destruction occurs, especially in full-thickness burns.

The pulse, blood pressure, central venous pressure, urine output and haematocrit must be carefully monitored in all patients with major burns. Failure to maintain an adequate circulation may be followed by renal failure and eventually multiorgan failure. The latter is often follows septicaemia from secondary infection in and around the burns.

Circumferential burns of the limbs or digits may cause peripheral ischaemia, and need urgent release.

Depigmentation This is a rare problem that can occur in black races after extensive scarring and burns.

Electrical burns

Most electrical burns come from faulty home appliances or the careless touching of electrodes. In high-voltage burns, such as lightening strikes, survival is uncommon because the depolarization usually causes severe cardiac arrhythmias and arrest.

A severe local burn develops at the point of entry, and adjacent nerves and muscles are often damaged (see *Investigation and Management*, Chapter 5).

Deep tissue damage can lead to metabolic derangements, compartment syndromes, arterial and venous thrombosis and even visceral damage if the entry point is over the torso.

Radiation injury

The initial skin injury caused by radiation often resembles a standard thermal burn. The clinical evidence of the commonly associated lung and bowel damage and bone marrow depression appears later.

Many patients exposed to high doses of radiation die from pulmonary complications or aplastic anaemia, and those who survive the early systemic effects may die later from radiation-induced malignant change in organs such as the thyroid gland.

Chemical burns

Most chemical burns are caused by contact with acids or alkalis; a few are caused by phosphorus and phenols. Chemical burns of the skin can be avoided by wearing protective clothing and washing off the contaminant as quickly as possible. They have the same clinical appearance as full-thickness and partial-thickness thermal burns.

The *oral ingestion* of corrosive chemicals may destroy the lining of the oesophagus and cause life-threatening complications and serious long-term morbidity (see *Investigation and Management*, Chapter 18).

INFECTIONS OF THE SKIN

Skin and subcutaneous infections are common, especially when the skin is breached. The cardinal signs of rubor, calor, dolor and tumour are usually present in all infections, and patients are invariably pyrexial.

Bacterial infections

Impetigo

This a relatively rare staphylococcal infection that causes blistering of the hands and face. Vesicles form and rupture, and are covered with a honey-coloured crust. They may form circinate or gyriform patterns. Fresh blisters form daily, and many develop inflammatory halos. A microbiological swab should be sent for culture. Patients are usually referred to dermatology clinics.

Furunculosis
(Boils)

Furuncles and boils are caused by infection entering a hair follicle. This first produces pus and then a central core of necrotic tissue. When only pus is present, it is called a furuncle; when it contains a solid core, it is called a boil.

Boils are often multiple and associated with general debility, or an underlying disease such as diabetes. They can occur on any part of the body, but are common in the skin of the head and neck, axillae and groins. They begin as a hard, red, tender area, which gradually enlarges and causes a throbbing pain. The tissue in the centre of the infected area eventually dies and forms a thick yellow slough. The lump then becomes fluctuant, the centre of the covering skin sloughs, and the pus and necrotic core are discharged.

Subcutaneous abscess

Abscesses in the subcutaneous tissue are common and usually follow the implantation of bacteria by a penetrating injury, or infection in a haematoma.

The common infecting organism is *Staphylococcus aureus*, but almost any organism can cause an abscess if the local conditions are favourable to its growth. An abscess is a pocket of pus (dead cells, exudate and bacteria) surrounded by granulation tissue.

History

Age They occur in all ages and both sexes.

Hygiene Poor social conditions and poor bodily hygiene increase the chances of an infection following a minor injury such as a pinprick.

Symptoms The principal complaint is of a throbbing pain that gets steadily worse and keeps the patient awake at night.

The patient notices an area of thickening and tenderness at the site of the pain, which slowly turns into a hard mass. The mass may discharge spontaneously, with relief of the symptoms, before the patient attends the doctor.

Previous history Patients who are debilitated, diabetic or drug addicts may have had previous abscesses as a result of their underlying disease and frequent injections.

Habits Enquire about the drug-taking habits of the patient if you have cause to think that the abscess might have followed a self-administered injection.

CHAPTER 4 | THE SKIN AND SUBCUTANEOUS TISSUES

Examination

The four classical signs of an abscess (the *signs of Celsus*) are *tumour*, *rubor*, *calor* and *dolor* (swelling, redness, heat and pain).

Site Areas subjected to trauma are more susceptible. The hands are common sites for subcutaneous infection (see Chapter 7).

Injections are usually given into the buttock or thigh, so these are also common sites for abscesses.

Self-administered injections by drug addicts are usually given into the veins in the cubital fossa and groin.

Shape and size The initial change is the development of a patch of induration. As the pus forms, this patch turns into a definite mass that is usually spherical. The mass may become large, and lose its spherical shape if the pus begins to spread through the subcutaneous tissues.

Surface The inner surface of an abscess is a layer of granulation tissue that is inseparable from the indurated inflamed tissues around it. Thus, an abscess does not have a definable outer surface, even though its contents may be easy to feel.

Colour The overlying skin is red.

Temperature The skin over an abscess is hot.

Tenderness Abscesses become increasingly tender as the tension in the pocket of pus increases.

Edge The edge is not palpable, as the induration and oedema gradually merge into the normal tissues.

Composition In the early stages, an abscess feels hard and solid. As the pus forms, the centre of the area becomes soft and, if it is not too tender to press, fluctuant.

Relations The skin over a subcutaneous abscess is invariably involved in the inflammatory process, so it is red, oedematous and fixed to the underlying mass.

The skin becomes white and then black as it dies and sloughs away if the pus points towards the skin. When the dead skin separates, the pus can escape from the abscess. Deep fixation depends upon the size and direction of spread of the abscess.

Local lymph glands The lymph glands that receive lymph from the infected area are likely to be enlarged and tender. They may even suppurate.

Local tissues The local tissues should be normal, apart from those close to the abscess that are involved in the inflammation. There may be scars from previous abscesses.

General examination A large abscess can cause considerable systemic disturbance. The patient looks pale and ill, but may be sweating and having rigors and episodes of flushing. The temperature and pulse are elevated.

Carbuncle

A carbuncle is a spreading necrotizing infection in the subcutaneous tissues, with pus and slough formation, similar to the changes that occur in a boil, but with many points of discharge through holes in the skin that appear when patches of necrotic skin slough. The subcutaneous tissue necrosis is much more extensive than the reddened area of overlying skin (Fig. 4.25).

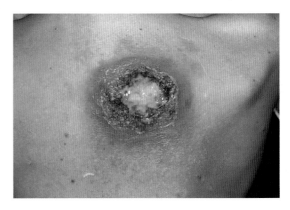

Fig. 4.25 A carbuncle.

Sinuses and fistulas

Sinus

A sinus is a tract lined by granulation tissue that connects a cavity (usually an old abscess) with an epithelial surface, for example the skin (Fig. 4.26).

A sinus produces a serous or purulent discharge and fails to close if:

- the cavity is inadequately drained;
- it is caused by a specific chronic infection (e.g. actinomycosis, tuberculosis, syphilis);
- a foreign body (e.g. stitch material) is present at the bottom of the sinus;
- the cavity has epithelialized;
- the cavity has undergone malignant change;
- the surrounding tissues have poor vascularity or have been irradiated.

Sinuses commonly follow surgical wound infections and necrosis of tumours (see Revision panel 4.5)

(a) A sinus is a connection between a cavity lined with granulation tissue and an epithelial surface.

(b) A discharging sinus from the centre of a groin wound.

(c) The same wound 3 weeks later. The sinus has opened widely to reveal its cause – an infected Dacron arterial graft.

Fig. 4.26 SINUS

Fistula

A fistula is a pathological connection between two epithelial surfaces (Fig. 4.27). For example, it is possible to have a fistula between the bowel and the skin, the bowel and another loop of bowel, or the bowel and the bladder.

Fistulas are usually lined with granulation tissue, but the tract can become epithelialized.

> ### Revision panel 4.5
> ### The causes of a chronic abscess or persistent sinus
> Inadequate drainage
> Specific chronic infection, e.g. tuberculosis
> Foreign body, e.g. a stitch
> Epithelialization of the cavity
> Malignant change in the wall of the cavity
> Arises in irradiated or ischaemic tissues

They form when a chronic abscess bursts in two directions, connecting two epithelial surfaces. They persist if they have to transmit the contents of one of the epithelium-lined cavities to the other if the former's normal outflow is obstructed.

They do not resolve until the cause of the abscess has been eradicated (see above for the factors that delay abscess closure) or the obstruction to the emptying of the viscus has been removed.

CHAPTER 4 | THE SKIN AND SUBCUTANEOUS TISSUES

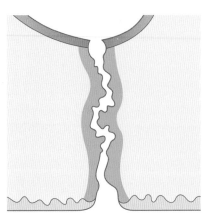

Fig. 4.27 A fistula is a connection between two epithelium-lined surfaces.

Fig. 4.28 Hidradenitis suppurativa. Infected and inflamed apocrine glands.

The common fistulas seen in surgical practice are between the anal canal and the perianal skin and the bowel (see Chapter 16).

Hidradenitis suppurativa

Whereas boils are infections in the hair follicles, hidradenitis is an infection of the apocrine sweat glands. It is most often seen in the axillae and groins. White individuals living in tropical countries are especially prone.

The patient presents with multiple tender swellings in the axillae or groins (Fig. 4.28), which enlarge and then discharge pus. The condition is made worse if there is an underlying systemic disease, such as diabetes. The site and the chronic recurring nature of this condition make it unpleasant and disabling.

Erysipelas and cellulitis

Erysipelas is an infection in the skin and subcutaneous tissues caused by a pathogenic *Streptococcus*. Whereas *Staphylococcus* commonly causes a localized infection and pus formation, *Streptococcus* spreads easily through the skin and produces a diffuse cellulitis. The erythrotoxins produced by *Streptococcus* make the infected area red, hot, tender and oedematous (Fig. 4.29). Oedema of the reddened skin gives the involved area a raised border – a diagnostic clinical appearance. The patient has a high temperature, tachycardia and general debility. Streptococcal infections rarely form thick pus.

Fig. 4.29 Erysipelas.

Careful examination may reveal a source of entry for the organism, such as a small cut or a scratch. Erysipelas is especially common when there is pre-existing oedema caused by venous or lymphatic insufficiency.

Infection of the skin and subcutaneous tissues caused by other organisms, without the bright red discolouration of the skin and the raised border, is called **cellulitis**. A patch of cellulitis may necrose and suppurate.

Erysipeloid

This is a Gram-positive coccal infection that is present in *shellfish, meat and poultry*. It commonly affects fishermen, fishmongers and butchers. It occurs in the hands, usually as a purple–red papule with a well-defined edge, and may spread to other fingers.

Anthrax

This is a spore-forming, highly resistant bacterium that is found in animal carriers and is present in wood, hide and bones. It causes a black, malignant-looking sore on the skin (Fig. 4.30), and patients may die rapidly from pulmonary complications.

Fig. 4.31 Lupus vulgaris: an apple jelly appearance.

Syphilis

Syphilis is rare in the UK, although its incidence has increased slightly in recent years.

The primary sore, or chancre This is acquired by sexual intercourse, biting or kissing, and develops between 3 and 6 weeks after inoculation. The common sites for chancres are the penis and the vulva, but they can occur on the cervix, lips, fingers, nipple or anus. A chancre is usually a 1 cm or less solid papular ulcer, with an indurated base that can be lifted up like a button in the skin (Fig. 4.32). Approximately 1 week after its appearance, one or more of the regional lymph glands become enlarged. Affected glands are not painful and feel rubbery. They are called **bubos**.

The secondary stage This develops 5–6 weeks later if the primary condition is not treated. This is the result of organisms disseminating through

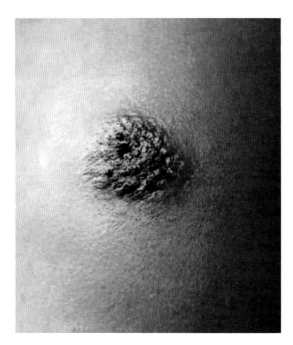

Fig. 4.30 An anthrax pustule.

Tuberculosis

Tuberculosis of the skin is a rarity. Primary tuberculosis of the skin produces a persistent ulcer with undermined edges. This is more commonly seen now in an unhealed BCG vaccination site. The associated lymph glands are enlarged and may suppurate.

Lupus vulgaris

This is the well-recognized cutaneous form of tuberculosis that often affects the head and neck of children. The skin is red, telangiectatic and scaly. When it is compressed with a glass slide, it appears to be composed of pale yellow-brownish nodules (apple jelly) (Fig. 4.31). It is a slowly progressive lesion that causes massive s carring.

Fig. 4.32 A syphilitic chancre.

CHAPTER 4 | THE SKIN AND SUBCUTANEOUS TISSUES

the bloodstream. A widespread polymorphic rash develops that is not itchy and consists of macules, papules and scaly lesions. Patients often complain of associated malaise, headaches and limb pains.

At first, the **macules** are pink or copper coloured and oval in shape, with an ill-defined edge. They are widely distributed on the trunk, limbs, palms of the hands and soles of the feet.

The **papules** have similar characteristics and become florid and scaly, appearing in groups, often with an annular pattern, which makes them look almost like psoriasis. This is associated with a **generalized lymphadenopathy**.

Enlargement of the **epitrochlear lymph glands** is said to be characteristic.

Superficial erosions may then develop in the buccal mucosa, appearing as tender, red patches. When these are covered by adherent mucus, they are likened to **snail tracks**. It is, therefore, always important to look in the mouth, and fold back the lips.

Flat, moist plaques that are purple in colour may appear in the perianal and vulval skin, at the angle of the mouth, and in any of the skin flexures (e.g. armpits and groins). These are called **condylomata lata**.

A patchy loss of hair often occurs that gives patients a **'moth-eaten' appearance**.

Tertiary syphilis This begins 2–10 years after the initial infection.

Serpiginous or arcuate nodules may develop that are either scaly or ulcerated. These leave central scars that may be mistaken for lupus vulgaris (see above), although the latter is usually much more chronic in its development.

Gummas can also develop at this stage. They start as a small nodule in the subcutis, but then enlarge and become red before ulcerating. The ulcer associated with a gumma is discrete, punched out (see above) and characteristically has a wash-leather slough in its base (Fig. 4.33).

Leukoplakia of the mouth and tongue is another manifestation of the tertiary stage of syphilis. The epithelium appears thickened and white. This condition is potentially premalignant (see Chapter 11).

Aortic aneurysms (see Chapter 10) and **tabes dorsalis** are other important complications of the tertiary stage. Tabes is the result of damage to the

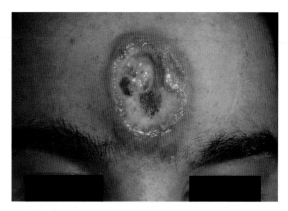

Fig. 4.33 A gumma.

posterior spinal columns causing loss of deep pain and proprioception, resulting in a 'stamping gait' (see Chapter 3).

The quaternary or final stage
This is **general paralysis of the insane**, in which insanity eventually develops in the unlikely event that the condition is left untreated.

Congenital syphilis
This is almost extinct in the home-born population of the UK because of routine serological screening in pregnancy. Affected children develop a bullous eruption on their palms and soles a few days after birth. The liver enlarges, and the affected neonate develops 'snuffles' from severe nasal discharge that obstructs the breathing. The bridge of the nose eventually 'caves in'. The long bones develop osteochondritis and periostitis, causing deformity.

Diagnosis
The diagnosis of primary syphilis is usually made by scarifying the chancre, transferring the resultant discharge onto a microscope slide and examining it with dark-ground illumination for the presence of spirochaetes. A number of serological tests are useful for detecting active or prior infection (see *Investigation and Management*, Chapter 5).

Leprosy
(Hansen's disease)
This is increasingly appearing in all parts of the world because of the ease of air travel and shifts

of large populations to seek asylum. It must always be considered in a patient from a tropical country presenting with an unusual rash. It is spread by prolonged contact.

The **'tuberculoid' form** is most commonly seen in the UK. The skin usually contains sharply defined asymmetrical areas of hypopigmentation with dry, scaly surfaces. Alternatively, there may be infiltrated, raised, hyperpigmented plaques with sharply demarcated erythematous edges. These may resemble vitiligo, but differ in that some pigment remains. These plaques or patches are insensate.

The ulnar, peroneal and greater auricular nerves are commonly thickened and easily palpable. Foot drop and ulnar palsy are common. Eventually, the insensate fingers are damaged by repeated trauma and disappear (Fig. 4.34).

Patients with **lepromatous leprosy** have no resistance to the spread of organisms. The early skin lesions are small, ill defined, erythematous macules that have a smooth and shiny surface. These become infiltrated to form plaques and nodules, especially in the face and pinnae. The polyneuritis described above is a late manifestation of this form of disease.

Fig. 4.34 Leprosy of the hands.

Diagnosis

The diagnosis is made by biopsy and nasal scrapings, when the microbacteria may be seen within the granulomas, consisting of epithelioid cells surrounding histiocytes and lymphocytes. Serological tests are also available (see *Investigation and Management*, Chapter 5).

Viral infections

Viral warts

These are papilliferous patches of overgrown hyperkeratotic skin whose growth has been stimulated by the human papilloma virus.

History

Age They can occur at any age, but are most common in children, adolescents and young adults.

Duration They grow to their full size in a few weeks, but may be present for months or years before a patient complains about them. Patients have usually made their own diagnosis and decided that there is no cause for concern.

Symptoms Warts are disfiguring. Multiple warts on the fingers can interfere with fine movements. They are painful only if they are rubbed or become infected.

Progression Once present, they may persist unchanged for many years, or regress and disappear spontaneously. 'Kiss lesions' may appear on adjacent areas of skin that make frequent contact. Warts occur in crops and may come and go spontaneously.

Family history They may occur in other members of the family.

Examination

Site Warts are commonly found on the hands, but may appear on other exposed areas that are frequently touched by the hands, such as the face, arms and knees.

Shape and size They arise as flat-topped, angular, smooth or hemispherical macules that are less than 1 cm in diameter (Fig. 4.35).

Surface Their surface is rough and hyperkeratotic, and often covered with fine filiform excrescences.

Colour Warts are greyish-brown.

Composition They are firm and not compressible.

Lymph drainage The regional lymph glands are not enlarged.

Differential diagnosis **Squamous papilloma**, **molluscum contagiosum** and **condylomata lata** are other conditions that may be considered in the differential diagnosis.

Plantar warts

Warts on the soles of the feet (**verrucas**) appear as flat tender plaques that are fundamentally the same as

Fig. 4.35 Viral warts.

Fig. 4.36 A plantar wart (verruca) (arrow).

any other wart, but they have a different appearance because they are pushed into the skin (Fig. 4.36). They must be differentiated from **callosities and corns** (see Chapter 8).

Molluscum contagiosum

These are discrete, pearly, rounded nodules with umbilicated centres; when squeezed, they release a white exudate that contains virus. They are usually grouped in one area of the trunk.

Herpes simplex

This is the most common skin virus, with more than 60 per cent of the population infected and remaining carriers throughout their lives. The primary infection often passes unnoticed, but it may cause a severe gingivo-stomatitis with fever and local lymphadenopathy. The mouth often contains a crop of 'aphthous' ulcers (see Chapter 11). Vesicles may be present over the face, the neck and even the eyes. The attack subsides in 10–14 days, but the virus remains latent in the epithelial cells of the buccal and nasal mucosa. The micro-organisms may proliferate again in response to a noxious stimulus such as a fever, sunlight, pneumonia or immune suppression.

History

Patients usually complain of a painful localized sore on their lip, which develops blisters that discharge and then crust over.

Examination

Site Most lesions occur at the mucocutaneous junctions, particularly on the lips and angle of the mouth, but they may appear on the nail clefts, trunk, genitalia, cheeks and natal cleft.
Shape and size A burning, uncomfortable papule develops that is usually oval or elliptical. It is slightly raised and very tender.
Surface The papular surface is smooth at first, but becomes covered in a crop of small vesicles (Fig. 4.37) that break to leave a crust. This heals in 7–10 days, and the skin returns to normal.
Lymph drainage The lymph nodes are rarely enlarged.

Fig. 4.37 Herpes simplex.

Herpes zoster

This skin rash is thought to be caused by reactivation of the chickenpox virus, which can lie dormant for many years in the anterior horn cells of the spinal cord.

History

Age It usually occurs after the age of 45 years.
Onset It can develop within a week of re-exposure to the varicella virus. Reactivation can be the result of tuberculosis or tumour.
Symptoms Pain occurs over the distribution of the nerve roots involved *before* the rash develops.

Examination

Site The rash can occur in any cutaneous dermatome or dermatomes. It appears in a continuous line, or as patches throughout these segments (Fig. 4.38). The trigeminal nerve may be involved, and if the virus enters the ophthalmic branch, the eye will be affected.
Rash Initially, there is a raised patch of erythema, which rapidly becomes covered with a cluster of umbilicated vesicles. These quickly become infected and haemorrhagic before necrotic crusts form. There may be severe photophobia, with a red, watering eye if the ophthalmic division of the trigeminal nerve is involved.
Resolution The pain improves as the rash clears. The rash starts to disappear after about 10 days, but, in some patients, severe cutaneous necrosis can leave disfiguring scars, and there may be persisting pain.

Fig. 4.38 Herpes zoster in the T12 dermatome.

Do not forget that herpes zoster may be the cause of severe abdominal pain before the rash develops and the diagnosis is clear (see Chapter 15).

Fungal infections

Candida

(Moniliasis)

This is a normal component of the body's flora and is present in the skin, mouth, vagina and gut of us all. Clinical problems only develop when there is a reduction in the normal defence mechanism that leads to infection.

It may present in a number of different ways.

Oral candida

The buccal mucosa and tongue of infants or adults on prolonged courses of antibiotics may become covered in white spots or plaques (see Chapter 11).

Flexural intertrigo

Scattered soft macules may appear in the skin flexures, especially in the submammary areas and axillae of obese females. Patients with these problems should be checked for coexisting diabetes.

Balanitis

Monilial balanitis can be a problem in uncircumcized males (see Chapter 18).

Chronic paronychia

Housewives, nurses and barmaids who frequently immerse their hands in water for prolonged periods have an increased risk of developing this problem. The prolonged immersion causes the quick to separate from the nail plate, which allows the fungus to gain access. Established infection causes a painful red swelling at the base of the nail, which may become thickened, opaque and soft.

The differential diagnosis of a chronic fungal paronychia includes herpetic or bacterial paronychia, collagen diseases and Buerger's disease (see Chapter 10).

CHAPTER 4 | THE SKIN AND SUBCUTANEOUS TISSUES

Tinea pedis

(Athlete's foot)

This is a common condition caused by one of three fungi. Damage to the protective barrier function of the skin caused by athlete's foot may predispose to the entry of bacteria that can cause cellulitis, especially in patients with chronic lymphoedema (see Chapter 10).

History

Age and sex It is common in fit, young male athletes and swimmers, who pick it up in showers and communal baths.

Symptoms Patients usually complain of itching, maceration and fissure formation in the interdigital spaces of the toes, most often in the space between the fourth and fifth toes. One foot is usually more affected than the other. It often improves in winter and worsens in summer. The sole of the foot may itch and develop vesicles, and a rash may arise on the palms. Lymphangitis and cellulitis may complicate the condition (see page 130).

Examination

Site Always inspect between the toes.
Rash Maceration, odour and fissure formation with desquamation may be present (Fig. 4.39). These may spread onto the dorsum of the foot. Asymmetry is characteristic. A vesicular eruption with bullae may be present on the soles of the feet and the palms of the hands. The nails may become distorted, white and soft.

The fungus may spread to the limbs and trunk, especially the groins, where annular lesions may develop.

Fig. 4.39 Tinea pedis.

Infestations

Scabies

This is the result of invasion of the epidermis by the *Acarus scabies* mite. The adult female is about 0.5 mm in length, and is only just visible to the naked eye (Fig. 4.40). The male is half this size.

The fertilized female moves over the warm body until it finds a place to burrow through the horny layer of the skin. The female remains here for the rest of her life, laying two or three eggs per day for several weeks. These hatch in 3–4 days, and the larvae leave the burrow and enter the hair follicles to mature. The adult mites then escape onto the skin, where mating occurs. This cycle then begins again, roughly every fortnight.

Sixty per cent of burrows are on the hands and wrists, the remainder being on the soles of the feet, the genitalia, the axillae, the elbows and the buttocks.

Fig. 4.40 A scabies mite.

History

In a patient who has never had scabies, an erythematous rash develops around the burrows 1 month after infestation. This is usually followed by a generalized urticarial reaction. The skin then begins to itch, especially at night. Other family members are often affected.

Examination

An urticarial rash is usually present, which in adults consists of wheals developing mostly on the trunk and limbs. Vesiculation may be present on the hands and limbs, which may become eczematous or infected.

Confirmation of diagnosis The diagnosis is confirmed by finding burrows (Fig. 4.41). A magnifying lens, a good light and a sterile needle are required. The mite is visible at the anterior end of the burrow as a white oval with a black dot at its front. The needle is inserted into the burrow, which is opened up, and the mite adheres to the tip of the needle. The mite is then put on a microscope slide and inked around, and the diagnosis is confirmed.

The differential diagnosis includes other causes of generalized itching (see below).

Fig. 4.41 A scabies burrow.

Pediculosis capitis

Infestation with head lice is common in schoolchildren. Severe infestation causes intolerable itching, and there is often secondary infection and enlarged cervical lymph glands.

Nits are present on the shafts of the hairs.

PRURITUS

This is itching of the skin caused by a local or general abnormality. The presence of multiple skin scratches (excoriation) is usually obvious. The causes include:

- Skin diseases:
  - ○ Urticaria.
  - ○ Eczema.
- Local irritation:
  - ○ Local allergy, e.g. washing powder.
  - ○ Parasites (see above).
  - ○ Discharge, e.g. rectal or vaginal.

- General disease:
  - ○ Jaundice from accumulation of bile salts.
  - ○ Hodgkin's disease.
  - ○ Uraemia.
  - ○ Thyrotoxicosis.
  - ○ Iron deficiency or polycythaemia.
  - ○ Diabetes.
  - ○ HIV infection.
- Psychogenic causes.

BENIGN SKIN LUMPS

Seborrhoeic keratosis

This is also called a senile wart, seborrhoeic wart, verruca senilis or basal cell papilloma. It is a benign overgrowth of the basal layer of the epidermis containing excess small, dark-staining basal cells, which raise it above the level of the normal epidermis (Fig. 4.42) and give it a semi-transparent, oily appearance.

Fig. 4.42 A seborrhoeic keratosis. The plaque consists of an excess number of basal cells and will peel off.

History

Age Senile warts occur in both sexes but, as the name implies, they become more common with advancing years. Most people over the age of 70 years have got one or two of these lesions.

Duration They are slow growing, beginning as a minute patch that gradually increases in area. Patients have invariably had the lesion for months or years before complaining about it.

Symptoms As it gets bigger, it becomes disfiguring, and may start to catch on clothes. It seldom bleeds, but may get infected. There is sometimes sufficient melanin in the lesion to make the patient think it is a mole.

Progression Senile warts gradually increase in area, but not in thickness. They can suddenly fall off, uncovering a pale pink patch of skin.

Examination

Site They occur on any part of the skin except those areas subjected to regular abrasion, such as the palms of the hands and the soles of the feet. The majority are found on the back of the trunk.

Shape and size They form a raised plaque of hypertrophic, slightly greasy skin, with a square-cut and distinct edge. They vary in size from a few millimetres to 2–3 cm in diameter (Fig. 4.43).

Surface They have a rough, sometimes papilliferous, surface.

Colour Their colour varies from pale yellow to dark brown, depending on the thickness of the epithelium and the quantity of melanin in the underlying skin (Fig. 4.44).

Fig. 4.43 A patient whose back was covered with seborrhoeic keratoses.

Fig. 4.44 The area outlined in the Fig. 4.43 is enlarged here.

Bleeding into a plaque after trauma makes the lesion swell and turn brown – changes that may be confused with malignant change in a **melanoma**.

An infected keratosis may become swollen and tender and be confused with a **pyogenic granuloma** or **squamous cell carcinoma**.

Consistency Seborrhoeic warts are a little harder and stiffer than normal skin. The surrounding tissues are healthy, but there are often other seborrhoeic warts nearby. They have a greasy, soapy feel.

Special diagnostic feature Because seborrhoeic keratoses are patches of thick squamous epithelium, they can be picked off. **They feel 'stuck on'.** When a wart is peeled off, it leaves a patch of pale pink skin, and one or two fine surface capillaries that bleed slightly. No other skin lesion behaves like this.

Never pick hard at the edge of any skin lesion for fear of damaging it. Interfering in this way with a malignant tumour may hasten its local spread.

Keratoacanthoma

(Adenoma sebaceum, molluscum pseudo-carcinomatosum)
This is a self-limiting overgrowth of hair follicle cells, which spontaneously regresses. *It is often mistaken for a squamous cell carcinoma because it grows so rapidly.*

History

The lesions occur in adults, who complain of a rapidly growing lump in the skin. They are not painful, but can be very unsightly. The lump takes 2–4 weeks to grow, and 2–3 months to regress. The cause is unknown. It may be a self-limiting benign neoplasm or an unusual response to a viral infection.

Examination

Site Keratoacanthomas are often found as solitary lumps on the face (Fig. 4.45), but they can occur anywhere where there are sebaceous glands.

Shape and size The lump is hemispherical or conical, and looks like a volcano when the central slough appears and the surrounding skin retracts (Fig. 4.46). The nodule is usually 1–2 cm in diameter by the time the centre of the lump begins to necrose.

Consistency The bulk of the lesion is firm and rubbery, but the central core is hard.

Colour The lump has a normal skin colour, but the necrotic centre is brown or black (Fig. 4.47).

Fig. 4.45 A keratoacanthoma is an overgrowth of hair follicle cells that produce a central plug of keratin. When the plug separates, the lesion usually undergoes spontaneous regression.

Fig. 4.46 A large keratoacanthoma on the face.

Fig. 4.47 A keratoacanthoma on the wrist. The slough is just beginning to separate.

Relations The lump is confined to the skin, and is freely mobile over the subcutaneous tissues.
Lymph drainage The local lymph glands should not be enlarged.
Natural history The central core eventually separates and the lump collapses, leaving a deep indrawn scar. In spite of this self-limiting natural history, keratoacanthomas are often excised to confirm the diagnosis.

Differential diagnosis A keratoacanthoma must be differentiated from a **squamous cell carcinoma**. The latter grows more slowly, and eventually becomes an ulcer. The diagnosis is confirmed by a pathologist after an excisional biopsy.

Hystiocytoma

(Dermatofibroma, sclerosing angioma)
This is a benign neoplasm of the fibroblasts of the dermis. Its name is derived from the many histiocytes that are present between the fibroblasts. The overlying epidermis is normal. It has also been suggested that it may be a haemangioma with a marked desmoplastic response.

History

Age Lesions appear on the skin of young and middle-aged adults.
Sex Both sexes are equally affected.
Symptoms The patient complains of a slow-growing lump on the skin.

Examination

Site They can occur anywhere, but are slightly more common on the skin of the limbs.
Shape As they grow, they form a hemispherical lump, which then flattens into a thick disc (Fig. 4.48). The edges of the disc may overhang its base.

Fig. 4.48 A large histiocytoma on the calf.

CHAPTER 4 | THE SKIN AND SUBCUTANEOUS TISSUES

Size Most patients complain of these tumours when they are 1–2 cm across, but they can grow to a considerable size if they are neglected.

Surface and colour The overlying skin is inseparable from the lump. The epidermis is usually a normal colour but may contain haemosiderin, which gives it a brown appearance like a mole.

Tenderness They are not tender.

Composition These tumours usually have a rubbery or spongy consistency.

Relations They are in the skin.

Lymph drainage The local lymph glands should not be enlarged.

Local tissues The surrounding tissues are normal.

Sebaceous cyst

The skin is kept soft and oily by the sebum secreted by the sebaceous glands. When an opening of one of these glands becomes blocked, it distends with its own secretion, and ultimately becomes a sebaceous cyst. These are more correctly called **pilar or trichilemmal cysts when they develop in the scalp**, as they arise from infundibular parts of hair follicles and have no function.

History

Age Sebaceous cysts occur in all age groups, but rarely present before adolescence, with the majority presenting in early adulthood or middle age.

Duration Sebaceous cysts are slow growing and have usually been present for some years before the patient asks a surgeon to remove them.

Symptoms Sebaceous cysts most frequently arise on the scalp, and the most common complaint is of a lump that gets scratched when the patient is combing their hair. Such scratches may get infected, and when infection develops in a cyst, it enlarges rapidly and becomes acutely painful.

A slow discharge of sebum from a wide punctum sometimes hardens to form a sebaceous horn.

Infection of the cyst wall and the surrounding tissues produces a boggy, painful, discharging swelling known as **Cock's peculiar tumour**. This only happens if an infected cyst is neglected.

Development Sebaceous cysts usually enlarge with time, but the increase in size is accelerated if the cyst becomes infected. A cyst will sometimes discharge its contents through its punctum (sebaceous gland opening), and then regress or even disappear.

Multiplicity Sebaceous cysts are often multiple (Fig. 4.49).

Fig. 4.49 Three sebaceous cysts on the scalp. Note that you cannot see a punctum, a common finding.

Examination

Site Most sebaceous cysts are found in the hairy parts of the body. The scalp, scrotum, neck, shoulders and back are the common sites, but they can occur wherever there are sebaceous glands. There are no sebaceous glands on the palms of the hands and soles of the feet.

Shape and size Most sebaceous cysts are tense and spherical. Even on the scalp, where there is the unyielding skull beneath them, they remain spherical by bulging outwards and stretching the overlying skin (Fig. 4.50). They can vary from a few millimetres to 4–5 cm in diameter, but most patients seek advice before they become very large.

Surface The surface of a sebaceous cyst is smooth.

Edge The edge is well defined and easy to feel, as it is usually lying in subcutaneous fat.

Colour The skin over the cyst is usually normal, although a 'punctum' or pit may be visible as a dark spot (Fig. 4.50).

Tenderness Uncomplicated sebaceous cysts are not tender. Pain and tenderness indicate infection.

Temperature The temperature of the skin over a cyst is normal except when the cyst is infected.

Composition Most sebaceous cysts feel hard and solid. They are occasionally so tense that it is not possible to elicit fluctuation, especially if there is no firm underlying tissue to press them against. On the scalp, the resistance of the underlying skull aids detection of fluctuation.

Fig. 4.50 A punctum of a sebaceous cyst.

They do not transilluminate because they are full of sebum.

Relations They arise from a skin structure but lie in the subcutaneous tissues, although they are attached to skin. Their point of discharge is usually along a hair follicle and, as the cyst grows, this point of fixation is often pulled inwards to become a small punctum (Fig 4.50). Only one-half of the cysts that you will see have a visible punctum, but when one is present it is a useful diagnostic sign. All sebaceous cysts are attached to the skin even if there is no punctum. The area of attachment may be quite small, but it prevents the cyst moving independently of the skin. Sebaceous cysts are not attached deeply.

Lymph drainage The local lymph glands should not be enlarged.

A sebaceous horn

This arises from a sebaceous cyst when the contained sebum slowly exudes from a large central punctum before drying and hardening into a conical spike (Fig. 4.51). The friction from clothes and washing normally removes the secretions of the gland as soon as they appear. A sebaceous horn can therefore only grow if the patient fails to wash!

Cock's peculiar tumour

Cock's peculiar tumour is an infected, open, granulating, oedematous sebaceous cyst. It looks angry, sore and malignant, and *is often mistaken for a squamous cell carcinoma of the scalp*. Granulation tissue arising from the lining of the cyst heaps up and bursts onto the skin, giving the lesion an everted edge (Fig. 4.52).

Fig. 4.51 A sebaceous horn on the ear. The 'horn' is simply the hardened sebaceous material (epithelial cells and sebum) extruding from the cyst.

Fig. 4.52 Cock's peculiar tumour. This is a mass of granulation tissue protruding from the base of a previously infected and ruptured sebaceous cyst.

CHAPTER 4 | THE SKIN AND SUBCUTANEOUS TISSUES

The infection in the cyst wall and surrounding tissues makes the whole area oedematous, red and tender. The regional lymph glands may be enlarged.

Pigmented naevi

(Moles)

The word 'mole' is a lay term used to describe a brown spot or blemish on the skin. The brown pigment is melanin. There are three ways in which an excess of melanin may be produced to colour the skin brown (Fig. 4.53):

- There may be a normal number of melanocytes, in their normal position, each producing excess melanin. This abnormality is called a **freckle or ephelis**. It is not called a mole because it does not contain an increased number of melanocytes.
- There may be an increased number of melanocytes, in their normal position, each producing normal amounts of melanin. This abnormality is called a **lentigo**.
- There may be an increased number of melanocytes, in abnormal clusters at the dermo-epidermal junction, producing normal or excessive amounts of melanin. This abnormality is called a **mole or pigmented naevus**.

A mole becomes **a malignant melanoma** if the melanocytes invade adjacent tissues or show signs of abnormal and excessive multiplication. It is called a **dysplastic naevus** if there are some nuclear abnormalities but no evidence of invasion.

The three benign pathological entities described above often have similar macroscopic features, and it is therefore safest to **call all benign melanin-producing lesions moles or pigmented naevi**, and to **call all malignant melanin-producing tumours malignant melanomas**.

Pathology

Whereas the clinical appearance of pigmented naevi is infinitely variable and almost unclassifiable, moles can be defined according to their microscopic appearance (Fig. 4.53). Melanocytes are normally found in small numbers among the cells of the basal layer of the epidermis. They first cluster in this layer, and then migrate into the dermis if they proliferate.

The mature adult mole consists of clusters of melanocytes in the dermis, and is therefore called an **intradermal naevus**. This can be flat or raised, smooth or warty, and hairy or non-hairy. Most of the moles on the arms, face and trunk are of this variety, and they hardly ever turn malignant.

There will be clusters of cells at various stages of maturity in the epidermis and the dermis if the growth and movement of the melanocytes stop before they have all migrated into the dermis. This lesion is called a **compound cellular naevus**.

The naevus is called a **junctional naevus** if the melanocytes remain close to the junction between the epidermis and dermis. These naevi are immature and unstable, and can turn malignant. The majority of malignant melanomas begin in junctional moles. Many of the moles on the palms of the hands, the soles of the feet and the external genitalia are of the junctional variety.

Melanocytes that have never reached the epidermis, and therefore lie in the deep dermis or subcutaneous tissues, may still proliferate and produce excess melanin. The resulting lesion has a blue appearance and is called a **blue naevus**.

History

Age Everyone, except for albinos, has a few moles at birth, but the number increases during life. It has been estimated that most white individuals have 15–20 moles. During childhood and adolescence, these may become more pigmented or completely regress. A mole on a child may be clinically and histologically difficult to distinguish from a malignant melanoma if it enlarges and becomes darker, but true malignant change is uncommon before puberty.

Ethnic group They are more common in white people living in hot countries, such as Australia,

Normal skin

Freckle (ephelis)
Normal number of melanocytes,
in normal position, producing excess melanin

Lentigo
Excess melanocytes, each in normal position,
producing normal amounts of melanin

Pigmented naevus/mole
Excess melanocytes, in clusters, variable but usually excess melanin production

Intradermal naevus   Compound naevus   Junctional naevus

Fig. 4.53 The histological varieties of pigmented spots and blemishes.

because the skin is exposed to more ultraviolet light. Moles occur in black individuals, particularly in the less pigmented areas such as the soles of feet and palms of the hands, but are rare.

Symptoms They rarely cause any serious symptoms, but may be disfiguring, protrude above the skin surface and catch on clothes. Itching or bleeding suggests the possibility that malignant change has occurred (see below).

Examination

Site Moles can occur on any part of the skin, but are most common on the limbs, face, neck and trunk.

Size Most are 1–3 mm in diameter.

Colour Their colour varies from light brown to black and does not fade with pressure. **Amelanotic naevi** do occur, but without their pigment they are unlikely to be recognized. Pigmented naevi may regress.

A mole surrounded by a white halo of regression is known as a **halo naevus** (Fig. 4.54).

Composition Moles usually have a soft consistency and are indistinguishable, by palpation, from the surrounding tissues.

Lymph glands The local lymph glands should not be enlarged.

Shape and surface There are four clinical varieties of mole:

- **Hairy mole** is a common variety. It is flat, or very slightly raised above the level of the surrounding skin, with a smooth or slightly warty epidermal covering, and has hairs growing from its surface (Fig. 4.55). The presence of hairs means that the mole also contains sebaceous glands that can become infected and cause changes such as swelling and tenderness, which may be indistinguishable from malignant change. Hairy moles are always **intradermal naevi**.

- **Non-hairy or smooth mole** is also a common variety. The epithelium is smooth and not elevated. The brown pigment looks as if it is deep in the skin (Fig. 4.56) – deeper than that of the hairy mole – but this is just an optical illusion. Non-hairy moles may be **intradermal, junctional or compound naevi**.

- **Blue naevus** is a mole deep in the dermis. The thick overlying layers of dermis and epidermis mask the brown colour of the melanin and make it look blue (Fig. 4.57). The overlying

skin is often smooth and shiny. This is an uncommon type of mole, more often seen in children. It usually occurs on the face, the dorsum of the hands and feet, and the buttocks.

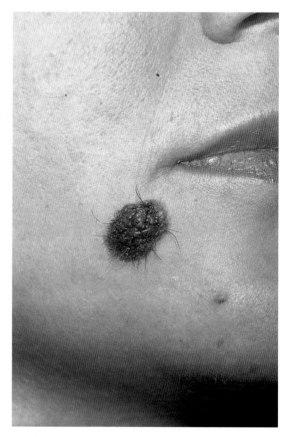

Fig. 4.55 A hairy mole.

Fig. 4.54 A 'halo' mole. This mole is regressing. It has faded and the skin around it has become depigmented.

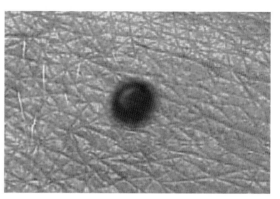

Fig. 4.56 A smooth mole.

- **Lentigo** is an area of pigmentation that appears in late adult life and is prone to undergoing malignant change (Fig. 4.58) (see below).

There are two other varieties of melanotic skin pigmentation: the café-au-lait patch (see page 115) and the circumoral moles of the Peutz–Jegher syndrome (see Chapter 11).

Fig. 4.57 A blue mole.

Fig. 4.58 A Hutchinson's lentigo on the face.

BENIGN SUBCUTANEOUS SWELLINGS

Lipoma

This is a cluster of fat cells that have become overactive and so distended with fat that they have become palpable lumps. They are never malignant. Liposarcomas, which often develop in the retroperitoneal tissues (see Chapter 15), arise *de novo*.

History

Age They occur at all ages, but are not common in children.

Duration They usually grow slowly for months or years before being noticed. They rarely regress.

Symptoms Most patients present because they have noticed a lump and want to know what it is. The lump may be unsightly or interfere with movement, especially if it becomes pedunculated or very large (Fig. 4.59).

Multiplicity Patients often have many lipomas, or have had others excised in the past. Multiple contiguous lipomas cause enlargement and distortion of the subcutaneous tissues. This condition is called **lipomatosis**. It usually occurs in the buttocks and sometimes in the neck.

Multiple lipomatosis (**Dercum's disease**) is a condition in which the limbs and sometimes the trunk are covered with lipomas of all shapes and sizes. These can be painful and may contain angiomatous elements (**angiolipomas**).

Examination

Site They are most common in the subcutaneous tissues of the upper limbs, chest, neck and shoulders, but they can occur anywhere.

Fig. 4.59 A large lipoma overlying the scapula.

CHAPTER 4 | THE SKIN AND SUBCUTANEOUS TISSUES

Colour The skin that overlies the lump is normal, and the veins crossing the lipoma may be visible as faint blue streaks.

Tenderness Lipomas are not usually tender, but angiolipomas are.

Temperature The temperature of the overlying skin is normal.

Shape and size They are usually spherical, but subcutaneous lipomas that develop between the skin and the deep fascia are usually discoid or hemispherical.

Most lipomas are lobulated, as fat in the body is in the form of lobules. The lobules can be seen and felt on the surface and at the edge of the lump (Fig. 4.60). Lipomas come in all sizes.

Surface The surface feels smooth, but firm pressure reveals the depressions between the lobules, which become more prominent with firm palpation or gentle squeezing. This increases the pressure within the lipoma and makes each lobule bulge out between the fine strands of fibrous tissue that surround it (Fig. 4.61).

Edge The edge is not circular but a series of irregular curves corresponding to each lobule. Because the edge is soft, compressible and sometimes quite thin, it slips away from the examining finger. This has been

Fig. 4.61 Lobulation.

described as the '*slip sign*'. It is not a very useful or diagnostic feature.

Evidence of lobulation on the surface and at the edge is the most significant physical sign.

Composition Most lipomas contain a soft but solid jelly-like fat when they are cut open immediately after removal. Lipomas often **give the impression of fluctuating**, but careful examination reveals that they are just yielding to pressure, spreading out in all directions because they are soft. They do not become more tense and prominent in the plane at right angles to the palpating finger. The larger the lipoma, the more it appears to fluctuate, but fat at body temperature is solid, not liquid.

Lipomas do not transilluminate in that they do not transmit light from a torch shone beside them, but they may light up if light is shone directly across them. They do not have a fluid thrill, and they do not reduce or pulsate.

The physical signs of pseudo-fluctuation and transillumination make them appear cystic, a false impression that emphasizes **the diagnostic importance of finding lobulation.**

Relations Lipomas may arise within deep structures, such as muscles. These lipomas are fixed deeply, and may become more prominent if they are pushed out of the muscle (Fig. 4.62), or disappear if they are drawn into the muscle when it contracts.

Subcutaneous lipomas are not attached superficially or deeply, and can be moved in all directions.

Lymph drainage The regional lymph glands are not be enlarged.

Local tissues The surrounding tissues are normal, but other lipomas may be present.

Fig. 4.60 A lipoma in the subcutaneous tissues of the upper arm. Note the lobulation.

Fig. 4.62 A lipoma in the forearm. This swelling became more prominent and fixed when the forearm muscles were contracted, showing that it was superficial to the muscle, but attached to its fascia.

Fig. 4.63 A soft multilocular ganglion on the back of the wrist.

Ganglion

A ganglion is a myxomatous degeneration of fibrous tissue. Ganglia can occur anywhere in the body, but they are common where there is a lot of fibrous tissue, i.e. around the joints.

History

Age The majority present between the ages of 20 and 60 years, and they are rare in children.

Duration They grow slowly over months or years.

Symptoms They are not painful. Most patients seek advice because they wish to know the diagnosis or because the lump is disfiguring. Some ganglia slip away between neighbouring bones, giving the false impression that they are reducing into the joint, but a true ganglion should not connect with or empty into a joint. Ganglia may rupture into the subcutaneous tissues and disappear.

Examination

Site Most ganglia are found near joint capsules and tendon sheaths, but they can occur anywhere. Ninety per cent arise on the dorsal and ventral surfaces of the wrist joint and hand (Fig. 4.63).

Shape and size Ganglia are spherical. Some are multilocular and feel like a collection of cysts. They come in all sizes. Small ganglia (0.5–1.0 cm) tend to be tense and spherical. Large ones, which can be up to 5–6 cm across, are flattened and soft.

Surface They have a smooth surface.

Composition Ganglia feel solid, but their consistency varies from soft to hard. The gelatinous material within them is very viscous, but most ganglia fluctuate, provided they are not very small or very tense.

They usually transilluminate brilliantly (Fig. 4.64).

Fig. 4.64 A ganglion transilluminating.

Reducibility A ganglion may slip away between deeper structures when pressed, giving the false impression that its contents have reduced into the joint.

Relations Ganglia are usually attached to the fibrous tissue from which they originate. They are not attached to the overlying skin, which should be freely mobile over them. The mobility of a ganglion depends on the extent and nature of its deep attachment. When the tissue of origin is part of a joint capsule, tendon sheath or intramuscular septum, the ganglion becomes less mobile when these structures are made tense. Therefore remember to palpate ganglia in all positions of the underlying joint, and with the surrounding muscles relaxed and tense.

Differential diagnosis The three common swellings found close to joints are:

- **bursae**;
- **cystic protrusions of the synovial cavity of arthritic joints**;
- **ganglia**.

The first two are usually soft; the ganglion is tense. With the first and third, the joint is normal.

Subcutaneous bursae

Bursae are fluid-filled cavities, lined with a flattened endothelium similar to synovium, that develop between tendons, bones and skin to allow tissues to slide easily. A considerable number of bursae are always present. Others called **adventitious bursae** develop wherever there is friction between two layers of tissue.

History

Age Bursae are uncommon in the young, and they usually appear in middle and later life as a result of prolonged friction between skin and bone, associated with the patient's occupation or with a deformity produced by injury or arthritis.

Symptoms Pain and an enlarging swelling at the site of repeated trauma are the common presenting symptoms, and may stop the patient working. A severe throbbing pain and a rapid increase in size indicate the presence of infection.

Development The swelling usually appears to develop rapidly, even though the bursa has probably been present for many years. The increase in fluid within the bursa is usually secondary to minor infection or trauma.

Multiplicity Bursae are often symmetrical, for example on both knees or elbows.

Cause The patient often knows the cause of the swelling (prolonged friction or a skeletal deformity), and may have had a similar complaint before.

Examination

Site Subcutaneous bursae occur where there is friction between skin and bone. The common sites are (Fig. 4.65):

- between the skin and olecranon – **student's elbow**;
- between the skin and patella – **housemaid's knee**;
- between the skin and patellar ligament – **clergyman's knee**;
- between the skin and the head of the first metatarsal – **bunion**.

Fig. 4.65 The common adventitious bursae.

Shape and size Bursae are usually circular in outline with an indistinct edge, but their depth, or thickness, can vary from a few millimetres to 3–4 cm.

Surface The surface feels smooth providing it is not attached to the skin.

Colour The overlying skin is usually thickened, and often appears shiny, white and cracked.

Tenderness They are only tender if they become very tense or inflamed. The overlying skin then turns red and hot.

Composition They contain a clear viscous fluid, similar to synovial fluid, which gives them a soft or spongy consistency.

They fluctuate, transilluminate and may have a fluid thrill.

These signs may be difficult to elicit if the wall of the bursa is thick, or the quantity of contained fluid small.

Relations The deep and superficial surfaces of a bursa are usually firmly attached to the two tissues it separates, so that the friction occurs between the lubricated inside surfaces of the bursa. This makes the bursa immobile and the walls impalpable.

Local tissues The bones and joints beneath the bursa must be carefully examined because a bursa may have developed to ease the movement of the skin over a skeletal abnormality such as an exostosis or deformed joint. The overlying skin is often thickened and cracked.

Complications Bursae can become inflamed by repeated trauma and by conditions that cause inflammation of the synovial surfaces, such as rheumatoid arthritis and gout. They also commonly become infected.

General examination Even though the patient complains of one lump, examine the same area on the other limb because symmetrical bursae are common. Also look for other skeletal abnormalities and joint diseases.

Sporadic neurofibroma

Multiple familial neurofibromatosis (von Recklinghausen's disease) has already been discussed on page 114.

Sporadic neurofibromas are benign tumours that contain a mixture of neural (ectodermal) and fibrous (mesodermal) elements. They are often multiple. Tumours that are derived from nerve sheaths (the

neurilemmoma, also known as the schwannoma), are very rare.

History

Age Neurofibromas can appear at any age, but usually present in adult life.

Symptoms Most cause no discomfort, and they rarely grow to be disfiguring. When they are related to a nerve trunk, they may be tender, and the patient may get tingling sensations in the distribution of the affected nerve.

Multiplicity They are often multiple.

Examination

Site They can occur anywhere in the skin and subcutaneous tissues. The forearms seem to be most often affected, perhaps because they are the part of the body most frequently palpated by the patient.

Shape and size Neurofibromas are usually fusiform, with their long axes lying along the length of the limb. They are rarely more than a few centimetres in length (Fig. 4.66).

Composition They have the consistency of firm rubber.

Relations The surrounding structures are normal. Subcutaneous neurofibromas are mobile within the subcutaneous tissues but move most freely in a direction at right angles to the course of the nerve to which they are connected.

Fig. 4.66 A neurofibroma on the leg of a patient with five other similar lesions.

Plexiform neurofibroma

Although this is a very rare condition, it is mentioned because it is one of those conditions that can cause considerable diagnostic confusion if the doctor has never heard of it.

It is an excessive overgrowth of neural tissue in the subcutaneous layers, which gives the tissues a swollen and oedematous appearance. It is sometimes called elephantiasis neurofibromatosis (Fig. 4.67).

It is often misdiagnosed as lymphoedema (see Chapter 10), so remember the condition when presented with a child with an apparent overgrowth of the soft tissues of the hand or foot. The diagnosis can only be made by the pathologist.

Fig. 4.67 A plexiform neurofibroma.

TUMOURS OF THE SKIN APPENDAGES

These arise from the sebaceous glands, sweat glands, eccrine and apocrine glands and hair gland cells. Most are benign and have exotic names. The majority are relatively benign, such as basal cell carcinomas (see page 152), but 5–10 per cent are malignant and liable to local recurrence. All arise as subcutaneous pink, brown or red/white nodules on different parts of the body, but mainly in the head and neck.

Sebaceous gland tumours

These include the **naevus sebaceous of Jadassohn**, **sebaceous adenoma** and **sebaceous carcinoma**, which is rare. They are all solitary subcutaneous tumours that are either soft and warty, or firm.

Eccrine (sweat) gland tumours

These include the **eccrine poroma**, the **spiradenoma** and the **acrospiroma**. These all present as solitary subcutaneous lumps, which can be reddish-pink or red–blue coloured.

Syringomas also arise from the sweat glands, and present as multiple flesh-coloured or yellow papules on the faces of females.

Cylindromas (turban tumours) are rare tumours that arise from the sweat glands of the head and scalp. They present as solitary or multiple, pink, spherical or slightly flattened nodules, which may coalesce to look like a turban, hence the common name (Fig. 4.68). They are soft with an ill-defined edge.

Fig. 4.68 A 'turban' tumour.

The apocrine gland tumours

These include **apocrine hidrocystomas** and the **syringocystadenoma papilliferum**.

The hair gland tumours

These include **trichofolliculomas, trichoepitheliomas, trichilemmomas** and **pilomatrixomas**, many of which are hamartomas.

PREMALIGNANT SKIN LESIONS

Solar keratosis

Prolonged exposure of the skin to sunlight can cause areas of hyperkeratosis of the skin, which may undergo malignant change.

History

The patient notices the gradual appearance of thickened patches of skin, which are not painful but can become unsightly.

Natural history Solar keratoses grow slowly, and the patients, usually elderly males who have worked out of doors for many years, ignore them. Any change in size or appearance should arouse suspicion.

Examination

Site They are commonly found on the backs of the fingers and hands, on the face and on the rim of the ears.

Shape and size Beneath their horny surface layer, there is a raised plaque of skin that may vary in diameter from a few millimetres to 1 cm and protrude above the skin surface (Fig. 4.69). The whole of the strip of skin along the rim of the pinna may be affected.

Colour The thickened patches of skin have a yellow–grey or red–brown colour.

Composition The keratinous layer is very hard, and clearly part of the underlying skin.

Relations They are confined to the skin, and if a nodule or patch is tethered to the underlying structures, it has already turned into a squamous carcinoma.

Lymph drainage The local lymph glands should not be enlarged unless one of the keratoses has become a squamous cell carcinoma.

Fig. 4.69 A solar keratosis on the back of the hand.

Bowen's disease

This also is a precancerous lesion. It presents as a cluster of flat, pink, papular patches that are covered with crusts. The patches and the adjacent skin have a pale brown, thickened appearance. (Fig. 4.70). Patients usually believe they have a patch of eczema.

When the crusts are removed, the papules can be seen to have a wet, oozy, slightly bloody, papilliferous surface.

Fig. 4.70 Bowen's disease on the skin of the chest.

CHAPTER 4 | THE SKIN AND SUBCUTANEOUS TISSUES

Hutchinson's lentigo

This is a large area of pigmentation that commonly appears and slowly enlarges on the face and neck in late adult life (after the age of 60 years). The surface is smooth, but there may be raised, rough nodules (see Fig. 4.58), which correspond to areas of junctional activity and become the sites of malignant change, alongside pale areas of regression. Areas of malignant change cause an increase in pigmentation that may pass unnoticed because the background pigmentation is so dark.

This mole is different from other moles because of two special features: its late development and its high incidence of malignant change. It may be 'premalignant' or 'frankly malignant' from the start: an example of malignant change 'in situ'.

MALIGNANT DISEASES OF THE SKIN

Basal cell carcinoma

(Rodent ulcer)

This is a locally invasive carcinoma of the basal layer of the epidermis. It does not metastasize, but can infiltrate adjacent tissues. It is common in exposed skin, especially in countries where there is a high incidence of ultraviolet irradiation, i.e. bright sunlight.

History

Age The incidence increases with age because it is related to the duration of exposure of the skin to ultraviolet light.

Geography It is the most common cancer in Europe, Australia and the USA, and is showing a worldwide increase in incidence.

Ethnic group It is rare in dark-skinned races.

Sex Males are affected more often than females.

Duration The lesions grow very slowly and have often been present for months or years before the patient seeks advice.

Symptoms The principal complaint is of a persistent nodule or an ulcer with a central scab that repeatedly falls off and then re-forms. The tumour eventually becomes disfiguring. It may itch or be painful, and if it is neglected, it eventually becomes a deep infected ulcer. A large, neglected ulcer destroying one side of the face is now rare.

Development These tumours grow very slowly and may have been present for months or years before the patient presents. The long history gives a false impression that the lesion is 'benign and unimportant'.

Persistence Some spread rapidly through the skin, leaving a central scar.

Multiplicity They are often multiple.

Predisposing factors The most significant aetiological factors appear to be a genetic predisposition and an exposure to ultraviolet radiation.

Examination (See Revision panel 4.6)

Site They are commonly found on the face above a line drawn from the angle of the mouth to the lobe of the ear (Fig. 4.71). This does not mean that they do not occur in other sites; all exposed skin is susceptible, particularly on the scalp, neck, arms and hands.

Size Most patients complain of the nodule or ulcer (Fig. 4.72) when it is quite small, but basal cell carcinomas can grow to a considerable size if they are neglected (Fig. 4.73). A few grow outwards from the skin to become a fungating mass on the skin surface (Fig. 4.74), but the majority erode deeply, destroying the underlying tissues and forming a deep cavity (see Fig. 4.73) – hence the name 'rodent'.

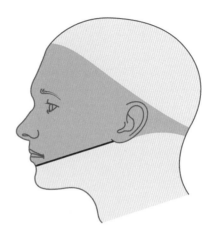

Fig. 4.71 Basal cell carcinomas commonly appear in the shaded area.

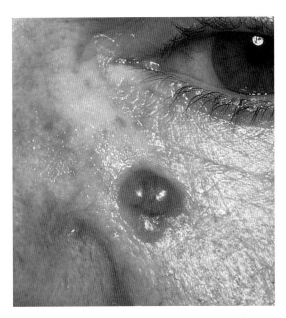

(a) An early nodule just below the eye. These nodules are sometimes mistakenly thought to be cystic.

(b) A recurrent basal cell carcinoma at the edge of a skin graft placed to cover the skin defect from a previous excision 7 years earlier.

Fig. 4.72 BASAL CELL CARCINOMA

Fig. 4.73 A true 'rodent ulcer'. The basal cell carcinoma has destroyed the orbit and the eye.

Fig. 4.74 A raised, wet, weeping basal cell carcinoma that was thought by the patient to be a patch of eczema.

Revision panel 4.6

The various clinical appearances of basal cell carcinomas

Nodule

'Cystic' (a large, seemingly transparent nodule)

Ulcer

Deeply eroding ulcer: the 'rodent' ulcer

Pigmented nodule

Geographical (advancing edge, healing centre)

CHAPTER 4 | THE SKIN AND SUBCUTANEOUS TISSUES

Shape Some of the many macroscopic appearances of basal cell carcinomas are shown in Figs 4.72–4.74. The tumour always starts as a nodule. When the central epithelium dies, the resulting ulcer develops **a rolled edge** (see Chapter 1). This means that the edge is raised up and rounded, but not everted. The nodule can become quite large and look like a cyst if the centre of the tumour does not necrose and ulcerate (see Fig. 4.72a). It is, however, not cystic, because it is solid and non-fluctuant, although the term 'cystic rodent ulcer' is unfortunately sometimes used to describe this appearance.

Colour The raised portion of the tumour – its edge if it is annular, or its centre if it is a nodule – is smooth, glistening and slightly transparent. This gives the impression that there are **pearl-white nodules of tissue** just below the epidermis (see Fig. 4.72b). These nodules also give the ulcerating variety its typical 'rolled edge'.

The whole lesion may be coloured brown by excess melanin (a **pigmented basal cell carcinoma**) (Fig. 4.75).

Surface The surface of the nodular variety is **covered by fine, distinct blood vessels**, which may give it a pink hue (see Fig. 4.72a).

Edge When the nodule first ulcerates, the rolled edge is circular, but as the malignant cells spread, its shape becomes irregular. The raised edge may be the only clue to the diagnosis if the ulcer heals. An irregular raised edge around a flat white scar is sometimes called a **'geographical' or 'forest fire' basal cell carcinoma** (see Fig. 4.72b). When the ulcer erodes into deeper structures, the edge becomes more prominent and florid, but not everted (see Fig. 4.72b).

Base The base of a small rodent ulcer is covered with a coat of dried serum and epithelial cells, and will bleed slightly if this layer is picked off. The bases of deeply eroding ulcers consist of fat, bone, muscle or other structures covered by poor-quality granulation tissue (see Fig. 4.73).

Depth Long-standing ulcers may erode deep into the face, destroying skin and bone, and exposing the nasal cavity, air sinuses and even the eye (see Fig. 4.73), *hence the name 'rodent' because the tissues look as if they have been gnawed by a rat.* Such extensive lesions are now uncommon.

Lymph drainage The local lymph glands should not be enlarged.

Relations A small tumour is confined to the skin, and is freely movable over the deep structures. Fixation of the ulcer indicates that it has invaded deeply.

Important differential diagnoses (Table 4.1) A rodent ulcer can resemble a **squamous cell carcinoma**. The long history and the rolled edge are the clinical features that indicate its basal cell origin.

A **keratoacanthoma** (see above) that is just beginning to slough at its centre can also look like an early rodent ulcer, but the short history and the deep slough should suggest the correct diagnosis.

Sweat gland tumours and **malignant melanomas** are other differential diagnoses that should be considered.

Squamous cell carcinoma

(Epithelioma)

This is a carcinoma of the cells of the epidermis that normally migrate out towards the surface to form the superficial keratinous squamous layer. The tumour cells infiltrate the epidermis, the dermis and adjacent tissues. Microscopic examination reveals tongues of tumour cells spreading in all directions, and clusters of cells with concentric rings of flattened squamous cells at their centre. These onion-like clumps of cells are often called '*epithelial pearls*', but are only seen under the microscope.

Fig. 4.75 A pigmented basal cell carcinoma.

Table 4.1   The diagnostic features of the four common surgical skin lesions

	Duration of growth	Physical features
Squamous cell carcinoma	Few months	Occasional bleeding Nodule or ulcer with everted edge
Basal cell carcinoma	Many months or years	Nodule or ulcer with rolled edge and permanent scab
Keratoacanthoma	Few weeks	Nodule with central hard necrotic core No bleeding Spontaneous regression
Pyogenic granuloma	Few days	Soft red nodule that becomes covered with epithelium Bleeds easily

History

Age The incidence of squamous carcinoma of the skin increases with age.

Causes The following are all associated with an **increased incidence of squamous carcinomas**:

- **Prolonged exposure to sunlight.**
- **Solar keratoses.**
- **Bowen's disease.**
- **Certain chemicals and irradiation.**
- **The presence of old scarring.**
- **Particularly following burns, or chronic ulcers.**

Cancer of the scrotal skin was once common in chimney sweeps (see Chapter 18).

Duration The ulcerating tumour has usually been present for 1 or 2 months before the patient presents. It may grow quite large before being noticed if it is in an inaccessible part, such as in the middle of the back.

Symptoms The patient complains of a lump, or of bleeding and discharge from an ulcer. Bleeding is more common with squamous cell than basal cell carcinomas. The tumour may become painful if it invades deep structures.

Patients occasionally notice enlarged lymph glands, and are unaware of the primary tumour. Dissemination of tumour cells throughout the body is a late event.

Development The ulcer or nodule enlarges steadily and inexorably. The edges become more prominent and florid (see Chapter 1).

Multiplicity There may be multiple tumours in skin affected by exposure to ultraviolet light or chemicals.

Examination

Site They can occur on any part of the skin, but are more common on the exposed skin of the head and neck, hands, forearms and upper trunk. They also develop in skin subjected to repeated chemical or mechanical irritation.

Colour The everted edge of a carcinomatous ulcer is usually a dark red–brown colour because it is very vascular (Fig. 4.76). The whole ulcer may be covered with old coagulated blood or serum.

Tenderness The ulcer is not usually tender.

Shape and size Squamous carcinomas begin as small nodules on the skin. As they enlarge, the centre becomes necrotic and sloughs, and the nodule turns into an ulcer. This is initially circular with prominent everted edges (Fig. 4.77), but can become any shape as it enlarges.

Fig. 4.76 A squamous cell carcinomatous ulcer on the face, with an everted edge and a necrotic base.

CHAPTER 4 | THE SKIN AND SUBCUTANEOUS TISSUES

Edge Squamous cell carcinomas have an **everted edge** because the excessive tissue growth raises it above and over the normal skin surface (see Figs 4.76, 4.77).

Base The base of the ulcer consists of necrotic tumour covered with serum and blood (Fig. 4.78). There is usually some granulation tissue, but this tends to be pale and unhealthy. Deep tissues may be exposed.

Fig. 4.77 A squamous cell carcinomatous ulcer on the hand, whose edge is not yet everted but is raised and almost everted on the proximal side.

Fig. 4.78 An extensive squamous cell carcinoma of the skin of the groin and scrotum.

Depth The depth of the ulcer is affected by the nature of the underlying tissues and the virulence of the tumour. Soft tissues are easily invaded, and when they slough they leave a deep ulcer (Fig. 4.78).

Discharge The discharge can be copious, bloody, purulent and foul-smelling. This is often the patient's most depressing and debilitating symptom.

Relations These vary according to the extent of the malignant infiltration. The tumour has spread beyond the skin and subcutaneous tissues into tendon, bone and muscle if the ulcer is immobile.

Local lymph glands The local lymph glands are often enlarged, but this does not always mean that they contain tumour. In about one-third of patients, the lymphadenopathy is caused by infection, which subsides after excision of the ulcer. Nevertheless, it should be assumed that palpable lymph glands contain metastases.

Local tissues The surrounding tissues may be oedematous and thickened, and there may be subcutaneous spread into nearby nerves. Invasion of local blood vessels can cause thrombosis and tissue ischaemia. These are features of the late stages of the disease.

Complications Infection and bleeding are the common complications. Bleeding can sometimes be massive and fatal.

General examination All the lymph glands that might contain metastases should be palpated (see Chapter 1). Distant metastases are uncommon, but hepatomegaly or a pleural effusion is indicative of systemic spread.

Differential diagnosis The differential diagnosis of squamous cell carcinoma is outlined in Revision panel 4.7.

Revision panel 4.7

Differential diagnosis of squamous cell carcinoma

Tumours of the skin appendages

Cutaneous secondary deposits

Basal cell carcinomas

Keratoacanthomas

Malignant melanomas

Solar keratoses

Pyogenic granulomas

Infected seborrhoeic warts

Marjolin's ulcer

(Squamous cell carcinoma)

This is an eponym for a squamous carcinoma that arises in a long-standing ulcer or benign burn scar. The most common ulcer to become malignant is a long-standing venous ulcer.

These carcinomas are very similar to an idiopathic squamous carcinoma, except that they may not be so florid. Their edge is not always raised and everted, and there may be pre-existing chronic ulceration or scarring (Fig. 4.79). Unusual nodules or changes in a chronic ulcer or a scar should be viewed with suspicion, especially if they increase in size and develop a very smelly discharge.

Fig. 4.79 A Marjolin's ulcer. The lipodermatosclerosis, pigmentation and scarring caused by long-standing venous hypertension and ulceration can be seen around the central neoplastic ulcer.

Malignant melanoma

Because of the confusion that has arisen from using the word 'melanoma' to describe a benign lesion and 'malignant melanoma' to describe a malignant one, *use the terms 'mole' or 'pigmented naevus' for benign lesions, and 'malignant melanoma' for malignant lesions.*

As the melanocyte originates from the neural crest and so is neuro-ectodermal in origin, it could be argued that malignant change in melanocytes should be called a carcinoma. Terms such as 'melanocarcinoma' and even 'melanosarcoma' only add to the confusion. It is therefore best to use the well-established descriptive term 'malignant melanoma'.

Cardinal symptoms of malignant change in a mole

- *Change in the surface.* One of the earliest signs associated with malignant change is a loss of the normal skin markings (creases) over the mole. The skin may also become rough and scaly (Fig. 4.80).
- *Itching.* This is an early and significant symptom, often associated with a pale pink halo around the mole (Fig. 4.81).
- *Increase in size, shape or thickness.* The patient usually complains that a long-standing mole, or a recently developed brown spot, has grown steadily over a period of a few weeks or months. The mole or part of the mole may become wider and thicker, often changing from a flat plaque to a nodule (Fig. 4.81). Alternatively, the mole may simply change in outline (Fig. 4.82).
- *Change in colour.* Malignant melanocytes usually produce more melanin, so the mole gets darker. The colour change is often patchy, with some

Fig. 4.80 Rough and scaly skin over a malignant melanoma arising in a Hutchinson's lentigo.

Fig. 4.81 A halo of pigment around a nodular melanoma.

Fig. 4.83 A superficial spreading melanoma with a 'pink' amelanotic area.

Fig. 4.82 A change in outline of pre-existing mole.

Fig. 4.84 Satellite nodules around a nodular melanoma.

areas becoming almost black, others turning blue–purple with the increased vascularity, and some areas not changing at all. Very occasionally, the malignant melanocytes do not produce melanin, so that the new growth is pink (Fig. 4.83).

- *Bleeding.* As the tumour cells multiply, the overlying epithelium becomes anoxic, and either ulcerates spontaneously or breaks down after a very minor injury. Bleeding is slight and a late sign.

- *Evidence of local or distant spread.* The pigment produced by the malignant melanocytes may spread diffusely into the surrounding skin to produce a brown halo around the primary lesion (see Figs 4.81–4.84). The malignant cells may also spread through the skin in the intradermal lymphatics. When they stop migrating and multiply, they become small intradermal nodules. Small nodules around the primary lesion are called satellite nodules (Fig. 4.84).

Patients occasionally notice enlarged lymph glands in the groin or axilla.

Not all malignant melanomas arise in pre-existing pigmented naevi.

All the changes listed above can develop in a few weeks or months (Revision panel 4.8).

History

Age Malignant melanoma is very rare before puberty, although it has been reported in children. Most cases occur in patients aged 20–30 years or more.

Sex Malignant melanoma occurs equally in both sexes, but is found more often in the lower limbs in females and on the trunk in males.

Ethnic group Malignant melanoma is common in white individuals and rare in black ones. People with fair complexions, red hair and a tendency to freckle are more susceptible.

Revision panel 4.8

The changes which suggest that a mole has turned malignant

Loss of normal surface markings (e.g. skin creases)

Change in size, shape or thickness

Change in colour

Itching

Bleeding/ulceration

Halo:

> Pink (inflammatory reaction) – early
> Brown (pigment) – late

Satellite nodules

Cause Melanocytes are stimulated by ultraviolet light. White-skinned people living in those parts of the world that enjoy abundant sunlight, such as Australia and the west coast of USA, have a high incidence of malignant melanoma. Those who work out of doors in these regions, especially those with a history of repeated episodes of sunburn, are particularly susceptible.

Symptoms The cardinal features have already been described. The common reasons for seeking medical advice are a change of size or colour, bleeding and the appearance of a brown halo or satellite nodules. It is usually the cosmetic disfigurement caused by an enlarging mole that brings the patient to the doctor, but more than 25 per cent of lesions arise *de novo*, i.e. in normal skin rather than in a pre-existing lesion. Malignant melanomas often itch, but are not painful.

The patient has sometimes observed the changes described above, but if the mole is on the sole of the foot or the back of the trunk where it cannot be seen, the patient may present with lymph gland enlargement or symptoms caused by distant metastases, such as weight loss, dyspnoea or jaundice.

Multiplicity Multiple malignant melanomas are very rare, but there are often multiple secondary nodules around a primary lesion Two concurrent primary lesions are very uncommon.

Examination

Site The majority of malignant melanomas are found on the limbs, head, neck and trunk. They are uncommon on the palms of the hands and the soles of the feet (except in black Africans). They may arise in the subungual tissues, at the mucocutaneous junction and in the mouth and the anal margin.

Shape and size When first noticed, the area of malignant change is usually quite small (0.5–2 cm in diameter), but the mole in which the change has begun may be of any size. When a malignant melanoma is neglected, it becomes a large, florid tumour, protruding from and overlapping the surrounding skin (Fig. 4.85).

Surface When the tumour is small, it is covered by smooth epithelium. When the epithelium dies, from ischaemic necrosis, the resulting ulcer is covered with a crust of blood and serum. Bleeding and subacute infection may make the surface of the tumour wet, soft and boggy.

Fig. 4.85 A large nodular melanoma.

Colour Malignant melanomas may be any colour from a pale pinkish-brown to black. If they have a rich blood supply, they develop a purple hue. Variations in the colour are common, some areas being very black and others pale. Amelanotic melanomas are rare but do occur (Fig. 4.86).

Temperature and tenderness A malignant melanoma is no warmer than the surrounding skin, and is not tender.

Composition The primary tumour has a firm consistency. Small satellite nodules feel hard.

Relations The malignant tissue is within the skin and moves with it.

Lymph drainage The local lymph glands may be enlarged.

Surrounding tissues There may be a halo of brown pigment in the skin around the tumour (see Figs 4.81–4.83), and satellite nodules in the skin and subcutaneous tissue between the primary tumour and the nearest lymph glands (Figs 4.84 and 4.87). It is important to feel all the subcutaneous tissues along the course of the lymphatics that drain the lesion, as nodules of melanoma may be palpable.

Clinical types

Although the above description indicates that a malignant melanoma may have many forms, there are four common clinical types:

- *Superficial spreading melanoma* is the most common variety (see Figs 4.82 and 4.83). It may occur on any part of the body, and is usually palpable but thin, with an irregular edge and a variegated colour.

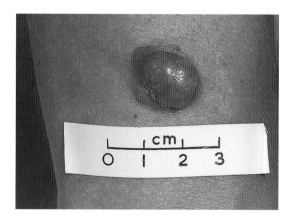

Fig. 4.86 An amelanotic melanoma.

Fig. 4.87 Multiple metastatic nodules of melanoma.

- *Nodular melanoma* is thick and protrudes above the skin (see Fig. 4.85). It has a smooth surface and a regular outline, and may arise *de novo*. It may become ulcerated, and then often bleeds.
- *Lentigo maligna melanoma* is a malignant melanoma arising in a patch of Hutchinson's lentigo (see Fig. 4.80). The malignant areas are thicker than the surrounding pigmented skin and usually darker in colour, but seldom ulcerate.
- *Acral lentiginous melanoma* is a rare type of malignant melanoma, but important to remember because it is often misdiagnosed as a chronic paronychia or a subungual haematoma. It presents as an irregular, expanding area of brown or black pigmentation on the palm or sole, or beneath a nail (see below).
- Amelanotic melanomas occasionally occur (see Fig. 4.86).

General examination Malignant melanoma spreads via the lymphatics to the regional lymph glands. It may then spread in the bloodstream to the lungs, liver and brain. Pleural effusions, hepatomegaly, jaundice and neurological abnormalities are indications of distant metastases. Blood-borne secondary deposits in the skin and subcutaneous tissues are not uncommon.

Mycosis fungoides

This is a rare skin lymphoma that occasionally presents in a surgical clinic. It begins as a patch of thickening and reddening of the skin, which enlarges into a plaque that may ulcerate. The tumours may be multiple. It is often associated with a generalized lymphoma.

Kaposi's sarcoma

Kaposi's sarcoma is a cutaneous sarcoma that, before the appearance of human immunodeficiency virus (HIV) infection, was a rare sporadic condition in Europe, but not uncommon and endemic in sub-Saharan Africa, particularly Zaire and Western Uganda.

The variety not associated with HIV infection runs a slow, indolent course, and is only very rarely associated with spread to the intestine or generalized malignant lymphoma.

The variety associated with HIV infection and acquired immunodeficiency syndrome (AIDS) runs an aggressive course, and is usually associated with systemic tumour infiltration of the lymph glands, intestine, mucous membranes, lungs and other organs.

History

Patients complain of the presence of painless nodules or plaques in and beneath the skin, which often appear first in the legs. There are likely to be a multitude of systemic symptoms if the patient has AIDS.

Examination

The nodules are red, hemispherical and painless (Fig. 4.88). They lie in the subcutaneous tissues, but the overlying skin is often red, adherent to and involved in the disease process. The overlying skin may break down into an ulcer.

OTHER COMMON SKIN CONDITIONS SOMETIMES SEEN IN SURGICAL PATIENTS

Hyperhidrosis

This an excessive quantity of sweat released without an appropriate heat stimulus. It most commonly affects the axilla, hands, feet and groins. It is closely associated with vasospastic disorders and is more common in females.

The skin becomes soggy, white, moist and macerated. Clothes may become saturated with sweat and offensive. It can cause social embarrassment when shaking hands, and interfere with writing.

Generalized hyperhidrosis can be associated with thyrotoxicosis, which must be excluded by careful examination and special tests (see Chapter 12).

Eczema/dermatitis

This is a red, weepy, vesicular rash that usually has an immune cause (Fig. 4.89). There are constitutional 'endogenous' factors in all patients with eczema, but 'exogenous' sensitizing factors are also very important. The condition may be inherited, when it is often associated with hay fever and asthma. It can also be initiated by an allergy, drugs or infection, or physical problems such as an injury, scratching or varicose veins.

Drug eruptions

A whole variety of different types of rash can occur in response to drugs, including maculopapular

Fig. 4.88 Kaposi's sarcoma.

Fig. 4.89 Eczema.

CHAPTER 4 | THE SKIN AND SUBCUTANEOUS TISSUES

rashes, eczema, purpura, urticaria and generalized desquamation. Patients occasionally develop severe malaise, pyrexia and generalized lymphadenopathy. A drug eruption must be considered in any patient who develops a rash (Revision panel 4.9).

> ### Revision panel 4.9
> #### Common causes of drug eruption
> Antibiotics
> Barbiturates
> Non-steroidal anti-inflammatory drugs
> Diuretics
> Chlorpromazine

Urticaria

This used to be called 'hives', and is the development of allergic wheals in the skin in response to a noxious stimulus. The condition is caused by the degranulation of mast cells, which release histamine. In some patients, the cause proves impossible to identify, and these cases are called idiopathic. Nettle stings, jelly-fish stings and insect bites are recognized causes, as are morphine and atropine.

The term **angioneurotic oedema** is used to describe a form of 'urticarial' swelling of the tongue, eyelids, lips and larynx that comes on intermittently and for which there is no known cause. A family history is occasionally present, indicating a genetic factor.

Acne and sycosis barbae

These are conditions in which the ducts of the sebaceous glands become blocked by overactivity. They may then become inflamed and secondarily infected. The condition causes comedos (blackheads) and blind cysts, which may turn into sebaceous cysts. Severe scarring may result. The condition declines after the age of 20 years.

Psoriasis

This condition occurs in 1–2 per cent of the white population, usually beginning between the ages of 5 and 25 years. About one-third of those affected have a family history of the condition, which may have an autoimmune cause.

It presents as sharply demarcated, red, raised, oval plaques mainly situated over the elbows, knees and scalp (Fig. 4.90). The plaques have a silver, scaly surface, and the pattern of distribution varies widely. Psoriasis is often associated with an arthritis of the hands, which has to be distinguished from rheumatoid arthritis. One-quarter of those affected develop pits in the nails, which are often thick, opaque and discoloured, and break easily.

Fig. 4.90 Psoriasis.

Pityriasis rosacea

This is the most common cause of a slightly itchy skin rash in a young person.

It usually starts with a single red, oval, scaly macule, which often develops over the lower abdomen or shoulder. Three or 4 days later, a characteristic rash appears over the trunk, consisting of both macules and papules. The rash does not involve the skin below the upper thighs and arms, and has a 'vest and pants' distribution.

The long axes of the macules are arranged along the line of skin cleavage (Langer's lines). They typically have a fawn centre with a pink surround. Scaling is often present at the junction with normal skin. The rash usually clears completely in 6–12 weeks.

The differential diagnosis includes **drug sensitivity**, **tinea pedis**, **guttate psoriasis** and **secondary syphilis**.

Lichen planus

An itchy rash develops on the wrists and forearms of adults before usually spreading to the trunk and legs. The face and scalp are almost never affected. The characteristic papules are flat-topped, shiny, purple and commonly polygonal in shape. They are often umbilicated and appear in scratch marks (the *Koebner phenomenon*). They may become warty and form larger plaques, which can coalesce.

Delicate, white striae, annular lesions or white dots may be present on the buccal mucosa, tongue or inside of the lips. Painless oral ulceration may also develop. Its course is very variable, but it usually lasts 3–6 months.

THE FINGERNAILS

Inspection of the nails often yields useful information about the patient's general health (see Chapter 1).

The nails are usually pale pink.

The most common cause of nail pallor is anaemia.

Another sign of anaemia in the hands of white-skinned races is a loss of skin crease colour. When the hand is relaxed, the palmar skin creases are slightly darker than the rest of the skin, but if the skin of the palm is stretched, the creases turn a deep red. This deep red colour is not visible if the patient is anaemic.

Splinter haemorrhages

Splinter haemorrhages are small extravasations of blood from the vessels of the nail bed caused by minute arterial emboli. They are long, thin, red–brown streaks, their long axis running towards the end of the finger. Their colour and shape make them look like splinters of wood beneath the nail (see Fig. 1.19).

The presence of splinter haemorrhages is an important physical sign because they are usually caused by emboli from a bacterial endocarditis or a fulminating septicaemia. They may also occur in rheumatoid arthritis, mitral stenosis and severe hypertension.

Revision panel 4.10

Some causes of clubbing

Congenital

Carcinoma of the bronchus

Chronic lung disease:

    Alveolitis

    Bronchiectasis

    Cystic fibrosis

    Congenital cyanotic heart disease

    Ulcerative colitis/Crohn's disease

Clubbing

Clubbing of the nails is a term used to describe the loss of the normal angle between the surface of the nail and the skin covering the nail bed. Some causes of clubbing are listed in Revision panel 4.10.

If you look at your finger from the side, you will see that the plane of the nail and the plane of the skin covering the base of the nail bed form an angle of 130–170° (see Chapter 1). In clubbed nails, there is hypertrophy of the tissue beneath the nail bed, which makes the base of the nail bulge upwards, and distorts nail growth so that the nail becomes curved. The planes of the nail and the skin covering the nail bed then meet at an angle greater than 180°.

It is possible to have a very curved nail but still have a normal nail–nailfold angle, so do not look only at the shape of the nail when assessing clubbing – look at the whole finger. The terminal phalanx may enlarge to make the end of the finger bulbous (Revision panel 4.11).

Revision panel 4.11

The signs of clubbing

Increased nail–nailfold angle

Increased longitudinal and transverse nail curvature

Bulbous terminal phalanges

Spongy nail bed

Spoon-shaped nails

(Koilonychia)

A normal nail is convex transversely and longitudinally, the degree of curvature varying considerably from person to person. Loss of both these curves produces a hollowed-out spoon-shaped nail (koilonychia) (see Fig. 1.17).

When a patient complains that their nails have changed from a normal to a spoon shape, it is very likely that they have developed anaemia following chronic loss of blood, usually from menorrhagia or haemorrhoids.

Subungual haematoma and melanoma

A blow on a nail can cause bleeding beneath it. A collection of blood beneath the nail is called a

subungual haematoma. If it appears at the time of the injury, the patient usually makes their own diagnosis, and only comes for treatment if it is painful.

Sometimes the patient does not notice the injury, and comes complaining of a brown spot beneath the nail. It is then important to decide whether the brown spot is haemosiderin or melanin – a haematoma or a mole. A **haematoma** is usually reddish-brown, with sharp edges. A **melanoma** is brown with a greyish tinge, and has indistinct edges (Fig. 4.91).

The presence of small blood vessels in the lesion, seen using a hand lens, indicates that it is cellular.

The patient may be able to tell you that it has moved down the nail with nail growth, or stayed still. **Haematomas move down the nail; melanomas do not move.**

If it is not possible to make a definite clinical diagnosis, the patient should be managed as if they have a melanoma until you prove otherwise.

Fig. 4.91 A subungual melanoma.

Glomus tumour

This is a very rare tumour, but is mentioned because it can cause a great deal of pain, and often occurs beneath the nail. It is an angioneuromyoma. The patient complains of severe pain every time the nail is touched. Examination usually reveals a small, purple–red spot beneath the nail (Fig. 4.92). The colour is

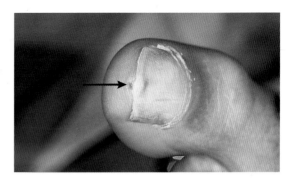

Fig. 4.92 A glomus tumour.

caused by the angiomatous nature of the tumour; the pain comes from its abnormally rich nerve supply.

Glomus tumours can occur in any part of the skin but are most often found in the hands.

Changes in the nails associated with generalized diseases (Revision panel 4.12)

- Psoriasis: pitting, ridges, poor growth.
- Myxoedema: brittle nails
- Cirrhosis of the liver: white nails.
- General debilitating illnesses: transverse furrows (*Beau's lines*)
- Anaemia: koilonychia
- Telangiectasia: Rendu–Osler–Weber syndrome.
- Gout (and pseudogout)

Revision panel 4.12
Common nail abnormalities

Loosening
Psoriasis
Fungal infections
Pitting
Psoriasis
Transverse ridges
Systemic illness
Local damage (paronychia)
Longitudinal ridges
Myxoedema
Thickening and twisting (onychogryphosis)
Trauma
Age
Clubbing (see Revision panel 4.11)

THE TOENAILS

The toenails may show the same changes in response to local or generalized disease that have been described for the fingernails. Paronychia and other forms of infection are far less common, but fungal infection (athlete's foot) between the toes and near the nails is very common (see above).

Onychogryphosis

The normal nail is a thin plate that slides along the nail bed (Fig. 4.93). When the sliding mechanism fails, the nail begins to thicken and heap up until it appears to be growing vertically out of the nail bed. It then curves over the end of the toe and looks like a '**ram's horn**' – an **onychogryphosis** (Figs 4.93, 4.94).

It can occur in young people after an injury to the nail bed, but is most common in elderly people, when the sliding mechanism presumably fails in old age.

Ingrowing toenail

This is a common condition in which the great toenail appears to be growing or digging into the soft tissues at the side of the toe An ingrowing toenail usually has an irregular jagged edge, which digs into the skin of the lateral fold. The damage is exacerbated when the skin at the side of the toe is forced upwards during walking. The precipitating factor is often an attempt by the patient to cut off the corner of the nail, which then gets torn off, leaving a jagged spike at the edge (Fig. 4.95).

History

Age and sex Ingrowing toenails are commonly found in adolescent and young adult males. Games

(a) Mild onychogryphosis.

(b) Severe onychogryphosis.

Fig. 4.94 ONYCHOGRYPHOSIS

Jagged spike on the side of the nail digging into the lateral fold

Fig. 4.95 Ingrowing toenail.

such as football, and less stringent hygiene in young boys and males, may contribute to the sex difference.

Symptoms The principal symptom is pain. The toe is sore and painful when walking. It throbs at night if it gets badly infected. There may be a purulent or serous discharge from beneath the lateral nailfold.

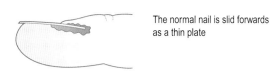

The normal nail is slid forwards as a thin plate

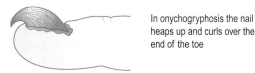

In onychogryphosis the nail heaps up and curls over the end of the toe

Fig. 4.93 Onychogryphosis.

The skin at the lateral nailfold becomes prominent, oedematous and soggy.

Examination

Site The lateral side of the nail (between the great and second toe) is affected more than the medial side, but both sides and both great toes are commonly affected.

Colour The skin of the lateral nailfold is reddish-blue, and red granulation tissue may be visible between the skin fold and the nail (Fig. 4.96).

Tenderness The swollen skin and the nail are tender. When there is extensive infection, the whole toe is tender, and movement of the interphalangeal joint is painful.

Shape The increase in the bulk of the lateral nailfold makes the great toe appear wide, but the nail itself does not look abnormal. It may be possible to see the extent to which the nail is digging into the tissues if the nailfold can be pulled away from the nail without causing too much pain.

Local lymph glands The inguinal lymph glands may be enlarged if there has been long-standing infection, but this is uncommon.

Complications Inadequate excision of the nail bed may result in the regrowth of spikes of nail.

Fig. 4.96 Ingrowing toenail.

5 The symptoms, signs and emergency management of major injuries

This is the only chapter in this book where basic 'management'(first aid and resuscitation) is discussed with the symptoms and signs of major injuries. This is a deliberate decision as resuscitation and assessment are carried out simultaneously in patients with major injuries. This combined approach has saved lives and is now well accepted.

The physical signs produced by injury are usually more evident and immediately significant than a detailed history, especially if the patient is unconscious. Obtaining a history of the type of injury and the possible forces involved, from the patient, family members, friends, onlookers or first-aiders who witnessed the event, is always helpful, but must not interfere with the initial rapid clinical assessment and resuscitation of the patient. Information on the injured person's habits, such as drug or alcohol addictions, may also be very helpful.

The Advanced Trauma Life Support course (ATLS) has established the value of a standardized approach to trauma assessment and management, especially for the lone practitioner faced with one or more patients who have sustained severe injuries. This chapter follows the ATLS approach using an 'ABCDE' mnemonic that is easy to remember in stressful circumstances.

Some injured patients are brought directly to the accident and emergency department by ambulance. Some severely injured patients may be brought in by private vehicles, or even walk into hospital, whereas others may be given treatment at the site of the accident. When an initial assessment has been made at the site of the injury, it must be repeated in the hospital. When ambulance staff are involved, they may radio ahead and warn of their casualty's likely injuries, a measure that allows the 'trauma team'

to be alerted and immediately available. Patients presumed to have sustained major injuries should be taken straight to the resuscitation area for their primary hospital survey.

Patients thought to have minor injuries should still be carefully assessed by an experienced doctor as soon as possible, as apparently stable patients may have sustained serious injuries, which may have passed undetected during the initial assessment, especially when an influx of many injured patients overwhelms local resources.

FIRST AID

First-aiders should ensure that there is no immediate danger to themselves before approaching a casualty. Many injured patients are best served by leaving them where they are until experienced help arrives, provided the environment is not continuing to damage or threaten them. Provided the injured patient has a strong pulse, is breathing normally and is not overtly bleeding, this is invariably the correct course of action. Patients should only be moved if there is a risk of further injury from leaving them where they are, for example if they are inside a burning car.

It is, of course, important to obtain help as soon as possible so that there is always someone available to stay with the patient to monitor their pulse and breathing, and provide moral support.

The widespread availability of mobile phones has improved the first-aider's ability to summon help.

Under no circumstances should an injured patient be given anything to eat or drink.

THE PRIMARY SURVEY AND MANAGEMENT AT THE SITE OF THE EVENT

This is carried out under the five easily remembered headings of 'ABCDE':

- **A**irway.
- **B**reathing.
- **C**irculation.
- **D**isability (neurological evaluation).
- **E**xposure/environmental control.

This approach is particularly important when assessing patients with multiple injuries.

Airway

The signs of an obstructed airway are **stridor (**noisy breathing**), increased respiratory effort**, **cyanosis** (a blue colour) and **apnoea** (not breathing).

It is essential to protect and secure an adequate airway. The lungs cannot oxygenate the blood if the airway is obstructed by the jaw and tongue falling back, swollen soft tissues, direct damage to the upper airway, false teeth, vomitus or blood.

The airway of unconscious patients lying on their back often becomes obstructed by their own intraoral soft tissues, but before they are rolled into the supine or semi-prone position, or the neck is extended, always consider, and if possible exclude, an **associated cervical spinal injury** (see Chapter 9).

All patients found to be unconscious after an injury must be treated as if they have an associated injury of their cervical spine, because abrupt or careless turning may further dislocate or sublux a cervical vertebra and injure the spinal cord when no injury originally existed. It is also possible to turn partial cord damage into a complete transection. The neck should therefore be immobilized in all unconscious injured patients by in-line longitudinal, manual support and stabilization, ideally using a hard cervical collar (Fig. 5.1), sand bags and tape until clinical examination and radiographs have excluded unstable fractures of the cervical spine.

Compromises are inevitable if an immobilizing collar is not available at the site of injury. The presence of two first-aiders may allow one to support the neck while the other assesses and manually clears the airway, feels the neck and jaws, and assesses the respiratory effort by palpating the chest during respiration.

Conscious patients with threatened airway obstruction will usually find a secure position

themselves, often sitting up and leaning forwards if there is significant facial trauma (see Chapter 11).

Airway obstruction in an unconscious patient can usually be relieved by lifting the jaw forwards, but it may require the insertion of a finger into the mouth to extract debris. Rarely, airway obstruction is associated with a fractured maxilla or mandible, and the jaw or palate may need to be pulled forwards, or the patient rolled into a semi-prone position.

When there is a low suspicion of a cervical spine fracture, the patient may be rolled into the semi-prone ('recovery') position to help maintain the airway, because the absence of a gag reflex in an unconscious patient makes aspiration of saliva, vomitus or blood into the lungs a major hazard. Alternatively, an oropharyngeal or nasopharyngeal airway (Fig. 5.2) should be inserted as soon as possible, and then, in an unconscious patient, replaced by an endotracheal tube inserted by an experience anaesthetist. The airway must be repeatedly reassessed to ensure that the measures you have taken are effective and secure.

Fig. 5.1 A hard collar.

Fig. 5.2 A nasopharyngeal airway.

Breathing

Mouth-to-mouth resuscitation should be started immediately if the patient remains cyanosed or apnoeic after the airway has been cleared. This is easier and safer (in terms of the risk of cross-infection) if a Brook's airway, a face mask, an Ambu bag and oxygen are available. Mouth-to-mouth ventilation combined with external cardiac massage may, however, be life saving in patients who have undergone a short period of respiratory arrest.

There are few indications for heroic attempts at inserting home-made 'tracheostomy' devices at the scene of the accident, and patients are probably better served by a rapid transfer to hospital by experienced ambulance staff who have been trained in resuscitation techniques.

Fig. 5.3 Tourniquet used by the armed forces to stop limb bleeding.

Circulation

Bleeding remains the most common preventable cause of death after trauma. It is absurd to concentrate on the detailed drills of assessment of the airway and breathing if the patient obviously has a normal airway but is losing vast amounts of blood – even to the point of literally bleeding to death.

Severe external bleeding at the scene of the accident requires manual compression directly over the wound or pressure proximal to the point of bleeding, where the feeding artery can be compressed against an underlying bony point. Direct pressure is usually the most effective technique for controlling blood loss. Remember that if the pressure applied to the outside of the injured blood vessels is greater than the blood pressure, the bleeding will stop.

Tourniquets should only be used to stop limb bleeding. Improvised tourniquets may exacerbate bleeding by obstructing the venous outflow, while failing to occlude the arterial inflow. Ambulance crews are now often trained and equipped with specially designed tourniquets that have also proved to be effective in military use (Fig. 5.3).

An effective tourniquet renders the whole limb ischaemic and will cause permanent muscle and nerve damage if it is kept in place for several hours. Tourniquets can also cause reperfusion problems when released, resulting in metabolic acidosis, myoglobulinuria and hypercalcaemia. Nevertheless, a tourniquet can sometimes be life saving if it is applied at the correct pressure to a mangled bleeding limb for a short period. The time of application must be carefully recorded and passed on to ambulance and medical staff.

Direct manual pressure, provided it is achieving its desired effect (i.e. stopping or reducing the blood loss), is usually preferable to a tourniquet. This can be very tiring because it may need to be maintained until the patient reaches the hospital's accident and emergency department.

Disability

(Neurological evaluation)
A brief note should be made of the patient's level of consciousness using the AVPU scale. Is the patient:

- **A**lert?
- Responding to **V**oice?
- Responding to **P**ain?
- **U**nresponsive?

The change in the level of consciousness over time is a very useful indicator of progress or evolving complications.

Exposure and environmental considerations

An unconscious or immobile patient can rapidly become hypothermic, which exacerbates coagulopathy and acidosis. It is important to keep the patient warm. In other situations, other environmental hazards need to be considered.

THE PRIMARY SURVEY IN THE ACCIDENT AND EMERGENCY DEPARTMENT

All patients who are unconscious or suspected of having multiple or serious injuries should be admitted directly to the resuscitation area of the accident and emergency department. While medical students are rarely required to have an active role in the management of acute trauma, the opportunity to witness assessment and resuscitation in this setting is extremely valuable, as the principles of the process are relevant to many other areas of medical practice.

The clinical assessment (history and examination) and resuscitation must occur simultaneously if lives are to be saved, hence the inclusion of treatment in this chapter.

The routine 'ABCDE' assessment must be repeated whatever happened before the hospital admission.

Airway

The neck must be protected by a collar and immobilized if the patient is unconscious, or if there is any suspicion of a cervical spine injury. An anaesthetist should assess the need for better control of the airway.

Look for the signs of inadequate oxygenation (see Chapter 2):

- Noisy breathing (stridor).
- Respiratory distress.
- Apnoea.
- Cyanosis.
- Loss of consciousness.
- The presence of major facial, neck or chest injuries that might obstruct the airway.

These may all indicate the need for endotracheal intubation.

Look for the signs of inadequate ventilation.

The chest should be uncovered, examined and palpated to assess the respiratory movements. The presence of air entry into the lungs should be confirmed with a stethoscope (see Chapter 2).

The neck and jaw should be palpated to check for deformity. Insert a finger into the mouth to extract any foreign bodies, and to check for jaw fractures (see Chapter 11). Occasionally, severe damage to the upper airways or trachea makes intubation impossible. An emergency cricothyroidotomy or tracheostomy is indicated if the patient's airway is compromised and an endotracheal tube cannot be safely inserted.

Breathing

Assess the condition and function of the thoracic cage (see Chapter 2).

Once you are certain that the airway is patent, assess the adequacy of ventilation by inspecting, palpating, percussing and listening to the chest for symmetry, movement, dullness and breath sounds.

Patients with multiple injuries or chest problems causing hypoxia should be given high-flow oxygen through a closed-circuit oxygen mask from the moment of their arrival in the accident and emergency department.

An oxygen saturation monitor is a valuable means of assessing the effectiveness of the patient's ventilation.

Inspection and palpation

Examination of the chest must include inspection of the back and sides of the chest wall up into the axillae.

Open chest wounds should be dressed with airtight dressings to prevent the development of a tension pneumothorax through a 'sucking' chest wound.

Flail segments occur where when several ribs are fractured in two places and the segments sink inwards during inspiration (Fig. 5.4). This indicates a high

Fig. 5.4 A flail segment.

likelihood of a severe underlying lung injury, and the patient is likely to need endotracheal intubation and ventilatory support.

Bruising over the chest indicates that rib fractures are likely, and the presence of **surgical emphysema** suggests that the pleura has been breached. Surgical emphysema presents as a 'crackling sensation' on palpation of the subcutaneous tissues.

Percussion

Characteristically, **a pneumothorax** is resonant to percussion, and a **haemothorax** is dull to percussion. These signs are, however, easy to miss in a noisy emergency room, and indeed may coexist in a mixed haemo-pneumothorax.

A chest radiograph is usually needed to confirm a diagnosis, except in the case of a tension pneumothorax, when clinical suspicion should prompt urgent treatment.

Uncomplicated pneumothoraces confirmed on chest radiographs do not necessarily require urgent chest drainage.

A **tension pneumothorax**, in which there is raised intrapleural pressure, must be suspected:

- if breathing is difficult;
- if the trachea is deviated to the contralateral side;
- if there is decreased air entry over the affected lung.

Urgent decompression is indicated if the patient is unstable, ideally with a chest drain.

Bilateral tension pneumothoraces are very rare, but cause severe cardiac and respiratory compromise, which manifests as cyanosis, severe air hunger, a weak pulse and hypotension. The trachea may, however, remain central.

The rapid insertion of a chest drain that is connected to underwater seal drainage bottles will relieve a tension pneumothorax (see *Investigation and Management*, Chapter 6). Needle thoracocentesis, in which a needle is inserted into the pleural cavity through the second intercostal space in the mid-clavicular line, may provide temporary relief while a chest drain is being prepared.

A large haemothorax may also cause respiratory and circulatory problems, which manifest as reduced breath sounds and a dull percussion note combined with reduced vocal fremitus and vocal resonance.

The diagnosis should be confirmed with an erect or decubitus chest radiograph, but a chest drain may occasionally have to be inserted as an emergency measure on the basis of the clinical signs.

A large amount of blood draining from a chest may destabilize the patient and demand urgent replacement into the circulation (see below), so intravenous lines should be inserted into both antecubital fossae before a haemothorax is drained. The chest drain may occasionally need to be clamped to prevent massive continuing blood loss. Lost blood should be replaced with a crystalloid solution at first, but subsequently with blood as soon as this is available (see below). Massive or ongoing bleeding from a haemothorax is an indication for surgery.

The blood pressure must be carefully and continuously monitored to confirm the adequacy of any blood volume replacement.

Circulation

In a clinical setting, assessment and restoration of the circulation can often be performed simultaneously with management of the airway and breathing if an experienced anaesthetist is available to manage ventilation.

There are two major causes of circulatory embarrassment:

- Haemorrhage.
- Cardiac damage/tamponade (see Chapter 2).

The former is the most common cause of potentially preventable death. The latter is rarer, but also life threatening and easily missed.

Tamponade must therefore be briefly considered in all patients with major injuries, especially in those with penetrating injuries of the chest (see below).

Revealed haemorrhage

Visible **arterial bleeding** presents as a pulsating stream of bright red blood coming from an open wound, whereas venous bleeding is dark and continuous. Arterial haemorrhage from an open wound can usually be controlled by direct digital pressure or proximal arterial compression, either manually or by using a medically approved tourniquet or pneumatic cuff.

Sterile vascular clamps can be applied directly to obvious bleeding arteries for temporary control before definitive surgery if these simple measures fail. Deep wounds in junctional areas (the groins, shoulder and neck regions) should not be explored in the emergency department.

Venous bleeding always responds to simple pressure and may be made worse by the application of an inadequate tourniquet.

Revealed bleeding should always be assessed and controlled as soon as possible. There is no point in pouring fluid and blood into the circulation through intravenous catheters when an equal amount is rapidly escaping.

Concealed (internal) haemorrhage

This is much harder to diagnose, and therefore must be suspected in all patients with multiple or serious injuries. It always accompanies major fractures of long bones and fractures of the pelvis. It must, if possible, be rapidly diagnosed and treated, as it is an important, potentially reversible, cause of death in an injured patient.

Clinical signs of haemorrhage

The diagnosis of haemorrhage is based on finding the signs of hypovolaemic shock, which are:

- a pale, anxious, sweaty patient with cold extremities;
- a rapid, thready pulse;
- tachypnoea;
- hypotension.

These signs occur when the body redistributes the circulation in an attempt to maintain the blood flow to the vital organs (heart and brain). Other organs, such as the skin, intestine and kidneys, become inadequately perfused and poorly oxygenated.

This homeostatic response is brought about by the sympathetic nervous system causing a tachycardia and vasoconstriction in the extremities. The skin becomes cool and clammy. The systolic blood pressure is usually maintained at first, but the pulse pressure (the pressure difference between the systolic and diastolic pressures) may be reduced by a rise in the diastolic pressure. The rate of respiration increases to try to improve oxygenation.

Patients who arrive in the accident and emergency department without overt haemorrhage but who exhibit these signs have almost certainly lost 1–2 L of blood. It is important to remember that young, fit patients can often tolerate a considerable blood loss before they develop, often very suddenly, any signs of hypovolaemic shock, whereas elderly patients, especially those on beta-blockers or digitalis, tolerate quite small amounts of blood loss do not.

All seriously injured patients must be continuously monitored for:

- Pulse rate.
- Blood pressure.
- Respiratory rate.
- Level of consciousness.
- Tissue oxygenation.

Patients with an associated head injury must be monitored using the **Glasgow Coma Scale** (see Chapter 3, page 97).

A urinary catheter and the measurement of central venous pressure provide additional valuable information for monitoring resuscitation when there are signs of hypovolaemia.

An intra-arterial pressure line is also very useful for continuously monitoring the blood pressure, and allows easy sampling of arterial blood for blood gas and acid–base measurement.

Intravenous access should be secured using two wide-bore cannulae inserted into the veins of the cubital fossae or, if ultrasound guidance and appropriate expertise are available, using a central venous catheter.

Blood must be sent for urgent grouping and cross-match.

Clinically stable patients may benefit from a crystalloid (normal saline) infusion, but unstable patients with ongoing bleeding are best resuscitated with red cell concentrate and plasma if this is available. Group O rhesus-negative blood and thawed fresh frozen plasma can be given if there is insufficient time for a cross-match.

Patients who fail to respond to the rapid restoration of their blood volume in the absence of cardiac or major respiratory problems, such as tamponade or tension pneumothorax, probably have severe continuing blood loss. In these circumstances, a blood transfusion should be started while a rapid assessment of the potential sites of concealed blood loss is made.

The most common sites of continuing concealed haemorrhage are the pleural or abdominal cavities. Fractures of the pelvis can also cause catastrophic blood loss.

The retroperitoneum can also accomodate litres of blood with few external physical signs.

A rapid clinical examination looking for chest dullness, abdominal distension and abdominal tenderness (if the patient is conscious) should be followed by chest radiography, the insertion of chest drains if indicated, focused ultrasound scans or computed tomography (CT) scanning of the torso where indicated (see *Investigation and Management*, Chapter 6).

The patient should be transferred to an operating theatre once the site of blood loss has been established.

Cardiac tamponade

This occurs when large quantities of blood collect within the pericardial sac around the heart, and embarrass its action (see Chapter 2). The cardiac output is reduced as a consequence, producing a weak pulse and hypotension.

The condition should be suspected:

- if the jugular venous pressure is markedly elevated and rises rather than falls with inspiration (**Kussmaul's sign**); remember, however, that jugular venous distension may not occur in a patient who has lost a large quantity of blood;
- if **pulsus paradoxus** is present, when the pulse volume decreases on inspiration rather than increasing (Fig. 5.5);
- if the **heart sounds are muffled and poorly heard**.

All of these clinical signs can easily be missed, and the most important thing is to consider the diagnosis

Chest radiographs may show an enlarged cardiac shadow (see *Investigation and Management*, Chapter 6)

An echocardiogram will confirm the diagnosis (see *Investigation and Management*, Chapter 6).

It may be possible to stabilize briefly the patient's condition by aspirating the blood from the pericardial sac under echocardiography, but definitive surgery is needed through either a left lateral thoracotomy or a sternotomy.

Echocardiographs and electrocardiographs (ECGs) can be helpful if cardiac injury or coincidental cardiac disease is suspected. The ECG leads should be kept connected to a monitor to detect any dysrhythmias. A cardiac contusional injury should be suspected if there is widespread ST segment elevation or depression.

Very occasionally, a **'clam-shell' thoracotomy** in the emergency department may be required to relieve a tamponade, to suture a penetrating wound of the heart or to clamp the hilum of the lung or the descending aorta to prevent massive blood loss. These heroic attempts are seldom successful (see *Investigation and Management*, Chapter 6, page 135). **Rapid transfer to an operating theatre with trained staff, proper instruments and adequate lighting increases the chances of success.**

THE SECONDARY SURVEY

Many injured patients do not deteriorate catastrophically. This provides time to carry out a full secondary survey to assess other systems and body parts that may have been injured and to assess the general fitness of the patient. **It is important to continue monitoring the patient while the secondary survey is being carried out to detect any further or new bleeding or chest problems.**

The whole patient must be examined from the top of the head to the toes. Other blood tests, investigations and diagnostic procedures should be undertaken as necessary after the secondary survey has been completed. Adequate analgesia may be needed before beginning the secondary survey, especially in fully conscious patients in whom the primary survey and resuscitation have been quickly completed.

History

A detailed history should be taken from a stable, conscious patient at this stage. It is helpful to ask the patient what they remember of the accident, and useful if they can describe what happened. The mechanism of the injury and the possible physical forces involved often give a useful indication of the site and severity of the damage.

It is often helpful to know about:

- the height of a fall;
- the speed of a car;
- the use of guns or knives;
- the presence of an explosion or fire;
- the use of protection devices such as seat belts or airbags.

Weaker during inspiration

Fig. 5.5 Pulsus paradoxus.

Obtain the observations and views of family, friends, bystanders or paramedics if the patient is unconscious.

Pain, dysfunction and malfunction

The conscious patient should be asked if they have any localized areas of pain or malfunction, which may indicate particular areas or systems that require more detailed examination.

Conscious patients must also be asked if they experienced any loss of consciousness during or after the injurious event. Their cognitive function should be quickly tested by asking a few questions about who they are, where they live and their occupation. The history from a third party of a lucid interval is also helpful if the patient is unconscious.

General and previous history

Take a full history of previous illnesses, operations, drugs and allergies (see Chapter 1). The patient's general fitness, occupation and tobacco and alcohol usage should be recorded following a full systematic enquiry.

Record the time that the patient last ate or drank. This is very important if the patient is to have a general anaesthetic.

GENERAL EXAMINATION OF A CONSCIOUS PATIENT

The head

Scalp This must be inspected and palpated for lacerations, swellings, bony depression and distortion.

Orbits Palpate the margins of the orbits for depressions or irregularities.

Eyes Examine the eyes for pupil size, reaction and the red reflex. Test the eye movements and visual acuity (see Chapter 1).

Occasionally, a corneal injury may lead to loss of the anterior chamber and prolapse of the iris, with an obvious collection of blood behind the cornea.

The presence of a **large subconjunctival haemorrhage** (Fig. 5.6) that spreads to the full extent of the conjunctival attachment suggests that there is a fracture of the base of the skull.

Panda eyes (black circumorbital haematomas around one or both eyes) (Fig. 5.7) also suggest the presence of a skull base fracture or a fracture of the upper jaw.

(a) A subconjunctival haemorrhage may arise from a subconjunctival vessel or be blood that has tracked forwards from behind the eye – usually from a fracture of the base of the skull. When this patient looked to the left, white sclera could be seen to the right of the haemorrhage, confirming that the bleeding was solely from the subconjunctival blood vessels.

(b) Extensive bleeding from a fracture of the base of the skull may cause a large periorbital haematoma as well as a subconjunctival haemorrhage.

Fig. 5.6 SUBCONJUNCTIVAL HAEMORRHAGE

Fig. 5.7 Panda eyes. Extensive periorbital extravasation of blood from a fracture of the base of the skull.

Diplopia, especially on looking up, is indicative of a blow-out fracture of the floor of the orbit, which often allows the eyeball to sink inwards, giving the upper face an asymmetrical appearance.

Signs of intracranial haemorrhage (see Chapter 3)

A **fixed dilated pupil** that fails to respond to light indicates IIIrd cranial nerve compression, by a contralateral extradural haemorrhage or a direct injury to the optic nerve.

Deterioration of the patient's score on the Glasgow Coma Scale – which quantifies eye opening, verbal response and motor response – and/or agitation indicate increasing cerebral compression. The patient is in 'coma' if their Glasgow Coma Score is less than 8.

Loss of upwards gaze, other cranial nerve pareses and the development of contralateral hemiplegia are indicative of a cerebral haemorrhage.

Observations should also be made on the patient's mental state, including whether they are agitated or confused.

A rising blood pressure, a falling pulse and slowing of respiration suggest **coning**, a condition in which the swollen brain is forced down into the medullary foramen, with subsequent loss of all vital functions. An urgent CT scan should be obtained.

The face (see Chapter 11)

Major facial injuries often cause considerable **orbital oedema**, but it is very important to retract the lids carefully, using two people if necessary, to look for any of the features described above.

The cheek bones should also be palpated for a 'step', and any **asymmetry** should be noted.

Fractures of the zygoma and blow-out fractures of the orbit have to be confirmed by radiographs, but **loss of sensation over the cheek** from damage to the infraorbital nerve strongly suggests a fracture of the cheek bones.

Instability of the maxillary zygomatic process (a Le Fort-type fracture) is tested by inserting a gloved finger or thumb into the mouth and attempting to pull the upper jaw complex forwards from the base of the skull (Fig. 5.8). A fracture is present if rocking occurs. This needs to be done

with care, as forceful rocking may cause a massive pharyngeal bleed, which can only be controlled by pushing the whole bony facial complex backwards to compress the bleeding vessels.

(a)

(b)

Fig. 5.8 LE FORT FRACTURE
(a, b) The maxilla being pulled forwards for the diagnosis of a Le Fort fracture.

CHAPTER 5 | THE SYMPTOMS, SIGNS AND EMERGENCY MANAGEMENT OF MAJOR INJURIES

The lower jaw and its stability on the temporomandibular joints must also be assessed. **Malocclusion** and **an open-bite deformity** suggest a fractured jaw, as does numbness of the lower lip.

Carefully palpate and inspect the mouth, teeth and gums, and record the number of missing or damaged teeth. **Missing teeth** indicate the need for a chest X-ray, if this has not already been performed, to exclude the possibility that they have been inhaled and are lodged in the lung.

The nose and ears

The nose should be palpated to exclude a fracture and detect the presence of any bloody or clear fluid discharge of cerebrospinal fluid, which would suggest the presence of a **fracture in the anterior cranial fossa** (often associated with panda eyes and an extensive subconjunctival haemorrhage).

The facial muscles (VIIth cranial nerve) and auditory acuity should be tested.

Blood or fluid coming from the ear suggests the presence of a posterior fossa fracture.

The tympanic membrane must be examined with an auroscope. Bruising behind the ear **(Battle's sign)** (Fig. 5.9) suggests a fracture in the posterior cranial fossa.

Fig. 5.9 Battle's sign. Bruising behind the ear suggests a fracture in the posterior cranial fossa.

Skull radiographs, specific facial views and CT scans are usually required to assess these injuries (see *Investigation and Management*, Chapter 6).

The neck (see Chapter 9)

Pain and local tenderness are suggestive of a cervical fracture, but there may be few, if any, physical signs, and further assessment may have to be delayed until the condition of the cervical spine has been established. The importance of not causing or exacerbating any spinal cord damage, especially during airway assessment, endotracheal incubation or moving the patient, is now well recognized.

If there are any concerns that the spine may have been damaged, a full radiological assessment of the cervical spine should be carried out as soon as the patient is relatively stable. A CT scan may be necessary if plain radiographic views are inadequate (see *Investigation and Management*, Chapter 6).

The neck can be carefully palpated for bruising and deformity and inspected for any penetrating wounds if the spine is normal. The position of the trachea in relation to the manubriosternal notch should be assessed to see whether it is central. Gentle palpation should detect the presence of any subcutaneous surgical emphysema in the neck or supraclavicular fossae.

Penetrating descending wounds of the root of the neck can be very dangerous, as they may cause damage to the supra-aortic blood vessels – the carotid, vertebral and subclavian arteries – as well as to the trachea, larynx, pharynx and oesophagus (Fig. 5.10). Major structures within the upper chest can also be damaged. The presence of neurological signs or ischaemia of the upper limb suggests a

Fig. 5.10 An entry wound in the neck.

major arterial injury, as does a rapidly expanding haematoma or a machinery murmur. Neck wounds should be explored in the operating theatre.

The clavicle should be palpated along its course. Severe compound clavicular injuries are often associated with injuries to the subclavian or axillary vessels, the brachial plexus and the apex of the lung. Examine the vascular supply and peripheral nerves of both upper limbs to exclude these possibilities.

The chest (see Chapter 2)

Although the chest was quickly assessed as part of the primary survey, it should now be carefully re-examined by inspection, palpation, percussion and auscultation to detect any minor signs that may have been missed at the time of the initial examination, when speedy resuscitation was essential. New signs may have developed, and subtle signs may have been missed. **Remember to check the back and sides of the chest**, including into the axillae.

Test again for rib fractures. A careful inspection may detect a small flail segment. The chest should be 'sprung' by compressing it with both hands, anteroposteriorly and from side to side, and then quickly releasing it. Pain on compression or release indicates the likelihood of rib fractures or costal cartilage separation from the ribs or sternum. Both can then be more accurately localized by detailed palpation. It should be remembered that rib fractures are often associated with injuries of the great vessels, lungs, spleen or liver.

The sternum must also be inspected and palpated. Sternal fractures are often associated with cardiac injuries.

Check again for the presence of a haemothorax, pneumothorax and cardiac tamponade, taking particular care to look for small pneumothoraces and an increase in the width of the mediastinum, which may be the only indication of an aortic dissection.

A chest radiograph should always be obtained if there is any question of a chest injury. CT chest scans are even more accurate in detecting minor abnormalities and rib fractures.

The abdomen (see Chapter 15)

The primary survey of the abdomen usually detects the signs of major intra-abdominal haemorrhage, but a secondary survey is essential to pick up continuing severe haemorrhage or further bleeding following the restoration of a normal blood pressure.

Increasing abdominal distension, **tenderness** and **guarding** are all significant signs, especially when associated with a rising pulse and other signs of hypovolaemia.

The bowel sounds may or may not be abolished by free blood or bowel contents in the peritoneal cavity.

Skin bruising over the abdomen (Fig. 5.11), penetrating wounds and associated rib fractures all indicate the possibility of abdominal organ damage.

When doubt persists, ultrasonography, CT scanning or peritoneal lavage may be indicated. A CT scan is very useful if there is an associated pelvic fracture.

Blood coming from the external urethral meatus or frank haematuria suggests kidney, bladder or urethral damage (see Chapters 17 and 18). Rectal and vaginal examination can confirm a high-riding and boggy prostate, or associated vaginal injuries. The presence of these injuries must always be excluded before allowing catheterization by inexperienced junior staff or nurses. It may be preferable to insert a supra-pubic catheter if palpation or percussion detects a large bladder, especially if the prostate feels abnormal or blood has been seen coming from the urethra.

Fig. 5.11 Abdominal trauma. This shows the impression and bruising made by a seat-belt, which is often associated with underlying abdominal trauma.

CHAPTER 5 | THE SYMPTOMS, SIGNS AND EMERGENCY MANAGEMENT OF MAJOR INJURIES

Pelvic fractures (see Chapter 9) are commonly associated with severe shock and with tenderness on springing the pelvis by pressing back on both iliac crests and releasing them.

The upper and lower limbs (see Chapters 7 and 8)

All surfaces of the limbs must be fully inspected, taking careful note of the presence of:

- Bruising.
- Lacerations.
- Instability.
- Deformity.

All the major bones should be carefully palpated along their full length to detect any bony deformity and swelling that were not appreciated by the inspection. The only indication of an undiagnosed, undisplaced fracture may be the detection of a localized point of tenderness. Major fractures are almost always associated with some deformity, together with swelling from the associated bleeding. **The radial and pedal pulses** should be felt and compared (see Chapter 10). The presence of equal symmetrical pulses indicates that a major vascular injury in the limbs is unlikely (see Chapter 7). Unfortunately, the peripheral pulses are often difficult to feel in a shocked, cold patient with severe limb bruising and concomitant fractures. When the pulses cannot be felt in an adequately resuscitated patient, it is helpful to measure the arterial pressure with a Doppler flow detector (see Chapter 7).

Persisting pallor, especially if it only affects one limb, is a sign of severe ischaemia.

The presence of a **compartment syndrome** must always be considered when there are combined bony and vascular injuries. This condition may also follow the successful surgical revascularization of an injured limb. Compartment syndromes begin with pain, tenderness and swelling over the anterior shin or calf muscles. The swelling can exacerbate the ischaemia, obliterate the pulses and lead to muscle and nerve death if left untreated.

The peripheral nerves (see Chapter 3)

These must be fully examined in both the upper and lower limbs if the patient is conscious. Test the power, tone, coordination, sensation and reflexes. Test the movement of joints controlled by the major muscle groups. Test sensation by the response to light touch and pinprick. Always test and document an examination of the peripheral nerves beyond any laceration. A more detailed neurological examination should be carried out if abnormal neurological signs are detected, or if the patient is unconscious (see below).

The back (see Chapter 9)

(Thoraco-lumbar spine)

The discovery of the paralysis or weakness of several muscles may be the first indication of a spinal cord injury. The patient must then be carefully immobilized and 'log-rolled' by a team of staff to allow examination of the spine. Log-rolling allows the patient to be turned in a coordinated manner that keeps the spine immobilized at all times (Fig. 5.12).

Palpation down the back over the spinous processes may detect a boggy swelling, a deformity or a 'step' in the regularity of the spinous processes. While the patient is on their side, take the opportunity to inspect and palpate the back of the head, neck, torso and limbs to exclude any major injuries to this surface of the body that may have passed unnoticed at the initial survey.

A rectal examination should be performed at this stage, and perianal sensation, motor function, sphincter tone and the bulbo-cavernosus reflex tested.

Fig. 5.12 The log-rolling technique.

Detailed radiographs and even CT scans are required if a spinal fracture or spinal cord injury is suspected (see *Investigation and Management*, Chapter 6).

THE SECONDARY SURVEY IN THE UNCONSCIOUS PATIENT

The secondary survey in an unconscious patient should begin with a reappraisal of the Glasgow Coma Scale score to discover whether the level of consciousness has changed from the initial assessment (see Chapter 3). This is important, as the whole purpose of resuscitation and assessment is to rectify factors such as hypotension or hypoxia that could cause neurological deterioration, while trying to detect the presence of an intracranial haemorrhage, which can usually be treated effectively.

Any suggestion of a '**lucid interval**' – a period of consciousness after the injury before the patient became unconscious – is an important sign of a developing intracranial haematoma.

Monitoring of the Glasgow Coma Scale score must be carried out at frequent intervals in comatose patients with a score of 8 or less. Patients must be frequently asked to open their eyes and move their limbs. Apply a painful stimulus by pressing hard on the bone of the upper orbit or the manubrium sterni if they do not respond. An ability to localize pain is accepted if the patient moves one or other hand to try to push away the painful stimulus, whereas flexion or, worse still, extension of the upper limbs indicates a severe brain injury.

Verbal responses are impossible to assess in patients who are anaesthetized or intubated, or have suffered severe facial injuries. It must also be remembered that some head-injured patients may have intellectual difficulties, some may have taken an overdose of drugs or alcohol, and some be unable to understand your language.

A detailed neurological examination should be carried out to discover if there are any focal neurological signs indicative of brain injury or an expanding intracranial haematoma. This should start with the examination of the size, symmetry and reaction to light of the pupils.

If the brain is shifted to one side by an expanding haematoma, the ipsilateral IIIrd cranial nerve becomes compressed against the rigid free edge of the tentorium cerebelli. At first, this causes slight constriction of the pupil, but then, later, dilatation and eventually a failure to respond to a bright light being shone directly into it.

The haematoma will continue to expand and force the brain down through the tentorium and into the foramen magnum if left untreated (see Chapter 3). The contralateral pupil then becomes dilated and unreactive. Compression of the medulla eventually causes bradycardia, a rising blood pressure and depressed respiration.

Do not forget that optic nerve injuries, previous eye disorders and drugs can also cause the pupil to be unresponsive.

Neurological examination of the limb should concentrate on detecting any evidence of hemiplegia. Unilateral paralysis, increased muscle tone, brisk reflexes and upgoing plantar reflexes on the contralateral side of the injury all indicate that a haematoma is present.

Intracranial haematomas outside the substance of the brain develop in two sites:

- Extradurally.
- Intradurally.

An **extradural haematoma** is usually the result of haemorrhage from the middle meningeal artery. This is often caused by a linear temporoparietal fracture of the skull. Patients are often briefly knocked unconscious or dazed by the initial injury, but then regain consciousness (the lucid interval) before becoming drowsy and eventually losing consciousness. As the intracranial pressure rises, patients may complain of a headache, blurred vision and vomiting. At this time, the localizing signs described above begin to develop.

It must be remembered that some patients develop an extradural haematoma without a lucid interval, and without the classic progression of neurological signs.

The certain indicator of deterioration is **a progressive reduction in their Glasgow Coma Scale score.**

A CT scan will confirm the diagnosis (see *Investigation and Management*, Chapter 6).

A **subdural haematoma** can be classified as either acute or chronic.

Acute subdural haematomas are invariably associated with a major brain injury when torn vessels on the surface of the brain continue to bleed into the subdural space. Patients are usually deeply unconscious and develop neurological localizing signs.

It is very difficult to differentiate an acute subdural haematoma from:

- An intracerebral haemorrhage.
- Cerebral oedema.
- Diffuse axonal injury.

A CT scan of the head is essential.

Chronic subdural haematomas usually occur in elderly patients after a minor injury that tears a vein on the surface of the brain, which bleeds slowly but persistently for days or weeks. They are also common in alcoholics and patients on anticoagulants. Patients often present with fluctuating levels of consciousness, worsening over several days or weeks. The raised intracranial pressure may cause headache, vomiting, blurred vision (papilloedema) (see Fig. 3.4), personality change and drowsiness. Pupillary changes and some neurological localizing signs are usually present.

The diagnosis is confirmed by a CT scan of the brain.

ASSESSMENT OF MULTIPLE CASUALTIES

All hospitals should have a major accident plan in which the roles of accident and emergency doctors, other medical staff, nurses, theatre staff, telephone staff, managers and press liaison officers are all clearly defined. These plans should be tested from time to time to assess their effectiveness and encourage familiarity.

Each patient must be carefully assessed by the techniques described above into:

- those who are dead;
- those with immediate life-threatening injuries;
- those with major injuries;
- the 'walking wounded'.

SCORING SYSTEMS

A number of scoring systems have been developed to try to improve the management and outcome of patients who have been injured. These allow the results of individual centres to be compared against one other. The **Revised Trauma Score** is probably the best measure. This allows an audit of outcome against expected recovery or likely death. Any variation from the expected outcome should be critically examined to discover whether earlier diagnosis or more efficient resuscitation or treatment would have achieved a better result.

6 Bones, joints, muscles and tendons

It is essential to learn how to examine the bones and joints properly, which must include an assessment of function, as well as the detection of any structural abnormalities that may be present. This is important because many patients who present to surgical or medical clinics have associated abnormalities of the musculoskeletal system, in addition to the increasing numbers presenting with such symptoms to an orthopaedic clinic.

COMMON SYMPTOMS

Pain

This is the most common symptom, and the additional questions related to it that should be asked (onset, character, duration, etc.) have already been discussed in detail in Chapter 1.

It is important to obtain the precise location of 'musculoskeletal pain', which is usually related to movement, whereas its severity and character are less helpful in coming to a correct diagnosis. Do not forget that pain **referral** is common; for example, hip pain may be experienced in the knee, and knee pain may be referred to the hip via the obturator nerve. Bone pain and joint pain are often 'diffuse' and poorly localized.

Musculoskeletal pain is usually improved by rest and aggravated by movement. The presence of 'night pain' is a strong indicator that treatment is required to improve the patient's quality of life.

Injury

Any history of problems, especially pain or loss of function after injury, suggests the possibility of bone fractures or joint dislocations. Soft tissue injuries such as muscle tears or tears of the joint capsules are also the result of trauma, and must also be considered. A pathological fracture should be excluded when the injury leading to a fracture appears trivial.

Deformity

This may be either congenital or acquired, and the latter may occur following a fracture such as the 'dinner fork' abnormality seen in a Colles-type wrist fracture.

Common congenital abnormalities include club feet (talipes), knock knees (genu valgus) and bow legs (genu varus).

Contractures of soft tissues and neuropathic damage can lead to deformity, as can large tumours arising from bone, cartilage and soft tissue. Some deformities can disappear with time, while others may progress, with serious consequences.

Stiffness

This may be 'generalized' or 'localized to a single joint or limb'. Early morning generalized stiffness in all joints, especially the hands, is a characteristic of rheumatoid arthritis, while short-lived stiffness of a specific joint, such as the hip, following inactivity, is indicative of osteoarthritis.

'Joint locking'

This occurs when there is a sudden inability to 'move' a single joint such as the knee, which may cause the patient to fall. This is usually followed by 'unlocking' when the structure responsible for the block shifts position.

Swelling

This may arise in a bone, soft tissues or a joint. The swelling may be the result of a congenital deformity, inflammation, fluid or blood accumulation, infection or neoplasm.

Inflammatory or infective swellings are usually painful and associated with pyrexia and malaise, while 'tumours' are commonly painless and progressive. Haematomas are usually sudden in onset, normally follow an injury and then improve, while joint effusions are mostly the result of arthritis and may fluctuate in volume.

Instability

This occurs when a limb 'gives way'. This can be repetitive as a result of ligamentous laxity (patellar dislocation in young females) or following a trauma (recurrent dislocation of the shoulder).

Weakness

This is usually the result of disorders of muscles or nerves, although joint disease can also result in muscle weakness. An assessment of which individual muscle groups are weak, combined with a full neurological examination (see Chapter 3), may indicate where the problem lies.

Loss of function

This is a combination of 'symptoms' and their 'effect on the patient'. Examples include an inability to work, run or bend over, which may be the result of disease in the hip, knee or back. The importance of functional loss varies with the occupation and hobbies of each individual.

Alteration in sensation

Numbness or tingling (paraesthesia) is often the result of nerve damage (e.g. a prolapsed intervertebral disc), ischaemia (e.g. Volkmann's contracture) or compression (e.g. carpal tunnel syndrome), although primary neuronal disease must always be considered and excluded. The presence of an upper or lower motor neuron lesion must be established by appropriate examination of limb tone and reflexes (see Chapter 3).

A GENERAL PLAN FOR EXAMINING THE MUSCLES, BONES AND JOINTS OF A LIMB

This can be broken down into five components:

- inspection;
- palpation;
- movement;
- percussion and/or auscultation when indicated;
- special tests.

Although moving the limb is normally part of inspection and palpation, it is such an important part of the examination that it should be regarded as a separate entity.

Note **Percussion, auscultation and special tests are not relevant to all joints or bones.**

Examination may be simplified into the four-letter words beloved of the late Alan Apley:

- **Look.**
- **Feel.**
- **Move.**

To these is added **X-ray**, which is discussed at length in *Investigation and Management*, Chapter 1.

Remember that the upper and lower limbs should be viewed from both the front and the back, which may require the patient to be both standing and supine. The normal limb should always be examined first.

Always ask the patient to perform active movements before performing passive movements, and then remember to check for any 'abnormal movements'.

Remember that the following is a general plan; the examination of individual joints, bones, tendons and muscles is considered in later chapters.

Inspection

Skin The skin should be assessed for discolouration, **erythema** and **oedema**. The presence of **bruising** may indicate recent trauma.

Look for **traumatic or surgical scars and sinuses** (Fig. 6.1) (see also Chapter 4). Observe **any abnormal or asymmetrical skin creases.**

(a, b) Sinuses and scars.

Fig. 6.1

Shape Observe the shape of the limb and consider whether there is a **true deformity** or a postural alteration in its appearance. Try to ascertain if the deformity is confined to a single joint (Fig. 6.2) or if it is more generalized (Fig. 6.3).

Fig. 6.2 Grossly deformed knees that are the results of neuropathic joints.

Fig. 6.3 Marked deformity of the lower limbs associated with rickets.

Consider whether there is any **swelling** present, and whether this is diffuse or localized. Finally, look for **muscular wasting** (Fig. 6.4).

Length Make a visual comparison of the length of each part of the limb with the other side.

Fig. 6.4 Charcot knee in valgus secondary to syphilis with associated quadriceps wasting.

Palpation

Skin Assess the temperature of the skin.

Palpate for oedema, and try to decide whether it is local or dependent.

There may be tenderness of the limb, which again may be diffuse or localized.

Shape Try to define the cause of any swelling; for example, a swelling confined to a joint may be:

- An **effusion**.
- **Haemarthrosis**.
- **Pyoarthrosis**.
- **Thickening of the synovium**.

Localized masses may be arising from the muscle or bone.

Note the relation of any swelling to the underlying or neighbouring anatomical structures, and elicit all its physical characteristics, as described in Chapter 1.

Record on a diagram any abnormality and degree of deformity of alignment.

Length Measure **the real and apparent length of each limb** and of each bone (see below).

Movement

Active Ask the patient to move each joint through its full range of movements and show you any tricks or abnormal movements. Watch the limb function on standing, walking, lifting, etc.
Passive Move all the joints of the limb through their full range.

A complete loss of all movement of a joint implies either **surgical arthrodesis** (fixation) or **fibrous or bony ankylosis** (consolidation or union), as it may be the result of a pathological process, such as infection (see below).

Note **any restriction to movement or fixed deformity**, which may result from contraction of the joint capsule, muscles or tendons. Locking or limitation may also occur as a result of the interposition of soft tissues, bone or loose bodies.

Record as accurately as possible the range of movements in degrees (e.g. 0–90° of flexion).

Test the strength of each movement against resistance (see page 91). Feel and listen for any **clicks or crepitations** (crackling sensations) in the joint on movement.

Abnormal movements Test for these by testing the integrity of the ligaments of each joint.

Other tests

It is essential to examine the structures that keep the limb alive and make it work – the arteries and nerves.

Arteries Palpate all the pulses (see Chapter 10).
Nerves Peripheral nerves may have **s**ensory, **m**otor, **a**utonomic, **r**eflex and **t**rophic (**SMART**) activity. The objective of the assessment is to identify the nerve root innervation of any pathology (see Chapter 3):

- *Sensory.* Check the appreciation of light touch, pinprick, temperature change, deep pain, vibration sense and position sense.
- *Motor.* During your examination of movement and strength, you will already have obtained some information on the ability of the muscles to contract. If weakness is present, determine which muscles are affected.

- *Reflexes*. Test all the limb's reflexes for reduced or increased activity (see Chapter 3).
- *Trophic/autonomic*. The skin may have an abnormal appearance, and may feel hot or cold and sweat excessively.

EXAMINATION OF THE MUSCLES

When a muscle appears to contain a definite lump, begin by examining the lump to ascertain its physical characteristics, as described in Chapter 1. It is better to examine the muscle first and the lump second if there is doubt about the relationship of a lump to the whole muscle.

Inspection

Observe the shape of the muscle at rest. Note any:

- **Wasting.**
- **Hypertrophy.**
- **Irregularity of shape** caused by a lump, or displacement of the muscle.

Always compare the abnormal muscle with the normal muscle of the other limb.

Observe the shape of the muscle when it contracts. Alterations in shape that appear when the muscle is contracting are caused by a lump either being concealed, or made more obvious by the muscle fibres either closing together or separating.

Look at the neighbouring bones and joints.

Palpation

Place the limb in a comfortable position so that the muscle is relaxed before feeling the muscle at rest.

Try to decide whether any abnormality is caused by:

- a **localized swelling**;
- an **abnormal muscle**.

Elicit all the features of any lump (see Chapter 1).

Feel the muscle when it is contracted, and record any changes in the position of the mass.

A lump inside or beneath the muscle becomes more difficult to feel when the muscle contracts (Fig. 6.5). A lump superficial to the muscle, or breaking through its fibrous sheath, becomes more prominent.

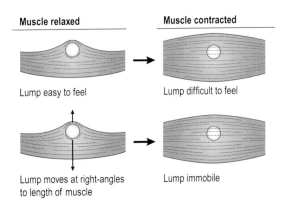

Muscle relaxed	Muscle contracted
Lump easy to feel	Lump difficult to feel
Lump moves at right-angles to length of muscle	Lump immobile

Fig. 6.5 Principal features of an intramuscular lump.

A gap or hollow that appears in the muscle when it contracts usually means that the fibres have ruptured (see below).

Strength

Muscle power can be classified according to the Medical Research Council scale. It is often better not to use numbers but to describe the strength:

- M0: No active contraction is visible.
- M1: Muscle contraction is visible but there is no movement of the joint.
- M2: Active movement is possible if gravity is eliminated.
- M3: Active movement can overcome gravity but not resistance applied by the examiner.
- M4: Active movement can overcome gravity and some resistance applied by the examiner.
- M5: There is full power against resistance.

Remember that muscle strength can be impaired by pain, wasting, denervation or other disease processes.

Innervation and blood supply

You will know if a muscle is innervated after testing its motor function, but you must also examine the integrity of the whole nerve and the spinal segment supplying the muscle by testing all of its other motor, sensory and reflex functions (see Chapter 3). This means that you must know which nerves and which spinal segments innervate the main muscle blocks in the body

The pulses in the limb must all be palpated (see Chapter 10).

CHAPTER 6 | BONES, JOINTS, MUSCLES AND TENDONS

EXAMINATION OF THE BONES

The basic plan follows the same format, namely:

- Look.
- Feel.
- Move.

Inspection

An **old tethered scar or a discharging sinus** in the overlying skin is indicative of old or active osteomyelitis (see Fig. 6.1).

Redness and oedema of the skin is suggestive of underlying infection, inflammation or a malignant growth.

When there is a **visible bony deformity**, its site and the overall alignment of the limb should be recorded (see Figs 6.2 and 6.3).

Palpation

Feel the whole length of the bone to assess its shape, and compare it with the normal side.

If there is **a localized swelling**, all its physical signs must be elicited (see Chapter 1).

The temperature of the overlying skin should be assessed, as conditions that increase the bone's blood flow, such as infection, tumours and Paget's disease, may raise the temperature of the surrounding tissues.

Measurement

There are three measurements that can be made of a limb and its constituent bones:

- The true length of individual bones.
- The apparent length of the whole limb.
- The true length of the whole limb.

The methods and principles of measurement are best described with respect to the lower limb; however, they apply equally to the upper limb, although these are less frequently utilized.

Bone length

Measurement of a single bone is straightforward as the measurement does not cross a joint.

Choose recognizable anatomical points at either end of the bone and measure between them.

Do the same on the other side and compare your findings.

Bony points have to be felt through the overlying skin and muscle, and it is difficult to get the end of the tape measure on identical points on both sides. The easiest method is to hold the tape measure between your thumb and index finger, and then press the back of the index finger firmly up against the bony point or edge that you are using as a landmark.

Apparent length of the limb

When a patient lies flat and 'straight' on a couch, the limbs may appear to be of different length (Fig. 6.6). This may be caused by a bone or joint abnormality. It is customary to record the apparent length, because when it is compared with the true length, it gives some indication of the degree to which the skeleton has adapted its position to keep both legs parallel and both feet flat on the ground when the patient stands up, or alternatively an indication of the effect of a joint deformity on the length of the limb.

Fig. 6.6 The apparent length of the limbs is measured from a central point with the patient lying comfortably straight. It is not possible with this measurement to tell whether any difference in limb length is caused by a bone or a joint abnormality.

Ask the patient to lie straight on the bed. Choose a point in the midline of the trunk – the umbilicus or xiphisternum – and measure from this central point to the tips of both medial malleoli (Fig. 6.7). These lengths will be the apparent lengths of the limbs.

Fig. 6.8 Measuring *real* limb length using the anterior superior iliac spine as the measuring point.

Fig. 6.7 Measuring *apparent* limb length using the umbilicus as the measuring point.

Real or true length of the limb

To find out the real length of the limb (i.e. the combined true length of the limb bones and joints, unaffected by the position of the spine, pelvis or hip joints), measure between fixed bony points at each end of the limb with the joints in identical positions. In the leg, the most commonly used points are the anterior superior iliac spine and the tip of the medial malleolus (Fig. 6.8).

The position of the joints profoundly affects this measurement. Figure 6.9a shows the measurements between the iliac spines and the medial malleoli in a patient, lying straight in bed, with disease of the left hip that has caused some fixed flexion and abduction. In order to lie straight in the bed, the patient has tilted their pelvis and adducted the other hip. There will be different measurements between the iliac spine and malleolus in this position, because one hip is abducted and the other adducted.

Before measuring the real limb length, the joints of both limbs must be placed in identical positions (Fig. 6.9b and 6.9c). The pelvis must first be set square to the sagittal plane, by checking that both iliac spines are in the same plane, at a right angle to the line of the spine. This may result in the hip and femur on the diseased side being

No
You cannot detect the real length of the limbs like this because the joints are in different positions

Yes
To measure the true length of the limbs you must put the joints in identical positions. This patient has a fixed abduction of the left hip so the right hip was abducted to the same degree before measuring

To detect the site of the bone shortening you must measure the length of each bone

Fig. 6.9 MEASURING LIMB LENGTH

abducted or adducted. The normal leg must be placed in the same position. Next check that the positions of the knee joints are identical – if one has some fixed flexion, flex the good side to the same degree (Fig. 6.10).

Fig. 6.10 A quick method of detecting difference in bone length is to put the patient's heels together, with the knees flexed, and look from the side and the end of the bed. This patient has shortening of the right tibia and femur.

Once the positions of the legs are identical, measurements on both sides, from anterior superior iliac spine to medial malleolus, can be made to establish a true comparison of the real leg lengths.

Joint deformities

Record the deformity of a joint in terms of the angle by which the distal bone is deviated from the sagittal plane (i.e. the angle of **varus or valgus** – see below). Bones may also be rotated on their long axis. Assess the angle of rotation from the displacement of the bony protuberances from their normal position.

Movement

Examine the joints at both ends of the bone. Also make certain that each bone moves as one piece. A fracture will clearly be painful, and it is seldom necessary to confirm the discontinuity. Sometimes a false joint (**pseudarthrosis**) may develop in the shaft of a long bone as the result of non-union of a fracture, and may produce pain-free abnormal movement.

EXAMINATION OF THE JOINTS

The two most common joint abnormalities that you will find are swelling and deformity.

Swelling of a joint must be caused by one or more of:

- bony enlargement;
- synovial thickening;
- an effusion.

Deformity of a joint is invariably caused by one or more of:

- skin contractures (e.g. a scar following burns);
- fascial contracture (e.g. Dupuytren's contracture);
- muscle spasm or weakness;
- tendon division or fixation;
- capsular fibrosis;
- bone deformity.

The basic plan of joint examination follows the same format as for the bones and muscles.

Inspection

Observe the colour of the overlying skin, and whether there are any **associated sinuses or scars** (see Fig. 6.1).

Consider the shape of the joint and any obvious deformity (see Fig. 6.2).

Malalignment of a joint in the coronal plane, the plane of abduction and adduction, is known as **a valgus or a varus deformity**:

- There is a **valgus** deformity if the limb below the joint is angled away from the midline (abducted) (Fig. 6.11).
- There is a **varus** deformity if the limb below the joint is angled towards the midline (adducted) (Fig. 6.11).

Assess whether there is any **general or localized swelling**, and whether there is any **muscular wasting** (see Fig. 6.4).

Also review the other joints in the limb and note the position in which the patient holds the joint.

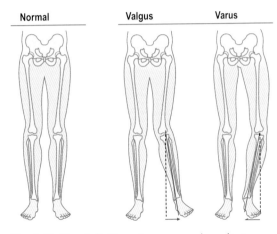

Fig. 6.11 The definition of a varus and a valgus deformity. In a valgus deformity, the distal bone forming the joint is abnormally abducted. In a varus deformity, it is abnormally adducted. Remember, knock knees = genu valgum.

Palpation

Feel the **temperature and texture** of the skin over the joint. The subcutaneous tissues may be normal or thickened.

Muscles Feel the local muscles for wasting and tone. The muscles may be in spasm if joint movement is painful.

Synovium The synovial membrane or capsule may be **thickened and palpable**. This is unusual, although there may be an **effusion** as a consequence of excess synovial fluid.

Bones Define the contours of the bones that form the joint. Check that they are in their correct anatomical positions.

Movement

Active movement Ask the patient to move the joint through its full range of movements. Record the degree of any limitation of movement and any associated discomfort.

Strength of movements Make the patient move the joint against resistance so that you can assess the strength of the muscles producing each movement. Record the power of such movements (see page 91).

CHAPTER 6 | BONES, JOINTS, MUSCLES AND TENDONS

Passive movements Move the joint through its full range of movement with the patient's muscles relaxed. Note any **crepitus** (grating sensations) felt during this passive movement, as well as any pain or discomfort.

Ligaments Check the integrity of each ligament associated with the joint by stretching it. This will also reveal any abnormal movements.

GENERAL EXAMINATION OF THE LIMB

Examine the arteries, nerves, lymph glands and other joints of the limb.

Examination of specific joints will be presented in the relevant chapters.

COMMON CONDITIONS AFFECTING MUSCLES

Ruptured muscle fibres and intramuscular haematomas

Muscle fibres usually rupture during an excessively strong or unusually sudden contraction. Rupture can also occur following a normal contraction if the muscle is weakened by a pathological process. The rupture may occur in the muscle belly or at the musculotendinous junction. As part of the healing process, an intramuscular haematoma forms within the muscle belly.

History

Age Muscle rupture can occur at all ages, but is most common in young males during exercise, and elderly males performing excessive or unaccustomed physical activity.

Symptoms There is usually pain, swelling and bruising at the time of the rupture.

Site Muscles commonly affected include the **quadriceps, hamstrings and gastrocnemius of the lower limb** and the **biceps of the upper limb**.

Examination

The diagnostic feature of a muscle tear is a **depression when the muscle contracts**, which is usually associated with a lump on either side from the torn ends of the muscle (Fig. 6.12). The lumps

Relaxed

May be a small depression

Contracted

A lump appears on one or both sides of a sharp depression

Fig. 6.12 The clinical features of ruptured muscle fibres.

cannot be felt when the muscle is relaxed because they have the same consistency as the adjacent muscle, but the hollow between the broken fibres may be visible and palpable.

As the muscle fibres try to heal, a haematoma will form, which is tender for a few days, before it is ultimately resorbed.

The local arteries, nerves, bones and joints are normal, as are the neighbouring bones and joints.

The strength of the muscle is reduced if a significant number of fibres are ruptured. The muscle action will be lost if all its fibres are ruptured, unless other muscles contribute to its function.

Muscle hernia

This occurs when a muscle bulges through its surrounding fibrous sheath. The hernia may be visible at rest, but when the muscle contracts, it is likely to become more apparent.

History

Symptoms The patient may notice the lump when looking at or feeling the muscle, or experience a slight ache in the muscle and find a lump when trying to pinpoint the source of the discomfort.

Examination

Site Although all muscles are surrounded by a fibrous sheath, only those with a thick covering are likely to cause symptomatic muscle hernias. A common muscle hernia is through the thick fascia that covers the anterior compartment of the lower leg.

Shape and size Muscle hernias can be of any size. Their characteristic feature is that they change in size according to the tension in the muscle. When the muscle contracts, it bulges through the fascial defect. When the muscle is relaxed, there is no lump – just a hole.

These signs are occasionally reversed. The muscle may bulge through the defect when relaxed, but be pulled back into its compartment when it retracts. Do not be confused by this variation. Provided the lump comes and goes as the muscle tension changes and there is a palpable defect in its covering fascia, it is a muscle hernia.

Intramuscular and intermuscular lipoma

Although there is little fat inside a muscle itself, there are often small collections of fat around the nutrient blood vessels and in the loose areolar tissue that separates groups of muscles. Lipomas can develop in this fat. Histologically, they are no different from any other lipomas, but the site gives them some distinctive physical signs.

History

Symptoms An intramuscular or intermuscular lipoma may interfere with the function of the muscle and causes pain when the muscle is being used, but it rarely makes the muscle weak.

The patient may have felt, or seen, a lump appear during exercise. The patient sometimes experiences a sharp pain and notices the sudden appearance of the lump if an intramuscular lipoma suddenly bursts out of a muscle during exercise. They often believe that the exercise caused the lump. The lump may change in size and shape as the muscle contracts.

Muscle lipomas are rarely multiple.

Examination

Site Any muscle can be affected. There is more fat between the flat muscles of the trunk than between the muscles of the limbs; hence lipomas are more common in this region.

Shape and size If there is only a thin layer of muscle or fascia covering the lipoma, its typical multilobular shape may be palpable (see Chapter 4).

These lipomas are often quite large (5–10 cm in diameter) because they grow unnoticed within or between the muscles for many years. They may become larger or smaller, or disappear, when the muscle contracts, according to their relation to the main bulk of the muscle.

Edge Their edge is difficult to feel. When a lipoma has herniated through the thick layer of fibrous tissue surrounding the muscle, you may feel a sharp edge, corresponding to the defect in the fascia, but there is usually a lot more of the lipoma deep to this edge that you cannot feel.

Composition The consistency varies with the tension in the muscle. When the muscle is relaxed, the lipoma has its typical soft consistency and may seem to fluctuate. When the muscle contracts, the lipoma becomes hard and tense if it is still palpable.

Relations Intermuscular and intramuscular lipomas are tethered to their site of origin and usually become fixed when the muscle contracts. An intermuscular lipoma may become impalpable when the muscle overlying it contracts.

Myositis ossificans

Myositis ossificans is calcification, or ossification, in part of a muscle. It is an uncommon condition that may follow an injury that has caused extensive intramuscular haemorrhage, sometimes associated with a fracture of the adjacent bone. Commonly affected muscles are the brachialis, after an elbow fracture, and the quadriceps femoris, after a fracture of the femur or a direct blow to the muscle. The patient often has an associated head injury.

History

Previous injury The patient will describe a recent fracture or previous injury.

Symptoms Stiffness is the principal symptom because the muscle cannot relax and contract normally, and the bone that forms may actually block movement. Ultimately, any joint that is involved may become fixed. While forced movements may be painful, the condition is usually painless once the original injury has resolved.

Examination

Site, size and shape The common sites for myositis ossificans are the lower part of the brachialis muscle and the lower part of the quadriceps femoris muscle. Its size and shape are very variable. The ossification tends to take the shape of the muscle in which it is occurring. It has an irregular outline.

Tenderness The mass of ossified muscle is not normally tender, but forced passive movements may cause pain.

Temperature The mass has a normal temperature.

Composition The mass is bony hard.

Relations The ossification in the muscle may be continuous with callus around an associated fracture, and hence it may be mistaken for a bony swelling.

The muscles over the callus of a healing fracture usually function normally, whereas ossifying muscles cannot work properly and cannot be moved over the callus.

Local tissues There may be other evidence of the previous trauma – bone and joint deformities, or nerve and artery damage – so it is important to examine the whole limb very carefully.

The diagnosis is confirmed by a plain X-ray (see *Investigation and Management*, Chapter 7).

Myosarcoma

Primary tumours of muscle are rare. There are two types:

- *Leiomyosarcomas* arise from smooth muscle.
- *Rhabdomyosarcomas* arise from striated muscle.

Almost all soft tissue sarcomas developing in the limbs will actually be **fibrosarcomas**, which arise from the intermuscular and intramuscular fibrous septae or the fibrous tissue at the origin or insertion of the muscles.

True rhabdomyosarcomas are rare, and clinically cannot often be differentiated from fibrosarcomas (Fig. 6.13).

The diagnostic features of a tumour arising in or from a muscle are that:

- it moves freely when the muscle is relaxed, especially in a direction at right angles to the length of the muscle;
- it becomes immobile when the muscle contracts, and its physical features may change.

Fig. 6.13 A large rhabdomyosarcoma of the thigh arising in the quadriceps muscles.

FIBROUS TISSUE

Fibrous tissue is tough, durable and stable. It covers muscles and links them to bone as tendons, fibrous insertions or aponeuroses. It generally causes little trouble during life, but is sometimes the site of malignant change.

Three tumours can arise from this tissue:

- *Benign fibroma* is very rare.
- *Fibrosarcoma* is a common mesodermal soft tissue malignant tumour.
- *Paget's recurrent desmoid tumour* is less common than fibrosarcoma, locally invasive and often recurrent.

Fibrosarcoma

This is a malignant tumour of fibrous tissue. It is locally invasive, and also spreads via the bloodstream to the lungs and liver. Spread to the lymph glands is uncommon. Distant spread is a late event, and the primary tumour often grows locally for years before metastasizing.

History

Age These tumours are more common in elderly patients, but they can occur at any age.

Duration The patient has often known of the existence of a lump for months – sometimes years – before they present to the doctor.

Symptoms The reasons for complaint include:

- growth of the lump, causing disfigurement or interference with muscle movements;
- pain in the lump itself or from invasion of nearby structures;
- muscle weakness caused by infiltration of nearby muscles;
- general debility, from multiple metastases.

Examination

Site Fibrosarcomas can occur anywhere in the body, but more commonly arise in the limbs.

Colour When a large vascular tumour lies just beneath the skin, it may make the skin shiny and pink. An advanced tumour can ulcerate through the skin.

Temperature Even slow-growing fibrosarcomas have an abnormal blood supply, and usually feel warmer than the surrounding tissue.

Shape Their shape depends upon their site of origin. They are roughly spherical if they grow in the middle of a soft tissue. When they arise close to a bone, they tend to be hemispherical, with their deep surface fixed to the bone (Fig. 6.14).

Surface The surface is usually smooth but may be bosselated (see Chapter 1).

Edge The edge of slow-growing tumours is well defined. Fast-growing and invasive tumours have an indistinct edge.

Composition Their consistency is firm or hard. They are rarely stony hard, because they do not ossify and their marked vascularity tends to keep them soft. They may be so vascular that they can pulsate and have an audible bruit and a palpable thrill.

Relations The relations of the tumour to the surrounding tissues depend entirely on its site of origin, size and invasiveness. Fibrosarcomas are usually firmly fixed to nearby structures and often invade neighbouring bones, nerves and arteries.

Fig. 6.14 A slow-growing fibrosarcoma of the arm. The overlying skin is stretched, and many distended subcutaneous veins are visible. There was no ischaemia or paralysis in the arm or forearm.

Lymph drainage On rare occasions, the local lymph glands may be enlarged by secondary deposits.

State of local tissues **Take particular care to test the integrity of any nerves running close to the mass of the tumour.** A nerve deficit is more likely to indicate infiltration than stretching of the nerve, and is almost diagnostic of a locally malignant lesion.

Paget's recurrent desmoid tumour

This is a rare condition that has the same features as a fibrosarcoma, but is less vascular and **very slow growing**. It occurs most often in middle-aged females, usually in the fascia covering the abdominal muscles, i.e. the rectus sheath and the external oblique aponeurosis (Fig. 6.15). These tumours can, however, arise in other sites, such as the plantar fascia of the foot or the palmar fascia of the hand. The malignant change affects a wide area. As a result, even after an extensive and apparently adequate excision of the presenting lump, **recurrences** may appear years later in fascia that was apparently healthy at the time of operation.

CHAPTER 6 | BONES, JOINTS, MUSCLES AND TENDONS

Fig. 6.15 A large Paget's recurrent desmoid tumour arising from the anterior sheath of the rectus abdominis muscle.

TENDONS AND TENDON SHEATHS

Ruptured tendons

When the tendon of a muscle is divided the muscle becomes ineffective. To assess the integrity of a tendon, you must know its site of insertion and the movement that contraction of its parent muscle would normally produce.

Tendons can be ruptured by direct violence, especially if they have been weakened by rubbing over a bone, which causes attritional wear. In most cases, however, tendon ruptures occur at a site that has been weakened by natural age-related changes (tendinopathy). The tendon of the biceps brachii, the Achilles tendon and various tendons in the hands are most frequently involved. These will be considered in subsequent chapters.

CONDITIONS OF BONES

FRACTURES

Definitions and subtypes

A fracture is a structural discontinuity of a bone and may be:

- complete or incomplete;
- open or closed;
- single or multiple;
- transverse, spiral, oblique or comminuted;
- pathological or stress;
- fracture–dislocation.

Bone is relatively brittle, but easily withstands the stresses of normal life. **The majority of fractures are caused by sudden and excessive direct or indirect force.**

An **incomplete fracture** is a crack or splintering of one side of a bone without displacement of the fragments, when it is classified as **complete** and the bone is broken in two (Fig. 6.16).

A **'greenstick' fracture** is a type of incomplete fracture that is common in childhood, in which the bone buckles like a bent green twig, but the periosteum and bone ends remain in continuity (Fig. 6.16).

Providing the overlying skin remains intact, the fracture is classified as **closed**, but any 'skin breach' or 'opening of a body cavity' makes the fracture **'open'**, which indicates that it is liable to infection because of potential contamination.

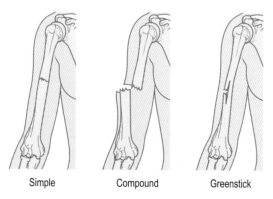

Simple   Compound   Greenstick

Fig. 6.16 A complete and an incomplete fracture, including a greenstick fracture.

Many fractures are confined to a **single bone**, but patients involved in high-speed accidents, falls from a height or battlefield injuries are liable to sustain **multiple fractures** (see Chapter 5). The latter are often associated with considerable blood loss and hypovolaemic shock, especially if the pelvis is fractured.

Direct force usually causes the bone to break at the point of impact in a transverse direction (a **transverse fracture**), although **comminution** can occur if the force is considerable. **Comminuted fractures** are defined by the presence of one or more fragments, and are usually the result of direct excessive force from, for example, missiles.

Indirect force, which is caused for example by 'twisting or excessive angulation', results in the bone breaking some distance from the point at which the force was applied. These fractures are often **oblique or spiral**.

Avulsion fractures, in which a fragment of bone is pulled off the main bone by the excessive action of a muscle, tendon or ligament, are also caused by indirect force.

Pathological fractures occur through diseased areas of bone, and are often spontaneous or caused by trivial force.

Osteoporosis (see page 201), **Paget's disease** (see page 199), **infections** (see page 202) and **bone tumours** (see page 206) are all well-recognized causes of pathological fractures.

Stress fractures occur in bones that are subjected to repetitive trauma (like a plane's fuselage) and low levels of stress. These fractures often develop in dancers, athletes and young soldiers sent on forced marches, and commonly occur in the **vertebral bodies**, **metatarsals**, **tibia** and **fibula**.

Fractures can involve a joint that can quite commonly become complexly or partially displaced. This is called **subluxation** (partial) or **dislocation** (complete) (Fig. 6.17). The injury can result in a combination of bone and joint injury when a '**fracture–dislocation**' occurs (Fig. 6.17). This can damage the articular cartilage, the metaphysis or the epiphysis, which will result in disordered bone growth.

Always remember that, despite the fact that the fracture appears to be the major injury, the soft tissues in the region are also severely damaged, and the nerves and blood vessels must always be carefully assessed.

Fracture displacement

The fragments of a complete fracture are displaced by the external force, by gravity and by the pull of the muscles attached to either side of the fracture line. The following need to be considered:

- *Shift.* The fragments can be shifted sideways, backward or forwards, but will usually unite.
- *Angulation.* The fragments are tilted from one another, causing malalignment.
- *Rotation.* One fragment is twisted over the other, causing a torsional deformity of the limb.
- *Length.* The fragments may overlap or be separated. This can result in shortening of the limb.

Symptoms

It is important to obtain a careful history of the injury, including the mechanisms and likely forces involved. It should, however, always be remembered that fractures can occur some distance from the point of impact.

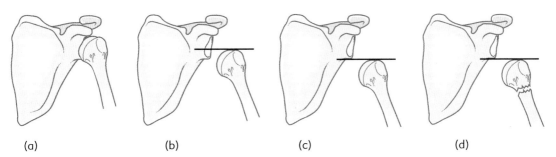

(a)   (b)   (c)   (d)

Fig. 6.17 SHOULDER GLENOHUMERAL JOINT (USED AS EXAMPLE)

The figure shows: (a) Normal joint; (b) Subluxation; (c) Dislocation; (d) Fracture–dislocation.

CHAPTER 6 | BONES, JOINTS, MUSCLES AND TENDONS

Pain, bruising and swelling are the common symptoms, but do not differentiate 'a fracture' from 'a soft tissue injury'.

The presence of a fracture is suggested by a history of **continuing pain especially on movement** or **'an inability' to use the injured limb**. The presence of a **deformity** is highly suggestive of a fracture, but in impacted fractures and greenstick fractures this will not occur and pain is often minimal.

Symptoms of associated injuries such as numbness, abdominal or chest pain, and loss of consciousness must always be enquired about (see Chapter 5), and a full history of past illnesses, family history, drugs and allergies must also be obtained (see Chapter 1).

The clinical signs of a fracture

The injured tissues must be carefully handled, and the general effects of trauma must be treated (see Chapter 5).

Inspection

Look for the following signs. **Swelling, bruising and deformity (Fig. 6.18) may be obvious and should be recorded.** Measure and record any:

- angulation;
- rotation;
- displacement;
- shortening.

This can sometimes be assessed clinically, but X-rays usually provide this valuable information (see *Investigation and Management*, Chapter 7).

Soft tissue swelling and injury must be assessed. This should be graded by the **Tscherne classification:**

Fig. 6.18 The classic dinner fork deformity.

- Grade 0: negligible soft tissue injury.
- Grade I: superficial abrasion or contusion of the soft tissues overlying the fracture.
- Grade II: significant contusion of the muscle with contaminated skin abrasions or both. The bone injury is usually severe.
- Grade III: significant injury to the soft tissues with significant degloving, crushing, compartment syndrome or vascular injury.

The presence of a compound wound should always be specifically looked for. This should be assessed and recorded using the **Gustilo classification.** There is a tendency for the Gustilo classification category to 'increase' with time as the patient moves through the management pathway:

- Type I: open fractures with a small, less than 1 cm clean wound with minimal injury to the musculature and no significant stripping of the periosteum from the bone. The bone injury is simple with minimal comminution.
- Type II: open fractures with 1–10 cm wounds but no significant soft tissue damage or avulsion. The fracture contains moderate comminution.
- Type III: open fractures with larger wounds and associated extensive injury to the muscle, periosteum and bone that is often associated with significant contamination of the wound. The fracture may be segmental. Such injuries can be subdivided into:
  - IIIa: extensive contamination or injury to the underlying soft tissues, but adequate viable soft tissue is present to cover the bone and neurovascular structures without muscle transfer.
  - IIIb: extensive injury to the soft tissues requiring a rotational or free muscle transfer to achieve coverage of the bone and neurovascular structures. These usually have massive contamination.
  - IIIc: open fractures with associated vascular injuries that require arterial repair.

Palpation

The site of the fracture is almost always **tender**.

Crepitus may be demonstrated if the patient is unconscious. This is a 'grating' sensation from the two sides of the fracture rubbing together. This can cause considerable pain in a conscious patient and should not be specifically elicited!

Movement

Movement is often very painful and is seldom required to prove a fracture. Remember that encouragement of abnormal movement may cause further soft tissue damage and further periosteal stripping.

Obtain an X-ray if a fracture is suspected.

X-rays

When ordering an X-ray, obtain the appropriate views, and follow the '**rule of twos**':

- *Two views*: usually an anterior–posterior view and a lateral view.
- *Two joints*: include the joint above and the joint below the bone under consideration.
- *Two sides*: which is useful for comparison, particularly in children, because it allows a comparison of the epiphyseal lines in immature bones and distinguishes them from the fracture line.
- *Two injuries*: one at a higher or lower level, for example the calcaneum with the pelvis or spine.
- *Two occasions*: another X-ray if the symptoms persist, for example a scaphoid fracture.

All X-rays should be centred on the area of maximal tenderness.

General examination

The **peripheral pulses** must be felt and recorded, and the skin circulation assessed (see Chapter 10).

The peripheral nerves must also be examined and defects recorded. Associated visceral injuries and any distal injuries must be excluded (see Chapter 3).

Remember that:

- **heart and lung injuries** are associated with **fractures of the ribs and sternum** (see Chapter 2);
- **the spinal cord** may be injured in patients with **spinal fractures** (see Chapter 9);
- **pelvic fractures** are associated with **abdominal visceral and urinary tract injuries** (see Chapters 9, 15 and 17);
- **pectoral girdle injuries** are often associated with **brachial plexus and subclavian vascular injuries** (see Chapters 3 and 10).

Revision panel 6.1
Complications of fractures

General
Blood loss
Deep vein thrombosis
Pulmonary embolism
Fat embolism
Acute respiratory distress

Immediate local
Bleeding
Vascular injury
Nerve injury
Visceral injury

Early complications
Local infection
Septicaemia
Gas gangrene
Compartment syndrome
Haemarthrosis
Fracture blisters/sores
Plaster sores
Nerve entrapment

Late complications
Malunion
Delayed union
Non-union
Myositis ossificans
Avascular necrosis
Joint instability
Joint stiffness
Algodystrophy
Osteoarthritis
Volkmann's ischaemic contracture
Complex regional pain syndrome

Joint injuries (Fig. 6.17)

A joint can be injured by either being:

- dislocated, where there is complete discontinuity;
- subluxed, where there is partial discontinuity;
- dislocated with an associated fracture.

If a joint dislocates, injuries to other structures can also occur. These include:

- soft tissue damage – ligaments, tendon and intra-articular structures;
- joint surface damage with chondral defects;
- neurovascular injury;
- chronic instability of the joint;
- recurrent dislocation;
- aseptic necrosis.

A dislocation may present with pain, loss of function or abnormal mobility.

The most commonly affected joints are the shoulder glenohumeral joint, the acromioclavicular joint and the elbow, finger, hip and knee joints. Dislocations and subluxations of specific joints are discussed in Chapters 7 and 8.

These complications are listed in Revision panel 6.1 and are covered extensively in *Investigation and Management*, Chapter 7.

BONE DISEASES AND DEFORMITIES

It is vital to make an accurate diagnosis of any bony lump, as bony swellings can be entirely benign or highly malignant tumours. The clinical presentation may provide some useful hints on the underlying nature of the pathological process, although radiological assistance is usually required. The actual site of a tumour in a long bone may give some clue as to its underlying pathology.

Exostosis

This is a lump that sticks out from the bone. An exostosis is mainly cancellous bone, with a covering of cortical bone and a cartilaginous cap (Fig. 6.19). Exostoses are usually single, but may be congenital and multiple (see below).

Solitary (diaphyseal) exostosis

These are derived from small pieces of metaphyseal cartilage that were not remodelled during the growth of the bone and have become separated from the main cartilaginous epiphyseal plate. Although isolated on the side of the bone shaft (diaphysis), they continue to grow and ossify, and

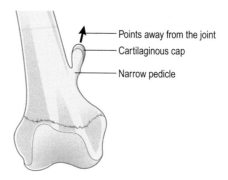

- Points away from the joint
- Cartilaginous cap
- Narrow pedicle

Fig. 6.19 The features of a solitary exostosis.

so produce a bony lump just above the epiphyseal line (Fig. 6.19).

They sometimes have an adventitious bursa over their cap, and they are not neoplasms.

History

Age Exostoses present when they are large enough to cause symptoms – usually in teenage and early adult life.

Symptoms The patient may have felt the lump, or it may have become noticeable and cosmetically disfiguring.

They sometimes interfere with the movement of the joint and its tendons because they arise near joints. Patients may find the movements of the joint limited, or associated with 'clicks' or 'jumps' as the tendons slip over the lump.

The overlying bursa, if present, may become enlarged and inflamed.

Examination

Position They are usually found adjacent to the epiphyseal line of the bone, just on the diaphyseal side. The majority occur at the lower end of the femur and upper end of the tibia.

Shape and size Initial palpation gives the impression of a sessile, smooth, hemispherical protuberance, but with careful palpation it is often possible to feel that the base is quite narrow, and that the exostosis leans away from the joint.

Exostoses are usually 1–2 cm in diameter when they are first noticed. As the cartilaginous cap ossifies, they may enlarge (4–5 cm across) and then interfere with joint movement.

Surface Their surface is smooth.

Composition They are **bony hard**, but their consistency may be masked by a soft, fluctuant bursa overlying their cap.

Relations They are fixed to the underlying bone. It is important to palpate the lump while the adjacent joint is moving to feel which muscles and tendons lie close to the lump, and to measure the range of joint movement.

Local tissues The rest of the bone and the nearby joint should be normal.

Multiple exostoses
(Diaphyseal aclasis)

This is a autosomal dominant hereditary condition, in which one-half of the patient's children can be expected to have the abnormality. It is more common in males. All the bones that ossify in cartilage can be affected, with the exception of the spine and skull. The long bones may be a little shorter than normal because this condition is caused by a widespread generalized abnormality of bone remodelling at the epiphyseal line, as opposed to the sporadic event that produces a solitary exostosis.

The clinical features of each exostosis are similar to those described for the solitary variety. They are multiple and especially common on the limb bones. They can grow to a considerable size of up to 5–10 cm in diameter.

Callus

Perhaps the most common cause of thickening of a bone is callus. Callus is the buttress of new bone formed around a fracture site to unite and strengthen it while the cortical bone is being slowly repaired.

History

In the majority of cases, the patient knows of the injury and the subsequent discomfort associated with the fracture that caused the callus, but this is not always the case. Some fractures are caused by repetitive stress. Furthermore, not every fracture causes severe pain, so the absence of a history of trauma or pain does not necessarily exclude the possibility that the lump might be callus. Clearly, however, this is unlikely.

Examination

Position The thickening of a bone by callus should be greatest at the site of the fracture, but it may be asymmetrical.

Tenderness Mature callus is not tender. Once a fracture has united, there is no local tenderness, and if an area of thickening in a bone is tender, it is unlikely to be callus around a united fracture. It may be provisional callus around non-union, but other signs of non-union will be present.

Shape Callus usually causes a fusiform enlargement of the whole bone – thickest at the site of the fracture.

Surface Callus becomes smooth as time passes. In young people, callus can be completely resorbed and remodelled.

ABNORMALITIES OF BONE METABOLISM

Paget's disease of bone
(Osteitis deformans)

Bone is usually continually repaired and replaced throughout life. This process follows the same pattern as the original ossification. The ossified cartilage that is reorganized into mature bone is called **osteoid bone**.

In Paget's disease, the repair process stops at the osteoid bone stage, with the healthy, mature bone being gradually replaced by thick, bulky, very vascular osteoid bone. The old bone, which is absorbed by the osteoclasts, is replaced by fibrous tissue. If the repair process stops a stage earlier, the bone is very weak. **The underlying cause of Paget's disease is still not known.**

Paget's disease occurs in later life and usually affects multiple bones, but can occasionally affect just one bone in the whole skeleton (monostotic Paget's disease). There is the potential for malignant change in the bone, and **osteogenic sarcoma complicates 1 per cent of cases**.

History

Age The patient is rarely under 50 years of age, often much older, and can be of either gender.

Symptoms **Pain is the most common symptom**, although patients may be symptomless. As the bones enlarge and become more vascular, the patient feels a deep-seated aching, gnawing pain in the bone. The back is the most common source of pain. Make a careful note of any change in the nature and severity of the pain. This may indicate malignant change. Headache may be the result of the increased vascularity of the bones.

Deformity The bone grows bigger and bends. The typical complaints are:

- enlargement of the skull, with the frontal bones becoming prominent;
- curvature of the spine, causing a kyphosis and increasing difficulty with fitting clothes; patients occasionally complain that they are getting shorter;
- bowing of the legs.

Deafness Paget's disease in the temporal bones may affect the middle ear and cause otosclerosis and deafness. The patient may also develop vertigo.

Examination

General appearance The patient with generalized disease has a **large head**, a **bent back**, **arms that seem too long** (because of the kyphosis) and **bow legs**.

Cardiovascular system Examine the cardiovascular system with care. The increased bone blood flow causes an increased cardiac output. The heart may be enlarged, there may be an aortic ejection murmur, and the blood pressure may be elevated. Paget's disease can cause a **high-output heart failure**, but this is very uncommon. The exacerbation of any myocardial ischaemia, secondary to coronary vessel disease, by the extra demands placed upon the heart of an elderly person is well recognized.

Respiratory system Rales and rhonchi may be present at both lung bases if the kyphosis is severe enough to interfere with movements of the chest wall.

Skeleton

- *Skull.* The enlargement occurs in the vault. The dome looks swollen, and the enlarged frontal bones make the forehead bulge forwards. Deafness is common.
- *Spine.* The disease usually affects the whole skeleton, producing an even **kyphosis**. The shoulders are rounded, and the head and neck protrude anteriorly.
- *Legs.* The femur and the tibia may bow in both anterior/posterior and lateral directions.

Fig. 6.20 'Sabre tibiae'. The anterior edge of the tibia is normally straight and sharp. In this patient, Paget's disease has made these edges thick and curved.

The sharp anterior edge of the tibia becomes so prominent that the description '**sabre tibia**' is apt (Fig. 6.20), although this expression is usually reserved for bowing caused by syphilis and yaws.

When examining the skeleton, look for any localized bony enlargement, especially in the areas where the pain is severe or has changed. A swelling of the bone that is painful, a little tender and warm to the touch suggests the presence of **sarcomatous change**.

Central nervous system The patient may have a **conduction deafness** and difficulty when standing, caused by middle ear and vestibular apparatus damage.

The function of other cranial nerves can be affected if the thickening of the bones reduces the size of the foramina in the base of the skull. **Blindness** can occur if the optic nerves are compressed.

Spinal nerves may also be damaged by collapse of the vertebrae.

Osteoporosis

In this disease, the bone mineral density is reduced, because **the balance of bone formation and resorption is disturbed**. This causes defects in the bone architecture in which the cortex is thinned with fewer trabeculae, and this leads to a **greater risk of fracture**. Osteoporosis may be primary, postmenopausal or secondary to, for instance, corticosteroids or heparin.

Risk factors for primary osteoporosis include:

- white or Asian ethnicity;
- family history;
- early-onset menopause;
- oophorectomy or hysterectomy;
- lack of exercise;
- smoking and alcohol abuse.

History

Age Females are usually perimenopausal or postmenopausal, usually between the ages of 45 and 50 years.

Symptoms **In the early stages, it is symptomless**, but symptoms arise from the development of **fragility fractures** or secondary to **pathological fractures**. Principal fracture sites include the vertebral body, wrist and hip.

Deformity Fragility fractures in the spine can result in increased **thoracic kyphosis** from wedging or compression of the vertebral bodies.

Examination

Other than the presence of a fracture, and its possible sequelae, the examination is normal.

Rickets/osteomalacia

These are the result of an inadequate mineralization of bone caused by inadequate absorption or utilization of calcium.

Osteomalacia is 'softening of the bones' in which thin bony trabeculae are covered by wide osteoid seams. The incomplete ossification process in children that occurs in **rickets** affects the physeal growth plate, leading to skeletal deformities.

In the past, the principal cause was often **lack of dietary vitamin D** or **insufficient exposure to sunlight**. Nowadays, any deficiency in vitamin D metabolism can result in the condition, including renal and liver disease.

Calcium deficiency and hypophosphataemia can result in similar mineralization defects.

History

Age Rickets occurs in children, while osteomalacia occurs in later life, and its effects become more apparent over a longer period of time.

Symptoms **Adults** present with **bone pain**, **muscle weakness** and even occasionally **tetany**.

Children may be **listless**, and have a '**failure to thrive**'.

Deformity **In rickets**, early bone changes include **deformity of the skull (craniotabes)**, thickening of the bones of the wrist, enlargement of the costochondral junction (**rickety rosary**; Fig. 6.21) and indentation of the chest (**Harrison's sulcus**). As the child begins to stand, **tibial bowing (coxa vara)** may become apparent, and increasing **spinal curvature** develops.

In **osteomalacia**, fragility fractures in the spine can result in increased **thoracic kyphosis**. There is also increased risk of traumatic fractures of the long bones.

Examination

Children may be small for their age because bone growth is stunted. Once the child stands, any deformity, particularly in the lower limbs, will increase. In adults, vertebral collapse can also cause loss of height, with mild deformities becoming more pronounced.

Fig. 6.21 A rickety rosary. Enlargement of the costochondral junctions and presence of Harrison's sulcus.

Hyperparathyroidism

This is discussed in Chapter 12. The elevated parathyroid hormone increases the osteoclastic resorption of bone.

Brown tumour-like masses develop in the bones that liquefy and become cystic. Less than 10 per cent, however, present with bone pains and pathological fractures.

INFECTIONS OF BONE

Acute osteomyelitis

Bone can become infected by organisms that reach it through the bloodstream or directly through a wound. Blood-borne organisms are probably trapped in thrombi or haematomas caused by minor trauma, usually in the capillary loops in the shaft adjacent to the epiphyseal line known as the **metaphysis**. The common infecting organisms are *Staphylococcus aureus* and *Streptococcus pyogenes*.

History

Age Patients with acute osteomyelitis are usually between 1 and 12 years old. When adults are affected, infection is often associated with immune suppression.

Symptoms The site of infection is painful, although in the early stages this is only a deep-seated ache. When pus forms and intramedullary tension increases, the pain becomes intense and throbbing.

A child will refuse to use a limb or allow it to be touched. Some swelling may be noted around the painful area, but this is not marked as it is caused by diffuse oedema of the overlying tissues, rather than swelling of the bone. The adjacent joint is often swollen and stiff.

Systemically, the infection causes a loss of appetite and general debility. Most patients feel hot and sweaty, and they may suffer from rigors.

Examination

Site The tibia, femur, humerus, radius and ulna are the most commonly affected bones.

Colour The skin over the painful area may be red or reddish-brown.

Temperature The skin becomes palpably hot when the infection has spread through the bone into the sub-periosteal layer.

Tenderness The swollen area is tender, and the whole bone is sensitive.

Consistency Any swelling is soft and indistinct because it is caused by oedema of the overlying structures. There may be an area that fluctuates when there is pus near the surface.

Lymph glands The local lymph glands are only enlarged if the infection has spread outside the bone.

Surrounding structures The overlying skin may be oedematous. The neighbouring joint may be swollen by an effusion, and its movements limited and slightly painful. The infection has probably spread into the joint and caused a septic arthritis if the joint movements are very restricted and painful (see below).

The subcutaneous veins of the limb are often dilated.

General examination The patient looks ill and feverish. Their face may be flushed, and their temperature raised. They may be hypotensive, sweating and possibly shaking, with a dry tongue and oliguria, if septicaemia has developed.

Chronic osteomyelitis

This often follows an open fracture or a surgical procedure or implant, but can also develop from acute osteomyelitis.

The common infecting organisms are again *Staphylococcus aureus* and **streptococci (especially *Streptococcus pyogenes*)**. *Staphylococcus epidermidis* is frequently isolated if there is associated metalwork from previous surgery. In children or patients with sickle-cell disease, chronic osteomyelitis can be caused by *Escherichia coli*.

As a result of the infection, bone is destroyed in areas around the focus of the infection or around a foreign implant. Cavities containing pus and dead bone (**sequestra**) become surrounded by vascular tissue and by areas of sclerosis. This may form an **involucrum** or bony sheath.

History

Age Patients can present at any age. It is more common in those who have either been inadequately treated or have immune suppression, for example elderly patients, those with diabetes or malnutrition, and those on steroid medication.

Symptoms Patients often present with recurrent bouts of pain around the infected area. They avoid using the limb. Systemic features of infection include feeling feverish from a raised temperature, associated with nausea and malaise. Episodes of infection are often interspersed with periods of quiescence.

Examination

Site The long bones of both the upper and lower limbs are most commonly affected. The spine may also be involved particularly after previous operations (see Chapter 9).

Colour The skin may appear red, with a flare.

Temperature This may be increased, but it may also be normal.

Tenderness The area is normally tender, and the bone is often very sensitive.

Surrounding structures A **surgical scar** may be present. **Sinuses** may also be noted in the skin, with discharging pus (Fig. 6.22). The skin itself is often thickened and puckered.

There may be deformity of the bone secondary to previous trauma. Despite surgical intervention, the bone itself may not have healed because of the infection. This can lead to further deformity.

The sinuses may wall off over a period of time, which suggests that they may have healed only to reopen again, either in the same place or elsewhere. The bone becomes brittle, and this can result in a **pathological fracture**.

Tuberculosis

Where pulmonary disease is endemic, the bones and joints of children and young adults may become infected. Elsewhere in the world, it tends to develop in **elderly adults with debilitating disorders or patients with immunodeficiency (AIDS)**.

It reaches the skeleton by haematogenous spread, and the acid-fast bacilli often lodge in the **bone metaphysis**, which has the greatest blood supply. Initially, there is a chronic inflammatory reaction with **granuloma formation and caseation**, which spreads into the soft tissues, where it liquefies to form a '**cold abscess**'. This can point some distance away, having tracked down through the tissue planes (Fig. 6.23).

It arises quite commonly in the anterior part of the vertebral body near the disc and can spread to the adjacent vertebra, which can lead to collapse and sharp angulation (a **kyphus**) (see Chapter 9).

Tuberculous arthritis is discussed on page 214.

Fig. 6.22 A sinus discharging pus associated with chronic osteomyelitis.

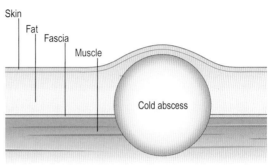

Fig. 6.23 A cold abscess.

CHAPTER 6 | BONES, JOINTS, MUSCLES AND TENDONS

MISCELLANEOUS CONDITIONS OF BONE

Osteonecrosis

(Avascular necrosis)

Osteonecrosis occurs when the blood supply to a bone is disrupted. This may be caused by:

- severance of the blood supply, or pathology in the lumen of the vessel or the vessel wall;
- external compressive forces causing occlusion of the blood flow (see Revision panel 6.2).

As a result, the bone cells die, but on reperfusion of the bone, there is attempted repair of the ischaemic areas. The necrotic bone collapses, and reactive new bone forms in the ischaemic boundary, with accompanying sclerosis.

History

Age Patients can present at any age, depending on the underlying cause.

Patients with **sickle-cell disease** present initially with an acutely painful crisis. Once vascular necrosis becomes established, they generally re-present in young adulthood, either from the pain associated with the condition or as the result of secondary joint changes.

Similar presentations occur following traumatic injury.

Revision panel 6.2

The causes of avascular necrosis

Trauma
Sickle-cell disease
Caisson disease (decompression sickness)
Coagulation disorders
Vasculitis
Gaucher's disease
Septic arthritis
Osteomyelitis
Corticosteroids
Excessive alcohol
Systemic lupus erythematosus
Ionizing radiation

Symptoms Pain is the common feature, although the early stages of cell death may be symptomless.

Examination

Site The shoulder, hip and knee are most often affected. The hip, talus and scaphoid may all develop osteonecrosis after a fracture.
Colour The skin appears normal.
Temperature The temperature is normal.
Tenderness The area may be tender, with sensitivity of the bone.
Movements There may be restriction in movement secondary to pain, with muscle wasting as a consequence of disuse. Deformities of the joint may arise.

The **diagnosis** is dependent on finding the typical changes on X-ray (see *Investigation and Management*, Chapter 7).

Osteochondritis

In this group of conditions, the **bone is usually compressed, fragmented or separated** near the bone ends or articular surfaces. The sclerosis and increased vascularity that occurs is very similar to the changes found in avascular necrosis.

The individual entities are dealt with in the chapters on the areas where they occur, for example **Perthes' disease** in the hip section of Chapter 8.

Benign tumours of bone

Benign tumours of bone fall into two categories:

- those arising from cortical bone (so-called **'ivory' osteomas**);
- those which are primarily cartilaginous tumours that arise within or on the surface of long bones (**enchondromas and ecchondromas**).

An exostosis (described earlier in this chapter) is not a benign neoplasm.

Osteoma
History

The patient complains of a lump that they have either felt or had drawn to their attention. These lumps are not painful, and they rarely occur in a site that interferes with joint or tendon movements.

Examination

Site Osteomas are common on the surface of the vault of the skull, frequently the forehead (Fig. 6.24).

Shape and size They are sessile, flattened mounds with a smooth surface.

Consistency Osteomas are bony hard – hence the name 'ivory' osteoma.

Relations Nearby muscles and fascia move freely over the lump, which is obviously fixed to and an integral part of the underlying bone.

Fig. 6.24 An osteoma of cortical bone – an 'ivory' osteoma on the forehead, which has been present for 40 years.

Chondroma

A chondroma can grow inside a long bone only if a piece of the cartilage from which the bone developed fails to become converted to bone:

- An **enchondroma** is a chondroma growing in the centre of the bone (Fig. 6.25).
- **An ecchondroma** is a chondroma growing on the surface of the bone (Fig. 6.25).

There is no pathological difference between these two varieties of chondroma.

When the chondromas are multiple and congenital (but not familial), the condition is called **dyschondroplasia or Ollier's disease**.

History

Age Patients usually present in teenage or early adult life.

Symptoms The patient notices either that a bone is gradually expanding or that a lump is appearing on the side of a bone.

Neither type of chondroma is painful, but an ecchondroma may interfere with joint and tendon movement.

Enchondroma

Ecchondroma

Fig. 6.25 The two varieties of chondroma that are found in long bones.

Examination

Site They are common in the bones of the hands and feet, but may occur anywhere. Large, long bones are rarely affected, except when the patient has congenital and multiple chondromas (Ollier's disease).

Temperature The overlying skin has a normal temperature.

Shape **Enchondromas cause a fusiform enlargement** of the shaft of the bone. **Ecchondromas form a sessile lump** on the surface of the bone (Fig. 6.26).

Surface The surface of both varieties is smooth.

Consistency They feel hard as they are usually covered by a thin layer of cortical bone.

Fig. 6.26 A large ecchondroma of the metacarpal bone of the thumb (arrow).

Osteoid osteoma

This is a very small bone tumour that can occur in any bone except the skull. It is usually less than 1 cm in diameter, and accounts for approximately 10 per cent of all benign bone tumours.

History

Age Patients usually present in teenage or early adult life. There is an increased incidence in males.

Symptoms The patient usually presents with **significant localized pain** in the bone. They do not want to use the limb or affected region, which can lead to **wasting and weakness**. Pain is typically severe at night, with a dull ache during the day, and is typically relieved by salicylates.

Examination

Site The most commonly affected bones are the tibia and femur.

Signs The patient may develop a limp with muscular atrophy.

Temperature The overlying skin has a normal temperature.

Shape The bone itself usually maintains its normal shape, as the tumour is located within the bone itself.

X-rays show the tumour as a radiolucent area known as a nidus, surrounded by a distinct zone of necrosis (see *Investigation and Management*, Chapter 10).

Conditions that present like benign tumours

Fibrous dysplasia

In this condition, normal bone is replaced by fibrous bone tissue. It can occur in childhood or early adulthood, and can affect one bone (**monostotic**), one limb (**monomelic**) or many bones (**polyostotic**).

Males and females are equally affected.

Symptoms In many cases, fibrous dysplasia is **symptomless**, and is an incidental finding when an X-ray is taken.

Bone expansion can cause **pain**, most often in the femur, tibia, humerus and ribs, and the patient may develop **a limp**.

Signs There may be **palpable tenderness** but no changes in temperature. There may be **bowing** of the upper femur or weight-bearing bones. **Pathological fracture** may occur.

Non-ossifying fibroma
(Fibrous cortical defect)

This is the most common benign lesion of a bone, in which **fibrous tissue appears and persists for some years before ossifying**. It is almost always symptomless, and is common in children as an incidental finding within the metaphyses of long bones.

Simple bone cyst

This is also known as a **solitary cyst or unicameral bone cyst**. It generally appears in childhood, usually in the metaphysis of a long bone, commonly in the proximal humerus or femur. It does not expand the bone.

It is usually **symptomless** and is an incidental finding on an X-ray, although it can present with a **pathological fracture**.

Aneurysmal bone cyst

This benign bone neoplasm is characterized by blood-filled spaces separated by fibrous septa. It can arise *de novo* or secondary to a pre-existing bone tumour. It may be intraosseous or extraosseous.

The tumour can arise at any position, but is most commonly found in the upper extremity, lower leg and femur. **Initially it is painless**, but as it expands it often causes **discomfort of increasing severity**. A large cyst may become visible or palpable. The skin temperature around the bone may increase. There may be a restriction of movement in the adjacent joints.

Malignant tumours of bone

These are either **primary or secondary**. A **metastasis** (a secondary deposit) is much the more common (see below).

There are **five principal primary tumours of bone**:

- Osteosarcoma.
- Chondrosarcoma.
- Reticulum cell sarcoma (Ewing's tumour).
- Giant cell tumour (osteoclastoma).
- Multiple myeloma.

The **five primary carcinomas** that commonly **metastasize** to bone, producing secondary metastatic tumours, originate in the:

- Lung.
- Breast.
- Kidney.
- Thyroid.
- Prostate.

Although these are the most common primary sites for bone metastases to originate, remember that any tumour can metastasize to bone.

The first four tend to produce lytic (dissolution of bone) metastases, while prostatic 'secondaries' are often sclerotic (hard).

The bones that most often contain secondary deposits are:

- the vertebral bodies;
- the pelvic bones;
- the ribs;
- the upper ends of the femur and the humerus.

These bones all contain red bone marrow and have a good blood supply.

History

General features Patients often give a history of previous malignancy (e.g. a mastectomy for a lump in the breast). They may also have symptoms related to the primary growth, such as a cough with haemoptysis, or difficulty with micturition.

Some patients develop bony secondary deposits with no signs or symptoms to indicate the site of the primary tumour.

Symptoms The most common symptom is **pain**. Low back pain or pain in the pelvis and hip is often the first indication of the existence of secondary deposits.

Acute pain will occur if there is a **pathological fracture**, such as the collapse of a vertebral body or a fracture of the femur.

Noticeable swelling at the site of a metastasis is very unusual unless it is in a superficial bone such as the vault of the skull, the clavicle or a rib.

Examination

Deep-seated bony metastases rarely produce any physical signs except pain on movement and tenderness on percussion.

When superficial, they may cause a swelling of the bone that appears rapidly and grows steadily.

The consistency of a secondary deposit in a bone may vary from hard and bone-like to soft and compressive.

Osteosarcoma

This is a malignant sarcoma of bone. It is seen in two groups of patients:

- the young;
- elderly patients with Paget's disease.

Sarcoma complicating Paget's disease has already been described (see page 199).

Osteosarcoma is a highly malignant spindle-celled tumour. It spreads locally into the surrounding soft tissues, and early and rapidly by the bloodstream.

History

Age It occurs in childhood and the teenage years.
Symptoms **Pain** is the predominant symptom. It usually begins before the patient notices a lump, and is a persistent ache or throb.

Swelling of the bone may be noticed, and in some instances this increases rapidly.

The development of **general malaise**, **cachexia** and **loss of weight** may precede or coincide with the appearance of local symptoms.

Pulmonary metastases may cause a cough and haemoptysis.

Abdominal discomfort and jaundice may follow the enlargement and destruction of the liver by metastases.

Patients often relate the onset of their symptoms to an injury, but there is no evidence that trauma causes sarcoma. The injury simply focuses their attention on symptoms that they had previously dismissed as trivial and insignificant.

CHAPTER 6 | BONES, JOINTS, MUSCLES AND TENDONS

Examination

Site The most common places to find an osteosarcoma (Fig. 6.27) are:

- the **lower end of the femur**;
- the **upper end of the tibia**;
- the **upper end of the humerus**.

Colour The overlying skin may be reddened, and the subcutaneous veins visibly distended.

Tenderness The swelling may be slightly tender but not exquisitely painful like osteomyelitis (see page 202).

Any red, warm, non-tender bony swelling should, in the first instance, be considered to be a tumour and not an infection.

Temperature The skin over the swelling is usually warm and sometimes quite hot.

Shape The swelling tends to appear on one side of the lower end of the bone, making it asymmetrical.

Surface Its surface is smooth unless it has spread into the surrounding tissues, when it becomes irregular.

Consistency Bony sarcomas feel **firm but not bony hard**.

It is a clinical aphorism that benign tumours of bone feel hard, whereas malignant tumours of bone feel soft.

A very vascular tumour may pulsate.

Relations The structures overlying a small osteosarcoma are mobile, but become fixed to it if the tumour spreads locally beyond the bone.

Lymph drainage The draining lymph glands are not enlarged in the early stages of the disease, which may be another indication that the red, warm swelling is not an infection. When the tumour invades the surrounding soft tissues, it may then spread to the local lymph glands.

Local tissues The nearby joint often becomes stiff and develops an effusion. The adjacent artery and nerves are only involved in advanced local disease.

General examination Take particular care to examine the chest and the abdomen, because the lungs and the liver are common sites for metastases. There may be generalized wasting, and wasting of the muscles of the affected limb.

Chondrosarcoma

This is one of the most common malignant tumours originating in bone. It may arise centrally in the

Fig. 6.27 The common sites to find osteosarcomas.

medullary cavity or peripherally from the cortex. It may develop *de novo* or by malignant change in a pre-existing benign lesion (secondary chondrosarcoma).

History

Age The incidence is greatest in the fourth to fifth decades, with males more commonly affected than females.

Symptoms The tumour is often **symptomless** in the initial stages. As it grows, the patient may become aware of a **dull ache** or a **gradually increasing lump**. Acute pain is associated with a 'pathological fracture'.

Examination

Site These tumours most commonly arise in the metaphyses of the long bones of the lower limb. They can also occur in the pelvis, ribs and upper limbs.

Colour The overlying skin is normal.

Tenderness There may be tenderness of the bone.

Temperature This is usually normal.

Shape The tumour may cause a swelling and enlargement of the bone with a smooth surface.

Lymph drainage The lymph glands are not usually palpable as most chondrosarcomas are slow growing and metastasize late.

Reticulum cell sarcoma

(Ewing's tumour)

This is a tumour that arises most often in the centre of long bones – a feature that helps to distinguish it from osteosarcoma and osteomyelitis.

This tumour occurs as large sheets of polyhedral cells that have a **distinct reticulate staining** and can be mistaken for a secondary deposit from an adrenal neuroblastoma.

The cell of origin is not known, but it may arise from the **endothelial cells of the bone marrow**.

History

Age This tumour occurs in childhood and the teenage years.

Symptoms The most common symptom is a **persistent ache or pain** made worse by movement.

Patients may also notice a **swelling** as the tumour enlarges, and many children with a tumour in the femur present with a **limp**.

These tumours can sometimes present as a **pyrexia of unknown origin** and cause rigors and night sweats.

There may be **weight loss and malaise**, especially if the lesion is a metastasis from a neuroblastoma.

Examination

Site The mid-shaft of the femur is the most common site to find these tumours, but the tibia and the humerus can also be affected.

Colour The overlying skin may be reddened.

Tenderness The swelling is usually a little tender.

Temperature The increased vascularity makes the whole area feel warm.

Shape The tumour causes a symmetrical **fusiform enlargement of the shaft of the bone**, the upper and lower limits of which are indistinct.

Surface The surface of the swelling is smooth.

Consistency When the bone is so expanded that the **tumour mass is palpable**, it feels **firm and rubbery, not bony hard**.

Relations The overlying structures can be moved over the mass because, although they are displaced, they are not usually infiltrated.

Lymph drainage The lymph glands should not be palpable.

Local tissues The arteries and nerves of the limb are rarely involved.

General examination There may be pyrexia and weight loss.

Examination of the lungs and liver may reveal evidence of secondary deposits.

Very rarely, a primary neuroblastoma may be palpable in the abdomen. This is palpable as a lobulated mass in the upper part of the abdomen, which may cross the midline (see Chapter 15).

Giant cell tumour

(Osteoclastoma)

These tumours are sometimes classified as having a **variable malignant potential** because approximately one-third are entirely benign, one-third invade nearby tissues, and one-third metastasize. The tumour has a red fleshy appearance and consists of multinucleate giant cells in a background of stromal cells that extend into the surrounding bone.

History

Age The patient is usually between 20 and 40 years old.

Symptoms The usual presenting symptom is **pain**. The pain is a dull ache, but it may become acute if there is a **pathological fracture**.

The patient may also notice **swelling of the lower end of the femur or the upper end of the tibia**.

The nearby joint may get stiff if the swelling disturbs the tendons around it, or if the tumour invades the bone just beneath the articular cartilage.

Examination

Site The common sites to find giant cell tumours are the **lower end of the femur and upper end of the tibia** (i.e. either side of the knee), and the **upper end of the humerus and lower end of the radius** (i.e. away from the elbow).

Colour The colour of the skin is normal.

Tenderness The swelling may be tender.

Temperature These tumours are not usually vascular, and the temperature of the overlying skin should be normal.

Shape Giant cell tumours usually cause a diffuse expansion of the end of a bone, but it may be asymmetrical and noticeable only on one side.

Surface Their surface is smooth.

Consistency The lump feels **bony hard** provided the outer layer of bone is reasonably thick. It may feel firm and slightly pliable if it is thin, and when it is very thin it crackles and bends when touched, and feels like **a broken egg shell**.

It does not pulsate unless very thin walled and malignant.

Relations The surrounding structures are usually freely mobile over the swelling.

Lymph drainage The local lymph glands should not be enlarged.

Multiple myeloma
(Plasmacytoma)

This is a malignant B cell lymphoproliferative disease of the bone marrow with multiple deposits of plasma cells. These cells have a large, eccentric 'cartwheel' nucleus.

The vertebral bodies, ribs, pelvis, skull and proximal ends of the femur and the humerus are the most commonly affected, and usually contain multiple lytic deposits.

History

The patient is usually aged 45–60 years and presents with **general malaise**, **loss of weight** and **intractable pain in the skeleton** – mostly in the back and chest wall.

Pathological fractures can occur and cause even more **severe acute pain**.

Hypercalcaemia may cause **polyuria**, **thirst** and **abdominal pain**.

A large single deposit (**plasmacytoma**) may become obvious as a bony '**lump**'.

Examination

A plasmacytoma may be palpable as a single bony lump.

There may be signs of involvement of other parts of the blood-forming tissues – enlarged lymph glands, hepatomegaly and splenomegaly.

The presence of **Bence Jones protein** in the urine is diagnostic, and an **abnormal band** of protein is usually present on the electrophoretic strip.

CONDITIONS OF JOINTS

Osteoarthritis

This common condition can affect any joint. It is believed to be caused by asymmetrical wear and tear, often exacerbated by injury and a disturbance of the normal stresses and strains associated with the transfer of weight across the joint. There may be an inherited genetic defect in the structure of type IV collagen that weakens the strength of articular cartilage.

The accepted causative factors are:

- age;
- previous fractures involving the articular surface and cartilage;
- previous joint diseases;
- malalignment of the skeleton following trauma or bone disease.

The **articular cartilage becomes thin and softened**, before it ultimately disintegrates and wears through.

This leads to joint space narrowing, with **subchondral cysts** and **sclerosis** developing in the sub-articular bone.

The joint synovium becomes inflamed, and the joint capsule becomes fibrotic.

This is accompanied by new growth of bone at the edges of the cartilage, causing **osteophyte formation**.

History

Age Most patients with osteoarthritis are over 50 years old, but secondary osteoarthritis following trauma or disease may begin in early adult life.

Symptoms The principal symptom is **pain**, which comes on gradually, but steadily increases until all movements of the joint are very painful. This is a very slow process. Associated with the pain is an **increasing stiffness** that may precede the onset of the pain.

Weakness The stiffness and pain lead to disuse atrophy, so **the muscles controlling the joint become weak and wasted**.

Deformity As the stiffness increases, the joint often develops a degree of fixed flexion, and the limb may lie with a degree of abnormal abduction or adduction.

Limping Pain, stiffness, weakness and deformity of the joints in the lower limb **interfere with walking**.
Swelling **The whole joint is often swollen** by bony osteophytes and an effusion. The synovium is not usually thickened.

Examination

Inspection

Colour The skin should not be reddened or discoloured.
Contour The joint is usually swollen (see Fig. 8.30).
Deformity The joint may be fixed in an abnormal position. Nearby muscles are wasted (see also Fig. 6.4).
Relations Other joints in the same limb, and the same joint in the other limb, may be similarly diseased.

Palpation

Skin The skin temperature is normal, not hot.
Tenderness Pressure on the joint, especially if it is swollen, may cause pain, but local tenderness is uncommon except during an acute exacerbation when there is an effusion.
Synovium The synovium is not usually palpable.
Muscle bulk The bulk of the muscles that control the joint is reduced (see Fig. 6.4).
Bony contours The bone at the edge of the articular cartilage may feel irregular and protuberant.

Movement

All movements of the joint are painful at their extremes, and some movements are reduced. Affected joints may eventually become unstable.

Not all movements of the joint will be equally affected. For example, early osteoarthritis of the hip may cause limitation of abduction and medial rotation long before it affects flexion, extension, adduction and lateral rotation.

Note **Make sure that you assess the limitation of movement accurately by asking the patient to do active movements before you perform passive movements.**
Crepitus The joint often crackles and clicks during movement. Although the patient can feel a grating sensation associated with the crepitus, it is not usually painful.
Abnormal movements There should be no abnormal movements because all the ligaments should be intact.

Arteries and nerves in the limb

These structures should all be normal.

Other joints

Osteoarthritis is often bilateral and symmetrical. The joints most often affected are the hip, knee, spine and fingers.

General examination

Osteoarthritis is not associated with any other generalized disease, so the rest of the examination should be normal.

As many of the patients with osteoarthritis are old and overweight, they frequently have unrelated diseases such as coronary, cerebral and peripheral artery disease. The detection of these diseases is important because their existence may alter the patient's management.

Rheumatoid arthritis

Rheumatoid arthritis is a generalized inflammatory joint disease that may have a genetic predisposition.

It is considered to be **an autoimmune disease**, perhaps initiated by a viral infection, although the exact cause remains **unknown**.

The synovial membrane becomes thickened by hyperaemia and a lymphocyte infiltration. As the disease progresses, the cartilage becomes damaged and eroded, and eventually the joint is destroyed, with progressive instability and deformity. There may be an **associated effusion**.

Near the joints, there may be **nodules** consisting of necrotic collagen surrounded by fibroblasts.

History

Age Rheumatoid arthritis may appear in patients of all ages, but the common time of onset is between the ages of 30 and 40 years.
Sex **Females are affected three times more often than males.**
Symptoms The first complaint is often of **early morning swollen, stiff fingers**. The main symptoms are **pain and swelling** of multiple joints. Occasionally, the condition can begin in a single large joint. The disease usually fluctuates between **remissions and 'flare-ups'**, and may eventually become quiescent. Occasionally, the onset is dramatic and the course relentless.

Wasting As the disease progresses, **the joint movements become restricted**, and the muscles that control the joint waste away and become weak. As the joints of the upper limbs are often the first to become affected, patients complain that they keep dropping things, and cannot carry a shopping basket.

General malaise The patient may **feel ill and listless** and **lose weight**.

The muscles ache, especially after exercise, and **tender, painful nodules** appear around the joints.

Skin rashes The patient may complain **of skin irritation and rashes**, especially if the joint changes are part of another generalized disease such as **Reiter's syndrome** or **systemic lupus erythematosus**.

Examination

Inspection

The disease, which is an **asymmetrical polyarthritis**, usually starts in the small joints at the end of the limbs – fingers, wrists, toes and ankles – before it moves to the larger joints of the limb, and ultimately to the joints of the trunk. The manifestations of the disease in the hands are described in Chapter 7.

Contour The joints are evenly enlarged. The finger joints become fusiform (Fig. 6.28).

Colour The skin overlying the joint may be red and, if there is much swelling, shiny and taut.

Deformity As the disease advances, it affects the ligaments and tendons around the joint as well as the articular surfaces, causing **a variety of joint deformities**. For example, there is often **ulnar deviation at the wrist joint** and **hyperextension of the proximal interphalangeal joints** (Figs 6.28a, b, 7.33). There may also be subluxation or dislocation of the metacarpal joints, with the development of **swan neck and boutonnière deformities**.

Wasting The muscles that control the affected joints are wasted.

Other joints Many joints are affected, and the condition is frequently symmetrical.

Palpation

Temperature The skin over the joint is warm.

Tenderness In the acute stage of the disease, the joint is tender to light palpation. The tenderness subsides

(a)

(b)

Fig. 6.28 RHEUMATOID HANDS

(a, b) Both show the typical features of fusiform swelling of the finger, muscle wasting and ulna deviation.

as the condition progresses, but the pain during movement persists.

Synovium Soft tissue thickening can often be felt around the joint. It is only possible to be certain that there is thickened synovium in those joints where it has a clearly palpable edge beyond the joint line. There may also be an **effusion** in the joint.

Muscle bulk The muscles that control the joint feel thin and atrophic.

Bony contours Until the joint surfaces are destroyed and **pathological dislocations** occur, the general bony contour of the joint remains normal, but it is often obscured by the synovial thickening.

Movement

- **Active movements** are limited by pain and reduced in power.

- **Passive movements** are limited by pain and fibrous contractures.
- **Abnormal movements** appear when the disease has weakened the ligaments, or tendons have ruptured.

Arteries and nerves in the limb

The other structures in the limb should be normal. Patients with long-standing rheumatoid arthritis sometimes get a peripheral arteritis, which causes gangrene of the tips of the toes and fingers, and ulceration of the skin of the lower third of the leg. Swelling of the joints around the wrist may cause a carpal tunnel syndrome (see Chapter 7), and peripheral neuritis can develop.

General examination

Apart from other joint involvement, there may be generalized wasting and anaemia. Three systemic diseases are associated with rheumatoid joint disease:

- *Still's disease*, a disease in which adults develop arthritis, splenomegaly and lymphadenopathy. A similar condition can occur in children, known as systemic onset juvenile idiopathic arthritis.
- *Reiter's syndrome*, in which there is urethritis, conjunctivitis, skin rashes and arthritis.
- *Systemic lupus erythematosus*, a collagen disease in which there is a scaly, red rash on the face, debility and manifestations in all tissues of a small vessel arteritis.
- Other conditions, which may also present in a similar fashion to rheumatoid arthritis (Revision panel 6.3)

Gout and pseudogout

(Pyrophosphate crystal deposition)
These two conditions are considered together as their symptoms are very similar. Gout is the result of deposition of **uric acid crystals**, while in 'pseudogout' **calcium pyrophosphate crystals** are deposited.

A disorder of purine metabolism is responsible for gout, in which there is often 'hyperuricaemia', deposition of urate crystals in the joints causing acute synovitis, and the formation of renal stones (see Chapter 17). Secondary gout can be caused by renal failure and cytotoxic treatment of malignancy,

> ### Revision panel 6.3
> #### Differential diagnosis of rheumatoid arthritis
> Seronegative polyarthritis
> Systemic lupus erythematosus
> Gout and pseudogout
> Ankylosing spondylitis
> Reiter's disease
> Polyarticular osteoarthritis
> Polymyalgia rheumatica
> Systemic onset juvenile idiopathic arthritis
> Adult onset Still's disease

with massive cell death resulting in an increased purine load.

Pyrophosphate is generated in cartilage, where it combines with calcium to form crystals in the collagen. These are extruded into the joint from time to time, where they cause an acute local inflammatory reaction that is almost identical to gout.

History

Age **Gout** usually occurs in middle-aged or elderly males, often with a family history of the disorder.

Pseudogout tends to occur in middle-aged females.

Symptoms The onset of gout is often heralded by the development of an **acute painful red first metacarpal joint**. The attack begins spontaneously, but can follow an 'alcoholic binge', a minor injury or excessive exercise, and usually takes several days or a week to abate. It can also arise in the ankles, knees, finger joints and bursae, and can occasionally present with acute pain in the heel or sole of the foot.

Patients may notice '**tophi**', which are clumps of crystals in tendons, in bursae and 'classically' in the subcutaneous tissues of the pinnae of the ears. They may also present with '**colic**' from renal calculi (see **Chapter 17**). The condition can become chronic, with recurrent bouts of acute pain that may become continuous, leading to stiffness of many joints. Large tophi may form, which may ulcerate.

The onset of pseudogout is also usually heralded by sudden pain and swelling in a joint, but this is usually in the knee rather than the foot, and is seldom as severe.

Other conditions may also present in similar fashion to gout, especially involving the first metatarsal phalangeal joint (Revision panel 6.4).

Revision panel 6.4

Differential diagnosis of gout/pseudogout

Septic arthritis

Infected bunion

Rheumatoid arthritis

Osteoarthritis

Examination

Inspection

Colour The gouty joint is red (Fig. 6.29), but the joint affected by pseudogout is not.

Contour Both conditions cause joint swelling.

Palpation

Tenderness The joint feels tender and hot in both conditions.

Movement

All joint movements are painful and restricted. Gout makes weight-bearing and walking very difficult.

The diagnosis of both conditions is made by identifying their characteristic crystals on joint aspirates.

Fig. 6.29 Gouty tophi occurring in a thumb (arrow).

Tuberculous arthritis

Any joint can become infected with the human or bovine tubercle bacillus, either directly from the bloodstream or more commonly from the adjacent bone (see page 203).

The infection produces typical pathological changes in the synovium, with 'granulomas' containing giant cells, lymphocytes and macrophages, before caseation occurs. The articular cartilage and bone are destroyed as the disease progresses.

The joints of the **vertebral column** are most often affected, but it can also occur in the hip or knee, and occasionally in the joints of the upper limb.

History

Age Tuberculous arthritis tends to occur in young adults and children. Mild symptoms may be present for many years before the patient complains or seeks advice.

Symptoms The common joint symptoms of **pain and swelling** usually begin simultaneously, but in the hip or the spine where the swelling is not apparent, pain is the presenting feature.

The pain **limits movement of the joint**, and this usually interferes with **walking, bending** and **stooping**.

An abscess can form in the joint, which may point onto the skin and then discharge. The resulting **chronic sinus**, with a sero-purulent discharge, persists until the disease is cured or dies out.

General malaise and **loss of weight** are common associated non-specific symptoms.

Social history It is important to enquire about social conditions, such as diet, housing and international travel, as well as the existence of any family history of tuberculosis.

Local examination

Inspection

Contour The joint (especially the knee) is diffusely swollen.

Colour The colour of the skin over the joint is normal.

Sinuses There may be a **discharging sinus near the joint, or the scars of healed sinuses** (see Fig. 6.1).

Muscle wasting There is usually marked muscle wasting, especially of the quadriceps femoris muscles when the knee joint is diseased (see Fig. 6.4).

Palpation

Skin The skin over the joint is not hot, but the inflammatory hyperaemia in the underlying synovium may make it slightly warmer than normal.
Tenderness The joint may be tender for a short period in the early acute phase of the disease, but once the infection is established, the joint is not usually painful.
Synovium The swelling around the joint feels soft and pliable – something like unbaked dough. There is always an effusion in the joint.
Bony contour The bones are only deformed or destroyed in long-standing severe disease.

Movement

This is only limited if the joints are painful, usually as a consequence of pronounced protective muscle spasm.

There should be no abnormal movements.

When the disease is advanced and has destroyed the joint, it becomes fixed by a **fibrous ankylosis** (Fig. 6.30).

Fig. 6.30 The end result of severe tuberculosis of the left knee joint: a fibrous ankylosis, shortening and wasting of the limb and healed sinuses.

General examination

There may be evidence of tuberculosis elsewhere, such as in the lungs or the kidneys, so **the general examination must be thorough and complete**.

Haemophilic arthritis

Intra-articular haemorrhage is a common complication in patients with deficiency of clotting factor VIII (**haemophilia**) or of factor IX (**Christmas disease**). These are X-linked recessive disorders and are therefore manifest in males, although females are the carriers of the conditions.

Recurrent episodes of bleeding leads to progressive articular cartilage destruction, with subchondral bone changes, including cyst formation.

History

Age Initial bleeding into the joint usually starts when the child begins to stand and walk. The arthritis usually develops in young adults.
Symptoms **Pain and swelling of the joints occurs often after relatively trivial trauma**, although the degree of bleeding also depends on the severity of the disorder.

The most commonly affected joints are the ankles, knees, shoulders, elbows and hips.

Bleeding can also occur into muscles, causing a painful swelling, with restriction of movement in the joints adjacent to the muscle.

Secondary compression of a peripheral nerve can cause neurological symptoms if the swelling is large. Bleeding into the nerve can also cause intense pain.

Examination

Inspection

Contour The joint is diffusely swollen.
Colour The colour of the skin over the joint may be normal, or **bruising may be apparent.**
Muscles There may be muscle wasting, when arthritis has become established. In an acute bleed, the muscles may contain a lump or become swollen.

Palpation

Skin The skin over the joint will be warm when bruising is present, and slightly warmer than normal in established chronic synovitis.
Tenderness The joint is painful following a bleed and becomes progressively more tender, as cartilage degeneration follows recurrent episodes.

Movement

Movements are limited by pain. When the disease is advanced and has destroyed the joint, it may become ankylosed.

Neuropathic joints

(Charcot's joint)

The brain is unable to protect a joint that has lost its 'pain and position sense' from harmful stresses and strains. The frequent minor injuries that result ultimately destroy the bones and the ligaments of the joint.

A neuropathic joint is therefore a painless, disorganized joint.

The possible causes of loss of joint sensation are:

- diabetic neuropathy (the most common cause nowadays);
- tabes dorsalis (rare today);
- syringomyelia;
- leprosy;
- cauda equina lesions such as a myelomeningomyelocele.

History

Age Neuropathic joints usually occur in middle and old age. In syringomyelia, the condition often dates from an earlier age, and there is often dissociation of sensory loss, with loss of pain and temperature sense, but not of touch.

Symptoms The patient notices that the joint is becoming **swollen and deformed** and **gives way frequently** but *is not painful*.

The mechanical weakness of the joint together with the sensory defects of the neuropathy make the patient's **gait unstable**.

Previous illness The patient will probably know if they have had **diabetes** for many years, but may not know if they have had syphilis.

Other neurological conditions may be present.

Examination

Inspection

Colour The colour of the skin over the joint is normal.

Contour The joint is usually **swollen and obviously deformed** (Figs 6.31, 6.4). There is no common pattern of deformity for any particular joint.

(a)

(b)

Fig. 6.31 TWO VIEWS OF A CHARCOT JOINT

(a, b) A totally disorganized, but painless, left ankle and foot. This Charcot ankle and foot was caused by diabetic peripheral neuropathy.

Palpation

Tenderness The joint is not tender, and movements in any direction do not usually cause pain.

Synovium The synovium is not thickened, but there is always an effusion.

Bony contours **The bones are displaced and deformed.** The normal shape of the bones forming the joint may completely disappear as a result of a combination of bone destruction in some areas, and new bone formation and hypertrophy in others.

The joint may be **subluxed or dislocated**, and there is gross bone erosion with irregular calcified masses in the capsule.

Movement

Normal movements may be impossible because of the destruction of the joints and ligaments.

Some passive movements may be limited by the bony deformities.

Grossly abnormal movements may be possible. It may also be possible to dislocate and then reduce the joint, which can usually be moved in a variety of abnormal ways **without the patient feeling any pain or discomfort**.

The knee and elbow joints may become so disorganized that the limb becomes **flail-like**, with grossly abnormal but painless movements.

Nerves of the limb

These must be examined with great care. **Vibration sense**, **position sense** and **deep pain sensitivity** are usually all reduced or absent. The motor innervation should be normal.

General examination

Look for the signs of diabetes and syphilis. Take particular care to examine the whole of the nervous system for evidence of any other neurological disease processes, such as syringomyelia, and test the urine for sugar.

Acute septic arthritis

This is usually caused by *Staphylococcus aureus* (like osteomyelitis; see page 202), but *Haemophilus influenzae* can also cause joint infection in young children. The organisms obtain access to the joint from the bloodstream, from a penetrating joint injury or from direct spread from an infected bone (osteomyelitis).

The infection destroys the joint, and the pus may then track into the soft tissues before discharging onto the skin as one or more **sinuses**.

The infection will eventually settle, and a **fibrous or bony ankylosis** will occur (see below).

History

Age Children of both sexes are most commonly infected, but septic arthritis is also seen in adults of all ages.

Symptoms **Acute pain and joint swelling** are the two most common symptoms, and these limit joint movement, leading to immobility and loss of function.

The patient will feel hot and sweaty, which may be accompanied by loss of appetite, general malaise and sometimes even rigors.

In neonates, the symptoms of sepsis predominate − irritability and failure to feed. Likely portals of entry include the umbilical cord and intravenous access sites.

Examination

Inspection

Colour The overlying skin may be red.
Contour The joint will usually appear swollen, and the limb may be held in flexion.
Overlying skin One or more discharging or healed sinuses may be present depending on the stage of the disease.

Palpation

Skin This may feel warm.
Tenderness This will be present over the joint, and there may be fluctuation if an abscess has formed.

Movement

Both active and passive movements will be severely restricted and very painful.

Ankylosis

An ankylosed joint is a fixed joint.

A **bony** ankylosis is present if the bones that form the joint are fixed together by bone. This is absolutely fixed and painless even when stressed.

A **fibrous** ankylosis occurs when the bones are fixed by dense fibrous tissue. This moves a little, and forced movement cause pain.

CONGENITAL/GENETIC DISORDERS OF BONES AND JOINTS

There are numerous disorders of cartilage and bone development, most of which cannot be discussed in a book of this type. Some (e.g. Marfan's syndrome) are the result of single defective genes, others are probably polygenomic, and some result from damage to the fetus in utero (e.g. phocomelia from thalidomide). The common conditions are covered in different anatomical sections of this book but are summarised in Revision panel 6.5.

Revision panel 6.5

Genetic skeletal disorders

Multiple exostoses (see above)

Dyschondroplasia (see above)

Achondroplasia (see Chapter 1)

Multiple epithelial dysplasia (abnormal metaphyses of long bones)

Osteopetrosis (marble bone disease)

Candle/spotted or striped bones

Osteogenesis imperfecta (brittle bones)

Extra/absent/hypoplastic or fused bones

Hemi- or fused vertebrae (see Chapter 9)

Congenital pseudo-arthrosis

Ehlers–Danlos syndrome (joint laxity and aneurysms)

Marfan's syndrome (see Chapters 1 and 9)

Hurler's syndrome (gargoylism)

Gaucher's disease (mucopolysaccharidoses/ excessive storage of glycosaminoglycans)

Neurofibromatosis (see Chapter 3)

Down's syndrome (see Chapter 1)

Sprengel's deformity (see Chapter 7)

Phocomelia (hypoplastic/absent limb)

Upper limb symptoms and signs

SHOULDER

The shoulder is one of the most mobile joints in the human body. This allows the arm and hand to be positioned for maximum reach. There are three principal joints of the shoulder:

- the glenohumeral joint;
- the acromioclavicular joint;
- the sternoclavicular joint.

The scapulothoracic articulation, together with a pseudo-joint between the humerus and the coracoacromial arch, is also required to facilitate movement.

The shoulder is made up of three principal bones:

- the clavicle (collar bone);
- the scapula (shoulder blade);
- the humerus (upper arm bone).

The principles of examination of the shoulder joint are the same as for any other joint:

- Look.
- Feel.
- Move.

Additionally, there are special tests for anatomical structures and pathological conditions that can be used. As in any orthopaedic examination, it is important to assess the joint above and below that principally being examined, in this case the cervical spine and the elbow.

The symptoms encountered are most commonly:

- *pain*, which may be located to a particular region of the upper limb such as the shoulder, elbow or hand, or may be referred into the upper limb from the neck (see Chapter 9); the pain may be present at rest, nightime or on movement;
- *deformity*, which is the result of congenital anatomical abnormalities, tumours, trauma or wasting;
- *disability*, caused by loss of function and stiffness, which may result from joint problems, nerve damage or muscular weakness.

PLAN FOR EXAMINATION OF THE SHOULDER

Inspection

The patient should be stripped to the waist and examined from both the front and the back. The upper torso, neck, shoulder, scapula and both upper limbs can then be examined and compared.

The skin should be inspected for evidence of **scars**, **sinuses** and **discolouration**.

Arthroscopic surgical scars are small and can be easily missed. Arthroscopic assessment of the shoulder is carried out through a scar positioned approximately 1 cm medial to and below the posterior lateral border of the acromion, i.e. on the posterior aspect of the shoulder joint. Further arthroscopic portals can be positioned laterally and anteriorly. Open surgical procedures usually involve an incision placed in the deltopectoral groove.

Shape

Wasting may be present in the muscles of the shoulder girdle.

- *Deltoid* wasting can occur secondary to an axillary nerve palsy.

- Wasting of the *rotator cuff muscles* – supraspinatus, infraspinatus, teres minor and subscapularis – can also be associated with a nerve palsy, for example of the suprascapular nerve affecting supraspinatus and infraspinatus, or with tendon tears.
- Wasting of the *trapezius muscle* can be seen following injury to the spinal accessory nerve during surgery to the neck, or following blunt trauma or traction injury.

(a) Acute rupture.

(b) Chronic rupture.

Fig. 7.1 RUPTURE OF PECTORALIS MAJOR

A 'Popeye sign' is associated with a rupture of the long head of biceps (see below).

In addition, the overall shape of the shoulder may be altered by a rupture of the pectoralis major tendon (Fig. 7.1).

The shape of the shoulder can also be significantly altered by the size, shape and position of the scapula. The scapulae should be symmetrical.

Failure of descent of the scapula during development can result in the scapula remaining elevated, smaller than usual and more prominent (**Sprengel's deformity**). This is associated with a shorter neck, and often a kyphosis or scoliosis of the thoracic spine (Fig. 7.2).

More commonly, both scapulae fail to descend (**Klippel–Feil syndrome**). Patients appear to have no neck with a low hairline, bilateral neck webbing and limitation of neck movement.

Winging of the scapula can occur in association with **long thoracic nerve palsy**, resulting in wasting of serratus anterior. This can be demonstrated by asking the patient to raise both arms to shoulder height and press into a wall (Fig. 7.3).

Fig. 7.2 Sprengel's shoulder.

Fig. 7.3 Winging of the right scapula.

The shape of the shoulder can also be altered by abnormalities of the acromioclavicular joint. Degenerative change or previous trauma resulting in dislocation makes the joint more prominent, with the appearance of a raised bump at the outer end of the clavicle.

Occasionally, a glenohumeral joint effusion can be seen as an anterior swelling that rarely extends into the axilla.

Other soft tissue masses may be visible, particularly lipomas in the region of the deltoid and scapula. Cystic swellings of the superior aspect of the shoulder are also common, particularly in relation to the acromioclavicular joint, and in association with massive rotator cuff tears.

Palpation

Palpation should begin at the sternoclavicular joint and then proceed laterally along the clavicle. Clavicular deformity may be apparent if there has been a previous fracture. The acromioclavicular joint and acromion should both be examined. The acromion passes laterally and posteriorly to the spine of the scapula. The anterior and posterior glenohumeral joint should also be assessed.

Palpation of the greater tuberosity may reveal problems associated with the supraspinatus tendon at the site of its insertion, while palpation of the biceps in the bicipital groove may also reveal pathology. Palpation is principally to elicit tenderness rather than to assess a temperature change associated with inflammation, which is generally difficult to identify.

Movement

This can be divided into active and passive. The normal range of shoulder movement is shown in Revision panel 7.1.

The range of movement in the shoulder may be restricted because of stiffness, or increased as the result of laxity of the joints.

Active movements may be limited by pain or weakness, and hence passive movement must always be assessed.

Movements should be observed from in front of the patient and also from behind.

As well as the range of movement, the rhythm of movement also warrants consideration.

When assessing movement, it should be understood that the plane of the scapula is strictly 30° anterior to the frontal plane. It is, however,

> ### Revision panel 7.1
>
> ### Normal range of shoulder movement
>
> 0–175° forward elevation
>
> 0–175° abduction
>
> Less than 80° external rotation with the elbows at the sides
>
> 90° external rotation in 90° abduction
>
> 70° internal rotation in 90° abduction
>
> Internal rotation assessed by the patient reaching up the back to thoracic vertebrae 7–10

generally accepted that forward elevation is in the sagittal plane, and abduction is in the coronal plane.

The glenohumeral joint does not account for all the movement of the shoulder and shoulder girdle, as some movement occurs at the **scapulothoracic joint**. To assess this, the scapula should be fixed by placing the hand on the top of the shoulder. Early movement takes place almost entirely at the glenohumeral joint, but as the arm is raised, the scapula begins to rotate on the thorax. The final 60° of movement is almost entirely scapulothoracic. In abduction, approximately 100° of movement arises from the glenohumeral joint, and 80° at the scapulothoracic joint.

When there is pathology around the shoulder, this movement may become disturbed. Patients '*hitch*' to gain increased range, by using their trapezius muscle to help raise their arm. During forward elevation and abduction, patients may experience a **painful arc** suggestive of rotator cuff pathology.

Power

This should be assessed in the principal muscles around the shoulder girdle:

- The *deltoid* is assessed by abduction against resistance.
- The *serratus anterior* is assessed by asking the patient to push against a wall with both hands. The scapula should remain close to the thorax, but if there is weakness it becomes more prominent.
- *Pectoralis major* may be assessed by asking the patient to push both hands into their waist.

Specific tests for the rotator cuff complex will be described below.

Neurological examination

A formal neurological examination should be performed, including for sensation (see Chapter 3). The most common abnormality is altered skin sensation in the C5 distribution overlying the deltoid. This region is known as the '**regimental patch**'. Birth trauma palsies such as **Erb's** (C5/6) and **Klumpke's** (C8/T1) neurological deficits may also be apparent.

Special tests

A number of special tests have been developed to assess the anatomy and function of the shoulder.

Rotator cuff tendons

Supraspinatus – the empty can test

The arm is placed with the thumb pointing to the floor in the plane of the scapula with 90° of elevation, as if 'emptying a can' (Fig. 7.4). Patients are assessed for pain and weakness as the examiner applies downward pressure on the arms.

Infraspinatus/teres minor

The elbows are placed at the sides in 90° of flexion. The patient is then asked to externally rotate against resistance. If weakness is perceived, the elbow is then placed in maximum external rotation, and the patient is asked to maintain this position (Fig. 7.5). When there is a major tear in these tendons, this position cannot be maintained, and the arm drifts back towards the midline (the **lag sign**).

Patients with a massive cuff tears cannot externally rotate the elevated abducted arm (**Hornblower's sign**).

Subscapularis

The patient is asked to stand with their hands in front of their belly, with their elbows forward in the coronal plane. The examiner pushes against the patient's elbow to elicit pain and weakness (the **belly press test**) (Fig. 7.6).

Alternatively, the patient places their arm behind their back in the mid-lumbar spine region. The examiner then lifts the patient's hand away from their back, and the patient is asked to maintain this position. This is impossible if there is pain or weakness from a tear (**Gerber's lift-off test**) (Fig. 7.7).

Long head of biceps

The arm is placed in 90° of forward elevation and external rotation. The patient is asked to resist flexion (**Speed's test**) (Fig. 7.8).

Fig. 7.5 The infraspinatus external rotation test.

Fig. 7.4 The supraspinatus empty can test.

Fig. 7.6 The subscapularis belly press test.

Alternatively, the elbow is flexed at 90°, and the patient is asked to supinate actively against resistance from a pronated position (**Yergason's test**) (Fig. 7.9).

Fig. 7.7 The subscapularis Gerber lift-off test.

Impingement tests

There are a number of tests that can be used to assess for impingement, which occurs when the patient experiences pain, usually in the anterolateral aspect of the shoulder, from compression of the subacromial bursa and rotator cuff tendons as they pass under the coracoacromial arch.

The painful arc

When moving the arm in abduction, the patient classically experiences pain between 60° and 120° (Fig. 7.10).

Neer's impingement sign

The scapula is stabilized, and the affected arm is raised and placed in flexion, abduction and internal rotation (Fig. 7.11). The test is positive when pain is elicited as a consequence of the greater tuberosity passing under the coracoclavicular arch.

Fig. 7.8 Speed's test for the biceps.

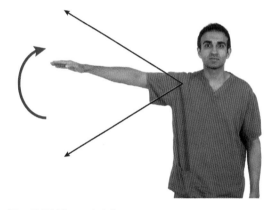

Fig. 7.10 The painful arc.

Fig. 7.9 Yergason's test for the biceps.

Fig. 7.11 Neer's impingement test.

CHAPTER 7 | UPPER LIMB SYMPTOMS AND SIGNS

Local anaesthetic may be injected into the subacromial space as a diagnostic test, which is considered positive if it relieves the patient of their symptoms.

Hawkin's test

The arm is placed in 90° of forward flexion with the elbow flexed to 90°, and the arm is then rotated internally. A positive test occurs when pain is elicited and is experienced in the anterolateral aspect of the shoulder (Fig. 7.12).

Acromioclavicular joint

The arm is placed in maximum adduction and pulled forcibly across the chest (the **scarf test**) (Fig. 7.13).

Fig. 7.12 Hawkins test for impingement.

Fig. 7.13 The scarf test.

Instability tests

The three major causes of shoulder glenohumeral joint instability are:

- Trauma.
- Hyperlaxity.
- Muscle patterning disorders, either in isolation or in combination.

These can result in anterior, posterior or multidirectional instability.

The tests described below aim to qualify the degree and nature of the instability.

General instability – the load shift test

The examiner places one hand over the shoulder and the scapula to stabilize the shoulder girdle, and uses the other hand to grasp the humeral head. The humerus is then loaded into the glenoid and pulled (translated) anteriorly and posteriorly. The humeral head may be felt to ride up on the glenoid rim.

The patient is placed in different positions to assess different components of the shoulder stabilizing structures. Grading is based on the position:

- mild: 0–1 cm translation;
- moderate: 1–2 cm translation;
- severe: greater than 2 cm translation up to the glenoid rim.

Anterior instability – the anterior apprehension test

The patient is asked to lie on the examination couch. The arm is placed in 90° of abduction. External rotation is then performed from the neutral position. The examiner observes the 'apprehension' of the patient, i.e. the patient becomes worried that the shoulder is unstable and may dislocate (Fig. 7.14).

Anterior instability – Jobe relocation test

The examiner repeats the apprehension tests and then returns to the start position, having noted the degree of external rotation. This is then repeated, and a posterior stress is applied over the humeral head, so that the escaping humeral head is pushed back into the joint. An increase in the external range before symptoms of apprehension are reproduced indicates a positive result (Fig. 7.15).

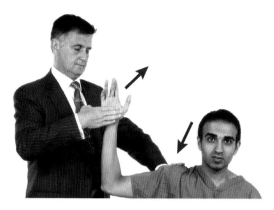

Fig. 7.14 The apprehension test.

Fig. 7.15 The Jobe relocation test.

Posterior instability

Posterior labral shift tests are assessed in the same manner as the anterior load and shift.

Posterior instability – the posterior apprehension test

The arm is held in an adducted and flexed position. The examiner pushes posteriorly to elicit apprehension.

Inferior laxity – the sulcus sign

The patient sits or stands with the shoulder in the neutral position. An inferior traction is applied by grasping the arm. The examiner observes for dimpling of the skin below the acromion, which indicates a widening of the subacromial space between the acromion and the humeral head. This may be graded I, II, or III depending on the degree of laxity.

CAUSES OF SHOULDER PAIN

The most common causes of shoulder pain are listed in Revision panel 7.2.

Impingement syndrome

This is pain in the subacromial space when the humerus is elevated or internally rotated, and is

---

Revision panel 7.2

Common causes of shoulder pain

Rotator cuff disorders
Impingement syndrome
Supraspinatus tendinitis
Subacromial bursitis
Tendon tears: partial or complete
Calcific tendinitis
Biceps tendinitis
Adhesive capsulitis (frozen shoulder)

Arthritis
Glenohumeral joint
Acromioclavicular joint

Bone lesions
Infection
Tumour
Avascular necrosis

Instability
Dislocation
Subluxation

Trauma
Fracture

Neurological pain
Brachial plexus neuritis
Suprascapular nerve compression

Referred pain
Cervical spondylosis
Cardiac ischaemia
Mediastinal pathology

---

classically seen between 60° and 120° in abduction. This is generally considered synonymous with supraspinatus tendinitis or subacromial bursitis.

History

Age and sex Impingement syndrome is usually seen in middle-aged patients, from 30 to 55 years of age. Both males and females can be affected. Instability should be considered as an associated factor when the syndrome is present in patients under 30 years.

Cause Often no cause is elicited, although it may be because of recurrent or unaccustomed activity, for example decorating or exercising at the gym. Symptoms can also arise and persist following an injury.

Symptoms **Pain and weakness** are noted during shoulder movement. The pain may be related to activity or may occur at rest, and is usually centred on the anterior and lateral aspects of the shoulder, radiating to the deltoid insertion.

Night pain can occur, particularly when lying on the shoulder.

Activities of daily living become inhibited, with difficulty reaching high (e.g. into a wardrobe) and behind the body.

Examination

The patient exhibits a painful arc in abduction. This may be associated with weakness of the rotator cuff, particularly the supraspinatus and, to a lesser extent, infraspinatus muscles. The patient will demonstrate **a positive impingement sign**, and a positive **Hawkin's test** (see above).

The pain is often relieved by injection of local anaesthetic into the subacromial space.

Rotator cuff tears

These occur in one or more of the four rotator cuff tendons, which attach to the supraspinatus, infraspinatus, subscapularis and teres minor muscles. The supraspinatus is the most commonly affected tendon, with a tear occurring at its insertion on the greater tuberosity of the humeral head.

The tears may be partial or complete. They can be caused by trauma, or more commonly are the result of degenerative age-related changes to the tendon; hence they may be either acute or chronic.

History

Rotator cuff tears are usually characterized by the acute onset of pain following trauma, or gradual persistent pain (chronic) with progressive pain and weakness.

Age and sex Patients are usually over the age of 40 years. Partial tears are more common initially, but full-thickness tears become increasingly common with age, especially after the age of 65 years. Tears can occur in both males and females.

Symptoms These usually consist of **pain** and **reduced function**, particularly when lying on the shoulder and reaching forwards trying to lift a weight.

Weakness eventually leads to **difficulty in raising the arm**, and **muscular wasting** can occur (Fig. 7.16).

Rotator cuff tears may also be symptomless.

Examination

Movement is restricted by pain and there is weakness in all planes, particularly forward elevation and abduction (supraspinatus). Passive movements

Fig. 7.16 Rotator cuff wasting of supraspinatus and infraspinatus.

are, however, largely preserved. Rotation may also be compromised by involvement of the infraspinatus and teres minor (external rotation) and subscapularis (internal rotation). Each tendon can be assessed by the special tests described above. Patients may also have positive impingement signs.

Calcific tendinitis

This is the result of a deposition of calcium hydroxyapatite in the tendons of the rotator cuff causing pain and inflammation. The most commonly affected tendon is the supraspinatus tendon. The cause is unknown. It may occur in an acute or a chronic form.

History

Age and sex The majority of patients will be aged 30–50 years. The condition can affect both males and females.

Symptoms In the acute disorder, the patient develops **severe pain** over a period of a few hours, which often causes them to seek urgent medical advice. The pain usually lasts 7–10 days, and then the shoulder generally returns to normal over a 6-week period.

In chronic calcific tendinitis, the patient may be symptomless, and the calcification may be an incidental finding on a shoulder X-ray. When the calcification is painful, it is generally less marked than in acute calcific tendinitis, and is more consistent with the presentation of an impingement.

Examination

The arm is often held immobile in an acute presentation because the pain causes limitation of movement. Even passive movements are likely to cause great pain.

Palpation 'about the shoulder' may reveal generalized tenderness, which is usually most marked over the greater tuberosity.

In chronic calcific tendinitis, patients have pain on movement, but this is generally relatively well preserved, often with an impingement arc. When the calcification is within the supraspinatus tendon, patients have a positive empty can test and signs of impingement (see above).

Adhesive capsulitis (Frozen shoulder)

This condition is caused by the capsule of the shoulder joint becoming contracted, thickened and inflamed secondary to an ill-defined process that appears to involve fibroblastic proliferation, similar to Dupuytren's disease of the hand (see below).

History

Age and sex This condition occurs mainly in patients aged 40–60 years, and is seen more frequently in females.

Cause There is often no obvious cause for the development of adhesive capsulitis. There is, however, an association with diabetes and possibly thyroid disease. The condition can also occur following a stroke or arterial or cardiac catheterization, and after trauma or surgery to the shoulder.

Symptoms The condition is characterized by an **initial phase of increasing severity of pain**, leading to difficulty in lying on the shoulder and marked sleep disturbance. Even at rest, there is a 'toothache-like' discomfort with significant positional exacerbation, particularly if a sudden movement is attempted.

Examination

The shoulder becomes increasingly stiff, with a **restricted range of both active and passive movement**, classically below 90° of forward elevation and 90° of abduction. Additionally, rotation is reduced, with external rotation of 0° and limited internal rotation, the arm often only reaching to as high as the buttock – indeed, **the loss of rotation is the key feature**.

The condition is generally self-limiting. The initial painful and stiff (freezing) phase, progresses through to a stiff but relatively painless (frozen) phase, before finally there is a recovery of movement (thawing) phase. The whole process can take 18 months or more. During these periods, the signs can vary, but the characteristic of reduced passive movement, especially of external rotation, remains the key feature.

CHAPTER 7 | UPPER LIMB SYMPTOMS AND SIGNS

Biceps tendinitis

The long head of biceps is often considered to be part of the rotator cuff, and can become inflamed as part of an impingement syndrome. It can also be present as an isolated inflammation, particularly in association with lifting heavy weights or gym activity. In the majority of cases, the tendon remains constrained in the bicipital groove, but if the supporting structures on either side are deficient, the tendon may become unstable.

History

Age and sex The patient is usually 30–55 years of age. It can occur in both sexes, although it is slightly more common in males.

Symptoms The patient presents with **pain on activity**, and will often trace a line of pain along the course of the biceps tendon, into the muscle belly. The symptoms are similar to those of impingement syndrome.

Examination

There may be localized tenderness along the bicipital groove.

The patient may have **positive Speed's and Yergason's tests** (see above).

They are likely to have positive impingement signs (see above).

Long head of biceps tendon rupture

Occasionally, a patient presents with chronic symptoms of bicipital tendinitis, prior to a rupture of the long head tendon. The tendon arises from the superior glenoid tubercle, where it attaches to the glenoid labrum.

History

Age and sex Patients are usually aged over 50 years, and the condition is more common in males.

Cause The injury can occur spontaneously, but can also be related to lifting a heavy object.

Symptoms The patient may have chronic pain in the proximal biceps region, which may be alleviated by the rupture. There is often a **snapping sensation**, particularly if the rupture occurs when lifting a heavy weight. Sometimes, however, the rupture

is relatively painless, and the patient is unaware of its occurrence.

Examination

The patient develops a lump in the lower part of the upper arm, which is particularly prominent when the elbow is flexed (Fig. 7.17). This is commonly known as the '**Popeye sign**' and may, in the initial stages, be associated with bruising.

Unless there are other pathological conditions, such as impingement syndrome or rotator cuff tears, the remainder of the examination is usually unremarkable.

During surgery on elderly patients, a biceps tenotomy (deliberate cutting of the tendon) is occasionally performed to relieve the symptoms.

The biceps tendon can sometimes hypertrophy and enlarge, making it unable to slide in and out of the bicipital groove. The tendon becomes trapped between the humeral glenoid when the arm is elevated. This can lead to pain and a loss of the end range of movement, particularly in forward elevation. The condition is sometimes called the '**hour-glass**' biceps.

Fig. 7.17 The 'Popeye sign' of a ruptured biceps tendon.

Osteoarthritis of the glenohumeral joint

This is a well-recognized cause of shoulder pain. It may follow previous trauma, instability or long-standing rotator cuff lesions. It may also occur after avascular necrosis of the proximal humerus (see Chapter 6).

History

Age and sex The patient can be of either sex, and is usually over the age of 50 years.

Symptoms The patient complains of **progressive pain and stiffness in the shoulder**, particularly in abduction and forward elevation. Rotational movements may also become reduced.

Occasionally, a more aggressive and destructive form of osteoarthritis may develop in the presence of long-standing or massive rotator cuff tears, leading to severe erosion of the glenohumeral joint. The humeral head migrates to lie directly beneath the acromion, where further erosion occurs. A rapidly destructive arthropathy with hydroxyapatite crystal formation has been called '**Milwaukee shoulder**' (Fig. 7.18).

Fig. 7.18 Milwaukee shoulder.

Examination

Active and passive movements become progressively more limited, although the speed of the restriction is slower than for adhesive capsulitis, and the pain is comparatively less in the early stages. Other tests are likely to be normal, unless there is associated rotator cuff pathology.

Osteoarthritis of the acromioclavicular joint

This is a relatively common problem but should not be confused with age-related changes in the acromioclavicular joint. These occur from the age of 20 because of an alteration in the structure of the fibrocartilaginous disc. The latter can result in expansion of the joint, with a symptomless lump developing.

History

Age and sex Both sexes can develop the condition over the age of 40 years.

Symptoms They present with **pain and tenderness directly over the acromioclavicular joint**. There may be associated bony or soft tissue swelling. The pain may radiate into the neck muscles or into the upper arm.

Examination

Movements of the shoulder become painful, particularly in the end range, but the passive range should be maintained. Most notably, there is pain and restriction in cross-arm activity (adduction).

A bony/soft tissue swelling may be palpable over the joint.

Rheumatoid arthritis of the shoulder joint

This can affect both the glenohumeral and acromioclavicular joints. Previously, this was suggested to be the most common arthropathy to affect the shoulder joint, but because of advances in the medical management of this rheumatoid arthritis, it is now much less common.

A severe synovitis within the glenohumeral joint can cause rupture of the rotator cuff with secondary migration of the humeral head, leading to the development of a rotator cuff arthropathy. The acromioclavicular joint can also develop erosive changes.

CHAPTER 7 | UPPER LIMB SYMPTOMS AND SIGNS

History

Age and sex Rheumatoid arthritis can arise in patients of all ages, but most commonly between 30 and 40 years. Females are more commonly affected than men (see Chapter 6).

Symptoms Patients present with **pain** and **restricted function** from loss of movement.

There may be **swelling around the joint**, particularly anteriorly, and the swelling may also extend into the axilla.

Examination

The patient may be known to have generalized rheumatoid arthritis affecting other joints.

Active movement becomes progressively more restricted, and while greater passive movement may be maintained initially, this also eventually becomes restricted. Impingement signs and special tests of rotator cuff function are positive if the rotator cuff tendons are involved (see above).

Shoulder instability

Glenohumeral joint stability is provided by static and dynamic stabilizers. The static stabilizers consist of the glenoid and the capsular ligaments, while the dynamic stabilizers are principally the muscles of the rotator cuff, but also include the shoulder ligaments. The negative intra-articular pressure within the joint also helps to maintain stability.

Instability of the joint may occur as a consequence of trauma, hyperlaxity or muscle patterning conditions, and all these may contribute independently to the problem. The instability may be acute, chronic or recurrent.

The joint is considered to have **dislocated** if there is complete separation of the articular surfaces, while a partial disruption of the joint alignment produces **subluxation** (see Chapter 6).

History

Age and sex The most common type of shoulder instability is '**traumatic anterior instability**'. This develops after an injury when the arm is in an abducted and externally rotated position. This is most common in males aged 16–25 years, and is often related to sporting activity.

Symptoms The patient may have **a single dislocation** or develop **recurrent problems** because of a tear of the anterior labrum (a **Bankart lesion**) around the glenoid, together with a bony injury to the posterior superior humeral head (a **Hill–Sachs lesion**).

The patient may also develop episodes of subluxation (partial dislocation). Even after the joint has been reduced and made congruent, these episodes may be associated with a period of pain and reduced movement before normal function is restored.

Patients often complain of **a lack of confidence** and are apprehensive in placing the shoulder in certain positions, particularly abduction and external rotation. As a consequence, they often avoid certain activities, for example throwing a ball or serving at tennis.

Examination

The special tests for shoulder instability, described above, are utilized to assess for increased movement of the humeral head in the glenoid (**anterior draw test**) and evidence of apprehension (the **anterior apprehension and Jobe relocation tests**) (see above).

Posterior instability of the glenohumeral joint is far less common but may be demonstrated by special tests (the **posterior draw and posterior apprehension tests**).

The patient should be assessed for signs of generalized ligamentous laxity, which may be contributing to the problem.

Superior labrum anterior posterior tear (SLAP lesion)

The labrum that surrounds the glenoid in the glenohumeral joint can be damaged not only by a dislocation, but also from loading of the arm in a flexed and abducted position, for example falling with the arm outstretched. This can cause a tear of the superior aspect of the labrum at the insertion of the long head of biceps tendon: a superior labrum anterior posterior tear. Different configurations of the tear can occur, but generally all present in a similar manner.

History

Age and sex The patient is usually less than 30 years old, and the condition is more commonly seen in males involved in sporting activity.

Symptoms After the initial pain of the injury subsides, the patient continues to have **discomfort when lifting the arm above shoulder height**. There is also a functional restriction from loss of power, particularly when trying to throw an object.

Examination

Pain may be elicited by stressing the biceps tendon.

O'Brien's test should be carried out. In this the arm is adducted medial to the sagittal plane with the elbow extended and the arm flexed to 90°. The patient is then asked to resist the downward force with the arm internally rotated, before this is repeated in supination. Pain is usually elicited with the first manoeuvre, but reduced or eliminated by the second.

ELBOW JOINT

This is a synovial hinge joint between the humerus in the upper arm, and the radius and ulna in the forearm. This allows the hand to be moved towards and away from the body. The proximal radio-ulnar joint also lies within the capsule of the elbow joint.

PLAN FOR EXAMINATION OF THE ELBOW

Inspection

Both upper limbs should be exposed. The elbows should be viewed from both the front and behind.

The joint above (the shoulder) and below (the hand and wrist) the elbow should also be examined.

The skin should be inspected for **scars and sinuses**, including small arthroscopic portal incisions, which are usually sited on the medial and lateral aspects of the joint.

Look for **generalized swelling** of the joint or **muscular wasting**, which may be associated with arthritis.

Swelling may be caused by an effusion filling out the hollows seen in the flexed elbow above the olecranon, or swelling about the radiohumeral joint.

Localized swellings may also be associated with olecranon bursitis and rheumatoid nodules (see below).

Shape

The two elbows should be compared. In the normal elbow, if the patient holds their arms with the elbows extended and the palms facing forwards or up, the bones of the humerus and forearm are not perfectly aligned. This deviation away from a straight line in the direction of the thumb is called the **carrying angle**. The normal carrying angle is approximately 5–15° of valgus.

The carrying angle may be increased, resulting in deformity, known as **cubitus valgus** (Fig. 6.11, page 189). The most common cause is from a previous fracture of the lateral condyle of the elbow (see page 250). Patients may develop an ulnar nerve palsy because of a change in the carrying angle.

If the carrying angle is less than 5–15°, such that the elbow is more angulated towards the midline, this is known as **cubitus varus** (a **gunstock deformity**). The most common cause is the result of malunion of a previous supracondylar fracture (Fig. 7.19).

Fig. 7.19 Cubitus varus.

Palpation

The joint should be **palpated along the bony landmarks**, starting at the olecranon process posteriorly, and proceeding to the medial and lateral epicondyles, the head of the radius and the joint line. The bony landmarks of the epicondyles and the olecranon should form an equilateral triangle, which may be disturbed if there has been previous elbow trauma.

The **soft tissues** should also be assessed, including the **olecranon bursa**. The anterior joint line, extending about the biceps tendon in the antecubital fossa and radiohumeral joint, should be palpated during movement. The **ulnar nerve** can be palpated behind the medial epicondyle.

Movement

Both active and passive movement should be compared in the two elbows. Normal extension of the elbow is to 0°. Patients with generalized ligamentous laxity may hyperextend beyond this. Normal flexion of the elbow is approximately 140°. The functional range of movement at the elbow joint, without a significant restriction in the ability to perform tasks, is generally accepted to be 30–120°. Restriction of movement may occur as the result of either a bony block or soft tissue contraction.

Pronation occurs when the elbow is flexed to 90° and the palm maximally rotated towards the ground, with a normal range of 75°. Supination occurs with the elbow flexed to 90° and the palm facing maximally upwards, with a normal range of 80°.

Loss of supination and pronation can be associated with fusion when there is a bony connection between the radius and ulna (proximal radio-ulnar synostosis). This can be congenital or acquired secondary to trauma. The radial head can also be displaced as the result of a congenital dislocation or subluxation, as a consequence of other bone dysplasia or following an unreduced dislocation.

Instability

This can arise following a previous dislocation or injury to the medial or lateral collateral ligaments, which can be stretched or ruptured. An apprehension response can be obtained by supinating the forearm while applying a valgus or varus force during flexion.

Power

Power is assessed during **elbow flexion**, which is performed by the biceps brachii, brachialis and brachioradialis.

The action of elbow **extension** is performed by the triceps brachii.

Supination is achieved by the supinator muscle, together with a contribution from the biceps brachii, and to a lesser extent brachioradialis.

Pronation is performed by pronator teres and brachioradialis.

CAUSES OF ELBOW PAIN

Lateral epicondylitis (Tennis elbow)

This is a common tendinopathy that occurs at the insertion of the common extensor origin onto the lateral epicondyle of the elbow. Small interstitial tears can develop within the tendon, associated with neovascularization. Localized inflammation may also occur. While it can occur in tennis players, it is also seen in patients not involved in sporting activity.

History

Age and sex The condition is seen in middle age, and can occur in both sexes. The cause is unknown. It may be associated with everyday activities such as gardening and the repetitive lifting of heavy objects.

Symptoms The patient complains of **pain and tenderness over the lateral aspect of the elbow**. This is made worse when the common extensor origin is stressed during exercise or shaking hands. The patient may occasionally complain of a **localized swelling** over the lateral epicondyle.

Examination

There is **localized tenderness just below the lateral epicondyle**.

There may be a minor restriction in elbow extension.

The patient may have **a positive finger extension test**, in which the elbow, wrist and fingers are extended, and pressure is then applied to the extended fingers by the examiner. The patient is asked to resist the downward force, and pain is felt about the lateral epicondyle.

Radial tunnel syndrome from compression of the radial nerve in the region of the elbow can mimic the symptoms of tennis elbow. Extension tests involving all the fingers simultaneously are, however, less positive, while single stressing of the middle finger is usually comparatively worse. Tenderness is localized to the radial neck.

Medial epicondylitis (Golfer's elbow)

This condition is similar to tennis elbow, except that it affects the common flexor tendon origin, which inserts into the medial epicondyle of the humerus. The same pathological processes occur as those seen in other tendinopathies. Although it is common in golfers, it can also occur in patients without a sporting background.

History

Age and sex The condition usually occurs in middle age in both males and females.

Symptoms **Progressive pain is experienced around the medial epicondyle.** The patient has difficulty in lifting heavy objects because this causes pain. The patient may complain of ulnar nerve symptoms if there is associated inflammation irritating the nerve.

In javelin throwers or other sportsmen performing similar repetitive throwing activities, pain can occur on the medial aspect of the elbow that is similar to golfer's elbow. This is usually as a consequence of an injury of the medial collateral ligament.

Examination

Pain is reproduced by flexing of the fingers or by passive extension of the wrist. There may be some localized swelling around the medial epicondyle, and tenderness on palpation.

Olecranon bursitis

This occurs on the posterior aspect of the elbow overlying the olecranon (Fig. 7.20). The bursa can become enlarged from an accumulation of inflammatory tissue. The serum uric acid levels may be raised, and urate crystals may be seen in any aspirate if the bursa is swollen by gout.

Fig. 7.20 Olecranon bursa (student's elbow) (see also Fig. 4.65).

History

Age and sex This is normally seen in middle-aged and elderly males.

Cause It may be the result of recurrent trauma. Bursitis is also associated with **gout and pseudo-gout**, or **rheumatoid arthritis**. Infection is unusual but can occur.

Symptoms The patient complains of **pain at the elbow**. They may have an associated systemic illness.

They may also complain of **stiffness** and some **restriction in movement**.

Examination

There is a large **swelling on the posterior aspect of the elbow**, with associated erythema and localized tenderness (Fig. 7.21). The swelling may be hot, and the condition may be bilateral.

(a) Inflamed bursa.

(b) Chronic bursa.

Fig. 7.21 OLECRANON BURSA

Loose bodies

These can occur in the elbow joint and present with both pain and mechanical locking. The loose bodies may be a consequence of **trauma**, **osteochondritis dissecans**, **synovial chondromatosis** or **osteoarthritis**.

History

Age and sex Loose bodies can occur in both males and females, with the age of presentation being dependent on the underlying cause.

Symptoms The elbow becomes **painful** and **locked in a certain position**. Depending on the position of the loose body in the joint, there may be a limitation of extension, flexion, supination and pronation or a combination of movements. The elbow then frees itself, and the range of movement is gradually restored. This, however, can take several days depending on any swelling that might arise.

Examination

There may be joint swelling in the acute phase, but there may be few signs after the acute episode. Very occasionally, permanent restrictions in movement can develop depending on the underlying cause. Loose bodies are almost never palpable.

Osteochondritis dissecans

This is a condition in which the cartilage–bone interface is altered, with separation and necrosis of these structures, often as the result of an ischaemic cause (see Chapter 6). The capitellum is one of the common sites for this process to occur.

History

Age and sex The condition is common in adolescents and young male adults.

Symptoms The patient complains of a **generalized ache** in and around the elbow, which is made worse by activity, and relieved by rest.

Examination

Occasionally, there is some **localized tenderness** on the lateral aspect of the elbow, with **mild stiffness** of the joint with some **associated swelling and an effusion**.

Locking of the joint can occur if a cartilage fragment becomes detached and forms a loose body within the joint.

Osteoarthritis

This is relatively uncommon in the elbow joint. It can follow a previous injury or fracture, and may be the result of long-term occupational demands on the elbow joint.

History

Age and sex The condition can occur in both middle-aged and elderly males and females.

Symptoms Patients complain of **pain and stiffness of the elbow**, which is worse following periods of inactivity.

They may also complain of **locking of the elbow** if loose bodies have formed.

Examination

There is often **localized tenderness** around the joint line, **crepitus** and **restricted movement**.

Rheumatoid arthritis

Although joint manifestations of rheumatoid arthritis have been significantly reduced with the advent of new medical treatments, rheumatoid arthritis can still affect the elbow and superior radio-ulnar joint. In many cases, the condition is bilateral.

History

Age and sex It is more common in females, and usually presents in the fourth or fifth decade.

Symptoms Patients usually complain of an **insidious onset of progressive pain**. They may also complain of **swelling about the elbow and stiffness**. Other joints are often involved, and systemic pathology may be present (see Chapter 6).

Examination

There is usually **swelling** of the elbow joint, with tenderness along the joint line.

There may be **a restriction of flexion and extension**, and the elbow may become **unstable**.

There is usually a **limitation of supination and pronation** if the superior radiohumeral joint is involved.

In advanced cases, **deformity of the joint** becomes increasingly apparent.

Distal biceps tendon rupture

The distal biceps can separate from its insertion into the radial tuberosity, or the tendon can rupture, causing a painful swollen tendon with bulging of the biceps muscle belly. This usually occurs following a traumatic incident when the elbow is flexed against resistance.

History

Age and sex Injury is more common in males in middle age.

Symptoms The patient experiences **sudden pain in the arm** and complains of **weakness in flexion**.

Examination

The biceps tendon can usually be felt as a cord-like structure crossing the joint when the patient is asked to flex the elbow against resistance. When the tendon has ruptured, it cannot be felt, and the biceps muscle belly usually retracts superiorly (Fig. 7.22). A palpable gap can often be felt.

In addition to a reduction in **flexion strength**, the patient also **loses supination power**. Flexion and supination are, however, still possible even in the presence of a biceps tendon rupture because of the action of the brachialis and supinator muscles.

Triceps tendon avulsions can also occur, but these are far less common, and are likely to be associated with weight training and steroid abuse.

Fig. **7.22** Distal biceps rupture.

Congenital dislocation of the radial head

In this condition, the radial head is dislocated anteriorly, posteriorly or laterally to the capitellum. It is usually bilateral, and can be associated with the rare nail–patella syndrome.

History

Age and sex Both males and females are affected. Patients usually present in early childhood or adolescence. The dislocation is sometimes recognized following a minor injury when an X-ray is taken.

Symptoms The patient is often **symptomless** but often notices **a lump** at the elbow joint. **Pain is unusual**.

Examination

There may be slight loss of extension and supination. Examination is, however, often unremarkable.

Pulled elbow

This is a separation of the head of the radius from the annular ligament and often occurs when a child's elbow is 'jerked' by a parent pulling on the arm. This common condition is sometimes called 'nursemaid's' or 'temper-tantrum' elbow.

History

Age and sex It can affect both males and females, usually below the age of 6 years.

Symptoms The elbow is painful, and movements are restricted.

Examination

There is an inability to use the elbow, which is **held immobile in extension with the forearm pronated. Attempted supination increases the pain.** This manoeuvre combined with flexion of the elbow, however, allows the radial head to relocate within the annular ligament.

Ulnar nerve compression (see Chapter 3)

The ulnar nerve passes behind the medial condyle of the humerus through the cubital tunnel. It can become trapped or compressed in this region because of a **bony abnormality** (e.g. **cubitus valgus deformity**). It can also be damaged by **soft tissue or joint swelling**, or **by fascial bands**. It may also be compressed as the nerve passes between the two heads of the flexor carpi ulnaris to enter the forearm.

History

Age and sex The condition can affect both male and female patients, usually in middle age.

Symptoms The patient complains of **pain, numbness and tingling in the little finger and ulnar half of the ring finger**. The pain may extend from the forearm into the hand.

The symptoms may be exacerbated when the elbow is flexed or held in position for a long period.

In the later stages, **weakness of grip and clawing of the fingers, together with muscle wasting**, may be observed.

Examination

A **bony abnormality** or **soft tissue swelling** may be apparent.

A **Tinel's sign** may be elicited by percussing over the ulnar nerve. This reproduces the sensory symptoms.

The patient may demonstrate **Froment's sign** if there is motor weakness, causing weakness of the adductor pollicis (see Chapter 3).

Radial nerve compression (see Chapter 3)

The radial nerve can be compressed at different points along its course through the elbow and into the forearm. Just above the elbow, it divides into the superficial branch and the posterior interosseus nerve. The superficial branch provides sensation to the skin over the anatomical snuff box. The posterior interosseus nerve passes between the two heads of supinator, and supplies motor branches to extensor carpi ulnaris and the extensors of the metacarpophalangeal joints.

History

Age and sex The condition affects both males and females, usually in middle age.

Symptoms The patient may experience pain if there is compression at the radial tunnel, similar to tennis elbow. This is generally worse at night or related to activity. The patient usually maintains strength.

There is a motor weakness of the wrist and finger extensors if the posterior interosseous nerve is compressed (see Chapter 3).

THE HAND

The hand is mankind's greatest physical asset and, anatomically, one of its most distinctive features. Everything that the doctor does to the hand should be aimed at restoring or maintaining its function.

PLAN FOR THE EXAMINATION OF THE HAND

Examine each system in turn, based on the principles of:

- Look.
- Feel.
- Move.

Inspection

Look for any abnormality of the **shape**, **size** and **contour** of the hand. Look for local discolouration, **scars** and **sinuses**. Look for **muscle wasting** by assessing the size of the thenar and hypothenar eminences, and the bulk of the muscles between the metacarpal bones (the interossei). Look at the wrist joint.

Palpation

Feel the bony contours, the tender areas and any localized swellings. Feel the finger joints to assess whether there is any swelling of these joints.

Movement

Check the range and ease of movement of all the joints:

- The *carpometacarpal joint of the thumb* (flexion, extension, abduction, adduction and opposition).
- The *metacarpophalangeal joints* of the fingers (flexion, extension, abduction and adduction).
- The *interphalangeal joints* (flexion and extension).

An inability to move these joints may be caused by joint disease, soft tissue thickening, divided tendons or paralysed muscles.

The circulation

Inspection

Pallor of the fingers indicates arterial insufficiency or anaemia. During an episode of vasospasm, the fingers may be white or blue (see Chapter 10). Observe the degree of filling of the veins on the back of the hands. Ischaemic atrophy of the pulps

of the fingers makes the fingers thin and pointed. Ischaemic ulcers, small abscesses and even frank gangrene may be visible (see Chapter 10).

Palpation

Feel the temperature of the skin of each finger. Feel both pulses (radial and ulnar) at the wrist (see Chapter 10). The digital arteries can sometimes be felt on either side of the base of the fingers.

Capillary return

A crude indication of the arterial inflow to the fingers can be obtained from watching the rate of filling of the vessels beneath the nail after emptying them by pressing down on the tip of the nail (see Chapter 10).

Allen's test

Ask the patient to clench one fist tightly, and then compress the ulnar and radial arteries at the wrist with your thumbs. After 10 seconds, ask the patient to open their hand. The palm will be white. Release the compression on the radial artery, and watch the blood flow into the hand.

Slow flow into one finger caused by a digital artery occlusion will be apparent from the rate at which that finger turns pink.

Repeat the procedure, but first release the pressure on the ulnar artery.

Auscultation

Listen with the bell of your stethoscope over any abnormal areas. Vascular tumours and arteriovenous fistulas may produce a bruit, and sometimes a palpable thrill (see Chapter 10).

Measure the blood pressure in both arms.

The nerves

The nerves should be examined in accordance with their anatomical distribution, remembering that each nerve has **s**ensory, **m**otor, **a**utonomic, **r**eflex and **t**rophic (**SMART**) function (see Chapter 3 and *Investigation and Management*, Chapter 7).

The skin and connective tissues

Much will have been learnt about the skin after studying its circulation and innervation. Be careful to note any colour changes and any inflammatory processes.

It is also important to palpate the palmar fascia, as thickening and contraction of this structure are a common cause of contraction deformities (**Dupuytren's contracture**).

Also note any change in the shape or configuration of the hand and digits, and any abnormal skin creases.

Hyperextensibility of the joints may indicate a connective tissue disorder such as Ehlers–Danlos syndrome.

The wrist, elbow, shoulder, thoracic outlet and neck

Examine the wrist, elbow, shoulder, thoracic outlet and neck because abnormalities at these sites can cause symptoms in the hand.

Recording data about the hand

Inadequate or misleading records of hand pathology can lead to serious errors. *It is imperative to state which hand you are describing and record in words: RIGHT or LEFT. A bad R can easily be confused with an L.*

Name the digits

Some people prefer to number rather than name the digits, the first digit being the thumb, the second digit the index finger and so on. But unless you remember to write the word 'digit' every time, you will eventually make a mistake because the first finger, which is the index finger, is the second digit.

Do not use this system; always use their proper names: thumb, index, middle, ring and little finger.

If you are marking a patient for surgery, ensure the arrow is directed to the digit involved. In addition, mark the radial or ulnar aspect of the digit if one side or the other is to be operated.

ABNORMALITIES AND CONDITIONS OF THE HAND

Congenital abnormalities

There are three common congenital skeletal abnormalities in the hand:

- Part of the hand (usually a digit) may be absent (*acheiria/adactyly*).
- There may be an extra digit (*polydactyly*) (Fig. 7.23).
- The digits may be fused (*syndactyly*) (Fig. 7.24).

Fig. 7.23 Polydactyly.

Fig. 7.24 Syndactyly.

All these abnormalities are rare, but immediately recognizable.

Dupuytren's contracture

This is a thickening and shortening of the palmar fascia and the adjacent connective tissues that lie deep to the subcutaneous tissue of the hand and superficial to the flexor tendons. The cause of this change in the fascia is not known. As the thickening increases, the fascia becomes attached to the skin of the palm.

The condition is known to occur in response to **repeated local trauma** and in association with **cirrhosis of the liver**, but in most cases there is no obvious predisposing cause.

History

Age Dupuytren's contracture usually begins in middle age, but usually progresses so slowly that most patients do not present until old age.

Sex Males are affected ten times more often than females.

Symptoms There is a **nodule in the palm**. The patient may notice a thickening in the tissues in the palm of the hand, near the base of the ring finger, many years before the contractures develop (Fig. 7.25).

Contraction deformities occur. The patient notices an **inability to fully extend the metacarpophalangeal joint of the ring finger, and later the little finger**. The finger can be pulled so far down into the palm of the hand that it becomes useless if the contraction of the palmar fascia becomes severe (Fig. 7.26).

There is usually no pain associated with this condition, but the nodule in the palm may be slightly tender.

Development The nodule gradually enlarges, and the strands of contracting fascia become prominent. Deep creases form where the skin becomes tethered to the fascial thickening, and the skin in these creases may get soggy and excoriated. The deformity of the fingers slowly increases.

Fig. 7.25 Dupuytren's contracture, showing puckering of the skin.

Fig. 7.26 Dupuytren's contracture – anterior view.

Multiplicity Dupuytren's contracture is commonly bilateral and can also occur in the feet.

Cause The known predisposing factors are shown in Revision panel 7.3. Dupuytren's contracture may follow repeated trauma to the palm of the hand, which is probably why it used to be found in shoe repairers and other manual workers, but nowadays it is uncommon to find a convincing cause.

Revision panel 7.3

Factors associated with Dupuytren's contracture

Alcoholism

Epilepsy

Diabetes

Repeated trauma

Family history

Systemic disease There may be symptoms of **epilepsy** or **cirrhosis of the liver**. There is a higher incidence of the condition in patients suffering from these diseases. The reasons for these associations are unexplained.

Family history Dupuytren's contracture can be familial. If so, it is inherited in an **autosomal dominant** manner.

Examination

Palpation of the palm of the hand reveals a firm, irregularly shaped nodule with indistinct edges, 1–2 cm proximal to the base of the ring finger. Taut strands can be felt running from the nodule to the sides of the base of the ring and little fingers, and proximally towards the centre of the flexor retinaculum. These bands get tighter if you try to extend the fingers.

The skin is puckered and creased, and tethered to the underlying nodule.

The deformity The metacarpophalangeal joint and the proximal interphalangeal joint are flexed because the palmar fascia is attached to both sides of the proximal and middle phalanges. The distal interphalangeal joint tends to extend. The ring finger is most affected and may be pulled down so far that its nail digs into the palm of the hand (Fig. 7.26).

CHAPTER 7 | UPPER LIMB SYMPTOMS AND SIGNS

The flexion deformity is not lessened by flexing the wrist joint.

Local tissues The rest of the hand is normal. There may be some thickening of the subcutaneous tissue on the back of the proximal phalanges of the affected fingers, sometimes called *Garrod's pads*.
General examination There may be evidence of liver disease (see Chapter 15), but this is a rare association.

The condition may be present in the feet (**lederhosen disease**) or penis (**Peyronie's disease**) (see Chapter 18).

Congenital contracture of the little finger

The patient is rarely aware of the fact that they have a deformity, accepting it as the normal shape of their little finger.

It is mentioned here because, although it is the opposite deformity to a Dupuytren's contracture, the student who is unaware of its existence may misdiagnose it.

Pick up a tea cup with your thumb and index finger and hook your little finger in the manner of the affected snob at a tea party. You will find that you have extended your metacarpophalangeal joint and flexed both of the interphalangeal joints. Someone with a congenital contracture of the little finger has this deformity all the time and cannot straighten the finger (Fig. 7.27).

Fig. **7.27** Congenital contracture of the little finger.

Volkmann's ischaemic contracture

This is a shortening of the long flexor muscles of the forearm, caused by fibrosis of the muscles, secondary to ischaemia. The common causes of the ischaemia are direct arterial damage at the time of a fracture near the elbow (most often a supracondylar fracture (see below), a tight plaster that restricts blood flow and arterial embolism.

History

Age Supracondylar fractures are common in children and young adults (see page 249), so Volkmann's contracture often begins between the ages of 5 and 25 years.
Cause The patient usually knows the cause of the deformity because they can clearly relate the loss of finger extension to their injury. Indeed, the loss of finger movements frequently begins while the arm is immobilized for the treatment of the fracture.
Symptoms When muscles become ischaemic, they are **usually painful**. If a patient complains of pain under their plaster at a point distant from the site of the fracture, **remove the plaster** and examine the muscles carefully.

Movements of the fingers, especially extension, become painful and then limited. This is more noticeable if there is no restriction of movement caused by a coexisting fracture. The patient soon discovers that they can extend their fingers if they flex their wrist when the forearm is not in a plaster cast.

The skin of the hand will be cold and pale as the blood supply of the hand is also diminished.

Ischaemia of the nerves in the anterior compartment (the median and anterior interosseous nerves) often causes **'pins and needles' (paraesthesia) in the distribution of the median nerve**, and sometimes the severe burning pain of ischaemic neuritis.

Development As the acute phase passes, the pain slowly fades away, but the restriction of finger extension increases, and the hand becomes claw-like. The patient may present with a fully developed deformity.

Examination

Inspection The skin of the hand is usually pale, and the hand looks wasted. All the finger joints are flexed, and the anterior aspect of the forearm is thin and wasted. The deformity is called a '**claw hand**' (Fig. 7.28).

Palpation In the acute phase, the forearm is swollen and tense, but once this has passed the forearm feels thin, the hand is cool and the pulses at the wrist may be absent. In the later stages, the fibrosis and shortening make the forearm muscles hard and taut.

Movement **Extension of the fingers is limited**, but improves as the wrist is flexed. This is an important sign, as it differentiates Volkmann's ischaemic contracture from Dupuytren's contracture.

Further flexion of the fingers (beyond the deformity) can occur, but the grip is weak. All other hand movements are present, but may be difficult to perform with the fingers fixed in an acutely flexed position.

Passive forced extension of the fingers is painful in the acute stage and uncomfortable in the established condition.

An important diagnostic feature of an ischaemic contracture is that all the muscles, even the damaged ones, have some function, whereas in a claw hand caused by a nerve lesion, some of the muscles are completely paralysed.

Fig. **7.28** Volkmann's ischaemic contracture.

Local tissues The abnormalities in the arteries and nerves of the forearm and hand have already been described. The vessels and nerves above the level of the fracture should be normal if the contracture follows a fracture.

The heart, great vessels, subclavian and axillary arteries must be examined carefully in case they are the source of an arterial embolus.

Palpate the supraclavicular fossa for a cervical rib (see Chapter 9) or subclavian artery aneurysm (see Chapter 10).

Carpal tunnel syndrome

This is a condition in which the median nerve is compressed as it passes through the carpal tunnel – the space between the carpal bones and the flexor retinaculum. The compression can be caused by skeletal abnormalities, swelling of other tissues within the tunnel, or thickening of the retinaculum.

It is often associated with pregnancy, rheumatoid arthritis, diabetes, myxoedema, previous trauma and osteoarthritis, which all reduce the change in pressure/volume relationship.

History

Age and sex Carpal tunnel syndrome is common in middle-aged females, especially at the menopause.

Local symptoms **Pins and needles in the fingers**, principally the index and middle fingers, is the common presenting symptom. The thumb is sometimes involved.

Theoretically, the little finger should never be affected, as it is innervated by the ulnar nerve, but occasionally patients complain that the whole of their hand tingles.

Pain in the forearm may also occur. For some (so far unexplained) reason, patients often complain of a pain that radiates from the wrist, up along the medial side of the forearm. This is usually an aching pain, not pins and needles.

There may be an associated **loss of hand function**. As the compression increases, the axons in the nerve are killed, and objective signs of nerve damage appear. Because the sensitivity of the skin supplied by the median nerve is reduced, the patient notices that she drops small articles and cannot carry out delicate movements.

Note that this is not caused by a loss of muscle power, but by the loss of fine discriminatory sensation.

Ultimately, if the nerve damage is severe, there may be a loss of motor function, which presents as **weakness and paralysis of the muscles of the thenar eminence and the first two lumbricals** (see median nerve palsy in Chapter 3).

Patients are often **woken in the middle of the night** by their symptoms. This feature is difficult to explain, but is so characteristic that it is considered to be pathognomonic of the condition.

General symptoms An increase in weight commonly exacerbates the symptoms of carpal tunnel syndrome. A change in weight may be secondary to another disease such as myxoedema, diabetes or steroid therapy, or to physiological water retention, as in pregnancy.

The patient may have symptoms of arthritis in the wrist and other joints if the condition is secondary to rheumatoid arthritis or osteoarthritis.

Examination

Inspection The hand usually looks quite normal, except in advanced cases, where there may be visible **wasting of the muscles forming the thenar eminence** (Fig. 7.29).

Palpation Pressure on the flexor retinaculum does not produce the symptoms in the hand, but **holding the wrist fully flexed for 1 or 2 minutes may induce symptoms**. Light-touch sensitivity and two-point discrimination may be reduced in the skin innervated by the median nerve (palm, thumb, index and middle finger). The loss of muscle bulk in the thenar eminence may be easier to feel when these muscles are contracting.

Fig. **7.29** Wasting of the thenar eminence.

The wrist pulses and the colour and temperature of the skin should be normal.

Movement All movements of the joints of the hand, active and passive, should be present.

Abduction, adduction and opposition of the thumb may be weak, but the muscles that cause these movements are seldom completely paralysed.

General examination There are two important aspects of the general examination.

First, you must exclude other causes of paraesthesia in the hand, such as **cervical spondylosis**, **cervical rib**, **peripheral neuritis** and **rare neurological disease**. This requires a detailed examination of the head, neck and arm.

Second, you must look for **evidence of the cause** of the carpal tunnel syndrome, such as pregnancy, rheumatoid arthritis, osteoarthritis or myxoedema.

Claw hand

This is a deformity in which all the fingers are permanently flexed (Fig. 7.30). Although an ulnar nerve paralysis makes the hand claw-like, because it causes flexion of the ring and little fingers, it does not cause a true claw hand, because only part of the hand is involved.

The causes of claw hand are neurological and musculoskeletal (see Revision panel 7.4 and Chapter 3).

Fig. **7.30** Ulnar claw hand.

Neurological causes

Remember these causes by thinking of the course of the nerve fibres from the spinal cord through the brachial plexus into the peripheral nerves. Although the deformity is caused by a loss of motor function, there is often an associated sensory loss:

- *Spinal cord* – poliomyelitis, syringomyelia, amyotrophic lateral sclerosis.
- *Brachial plexus* – trauma to the medial roots and cords, especially birth injuries of the lower cord, as in Klumpke's paralysis; infiltration of the brachial plexus by malignant disease.
- *Peripheral nerves* – traumatic division of the median and ulnar nerves; peripheral neuritis.

Musculoskeletal causes

- *Volkmann's ischaemic contracture* – this only causes a claw hand at rest, as the deformity can be reduced or abolished by flexion of the wrist.
- *Joint disease* – asymmetrical muscle tension, bone and joint deformities and subluxation of the finger joints caused by rheumatoid arthritis may produce a claw-like hand.

Trigger finger

This is a condition in which a finger gets locked in full flexion and will only extend after excessive voluntary effort, or with help from the other hand. When extension begins, it does so suddenly and with a click – hence the name trigger finger. The condition is caused by a thickening of the flexor tendon or paratenon, or a narrowing of the flexor sheath, preventing movement of the tendon within the flexor sheath.

History

Age and sex There are two groups of patients affected by this condition – middle-aged females and very young children. The thumb can be

affected in neonates and infants, but this is a rare condition.

Symptoms The patient complains that the **finger clicks and jumps as it moves**, **or gets stuck in a flexed position**.

A trigger finger is not usually a painful condition, even when force is required to extend it.

The disability gradually gets more severe, but a fixed, immovable flexed finger is uncommon.

Cause The patient can occasionally recall an injury to the palm of the hand, which may have caused the tendon or tendon sheath to thicken, but in most cases there is no indication of the cause.

Examination

Inspection The patient will show you how the finger gets stuck and how it snaps out into extension. The finger looks quite normal.

Palpation and movement The thickening of the tendon or tendon sheath can be felt at the level of the head of the metacarpal bone. During movement, the thickening can be felt snapping in and out of the tendon sheath.

General examination Trigger finger is not associated with any systemic musculoskeletal disease.

Mallet finger

This is a **fixed flexion deformity of the distal interphalangeal joint of a finger**, caused by an interruption of the extensor mechanism, either by a rupture of the extensor tendon, or by an avulsion fracture of its insertion. It is also known as **'baseball' finger** because the most common cause of the injury is a blow on the tip of the finger by a ball or hard object that forcibly flexes it against the pull of the extensor tendon, which then ruptures or pulls off the bone.

History

The patient usually remembers the original injury but, if the finger is not painful, may not complain about it until the deformity is established and a nuisance.

Symptoms The inability to extend the tip of a finger is not a great disability, but for a person with an occupation that requires fine finger movements, including full extension of the distal interphalangeal joints, the deformity can be a serious handicap. Some patients complain that the deformity is disfiguring.

Examination

When the patient holds out their hand, with the fingers extended, the distal phalanx of the affected finger remains flexed to 15–20° (Fig. 7.31). If you flex the distal interphalangeal joint to 90°, the patient can extend it back to the 20° position, but cannot get it straight.

Fig. 7.31 Mallet finger.

Ganglion

A ganglion is an encapsulated myxomatous degeneration of fibrous tissue. When a ganglion occurs on the anterior aspect of a flexor sheath, it can interfere with the grip, and cause pain and disability out of proportion to its size.

History

Age and sex Flexor sheath ganglia are most common in middle-aged males.

Symptoms The patient complains of a sharp pain at the base of one finger whenever they grip something tightly.

They may also notice a **lump at the site of the pain**.

Examination

Colour and temperature These are normal.

Site A small, tender nodule can be felt on the palmar surface of the base of a finger, superficial to the flexor sheath.

Tenderness Direct pressure on the lump is usually very painful.

Shape The nodule is spherical or hemispherical (Fig. 7.32).

Size Flexor sheath ganglia are usually quite small; some cause symptoms when they are only 2–3 mm in diameter.

Surface and edge The surface of the nodule is smooth, and the edge sharply defined.

Fig. 7.32 Soft multilocular ganglion on the back of the wrist.

Composition The nodule feels solid and hard. It is usually too small to permit the assessment of any other features such as fluctuation or translucency.

Lymph glands The local lymph glands should not be enlarged.

Local tissues The rest of the hand is normal.

Comment Benign giant cell tumours of the flexor sheath present in an identical manner, and are indistinguishable from flexor sheath ganglia.

Heberden's nodes

Heberden's nodes are bony swellings close to the distal finger joints. They are non-specific, and do not indicate any particular disease.

History

The patient complains of **swelling and deformity of their knuckles**. There may be a history of an old injury to the finger, or aching pains in both the lumps and the joints.

Examination

Heberden's nodes are commonly found on the dorsal surface of the fingers just distal to the distal interphalangeal joint. They are not mobile, and can be easily recognized as part of the underlying bone (Fig. 7.33).

The joint movements may be slightly restricted by osteoarthritis, and there may be radial deviation of the distal phalanx. The index finger is most often affected. Small adventitious bursae may develop between the skin and the nodes. Similar nodes may appear near the proximal interphalangeal joint.

Comment Heberden's nodes do not indicate any specific underlying bone or joint disease, and have no clinical significance. They should not be confused with rheumatoid nodules, which are areas of necrosis

Fig. 7.33 Heberden's nodes.

surrounded by fibroblasts and chronic inflammatory cells, and are found in all types of connective tissue. Patients with rheumatoid nodules invariably have other evidence of rheumatoid arthritis.

Rheumatoid arthritis in the hand

The symptoms and signs of rheumatoid arthritis are described in Chapter 6, but, as this disease so often affects the hand, its manifestations are described again here. All the deformities of rheumatoid arthritis result from the combination of an uneven pull by the tendons and destruction of the joint surfaces.

Thickening of the joints

The joints most affected are the metacarpophalangeal and the proximal interphalangeal joints. Swelling of these joints gives the finger a fusiform, spindle shape.

Ulnar deviation of the fingers

The fingers are pulled towards the ulnar side of the hand, causing a varus deformity at the metacarpophalangeal joints. In advanced disease, the varus deformity can be as much as 45–60°.

Flexion of the wrist

The wrist joint develops a fixed flexion deformity and usually some ulnar deviation (Fig. 7.34).

Fig. 7.34 Rheumatoid arthritis of the hands.

'Swan neck' deformity of the fingers

This deformity is hyperextension of the proximal interphalangeal joint, and flexion of the distal interphalangeal joint. It is caused by fibrotic contraction of the interosseous and lumbrical muscles (Fig. 7.35).

Fig. 7.35 Swan neck deformity.

Boutonnière deformity

The joint deformities of this abnormality are the opposite of those of the 'swan neck' deformity: flexion of the proximal interphalangeal joint, and hyperextension of the distal interphalangeal joint (Fig. 7.36).

It is caused by the projection and trapping of the flexed proximal interphalangeal joint through a rupture of the central portion of the extensor tendon expansion.

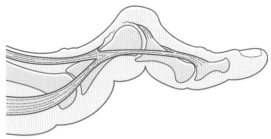

Fig. 7.36 Boutonnière deformity.

Tendon ruptures

In severe rheumatoid arthritis, any tendon may undergo attrition (damage from friction) and rupture. This causes a variety of deformities. The most common tendons to rupture are the long extensor tendons of the fingers and thumb.

CHAPTER 7 | UPPER LIMB SYMPTOMS AND SIGNS

Compound palmar 'ganglion'

This is a term that is applied to an effusion in the synovial sheath that surrounds the flexor tendons. It is not a ganglion. In the UK, it is now invariably secondary to rheumatoid arthritis, but in many other parts of the world it is almost always caused by a **tuberculous synovitis**.

History

The most common presenting symptom is **swelling on the anterior aspect of the wrist** and sometimes in the palm of the hand. **Pain is uncommon**.

The patient may notice crepitus during movements of the fingers.

Paraesthesia may occur in the distribution of the median nerve.

Examination

Distension of the flexor tendon synovial sheath produces a soft, fluctuant swelling that can be felt on the anterior aspect of the wrist and lower forearm, and in the palm of the hand. Because the swelling passes beneath the flexor retinaculum, compression of the lump on one side of the retinaculum makes it distend on the other side.

Crepitus may be felt during palpation and when the patient moves their fingers. This is caused by the presence of fibrin bodies within the synovial sheath – commonly called 'melon seed bodies'.

There are no local signs of inflammation.

General examination All the joints should be examined to exclude rheumatoid arthritis, and the chest should be examined (and X-rayed) to exclude tuberculosis.

The nails

Inspection of the nails often yields useful information about the patient's general health. Conditions of the nails are described in Chapter 4.

FRACTURES AND DISLOCATIONS OF THE UPPER LIMB

Fractures of the upper limb occur at all ages, the most common cause being a fall onto the outstretched hand. A history of the mechanism of injury suggests which bones and joints are likely to have been injured. High-energy trauma indicates that other possible injuries must be assessed. Conversely, patients with multiple injuries should have their upper limbs included in the secondary survey (see Chapter 5).

FRACTURES OF THE CLAVICLE

These common injuries can occur in children and adults. Most are the result of a fall directly onto the shoulder, although some result from a direct blow and less commonly a fall onto the outstretched hand.

The site can be the:

- middle third (80 per cent);
- lateral third (15 per cent);
- medial third (5 per cent).

History

There is pain and tenderness. Arm movements hurt, especially cross-arm abduction.

Examination

Distortion and swelling are apparent at the fracture site (Fig. 7.37).

The overlying skin may be lifted and give the appearance that it will be pierced by a spike of bone, although this is event is very unusual.

The shoulder is rotated anteriorly and inferiorly, and the arm is often held supported by the other hand.

Associated injuries of the brachial plexus and blood vessels (see Chapters 3 and 10) must be excluded in all cases.

Fig. 7.37 Fractures of the clavicle and scapula.

FRACTURES OF THE SCAPULA

Considerable direct force (such as a blow on the back of the shoulder from a fall) is required to cause a scapular fracture as the bulky surrounding muscles protect the bone. Additional injuries to the ribs and chest are common.

Scapular fractures can be subdivided into those of the body, spine, neck, glenoid, acromion and coracoid process:

- *Fractures of the body and spine* cause pain and bruising. The arm is held adducted, and all shoulder movements are restricted.
- *Fractures of the neck* are often associated with fractures of the humerus or clavicle. The glenoid, which is effectively lying free, is usually displaced inferiorly by the weight of the arm.
- *Fractures of the glenoid* may be minor and associated with shoulder dislocation (see below), or more severe and comminuted, when there is severe bruising and swelling with restriction of all shoulder movements.
- *Fractures of the acromion and coracoid* are caused by direct blows and produce local pain and tenderness with restricted shoulder movements.

INJURIES OF THE ACROMIOCLAVICULAR JOINT

Dislocation and subluxation of this joint is a common sports injury from a fall onto the shoulder or less commonly the outstretched hand. The acromioclavicular and strong costoclavicular ligaments are disrupted to a varying extent.

This may be a simple sprain involving only the acromioclavicular ligaments, or involve a total disruption of all the ligaments. The position of the clavicle varies accordingly, and may be relatively well aligned, or severely displaced upwards, backwards or very rarely downwards (Fig. 7.38).

History

There is always pain and swelling over the joint. All shoulder movements are restricted and painful.

Examination

The joint appears swollen and is tender to palpation. The arm is held adducted.

The lateral end of the clavicle is usually displaced upwards relative to the downwards displacement of the shoulder; hence there is an altered contour. It may be reduced back into place, but springs back when the pressure is released.

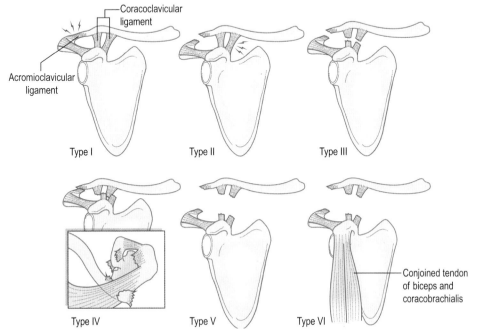

(a) Types of ACJ injury.

Fig. 7.38 DISLOCATION OF THE ACROMIOCLAVICULAR JOINT (ACJ)

CHAPTER 7 | UPPER LIMB SYMPTOMS AND SIGNS

(b) Clinical appearance of a type V ACJ injury.

Fig. 7.38 DISLOCATION OF THE ACROMIOCLAVICULAR JOINT (ACJ) (CONTINUED)

INJURIES OF THE STERNOCLAVICULAR JOINT

This joint is injured much less commonly, and can be damaged without a history of trauma. The grade of injury again varies between a partial ligamentous tear (a sprain) to total disruption with anterior, or less commonly posterior, displacement of the medial end of the clavicle.

A direct blow in a road traffic or sporting accident applies medial force to the lateral aspect of the shoulder.

The injury can also occur from a fall onto an outstretched hand.

History

The pain is made worse by shoulder abduction and adduction.

Examination

There is localized tenderness over the swollen joint. The medial end of the clavicle is prominent with an anterior dislocation, and lies downwards and forwards. With posterior dislocation, the normal anterior bony clavicular contour is lost.

Associated injuries Venous congestion and arterial damage to major blood vessels, or dyspnoea from a pneumothorax or tracheal injury, can all occur.

DISLOCATION OF THE GLENOHUMERAL JOINT

The shoulder is the most mobile joint in the body, but with the least bony stability. This makes it very likely to dislocate.

There are two peaks of incidence, the first between 16 and 25 years, associated with trauma, and the second much later in the elderly, when the stability is impaired by muscle weakness and falls become more frequent.

Anterior dislocation

This is far more common, usually caused by a fall with the shoulder in an abducted and externally rotated position.

There is severe pain and loss of shoulder movements.

On examination, the shoulder contour is flattened or lost, and the arm, often supported by the opposite hand, is held in slight abduction and internal rotation. The acromion and humeral head appear prominent (Fig. 7.39), and all movements are limited and painful.

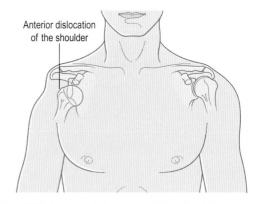

Anterior dislocation of the shoulder

Fig. 7.39 Anterior dislocation of the shoulder.

Posterior dislocation

Posterior dislocation is less common. It is caused by a fall onto an outstretched internally rotated arm.

This can also occur during an epileptic fit, or can follow a direct blow on the front of the shoulder.

On examination, the shoulder appears normal in contour, but the arm is held adducted and internally rotated. Abduction is limited, and external rotation beyond the neutral position is very difficult.

Inferior dislocation (luxatio erecta)

This is rare. The patient is in great pain, and the arm is held above the head. The humeral head may be palpable over the lateral chest wall. There is a high incidence of associated neurovascular injury.

Complications

There is a high rate of recurrent shoulder dislocation, particularly in the younger population. Associated humeral fractures can occur. The axillary nerve is injured in 10–20 per cent of cases, and can be assessed by testing pinprick sensation over the 'regimental patch' area on the lateral aspect of the proximal humerus. Other brachial plexus injuries occur less frequently. The rotator cuff tendons can be torn during the injury, especially in the elderly.

FRACTURES OF THE HUMERUS

The site can be:

- Proximal.
- Shaft.
- Distal/supracondylar.

Proximal fractures

These are the most common and occur in all age groups, especially in elderly patients with osteoporosis and in young children. A fall onto the outstretched hand is the most common cause, but a direct blow on the outer arm can also be responsible. Fractures may involve the surgical neck, the anatomical neck, the greater tuberosity, the lesser tuberosity or a combination, whereby they are described as two-part, three-part or four-part fractures.

History

Pain, swelling and restriction of shoulder movement suggest a fracture.

Examination

There is tenderness, swelling and restricted arm movement with crepitus. Significant bruising may develop down the arm. There may be an associated neurovascular injury, especially to the axillary nerve, and shoulder dislocation.

Humeral shaft fractures

These occur at all ages, usually caused by a direct blow from a motor car accident or a fall. They can also follow a fall onto the elbow or outstretched hand. Twisting injuries, caused by arm wrestling, can result in spiral fractures.

History

There is pain and loss of use of the arm.

Examination

Tenderness, swelling/bruising and deformity with crepitus are seen. The deformity depends upon the force applied and the relationship of the muscle insertions to the site and direction of the fracture (spiral or transverse).

In upper third fractures, the proximal fragment is pulled into adduction by the action of the pectoralis major muscle, while in the middle third the proximal fragment is abducted by the deltoid.

A radial nerve injury complicates 20 per cent of humeral shaft fractures and results in a wrist drop.

Distal/supracondylar fractures

In children, fractures around the elbow are common. Supracondylar fractures have a peak incidence at 8 years and result from a hyperextension of the elbow, with the olecranon levering on the back of the humerus, during a fall onto an outstretched hand.

History

A painful swollen elbow occurs, with restricted movement.

Examination

The inferior fragment is *usually* displaced backwards, and the humeral shaft appears prominent and may tent the overlying skin. The olecranon is palpable posteriorly and appears displaced upwards

CHAPTER 7 | UPPER LIMB SYMPTOMS AND SIGNS

(Fig. 7.40). Occasionally, the distal fragment is displaced anteriorly.

Neurovascular injuries are commonly associated. The radial, median and ulnar nerves may all be damaged, but injury to the brachial artery is especially important. The vessel may be torn, stretched, lacerated or trapped in the fracture fragments. It may be transected or thrombosed, or the intima may be torn. Look carefully for the radial pulse and signs of arterial compromise (pain, pallor, paraesthesia, paralysis and perishing cold).

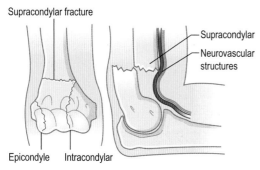

Fig. 7.40 Supracondylar and intracondylar fracture of the humerus.

Fractures of the medial epicondyle

These are much more common in children than adults, and are caused by a direct blow, a fall onto the outstretched hand with the wrist hyperextended, or avulsion by the ulnar collateral ligament during elbow dislocation. The pain is made worse by elbow flexion, and the medial epicondyle is tender, swollen and bruised.

Fractures of the lateral epicondyle are less common but present in a similar manner to medial epicondyle fractures, although they involve the outer aspect of the joint.

In the adult, *distal humeral fractures* occur following a fall on the outstretched hand. The clinical features are as for children, but there may be more comminution and angulation of the fracture fragments.

Intracondylar fractures

Intracondylar fractures, which are T- or Y-shaped fractures extending into the articular surface, can also occur (Fig. 7.40). They cannot be differentiated clinically from supracondylar fractures.

DISLOCATION OF THE ELBOW

The elbow is the second most common large joint to dislocate, and this can occur in children and adults. It can be confused with a supracondylar fracture.

The majority of dislocations are in a posterior direction. Disruption of the ulnar collateral ligament or fracture of the medial epicondyle allows the radial head and olecranon to displace backwards behind the lower end of the humerus.

Anterior dislocation can occasionally occur following a blow on the back of the elbow.

History

A fall onto the outstretched hand in a teenager or young adult is the usual cause.

Examination

In posterior dislocation, the elbow is swollen and held in 45° of flexion. The olecranon appears very prominent, and its relationship with the medial and lateral epicondyles is disrupted, unlike in supracondylar fractures, where the relationship is maintained (Fig. 7.41).

In anterior dislocation, the elbow is extended, and the olecranon cannot be felt in its usual position. The forearm appears elongated and is held supine.

Neurovascular injuries of the median and ulnar nerves and brachial artery must be carefully excluded in all patients with elbow dislocations.

Associated fractures are common, especially of the medial epicondyle and coronoid process.

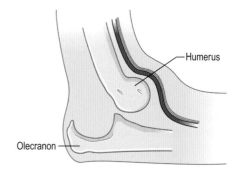

Fig. 7.41 Posterior dislocation of the elbow.

FRACTURES OF HEAD AND NECK OF RADIUS

These occur at all ages, in isolation or with other fractures and elbow dislocation. They may be displaced or undisplaced, comminuted or simple, and may involve the articular surface. A transverse fracture across the neck of the radius can lead to the radial head lying free from the shaft. The fracture line may alternatively run through the head itself.

The mechanism of injury is usually a fall onto the outstretched hand, which causes the radial head to impact against the capitellum, disrupting the distal radio-ulnar joint and the interosseous membrane, and fracturing the radial head.

History

The elbow joint is swollen and painful.

Examination

The joint is swollen by haemarthrosis, and there is localized tenderness over the head of the radius. Elbow movements and forearm rotation are painful and diminished. During recovery, elbow extension is usually the last movement to be restored. The distal radio-ulnar joint and interosseous membrane may also be tender, with subluxation of the distal end of the ulna (an **Essex-Lopresti** fracture–dislocation).

FRACTURES OF THE OLECRANON

Rare in children, the fracture can be displaced or undisplaced, transverse, oblique or comminuted. The mechanisms of injury may be a direct blow, or a fall onto the elbow or outstretched hand when the elbow is flexed and the triceps is forcefully contracted.

History

There is pain and swelling over the back of the elbow.

Examination

It may not be possible to extend the elbow and there is tenderness and a palpable swelling over the point of the elbow. A gap can sometimes be felt between the bone fragments.

Complications

The ulnar nerve is at risk and must be tested (see Chapter 3).

FRACTURES OF THE SHAFTS OF THE RADIUS AND ULNA

These bones articulate at each end, bound by the annular ligament and inferior radio-ulnar ligaments, and are further held together by the strong interosseous membrane. This allows the curved radius to rotate around the straight ulna, such that they act as a single unit. It means that fractures or dislocations of the shafts of either bone are often accompanied by similar injuries in the other.

A **Galeazzi fracture** occurs when there is a fracture between the middle and distal thirds of the radius, accompanied by a subluxation/dislocation of the distal radio-ulnar joint (Fig. 7.42a).

A **Monteggia fracture** occurs when there is a fracture of the proximal third of the ulna, accompanied by a dislocation of the radial head (Fig. 7.42b).

Most commonly, these injuries are the result of a fall onto the front or back of an outstretched hand. Direct trauma can also fracture both bones, such as in road traffic accidents. In a Monteggia fracture-dislocation, there may be forced pronation of the arm at the moment of impact.

When the arm is raised to protect the head from attack, a direct blow from a blunt instrument can cause an isolated ulnar fracture (a **nightstick fracture**).

(a) A Galeazzi fracture.

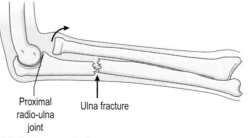

(b) A Monteggia fracture.

Fig. 7.42 FRACTURES OF THE SHAFTS OF THE RADIUS AND ULNA

CHAPTER 7 | UPPER LIMB SYMPTOMS AND SIGNS

In children, greenstick fractures are very common, and displacement is often minimal.

History

There is pain, swelling, deformity and an inability to rotate the forearm. Associated injuries may interfere with movement of the wrist or elbow.

Examination

There is an obvious deformity if both bones are broken, with localized tenderness and swelling over the fracture lines. Examine the elbow and wrist to exclude dislocation of the radial head (see above) and distal radio-ulnar joints. Pronation and supination are prevented by severe pain.

Complications

Open fractures are not uncommon, but they are often associated with neurovascular complications (especially the posterior interosseous nerve) and other soft tissue damage. Compartment syndrome of the forearm can occur, and is a very important diagnosis not to miss.

FRACTURES OF THE DISTAL RADIUS AND ULNA

These are the most common fractures in both adults and children, with age peaks at 5–10 and over 50 years of age.

A **Colles' fracture** is an impaction fracture through the distal radial metaphysis within 2.5 cm of the wrist joint, with dorsal angulation, dorsal displacement, radial angulation and radial displacement. It was originally common in elderly patients, but is now recognized in all ages. It can be accompanied by a fracture of the ulnar styloid in 60 per cent of cases (Fig. 7.43a).

A **Smith's fracture** is also through the distal radius, but with volar displacement of the distal fragment. The fracture can extend into the joint (Fig. 7.43b). Smith's fractures are less common than Colles' fractures.

A **Barton's fracture** is subluxation or fracture–dislocation of the wrist accompanied by an intra-articular fracture of the distal radius. This causes the carpus and hand to displace backwards or forwards (Fig. 7.43c).

Fractures in children occur through either the metaphysis or the epiphysis. They can be minimally

(a) A Colles' fracture.

(b) A Smith's fracture.

Radius

(c) A Barton's fracture.

Fig. 7.43 FRACTURES OF THE DISTAL RADIUS AND ULNA

displaced greenstick fractures, where there is only slight buckling of the cortex (see Chapter 6), although complete fractures do occur.

Mechanism

Wrist fractures usually result from a fall onto the outstretched hand, common in snowy and icy conditions. Direct blows and motorcycle injuries are other causes. The direction of force often determines the type of fracture.

A Colles' fracture usually occurs when there is a fall onto an outstretched arm with the wrist in extension. In a Smith's fracture, the wrist is flexed on impact.

History

There is pain, deformity and an inability to move the wrist following a fall or injury.

Examination

A *dinner fork deformity* is typical of a Colles' fracture (Fig. 7.44), while in a Smith's fracture the hand is displaced forwards, with a swelling in front of the wrist. The fracture site is tender, and wrist movements are restricted.

Fig. 7.44 Dinner fork deformity from a distal radial fracture.

Complications

Open fractures following falls are rare. They happen when considerable force is involved, and the bones puncture the skin from within.

Injury to the median and ulnar nerves should always be excluded.

Forearm compartment and acute carpal tunnel syndromes can occur, and carpal tunnel syndrome can also develop once healing has been completed.

Reflex sympathetic dystrophy (Sudek's atrophy) complicates up to 40 per cent of wrist fractures, causing, pain, swelling, loss of joint mobility and vasomotor instability.

Rupture of the extensor pollicis tendon and osteoarthritis of the wrist joint are late complications.

FRACTURES OF THE SCAPHOID BONE

The scaphoid is the largest carpal bone, linking the two rows of carpal bones and the radiocarpal joint. The majority of its surface is articular, and most of its blood supply enters distally, so that fractures can cause devascularization of the proximal fragment.

The most common site for a fracture is through the waist of the bone (50 per cent), followed by the proximal half (38 per cent) and the distal half (12 per cent).

Mechanism

Fractures of the scaphoid account for three-quarters of all carpal injuries. They are usually caused by a fall onto the outstretched hand with the wrist extended. As the wrist hyperextends, the scaphoid is compressed by the distal radius.

The fracture may be complete or incomplete, angulated or rotated, displaced or undisplaced and occasionally comminuted.

History

The pain may be mild, and patients often think that they have only sprained their wrist.

Examination

The signs may be minimal. There is often some subtle swelling and localized tenderness in the anatomical snuff box (Fig. 7.45). Maximal passive radial and ulnar deviation of the wrist produces pain in the radial side of the wrist. Thumb compression may also induce pain.

Complications

Avascular necrosis of the proximal fragment is an important and not infrequent complication that leads to progressive bony collapse and late osteoarthritis.

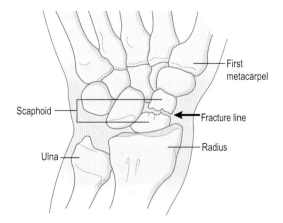

Fig. 7.45 Fracture of the scaphoid: tenderness in the anatomical snuff box.

Non-union of the fracture is also a common complication.

PERILUNATE AND LUNATE AND DISLOCATION OF THE WRIST

Dislocations of the carpus are an uncommon group of injuries. A perilunate dislocation occurs when the metacarpals, distal carpal row and part of the proximal row are dislocated (Fig. 7.46a). The term 'peri' is used to describe the bones that remain undisplaced in the proximal row. The lunate remains attached to the radius through a strong volar ligament, while the rest of the carpus dislocates posteriorly. These injuries may be associated with fracture of the scaphoid.

The distal row may alternatively realign with the radius, and part of the proximal row is extruded, causing a lunate dislocation (Fig. 7.46b). This is the most common carpal dislocation.

The injuries are usually caused by a fall onto an outstretched hand, or a road traffic accident causing extreme dorsiflexion of a radially deviated wrist.

History

Pain is often surprisingly mild, but wrist movements are uncomfortable.

Examination

Physical signs are subtle and the diagnosis, like that of a scaphoid fracture, is easily missed. There is usually some swelling, diffuse tenderness and discomfort on wrist movement. The median and ulnar nerves and wrist tendons may be damaged.

METACARPAL FRACTURES AND DISLOCATIONS

These bones can fracture at the shaft, base or neck. The usual mechanism is punching a hard object, either deliberately or in a fall. A direct blow on the back of the hand may also be responsible. Deformity is often minor, as the metacarpals are splinted by their fellows and surrounding muscles. Rotational deformity can interfere with hand function. The most common fracture is to the fifth metacarpal (a **Boxer's fracture**).

(a) Perilunate.

(b) Lunate.

Fig. 7.46 DISLOCATIONS OF THE WRIST

History

There is local pain, swelling and loss of hand function.

Examination

Local tenderness and swelling are seen, and occasionally a dorsal hump or a flattened knuckle.

Bennett's fracture–dislocation is an oblique fracture at the base of the first metacarpal bone extending into the carpometacarpal joint, making it unstable, with proximal and lateral subluxation of the thumb (Fig. 7.47b). The usual cause is a punch. The thumb is shortened because of posterior subluxation, and is swollen around its base.

In a *Rolando fracture*, there is a fracture at the base of the thumb metacarpal with a T- or Y-shaped extension (Fig. 7.47c). Its presentation and signs are similar to those of a Bennett's fracture.

FRACTURES AND DISLOCATIONS OF THE PHALANGES

Direct violence is the most common cause, and fractures may often be compound.

There is pain, loss of function, swelling, deformity and local tenderness.

Dislocations of finger joints are usually obvious from the deformity and loss of function. In the presence of significant swelling, however, they can be missed.

(a) Normal metacarpal bones.   (b) A Bennett's fracture.   (c) A Rolando's fracture.

Fig. 7.47 TYPES OF FIRST METACARPAL FRACTURES

CHAPTER 7 | UPPER LIMB SYMPTOMS AND SIGNS

8 Lower limb symptoms and signs

THE HIP

This is a very mobile ball and socket joint that articulates between the lower limb and the pelvis, supporting the weight of the body in both static and dynamic movement. It comprises:

- the head of the femur;
- the three bones that form the pelvis and acetabulum: the ilium, ischium and pubis;
- a tough membranous capsule lined by synovium;
- a labrum surrounding the socket;
- synovial fluid, which lubricates the joint;
- muscles and tendons, which assist in movement.

As with any joint, examination is based on the principles of:

- Look.
- Feel.
- Move.

These principles are followed using specific tests of anatomical structure and pathological conditions.

Remember that the examination of the hip is not complete until the joints below and above have also been assessed, namely **the knee** and **lower back**.

SYMPTOMS

The main symptoms caused by hip diseases are **pain** and **stiffness**.

Pain is classically experienced in the groin region, and the patient often points to or places their hand in this region. Pain from the hip joint can also be referred to the knee, and hip pathology can then be missed if the focus is on the other joint.

Equally, pain from the lower lumbar spine and sacroiliac joints can be experienced in the hip region, which is a consequence of their shared nerve supply from the L2, L3 and L4 nerve roots. This highlights the importance of always examining the joints above and below the joint under investigation.

Hip pain may be present at rest or can be related to activity. It becomes debilitating when patients experience night pain with sleep disturbance.

In the degenerate hip, stiffness in the morning is a common complaint, coupled with restriction of movement during the day. This results in **disability** and loss of functional capacity, such as the ability to put on socks and shoes. The patient may walk with a limp, using a walking stick for support.

Deformity of the hip can arise from congenital or acquired conditions, including trauma, infection and degenerative, neurological and neoplastic conditions, which affect the anatomical structures (Revision panel 8.1).

Revision panel 8.1

The causes of joint deformities

Skin – contractures

Fascia – contractures

Muscle – paralysis, fibrosis, spasm

Tendon – division, adhesion

Ligament – rupture, stretching

Capsule – rupture, fibrosis

Synovium – inflammation

Bone – changes in shape, trauma, pressure atrophy

PLAN FOR EXAMINATION OF THE HIP JOINT

Inspect the patient's surroundings, paying particular attention to any walking aids. If the patient's footwear is available, a quick inspection will demonstrate whether there is a heel raise and alert you to a limb length discrepancy.

First examine the patient standing up if possible. This gives you the opportunity to inspect the patient from the front, the side and then the back.

Next perform Trendelenburg's test and assess the patient's gait (see below). Then ask the patient to lie flat and straight on the couch, and check that the pelvis is square to the midline by feeling the positions of the anterior superior iliac spines. By examining a hip in this manner, unnecessary position changes are avoided during the examination.

Inspection

Skin

Remember that sinuses and scars from the hip joint are often found on the buttock and posterior aspect of the upper thigh, so look at the skin over the back of the joint as well as the front.

Shape

Check the contours of the thigh and buttock. Asymmetrical skin creases indicate joint displacement. Note any muscle wasting or rotational deformity. Also observe any increased lumbar lordosis or scoliosis (see Chapter 9).

Position

When the hip joint is painful or distended by an effusion, it is held slightly flexed and abducted. This flexion deformity may also be fixed. In cases of true shortening, once the anterior superior iliac spines are level, a degree of shortening may be apparent by noting that the heels are not level. This should stimulate an accurate assessment of shortening and limb length measurement (see Chapter 6).

Palpation

The capsule and synovium of the hip joint **cannot** be felt, but the bony contours of the pelvis and trochanter can be palpated. It is important to note any tenderness posterior to the greater trochanter

as this is indicative of trochanteric bursitis, which is often confused with hip joint pathology.

Relationship between the pelvis and femur

In cases of shortening, the position of the greater trochanter with respect to the pelvis (i.e. acetabulum) can be checked in three ways:

- *Bilateral palpation.* To compare the two sides, put your thumbs on the anterior superior iliac spines and your fingers on the tops of the greater trochanters. You will appreciate any difference in the distance between these points through the position of your fingers (Fig. 8.1).
- *Nélaton's line.* Turn the patient on their side, and imagine a line drawn from the anterior superior iliac spine to the ischial tuberosity (Fig. 8.2). The top of the greater trochanter should just touch this line. If it lies above the line, there is shortening of the neck of the femur or a dislocation of the hip.
- *Bryant's triangle.* This gives a measurement of the distance between the top of the greater trochanter and the coronal plane of the iliac spine. Lie the patient supine. Imagine a horizontal line passing through the anterior superior iliac spine. Measure the vertical distance between this line and the top of the greater trochanter (Fig. 8.3).

Nélaton's line and Bryant's triangle are now very rarely used clinically (as radiographs are much more accurate), but they are useful ways of remembering the normal relationships of the bony landmarks.

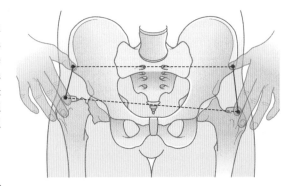

Fig. 8.1 Bilateral palpation. Thumbs placed on anterior superior iliac spines, index finger on greater trochanters. Length differences indicate pathology in femoral head or neck, e.g. developmental dysplasia of hip or fractures of the femoral neck.

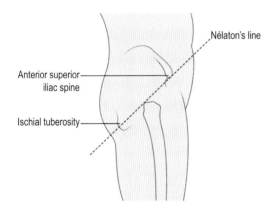

Fig. 8.2 Nélaton's line is a line drawn through the anterior superior iliac spine and the ischial tuberosity. It should just touch the top of the greater trochanter.

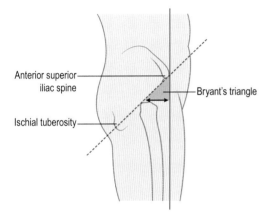

Fig. 8.3 Bryant's triangle measures the vertical distance from the anterior superior iliac spine to the greater trochanter, and the horizontal distance between the coronal planes of the iliac spine and the trochanter.

Movement

This can be divided into active and passive. The passive range is generally more useful in determining pathology in the hip joint.

The **normal range of hip movement** is:

- Flexion 0–130°.
- Extension 0–10°.
- Internal rotation 45°.
- External rotation 45°.
- Abduction 45°.
- Adduction 30°.

The range of movement in the hip can be restricted by stiffness, but unlike the glenohumeral (ball and socket) joint of the shoulder, it is less likely to present with instability problems because of increased movement.

Test for fixed flexion

When the hip joint is stiff, the range of movement may appear to be preserved by compensation from the surrounding joints. Fixed deformities of adduction and abduction will be clearly visible from the position of the thigh when you set the pelvis square with the spine, but fixed flexion can be masked by a lumbar lordosis.

To assess for fixed flexion, place your left hand underneath the hollow of the lumbar spine. Ask the patient to bring both knees up to their chest as far as possible. At this point, you can assess hip flexion of both hips and note any discrepancies between the limbs. The lumbar lordosis should be obliterated at this point.

Next ask the patient to let one leg lie back on the couch. The thigh on that side will remain flat on the couch if the hip joint is normal. If the hip lifts off the couch, this indicates a loss of extension in that hip, which is referred to as a **fixed flexion deformity** (Fig. 8.4), and the angle of elevation, or fixed flexion, should be recorded. This is called *Thomas' test* for fixed flexion. Now flex the other leg to check the opposite joint.

Passive movements

You can only test the movements of a joint by keeping one of the bones that forms the joint still, and moving the other bone. A false impression of hip movement may be obtained if the pelvis moves during the examination. Therefore, during all passive movements of the hip, you must continually check that the pelvis is not moving by keeping the thumb and little finger of one hand resting upon the two anterior superior iliac spines.

Flexion Flex the good hip and knee until the thigh presses against the abdomen, and get the patient to hold the leg in this position. Then flex the hip under consideration, using your other hand to check that no further pelvic movement takes place. Record the degree of flexion, and any fixed flexion deformity that is present (Fig. 8.5).

Abduction and adduction Keeping one hand firmly on the anterior superior iliac spines, abduct or adduct each leg until the pelvis begins to move, and record the range of movement (Fig. 8.6).

(a)

(b)

Fig. 8.4 THOMAS' TEST FOR FIXED FLEXION
Measure the degree of fixed flexion by flexing the good hip until the lumbar spine straightens and presses on your other hand placed beneath the lumbar spine. There is no fixed flexion in the left hip (a) but there is 25° of fixed flexion in the right hip (b).

Fig. 8.5 When testing hip movements such as flexion, place your fingers on the greater trochanter and your thumb on the iliac spine so that you detect any tilting of the pelvis.

Fig. 8.6 Keep your fingers and thumb stretched across the iliac spines when testing abduction and adduction to detect any movement of the pelvis.

Rotation Both internal and external rotation can be assessed by rolling the whole limb, but the best way is to flex the hip and knee to 90°. The foot can then be moved laterally to assess internal rotation, and medially to assess external rotation (Fig. 8.7). The range of movement can then be measured by comparing the position of the leg to the midline.

Abnormal movements The only abnormal movement you are likely to meet, except those caused by acute trauma, is '**telescoping**' of the joint, caused by a dislocated head of the femur sliding up and down the outer aspect of the ilium. This abnormal movement is detected by pushing and pulling the femur along its long axis while steadying the pelvis and feeling the top of the greater trochanter. It is sometimes easier to do this by flexing the hip to 90° and pulling the thigh upwards.

Extension Do this last, as you need to turn the patient onto their face. Put your hand under the knee and lift up the thigh, again steadying the pelvis with your other hand (Fig. 8.8). A normal hip extends only 2–5°.

With the patient standing

Look for deformities and abnormal skin creases from the front side and back if this has not already been done.

Trendelenburg test

With the patient standing, ask the patient to hold onto your forearms to provide support. Now ask the patient to stand on one leg, ensuring they do

Fig. 8.7 Rotation is measured by flexing the hip and the knee to 90° and rotating the femur by moving the foot back and forth across the line of the limb.

Fig. 8.8 With the patient lying on their front, lift each thigh and assess hip extension.

(a)   (b)

(a) Ask the patient to stand on one leg. There should be a raising of the pelvis on the opposite side, a negative Trendelenburg test.

(b) When the pelvis drops, the sign is positive.

(c) The pelvis remains parallel to the floor as the leg is raised, hence this is a negative test for pathology.

Fig. 8.9 TRENDELENBURG'S TEST

not flex the hip on the raised leg. The unsupported side of the pelvis should rise to help balance the trunk on the standing leg by bringing the centre of gravity over the weight-bearing foot (Fig. 8.9). This involves the use of the hip abductors – gluteus medius and minimus. The test is positive if the unsupported side of the pelvis falls and the patient has difficulty standing and leans on one of your forearms. A positive test means one of the following:

- The abductor muscles are paralysed.
- The joint is unstable (e.g. a congenital dislocation of the hip or a fracture of the neck of the femur).
- The insertion and origin of the abductor muscles are approximated, preventing their proper function, which is produced by a severe coxa vara or a dislocation of the hip.

CHAPTER 8 | LOWER LIMB SYMPTOMS AND SIGNS

Assessment of the gait

Ask the patient to walk. Observe their gait from the front, the rear and the side. Different patterns of gait can be recognized depending on the underlying pathology. An *antalgic or painful gait* occurs when there is a shortened stance phase and a lurch of the trunk towards the painful side during the stance phase.

This moves the centre of gravity of the body towards the painful hip, and decreases the moment arm of the body weight to the hip joint. This reduces the total force on the hip.

This is different from a *Trendelenburg gait*, which arises for the reasons outlined above, most commonly from adductor insufficiency, which can follow polio. The weakened gluteus medius allows the opposite side of the pelvis to tilt downwards during the stance phase on the weakened side. In an effort to compensate, the trunk lurches towards the weakened side (an abductor lurch) during the stance phase. In moving the centre of gravity towards the hip joint, there is a reduction in the effort that is required of the adductors.

Any instability of a joint becomes more noticeable during the stresses of walking.

Examination of the nerves and arteries of the limb

(see Chapters 3 and 10)

Joint disease is often secondary to neurological abnormalities).

CAUSES OF PAIN IN THE HIP

Trochanteric bursitis

There are two bursae that lie between the gluteus medius, gluteus minimus and tensor fascia lata muscles and their attachments to the greater tuberosity. These bursae can become inflamed, resulting in pain and disability.

History

Age and sex Trochanteric bursitis is usually seen in middle-aged patients, from 30 to 55 years. It is more common in females.

Cause Often no cause is elicited, although it may occur because of recurrent or unaccustomed activity, for example exercising at the gym or running. Symptoms can also arise and persist following an injury. Patients may have a previous history of other sites of bursal inflammation, such as the shoulder or knee.

Symptoms **Pain and weakness** are noted during hip movement. The pain may be activity related or occur at rest, and is usually centred over the lateral aspect of the hip joint. Patients are unable to lie on the affected side and have difficulty getting out of a chair and going up stairs.

Examination

There may be no visible swelling as the trochanteric bursa lies deep under the iliotibial band. *Palpation* is often painful, and *tenderness* is often localized over the greater trochanter.

Movements of the hip, particularly maximal flexion and then extension, may reproduce the pain. A clicking sound may be present, if the iliotibial band is also inflamed, as it moves over the greater tuberosity and the bursa.

Adductor tendinitis

Inflammation of the principal adductor muscles – pectineus, adductor magnus, adductor longus and adductor brevis – can occur.

History

Age and sex The majority of patients will be aged 30–50 years. The condition can affect both males and females. It is common in athletes, especially horse riders.

Symptoms **Pain** is classically centred in the groin in the region of the adductor muscles, and is exacerbated by exercise.

Examination

There are no visible manifestations of the inflammation, but palpation reveals tenderness over the insertion of the adductor muscles and down the inside of the thigh. Adduction of the hip causes localized pain in the groin and around the adductor tendon insertions on the medial aspect of the femoral shaft.

Iliopsoas tendinitis

The iliopsoas comprises two muscles that merge to form a single large tendon that inserts into the lesser trochanter. The iliacus arises from the ischium, and the psoas originates from the first to the fifth lumbar vertebrae.

History

Age and sex The condition arises in both males and females, most commonly from 20 to 50 years of age.
Symptoms Pain in experienced in the groin and can extend down the leg, sometimes to the knee. It increases with activity, and stiffness of the hip may develop. Some patients complain of a loud clicking sound in the groin.

Examination

Tenderness is felt on palpation of the groin, and flexion of the hip increases the pain. As the hip is flexed and then extended, the psoas tendon may, if it is inflamed and thickened, catch on the anterior superior iliac spine, lesser trochanter or iliopectineal ridge, giving a clicking sound.

Developmental dysplasia of the hip

Congenital dislocation of the hip is now known as developmental dysplasia of the hip. This describes the displacement of the femoral head relative to the acetabulum as the result of abnormal development, encompassing a spectrum of disorders of acetabular dysplasia and femoral head subluxation and dislocation.

History

Age and sex The condition occurs in 1.5 per 1000 live births, and usually presents from 0 to 4 years of age. It is more common in females than males (7 to 1). The left hip is more commonly affected. Other risk factors include being a first born, breech presentation, caesarean section, oligohydramnios and a positive family history.
Geography It is more common in the North and Eastern Mediterranean, because of a genetic predisposition. It is also more common in Lapp and North American Indian populations, who swaddle their babies with their legs together.

Examination

Every newborn child should be screened for hip instability.

   In **Ortolani's test**, the baby's thighs are held with the thumbs medially and the fingers resting on the greater trochanters; the hips are then flexed to 90°, which should normally be a smooth movement (Fig. 8.10). In the presence of dysplasia or dislocation,

(a) The hips are abducted and the joints are pushed forwards to demonstrate 'dislocation click'.

(b) The dislocation is reduced.

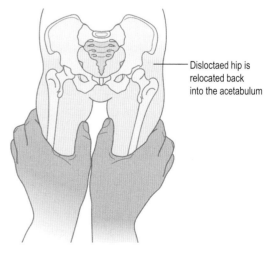

Disloctaed hip is relocated back into the acetabulum

(c) The lower limbs are pushed together and apart by the examiner.

Fig. 8.10 ORTOLANI TEST

CHAPTER 8 | LOWER LIMB SYMPTOMS AND SIGNS

there is resistance that is overcome when pressure is applied to the greater trochanter. There is a soft clunk as the hip is reduced.

Barlow's test is performed in a similar manner, but in this instance the examiner's thumb is placed in the groin and the thigh is then held (Fig. 8.11). By

(a) Forced adduction.

(b) Forced abduction.

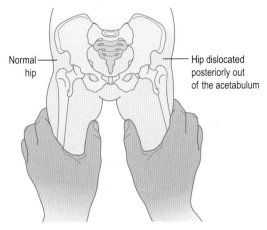

Normal hip —   — Hip dislocated posteriorly out of the acetabulum

(c) Forced abduction and adduction applied. Hip on left dislocates.

Fig. 8.11 BARLOW'S TEST

applying pressure with adduction and abduction, the examiner tries to dislocate the femoral head from the acetabulum.

A child may present later in life if the diagnosis was missed when he or she was newborn. Symptoms include clicking and gait disturbance because of a shortened leg and limitation of abduction. Affected individuals may have asymmetrical buttock skin creases.

Legg–Calve–Perthes' disease

This is an osteochondritis of the proximal femoral epiphysis caused by a vascular disturbance (see Chapter 6). The femoral head undergoes a form of avascular necrosis with remodelling.

History

Age and sex This occurs in 1 in 10 000 children and usually presents from 4 to 9 years of age. It is more common in males than females (4 to 1) and it is bilateral in 15 per cent of cases. There may be a family history.

Geography The condition is more common in Japanese and central European individuals. It is less common in native Australians, native Americans, Polynesians and black races.

Symptoms The child complains of **pain in the hip**, which is worse on activity. Although the pain is centred in the groin, it can radiate to the knee and cause a **limp**.

Examination

There is often little to find on examination, especially in the early stages, but the hip may be irritable with all movements. When the child is seen late in the progression of the condition, abduction is always limited, and this is often associated with a restriction of internal rotation. The older the child at the time of onset, the worse the prognosis.

Slipped upper femoral epiphysis

This occurs because of a slip in the hypertrophic zone of the cartilaginous growth plate of the upper femoral epiphysis. The head of the femur remains in the acetabulum, but the femoral shaft displaces anteriorly and rotates externally.

History

Age and sex This occurs in 1 in 10 000 children, and the condition usually develops between 10 and 14 years of age. Males are more affected than females, and generally present 2–3 years later than females. The left hip is more commonly affected, and 35 per cent of cases are bilateral.

Symptoms The child presents with pain in the groin radiating to the knee that is made worse by exercise, and begins to limp. There are often a series of minor episodes of pain rather than a single event, although 'acute-on-chronic' and isolated acute slips can occur. Half the cases are associated with some form of trauma.

Examination The child may become aware that the leg is turning outwards, and examination reveals that the leg is externally rotated and shortened by 1–2 cm. As the hip is flexed, it rotates into further external rotation.

The hip is not normally painful on movement unless there has been a recent acute slip.

Many of the children are fat or skeletally immature, and they may have an underlying hormonal imbalance, such as hypogonadism (Fröhlich child) or hypothyroidism.

Coxa vara

This condition may be congenital (noted at birth), developmental or acquired. It is usually the result of a defect in an ossification centre in the femoral neck, which leads to a decreased angle between the femoral head and neck. It is bilateral in 33 per cent of cases and occurs in 1 in 25 000 births.

Acquired causes include trauma, slipped upper femoral epiphysis and Perthes' disease (see above).

History

Symptoms The child usually presents aged 2–6 years with an altered gait, but otherwise they are relatively free of symptoms.

Examination

The gait may be waddling when the condition is bilateral, or a painless limp when the condition is unilateral.

The affected leg is shortened.

Movements of the hip are restricted in all directions, especially abduction and internal rotation.

Irritable hip

(Transient synovitis)

This is a condition in which there is a short-lived, nonspecific synovitis in the hip joint. The cause is often unknown, but it may follow a recent viral infection. A synovial effusion develops in the hip joint, and the condition usually resolves within 7 days.

History

Age and sex It occurs in 14 per 1000 children, and is more common in males than females (2 to 1). It usually occurs in 3–8-year-olds, and in 5 per cent of cases can affect both hips.

Symptoms The child presents with **acute pain in the hip**, **difficulty weight-bearing** and **a limp**. The pain may radiate to the knee, and is worse on activity.

Examination

All movements are painful and may be restricted.

Septic arthritis of the hip

Infection in the hip joint is relatively uncommon in adults, unless it is associated with a previous hip replacement.

History

It is more common in children, usually under the age of 2 years. Up to 50 per cent of neonates with the condition have adjacent infection in the bone metaphysis. The usual infecting organism is *Staphylococcus spp*.

Symptoms The child usually complains of localized pain in the groin and the medial aspect of the thigh. The pain is normally progressive and severe.

Examination

The child lies still with the hip flexed and externally rotated. All movements, especially internal rotation, are painful and resisted. The child does not want to weight-bear.

Palpation of the hip and groin is very tender.

Pyrexia, loss of appetite and sweating are usually present, and indicate the presence of systemic infection.

Tuberculosis of the hip

Chronic granulomatous infection caused by *Mycobacterium tuberculosis* usually arises in the hip from haematogenous spread. It can also develop from an osteomyelitis in an adjacent bone (see Chapter 6). The infection causes a synovitis and attacks both sides of the joint, leading to a rapid destruction of all the joint structures. It is usually monoarticular, and can initially be mistaken for other forms of arthritis.

History

Symptoms Pain in the groin is the usual presenting symptom.

Examination

The patient walks with a limp, and all joint movements are painful.

In chronic cases, muscle wasting is present and the limb may be shortened.

The hip may fuse (ankylosis) after gross joint destruction, when there will be no movement of the joint.

Osteoarthritis of the hip

The hip is one of the most common joints to be affected by osteoarthritis, which can be either primary or secondary (see Chapter 6).

History

Age and sex **Primary osteoarthritis** usually presents in patients over 50 years of age. The exact aetiology is unknown. It occurs in both males and females.

Secondary osteoarthritis can be predisposed to by developmental dysplasia of the hip, Perthes' disease, a slipped upper femoral epiphysis, avascular necrosis, a previous fracture or abnormal biomechanics. It often presents in a younger age group, with both males and females equally affected.

Symptoms Patients complain of **groin pain**, which is often accompanied by **pain in the knee**. Severe pain may cause **sleep disturbance**. Patients are usually **stiff in the morning** and often have **difficulty getting out of a chair**. They have **a reduced walking distance** and have to **stop frequently**. They complain of having **a limp** and may be helped by using a stick for support.

Dressing and washing becomes difficult, and they struggle to put their shoes and socks on and wash their feet.

Examination Deep palpation of the hip may elicit tenderness.

Hip movement produces variable pain. There may be a limited painless range of movement, followed by pain at the end of range.

There is often reduced flexion of the affected hip, and a positive Thomas' test. Abduction and adduction are also often restricted, with a loss of internal and external rotation.

The leg often lies in external rotation and adduction, and hence it may appear short. While there may be a true leg length discrepancy, you must measure both the true and apparent leg lengths to establish this. If the shortening is real, you must determine whether it is occurring above or below the hip joint (see Fig. 8.1).

When asked to walk, the patient will often have an **antalgic gait** and a **positive Trendelenburg test**.

Rheumatoid arthritis of the hip

As elsewhere in the body, rheumatoid arthritis attacks the synovium causing tissue destruction, articular cartilage erosion and progressive changes in the bones on either side of the hip joint, without osteophyte formation (see Chapter 6).

The signs and symptoms are similar to those of osteoarthritis, but the patient may also have other joints affected by the condition, especially in the hands (see Chapter 7).

Femoro-acetabular impingement

This is a relatively newly recognized condition, which is caused by a pinching mechanism in the hip joint. This may be the result of a **pincer** movement where the femoral head is over-covered by an acetabular rim prominence. During rotation, the femoral neck abuts against this prominence and the acetabular labrum, causing pain. The condition may also occur from a **cam** (shaft) mechanism that is the result of thickened bone at the junction between the femoral head and neck, which again causes impingement of the femoral neck against the acetabulum. It has been postulated that these pathologies can lead to osteoarthritis.

History

Age and sex The pincer type is more common in females and presents at age 30–40 years. The cam type is more common in athletic males between 20 and 30 years of age.

Symptoms Intermittent groin pain and limited movement are the usual presenting symptoms. The patient classically demonstrates a C-shaped distribution of pain over their hip (the C sign). The pain may be exacerbated by periods of prolonged sitting or be related to activity. It then can extend into the thigh, buttock and lower back. Patients may complain of a sudden catching and the hip giving way.

Examination

There is usually a painful restriction of internal rotation in flexion and adduction, known as a *positive hip impingement sign*.

Snapping hip

This is a snapping sensation experienced in the hip. It usually occurs in males aged 15–40 years, and is more common in athletes of both genders.

It is thought to be caused by the iliotibial band of the tensor fascia lata or the gluteus medius tendon sliding back and forth across the greater trochanter. It can also occur if the iliopsoas tendon catches on the anterior iliac spine or lesser tuberosity.

Intra-articular causes include loose bodies, acetabular labral defects and articular damage.

History

Symptoms Patients complain of a pop or snap when they move their hip, which may be associated with pain if the surrounding tissues become inflamed, The pain is usually relieved by rest and aggravated by activity.

Examination

When the hip is flexed and extended, the affected structures can be felt to snap across the bony prominence.

Avascular necrosis of the femoral head

This is also sometimes called 'osteonecrosis' or 'aseptic necrosis' and is caused by an occlusion of the microcirculation of the femoral head. This causes the bone and overlying articular cartilage to die, with subsequent collapse of the avascular portion, eventually leading to osteoarthritis (see above).

The causes are trauma (fractures of the femoral neck, acetabular fractures and hip dislocations; see page 290) and a number of systemic disorders including sickle-cell disease, decompression sickness and fat emboli. Other factors that may predispose to the condition include steroid treatment, excessive alcohol intake, radiation treatment, pregnancy, Perthes' disease, systemic lupus erythematosus and Gaucher's disease (see Chapter 6).

History

Age and sex Males aged around 40 years are most commonly affected, and in one-half the condition is bilateral.

Symptoms Deep pain in the groin is the usual presenting symptom, and patients may develop a limp.

Examination

All movements of the joint are painful, but they only become limited at a late stage in the disease.

THE KNEE JOINT

The joint is a synovial hinge joint between the femur and the tibia, and is the largest joint in the body. It has two articulations, one between the femur and the tibia, and the other between the femur and the patella. This allows flexion and extension of the lower leg and facilitates the transmission of loads when running, walking and jumping. Stability of the joint is provided by tendons, ligaments and muscles rather than bones.

SYMPTOMS

Adults with knee problems may present with pain, swelling, instability, locking, deformity or impaired function. The patient may point to a specific area of the knee or experience more diffuse symptoms. Remember that pain felt about the knee can arise from hip pathology and be referred to the region.

Knee pain can occur at rest or during movement and exercise. It can become debilitating and cause sleep disturbance.

In the degenerate knee, stiffness in the morning is a common complaint, coupled with restriction in of movement during the day. The patient may walk with a limp.

If the patient has injured the knee, they may state that the knee feels unstable and that it 'gives way'. This is usually due to disruption of the stabilizing ligaments. This is particularly common when ascending or descending stairs, or suddenly changing direction of travel.

The knee may also become locked in a position or significantly restricted in its range of movement; for example, the patient may state that they are unable to fully extend the knee. This may be a symptom of meniscal pathology.

PLAN FOR EXAMINATION OF THE KNEE JOINT

Inspection

Skin

Look at the skin all round the joint – front and back – for discolouration, scars, swellings and sinuses (see Fig. 6.1). Erythema may be associated with inflammation and infection, whereas bruising may indicate trauma. Note any skin conditions that are often associated with joint problems, such as psoriasis.

Shape

The contours of the knee joint are easy to see, and any bony or joint swelling distorts them at an early stage. The size of the whole joint should be compared with that on the other side. A swelling in the knee joint is usually first seen in the hollows either side of the patella.

Assess any swelling to determine whether it is confined to the limits of the synovial cavity or extends beyond the joint boundaries, which would suggest infection, tumour or injury.

Note any localized swellings that may indicate bursitis, a meniscal cyst or 'tumours' such as exostoses. Look for any evidence of muscle wasting, particularly of the quadriceps muscle (see Fig. 6.4).

Position

A knee joint that is swollen and painful is most comfortable when slightly flexed. Stand the patient up and look for any degree of genu valgus or varus (Fig. 8.12; see also Fig. 6.11).

Palpation

Skin

Note any increase in temperature that may indicate active arthritis or infection.

Synovium

The synovium of the knee joint can be felt on either side of the patella and in the suprapatellar pouch. In some diseases, it becomes thickened and rubbery, or 'boggy'. A thickened synovium is

Fig. 8.12 Knee effusion seen as a fullness on either side of the patella.

usually hyperaemic and makes the overlying skin warm.

Bony contour

Check the position of the patella. It should be in the patellar groove of the femur, but it may be displaced laterally or superiorly if there is lengthening or rupture of the patellar ligament. The size, shape and position of the patella should be noted. The bone should also be felt on its anterior surface, at its edges and at the sites of attachment of the quadriceps and patellar tendons.

Check the position of the knee joint. **When students are asked to put their index finger on the line of the knee joint, they invariably point to a spot 2.5–5 cm above the joint**. Remember that the main bulge of the knee is formed by the lower end of the femur. The easiest way to find the joint line is to flex the knee until you can feel the anterior curved edge of the femoral condyles and can slide your finger downwards over this edge until you reach the tibial plateau.

It is important to relate areas of tenderness to the joint line (Fig. 8.13a) and the points of attachment of the collateral ligaments.

(a) Joint line tenderness.

(a) Milking of fluid on the medial side of the knee. The fluid displacement test: compress one side of the knee and note the joint distending on the opposite side.

(b) Patellar tenderness.

Fig. 8.13 PALPATION FOR TENDERNESS ABOUT THE KNEE

Effusions

Effusions of the knee joint are common and easy to detect because the excess synovial fluid collects in the front of the joint where it can be seen and felt. There are three tests for detecting an effusion in the knee joint:

- *Visible fluctuation.* A small quantity of fluid does not make the whole joint look swollen, but if you press gently on one side of the joint, the other side may bulge outwards (Fig. 8.14a). Position the leg in a good oblique light so the hollows on either side of the patella are visible. Stroke the joint just to one side of the patella and watch the hollow on the other side of the patella to see if it gradually fills out as the effusion is pushed into it. This is the most sensitive way of detecting a small effusion (Fig. 8.14c). It cannot be used if the joint is full and tense.

(b)

(c) Milking of fluid on the lateral side of the knee. The fluid displacement test: compress one side of the knee and note the joint distending on the opposite side.

Fig. 8.14 TESTING FOR A KNEE EFFUSION

- *Palpable fluctuation.* When the knee joint is full of fluid, it is possible to press on one side and feel the increase in pressure transmitted over to the other side. Place the palm of the left hand above the patella, and the thumb and index finger either side of it (Fig. 8.14b). Press posteriorly and distally to squeeze any fluid in the suprapatellar pouch down into the joint behind and either side of the patella. Place the thumb and index finger of the right hand either side of the patella and see if you can feel fluctuation or fluid displacement between your thumb and finger.
- *Patellar tap.* When the joint is full of fluid, the patella is lifted off the femur. If it is pressed or tapped, it can be felt to move backwards and hit the femur (Fig. 8.15). This test is also helped by emptying the suprapatellar pouch into the space behind the patella with the left hand.

(a)

Fig. 8.15 The patellar tap text: squeeze any fluid out of the suprapatellar pouch using the right hand and then press down on the patella. A tap or click will indicate an effusion.

Surrounding tissues

Pay particular attention to the bulk and strength of the quadriceps muscle, but remember that the quadriceps of the patient's dominant leg will always be slightly bulkier. Any substantial wasting can be measured by comparing the circumference of the thighs at the same distance above the joint line (Fig. 8.16).

Movement

Ask the patient to move the joint themselves before checking passive movement. Record the extent of

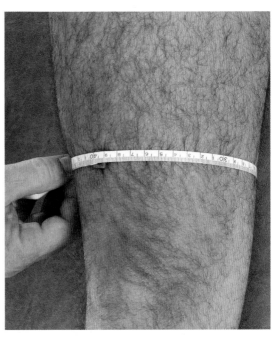

(b)

Fig. 8.16 QUADRICEPS MEASUREMENT
(a, b) Measurement of quadriceps muscle bulk for wasting from a fixed measurable distance from the tibial tubercle.

the active knee movements in degrees. Remember that when the leg is straight, the angle between the femur and tibia is 0°. The angle is usually 135–150° in full flexion, and between 0° and –10° in full extension.

Flexion

Bend the knee as much as possible (Fig. 8.17). When there is disease of the hip joint, you may have to turn the patient on to their side to see the full extent of knee flexion. Record the degrees of flexion from the zero position of normal extension.

Extension

Lift the leg off the bed by the heel, and ask the patient to relax (Fig. 8.18). Record any limitation of extension as well as any excess of extension. In females, the knee joint often extends 5° or 10° past the 0° mark.

Rotation

There are small degrees of rotation of the tibia on the femur, but these are not easy to detect unless the knee is slightly flexed.

Crepitus

This can be felt during movement and usually signifies patello-femoral pathology.

Abnormal movements

Abnormal movement can occur if the ligaments are ruptured or stretched, because the knee joint is a hinge joint that depends entirely on muscles and ligaments for its stability. Thus, by testing for abnormal movements such as abduction and adduction, and anteroposterior glide or sliding of the tibia on the femur, you are really checking the stability of the knee and the integrity of its ligaments.

Medial and lateral collateral ligaments Let the leg rest extended on the couch. Standing on the patient's left side, place the fingers of your right hand under the right knee joint, and the butt of your hand firmly against the medial aspect of the joint. Keep this hand firm and use it as a fulcrum to try to adduct the knee joint by pulling the ankle towards you with your left hand (Fig. 8.19). There should be only the slightest movement in the joint. If it moves easily, the lateral collateral ligament is ruptured. If you stay on the same side of the patient, the same action on the other leg will abduct the joint and test the medial collateral ligament.

To test the ligaments on the opposite side of the joint, change your hands around so that your right hand lies on top of the joint with the fingers resting on the side of the joint. Pull this hand towards you, and push the ankle away from you with the other hand.

An alternative method is to tuck the patient's leg under your arm and then, with your hands on

Fig. 8.17 Testing knee flexion.

Fig. 8.18 Testing knee extension.

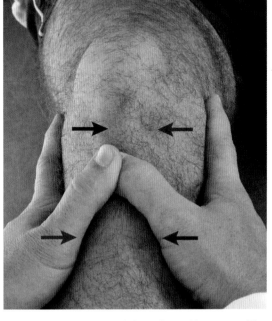

Fig. 8.19 Examination of the collateral ligaments. The blue arrows show forces applied to assess the medial collateral ligament, whilst the red arrows show forces applied to assess the lateral collateral ligament.

each side of the knee joint to detect movement, move the tibia from side to side with your body (Fig. 8.20).

Anterior and posterior cruciate ligaments

Remember that the anterior cruciate ligament stops the tibia sliding anteriorly. The posterior ligament stops the tibia sliding posteriorly.

Assess the resting position with both of the patient's knees flexed to 90° and their heels placed together on the couch. Observe the upper tibia from the side. If the upper end has dropped back, it can indicate a tear of the posterior cruciate ligament (the sag sign) (Fig. 8.21).

Then test the ligaments, with the patient's knee flexed to about 70°. Grasp the upper end of the tibia with both hands and pull it towards you. This is the **anterior draw test**, and any significant movement suggests a torn anterior cruciate ligament, possibly associated with damage to the lateral ligaments as well (Fig. 8.22).

Now repeat the test, but this time pushing the tibia backwards – the **posterior draw test**. Any significant displacement indicates rupture of the posterior cruciate ligament. Always compare the degree of movement between the two sides.

The **Lachman test** is difficult to perform if the patient has large thighs, but can also be used to assess the cruciate ligaments. The knee is flexed to 20° degrees. Grasp the lower thigh and the upper part of the leg. A translational force is then applied

(Fig. 8.23). The knee is unstable if the joint surfaces glide over each other. In normal knees, there should be little or no movement.

(a)

(b)

(c)

Fig. 8.21 POSTERIOR SAG
(a–c) Posterior sag of the knee occurs when the upper end of the tibia falls backwards from the normal contour.

Fig. 8.20 Varus and valgus stress of the knee with the leg supported. The red arrow shows varus stress and the blue arrow shows valgus stress applied to the knee with the leg supported.

Fig. 8.22 Anterior draw test (blue arrow) for the anterior cruciate ligament and posterior draw test (red arrow) for the posterior cruciate ligament.

Fig. 8.23 The Lachman test for cruciate insufficiency.

The knee may have rotational instability if there are combined injuries of the collateral and cruciate ligaments. This can be assessed by the **pivot shift test**. Lift the leg in full extension with the tibia internally rotated. Then apply a valgus force to the lateral side of the joint as the knee is flexed. If there is instability, the tibia will suddenly move posteriorly as the joint relocates.

Note It is not necessary to sit on the patient's foot and crush their toes to death to perform some of these procedures, but it does help if the foot is fixed by the pressure of your buttock as you sit beside the leg, facing the patient's head, so that both of your arms are in front of you and in line with the leg.

Clicks

There are some special tests that make the joint click if there is a torn cartilage. Do not try these tests. They are difficult to perform and to interpret.

Normal joints sometimes click. If the patient is complaining of clicking, find out exactly when it occurs, and whether it is painful. Then ask the patient to reproduce it for you, but do not indulge in excessive manipulation just to hear it.

Gait

Ask the patient to stand up and walk about. Observe the gait carefully. Look for a limp, use of a walking stick or shoe raise.

Alignment of the knees

The normal alignment of the knee is 5–7° of valgus.

Genu varus (bow legs) is diagnosed by measuring the distance between the knees with the malleoli placed together. This is usually less than 6 cm. In children, this can be a normal finding and corrects itself as the child grows. It may, however, also be associated with bone dysplasia or rickets. The distance between the knees increases if the deformity is progressive. This may be associated with Blount's disease, which is caused by abnormal growth of the proximal posteromedial tibia.

Genu valgum (knock knees) can be estimated by placing the knees together and measuring the distance between the malleoli, which is usually less than 8 cm. Again, this can be a normal developmental finding in children.

If abnormal alignment of the knees develops in adulthood, this is usually secondary to trauma or underlying degenerative change. Varus deformity is commonly associated with osteoarthritis, while valgus deformity is more commonly seen in rheumatoid arthritis.

CAUSES OF KNEE PAIN

Tendon ruptures

The quadriceps and patellar tendons form part of the knee extensor mechanism on either side of the patella. Tears can occur when there is resisted extension of the knee. This usually occurs during sporting activity, but can be caused by simple stumbling when active extension is not possible.

CHAPTER 8 | LOWER LIMB SYMPTOMS AND SIGNS

History

Age and sex The age of the patient has significant bearing on the level of injury. In the elderly, the injury is usually above the patella, either in the rectus femoris muscle or as an avulsion of the quadriceps tendon from the upper pole of the patella (Fig. 8.24). It is more common in males than females (8 to 1).

In middle age, fractures of the patella are more common (see below).

In the young, the patellar tendon is ruptured or avulsed from the inferior pole of the patella.

Partial rupture leading to tendinitis and calcification in the patellar tendon can occur (Sinding-Larsen–Johansson syndrome).

Quadriceps tear

Patella fracture

Patella tendon tear

Fig. 8.24 The quadriceps mechanism will fail with a quadriceps tear, patella fracture or patella tendon tear.

Symptoms The patient is likely to present with **severe pain** and an **inability to walk**.

Examination

There will often be a haemarthrosis of the knee joint. Depending on the level of injury, there may be a palpable gap in either the quadriceps or the patellar tendon. The patella will migrate proximally (a high-riding patella) if the patellar tendon is torn. The patient is usually unable to perform a straight leg raise.

Recurrent dislocation of the patella

The patella can dislocate acutely as the result of trauma (see below), resulting in chronic instability in 15–20 per cent of cases. The patella can, however, dislocate spontaneously, when the quadriceps contracts with the knee in flexion.

History

Age and sex This occurs from 10 to 30 years of age, and is more common in females. The condition may be bilateral. Predisposing factors include generalized ligamentous laxity, underdevelopment of the lateral femoral condyle, maldevelopment of the patella, valgus deformity of the knee and external tibial torsion.

Symptoms There is **acute pain** and the **knee becomes stuck in flexion**. The patient is unable to weight-bear.

Examination

The patella is dislocated laterally, exposing the medial femoral condyle and causing a **flattening of the front of the knee** (Fig. 8.25). A haemarthrosis develops. Once the patella has been reduced, the patient may have a positive **patellar apprehension sign**. Place pressure on the lateral aspect of the patella while flexing the knee. This causes the patient to worry that it is going to dislocate.

Fig. 8.25 Flattening of the front of the knee in patellar dislocation.

Chondromalacia patellae

This is softening of the cartilage on the articular surface of the patella.

History

Age and sex This is common in adolescents and in athletic young adults. It is especially common in teenage females. It can be bilateral.

Symptoms There is **anterior knee pain**, which is worse on walking up stairs and after sitting with the knee flexed for prolonged periods. The patient often complains that the pain is centred 'underneath the knee cap'. **The knee may give way or catch**.

Examination

Look for evidence of quadriceps wasting (see Fig. 6.4), fluid in the knee and tenderness on the edge of the patella. The patella may appear malaligned, tilted or high-riding. Crepitus of the patella femoral joint may be felt on flexing and extending the knee, and also by compressing the patella into the femoral trochlea.

Patellar tendinitis

(Jumper's knee)
This is part of the family of tendinopathies that can occur around the body.

Symptoms **Anterior knee pain** occurs principally over the patellar tendon and the inferior pole of the patella, particularly during running and jumping.

Examination

There is localized tenderness on palpation of the patellar tendon, and pain on extending the lower leg against resistance. The tendon may appear thickened.

Plica syndrome

This is caused by an embryonic remnant of a synovial partition that persists into adult life. It is usually found as a median infrapatellar fold. It only becomes pathologically significant if there is an acute injury or repetitive activity that causes it to become inflamed, when it acts like a bowstring, causing further inflammation in the joint.

History

Age and sex It can occur in both males and females, usually in adolescence or young adulthood.

Symptoms It presents as **anterior knee pain**, worse after activity or prolonged periods of inactivity. The pain may be an ache, or more acute when the knee is stressed. The patient may complain of **clicking**.

Examination

The may be **muscle wasting** (see Fig. 6.4) caused by disuse.

Palpation reveals **localized tenderness near the upper pole of the patella** and over the femoral condyle. A thickened band of tissue can occasionally be felt, which snaps during movement of the knee.

Osteochondritis dissecans

A segment of bone undergoes avascular necrosis (see Chapter 6) and separates from one of the femoral condyles, often appearing as a loose body in the joint. This may be the result of either direct trauma or repeated microtrauma, and is most frequently observed on the lateral part of the medial femoral condyle. Less commonly, the lateral femoral condyle or patella is involved.

History

Age and sex This is more common in males and presents between 10 and 25 years of age. Its incidence has increased in recent years, probably because of greater participation in sports. It can be bilateral in 25 per cent of cases.

Symptoms There is an **aching pain on the anterior aspect of the knee**.

The knee may **lock** or **give way**.

Examination

It is usually possible to observe **wasting of the quadriceps** and **a small effusion** in the joint. It may be possible to elicit tenderness of the femoral condyle.

Osgood–Schlatter disease

This is a traction apophysitis (inflammation) of the tibial tubercle, where the patellar tendon inserts into the tibia.

History

Age and sex This is a common disorder of teenagers, most often seen in males.

Symptoms **Pain** mainly occurs during activity such as running, football and cycling but can develop into discomfort at rest.

Examination

There is tenderness of the tibial tubercle, and a lump is felt on palpation. Active knee extension against resistance can be painful.

Bursitis around the knee

Fluid can collect in and distend the prepatellar (housemaid's knee (Figs. 8.26a, b)), infrapatellar (clergyman's knee) and semimembranosus bursae (Fig. 8.26, see Fig. 4.65).

The prepatellar bursa is a normal structure that allows the skin to slide over the patella as the knee is flexed. It can become inflamed when there is prolonged kneeling on the knee. It is associated with occupations such as carpet fitting, tiling and roofing.

The infrapatellar bursa lies in front of the tibial tubercle and can become inflamed when load is taken through this region rather than the patella.

The semimembranosus bursa lies at the back of the knee, medial to the joint line, and can become swollen in children and adults.

Symptoms The knee may be painful on movement, although the range of movement is preserved.

Examination

Prepatellar and infrapatellar bursitis presents with localized tenderness and swelling of the bursae, which may feel warm. The skin may become erythematous if there is associated infection. Swelling of the semimembranosus bursa is not usually tender. The lumps will transilluminate.

Baker's cyst

(Popliteal cyst)

This results from the passage of fluid or herniation of the synovial membrane through the posterior joint capsule. It is associated with degenerative joint disease and meniscal tears.

Symptoms The lump is usually painless, but if it ruptures there is significant pain behind the knee, radiating into the calf, with marked swelling. It can then be mistaken for a deep vein thrombosis.

(b)

Suprapatellar bursa

Subcutaneous prepatellar bursa (housemaid's knee)

Semimbranosus bursa

Subcutaneous infrapatellar bursa (clergyman's knee)

Deep infrapatellar bursa

Subsartorial (pes anserinus) bursa

(a)

Fig. 8.26 KNEE BURSITIS OR 'HOUSEMAID'S KNEE'

Examination

The swelling is usually in the popliteal fossa, either at the level of or just below the joint line. It is usually non-tender. It is fluctuant and transilluminates.

Haemarthrosis

This is caused by a bleed into the joint and can occur spontaneously, in patients with a bleeding disorder such as haemophilia, or when a patient is taking anticoagulation, for example warfarin.

More commonly, it is associated with a traumatic injury.

There has usually been either been an associated fracture, or an anterior cruciate ligament or meniscal tear if the swelling occurs almost immediately after injury.

Symptoms The joint is very painful and feels tense.

Examination

The knee is warm and tender to the touch. All movements are restricted.

Meniscal tears

These can occur as a result of trauma, or from degenerative changes with increasing age. The menisci are important as they distribute the load across the joint, help lubricate and facilitate the rolling and gliding actions of the joint, and provide proprioception leading to improved stability of the knee.

Both menisci are C shaped. The medial meniscus is larger and less mobile, and as a consequence tears of it are more common. Most tears are vertical, and if the fragment remains attached at the front and back, it is called a 'bucket handle' tear (Fig. 8.27). Where the tear emerges at a free edge, it is either an 'anterior horn' or a 'posterior horn' tear. Horizontal tears are more frequent in the degenerative knee. Tears can occur in combination with ligamentous injuries.

History

Age and sex Traumatic tears are common in young athletic persons, more often males, and are often associated with a twisting injury. Degenerative tears become increasingly common from 35 years onwards.

Symptoms **In an acute traumatic tear, the knee is painful and may be locked in a flexed position.**

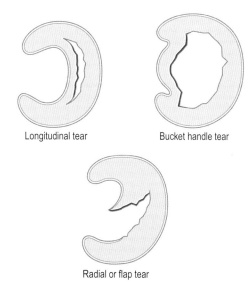

Longitudinal tear   Bucket handle tear

Radial or flap tear

Fig. 8.27 Line diagram of types of meniscal tear.

There is usually initial difficulty in weight-bearing, but this will improve in the absence of locking.

Degenerative tears may be relatively painless. These patients usually complain of the knee **locking or giving way**.

Examination

The knee **swells** within a few hours of the injury. It is often **held in flexion**. Full extension is not usually possible because of pain.

Palpation elicits **localized tenderness on the joint line**, usually on the medial side.

There are specific tests for meniscal pathology, such as McMurray's test, but these are painful and best avoided.

Meniscal cysts can occasionally develop at the site of a tear, most commonly of the lateral meniscus. Examination reveals a small lump at the side of the joint, most easily seen with the knee flexed. The lump may be tender.

The lateral meniscus may also be disc shaped (a **discoid lateral meniscus**) rather than semi-lunar. Young patients may complain that the knee gives way and clunks, typically at 110° of flexion and 10° from full extension.

Knee ligament injuries

There are four principal ligaments around the knee joint, namely the anterior and posterior cruciate ligaments, and the medial and lateral collateral ligaments. These provide support for the joint because the bony structures are inherently unstable.

All the ligaments are most commonly injured during sporting activity, and therefore they are more common in the younger, usually male population.

Anterior cruciate ligament injury

This ligament is intra-articular and prevents anterior translation and external rotation of the tibia on the femur. It has two bundles: the anteromedial bundle resists excess translation (forward–backward movement) in flexion, while the posterolateral bundle tightens as the knee is extended.

A tear of this ligament is often sustained when there is a sudden change in direction about an implanted foot, with a twisting motion. It can also occur after jumping and landing on a flexed knee. Injury is often associated with a medial meniscal tear.

Symptoms The knee is **immediately painful** and there is **difficulty weight-bearing**. The patient may have a **heard a 'pop' or feel the tear happen**. As the acute event settles, the patient feels the **knee is unstable**, and they have difficulty descending stairs. Changes in direction also cause anxiety, and the **knee may collapse**.

Examination

There is often a **large haemarthrosis** almost immediately after the injury. There is **tenderness** along the joint lines, as these injuries are often associated with meniscal damage. All movements are painful in the initial phase. The diagnosis is confirmed by a **positive anterior draw test**, **positive Lachman's test** and possibly a **positive pivot shift test** (see above).

In the chronic case, movements may be painless, but the special tests remain positive.

Posterior cruciate ligament injury

This ligament prevents posterior 'sliding' of the tibia on the femur. It has two bundles: the anterolateral bundle, which stabilizes the knee in 90° of flexion, and the posteromedial bundle, which stabilizes the knee when straight.

Injuries are usually caused by a blow to the knee while it is bent, for example when striking the dashboard in a road traffic accident, or falling directly onto the knee while it is flexed. The posterior ligament is stronger than the anterior and is less frequently injured.

Symptoms There is usually initial pain and swelling, but this often settles, and unless examined carefully these injuries can be missed. In time, the patient will complain of the knee **feeling unstable and 'wobbly'**.

Examination

There is often a small effusion, tenderness along the posterolateral joint line, and a **positive posterior draw test**. A **positive posterior sag sign** may also be present.

Medial collateral ligament injury

This protects the medial side of the knee from being bent open by a stress applied to the lateral side of the knee, which is a valgus force. Complete tears are usually associated with an anterior cruciate tear, although isolated tears can also occur.

Injuries are commonly sustained in football tackles or when skiing.

Symptoms The **knee will be painful**, and there may be initial **difficulty in weight-bearing**. Laterally, the knee may feel **unstable**.

Examination

Tenderness can usually be elicited along the course of the medial collateral ligament from the medial epicondyle of the femur to the medial tibial condyle. As this is extra-articular, there is normally no haemarthrosis, but there may be some **localized swelling**. Movements will be relatively preserved.

Tests for disruption of the ligament by applying a valgus strain will be positive. Both pain and opening of the joint as the result of joint instability may be recognized.

Lateral collateral ligament injury

This is seldom injured in isolation and it is usually part of a pattern of injury that results in posterolateral instability.

Osteoarthritis of the knee

The knee is the most common of the large joints to be affected by osteoarthritis. While it may be a primary pathology, a number of predisposing factors are recognized, including previous fracture, meniscal pathology and abnormal biomechanics caused by instability or deformity.

History

Age and sex Patients are usually over 50 years old. In white populations, there is an equal male to female distribution. Black African females are, however, more commonly affected than their male counterparts.

Symptoms This condition usually has a slow insidious onset, with patients complaining of **pain on weight-bearing** that is made worse by walking and exercise.

Subsequently, they develop **night pain** and often sleep with a pillow between their legs. The knee is generally very **stiff** when they awake in the morning or after prolonged immobilization. The knee **may lock or give way**.

Examination

There may be **wasting of the quadriceps** from disuse (see Fig. 6.4), with an obvious deformity, usually varus and fixed flexion (Fig. 8.28).

A small effusion may be present. Patello-femoral crepitus may be felt and heard, and the joint line is usually tender on palpation. The range of movement may be reduced, with **loss of extension** and pain elicited on all movements.

Rheumatoid arthritis

This can occur in the knee joint but, as in other joints, the presentation of significant pathology is now much less common as a result of advances in medical management.

Symptoms In the synovitic stage, the knee is painful and swollen. As the disease progresses, the knee becomes increasing unstable, with progressive pain. The patient has difficulty mobilizing, using the stairs and standing from a sitting position.

Examination

On inspection, there may be quadriceps wasting and deformity of the joint. Palpation reveals a palpable

Fig. 8.28 Knee deformity in osteoarthritis.

effusion and thickened synovium. Movements become increasingly restricted. Examination of the supporting ligaments may demonstrate instability.

Septic arthritis and tuberculosis

These can both cause infection in the knee joint but are relatively uncommon. They present in much the same way as the same infections of the hip joint with pain, loss of movement, swelling and signs of systemic infection.

Examination

The knee joint is swollen and tender, and its movements are restricted.

Bony swellings

These are common around the knee and vary from benign osteomas/diaphyseal achalasia through osteoclastomas to highly malignant osteosarcomas (see Chapter 6).

THE FOOT AND ANKLE

THE ANKLE JOINT

The ankle joint is a synovial hinge joint between the lower ends of the tibia and fibula and the upper part of the talus. The proximal articular surface comprises the distal end of the tibia, the medial malleolus and the lateral malleolus, which together form a deep socket. The socket is wider anteriorly than posteriorly, and articulates with the upper part of the talus, which is reciprocally wedge shaped. The lateral side of the talus is larger than the medial side.

The ankle joint is supported by:

- the lateral ligaments: the anterior and posterior talofibular and calcaneal fibular ligaments;
- the medial deltoid ligament;
- the transverse tibiofibular ligament;
- a fibrous capsule.

The movements are extension (dorsiflexion) and flexion (plantar flexion). The ankle is more stable in dorsiflexion than plantar flexion.

Distal to the ankle joint is the **subtalar joint**, which is the articulation between the talus and the calcaneum. This joint allows inversion and eversion of the foot, but does not contribute to dorsiflexion or plantar flexion. The other joints of the foot include those between the tarsal bones, the metatarsals and the phalanges. They are all synovial joints, and have shapes related to their movement.

THE FOOT ARCHES

The medial arch is higher and forms the instep of the foot. It comprises the calcaneum, the talus, the navicular, the cuneiforms and the medial three metatarsals.

The transverse arch runs in a medial to lateral direction on the plantar surface of the foot (concave). The distal tarsal joints make up the arch. The arch/bones provide stability across the midfoot.

These arches are important in promoting forward propulsion. Each arch is supported by ligaments, muscles and tendons.

SYMPTOMS

Adults with foot and ankle problems generally present with **pain**, **swelling**, **deformity** and **impaired function**. Pain is usually referenced to a well-localized structure, but pain symptoms are sometimes vague; for example, **metatarsalgia** is a poorly localized pain in the forefoot that has many causes (Revision panel 8.2).

Pain may be present at rest or be 'activity related' (Revision panel 8.3). It may also be associated with the wearing of shoes. The foot and ankle can often be **stiff in the morning**. This can result in **difficulty weight-bearing**. Ascending and descending the stairs can be problematic.

Deformities of the foot and ankle can be caused by either congenital or acquired conditions. Deformity may or may not coexist with pain.

The ankle or subtalar joints **can become unstable**, leading to episodes of the joint giving way.

Revision panel 8.2

Causes of pain in the ankle region

Commoner causes

Ankle osteoarthritis

Ankle impingement

Achilles tendinitis/tenosynovitis

Gouty arthritis

Rheumatoid arthritis

Rarer causes

Acute osteomyelitis

Chronic osteomyelitis

Pyogenic arthritis

Septic arthritis

Haemophilic arthritis

Tibialis posterior tendon dysfunction

Osteochondral defects of the talus

Revision panel 8.3

The painful foot

Heel

Traction apophysitis of the Achilles insertion

Calcaneal bursitis

Plantar fasciitis

Osteomyelitis

Neoplasms – benign and malignant – of the bones of the foot

Revision panel 8.3 (continued)

Midfoot

Osteochondritis of the navicular bone (Köhler's disease)

Midfoot osteoarthritis

Forefoot

Stress fracture of a metatarsal

Morton's metatarsalgia

Osteochondritis of the second metatarsal head (Freiberg's disease)

Hallux valgus

Hallux rigidus

Claw toes

Pes cavus

Gout

Rheumatoid arthritis

PLAN FOR EXAMINATION OF FOOT AND ANKLE

This follows the usual principles of look, feel and move. The examination includes the joints above and below the principle area of assessment, together with a neurovascular examination (see Chapters 3 and 10).

Observe for walking aids or supports. Ask to see the patient's footwear, the shape of which may be altered because of an underlying deformity. Observe the heel and sole for patterns of wear that may be altered as a result of changes in gait.

Ask the patient to stand and expose the lower limbs from the thighs down.

Ask the patient to walk, paying attention to all the phases of the walking cycle: heel strike, footflat, midstance to heel off and heel off to toe off. Patients may have an antalgic gait secondary to pain. Their gait may also be disturbed by muscular weakness, deformity or stiffness.

Patients may have a **foot drop** when the ankle dorsiflexors are weak, causing a slapping foot strike. The leg may be lifted higher than usual so the foot can clear the ground (a high-stepping gait), usually because of neurological conditions.

Patients may also walk on the inner or outer border of the foot because of deformity.

Push-off from the ground involves the first metatarsal joint and can be altered by joint pain or stiffness involving the great toe.

Inspection

During standing, the heels are normally in slight valgus alignment. When a person is on tip toes, there is inversion because of movement at the subtalar joint (Fig. 8.29).

(a) The heel is in valgus when viewed from behind.

Fig. 8.29 ANKLE INSPECTION

(b) As the patient goes onto tip toes, the heel swings inwards into varus.

CHAPTER 8 | LOWER LIMB SYMPTOMS AND SIGNS

Skin

Look all around the joints from front and back for scars, and for callosities caused by pressure from footwear or abnormal transmission of load. Erythema may be associated with inflammation and infection.

Shape

Deformity may occur in the ankle, foot or toes. Common deformities include:

- flat foot (pes planus);
- high instep (pes cavus);
- lateral deviation of the great toe (hallux valgus);
- fixed flexion of one interphalangeal joint in the toe (hammer or mallet toe);
- fixed flexion of both interphalangeal joints in the toe (claw toes).

Palpation

Any increased temperature of the skin may be indicative of arthritis or infection.

Feel for any localized tenderness, swelling and oedema of soft tissue or bone.

Ensure an assessment of sensation and motor function is performed (see Chapter 3).

Movement

Ask the patient to move their joints themselves before checking the passive range.

Ankle joint

Hold the heel in the left hand and the midfoot in the right hand (Fig. 8.30). Assess plantar flexion (0–40°) and dorsiflexion (usually 0–15°).

Subtalar joint

In order to assess inversion and eversion, the ankle joint must be locked. The ankle is placed in plantar flexion. Eversion is usually 0–15°, and inversion 0–30°.

Mid-tarsal joint

Grab the heel to stabilize the hindfoot and assess movement of the forefoot in both the vertical and horizontal planes.

Toes

Extension and flexion of the toes, in particular the great toe, should be assessed (Fig. 8.31).

(a) Ankle dorsiflexion.

(b) Ankle plantar flexion.

Fig. 8.30 ANKLE JOINT INSPECTION

Abnormal movements

To maintain stability, the ankle joint is reinforced by muscles and ligaments. Abnormal movement and instability can occur if the ligaments are injured.

Stability in the anterior posterior plane is tested with the patient sitting on the couch. Hold the distal tibia with both hands, and push firmly backwards and forwards on a fixed foot (draw tests). In normal ankle joints, there should be little or no movement. Stability to varus stress is a useful test for integrity of the calcaneofibular ligament (Fig. 8.32).

(a) Great toe dorsiflexion.

Fig. 8.32 Inversion stress for ankle instability.

(b) Great toe plantar flexion.

Fig. 8.31 EXTENSION AND FLEXION OF THE TOES

Fig. 8.33 An infant demonstrating polydactyly of both feet.

CONGENITAL AND ACQUIRED CONDITIONS OF THE FOOT AND ANKLE

There are many congenital abnormalities of the foot, such as polydactyly (too many toes) (Fig. 8.33), but the most important is club foot.

Club foot

(Congenital talipes equinovarus)

These deformities of the foot and ankle develop in utero and are usually present at birth. They are classified according to the skeletal deformity but are collectively known as talipes or club foot. Similar deformities can also develop in adult life after injury, paralysis and other musculoskeletal disorders.

The incidence is 1–2 per 1000 births, with males more often affected than females (2 to 1). The condition is bilateral in one-third of cases.

When a club foot abnormality is present, the infant must be examined for other associated disorders, especially developmental displacement of the hip and spina bifida (see Chapter 9) or arthrogryposis.

There are two main types of deformity (Fig. 8.34):

- The ankle may be abnormally extended so the weight-bearing is on the toes – an equinus deformity; or abnormally dorsiflexed so that the weight-bearing is on the heel – a calcaneous deformity.
- The foot may be deviated into a varus or valgus position, which usually means there is some associated inversion and eversion, respectively.

Of these eight variations, only two are common: **talipes equinus**, caused by a short Achilles tendon, and **talipes equinovarus** – the true club foot (Fig. 8.35).

The obvious deformities of the true club foot would be equinus at the ankle, so the ankle keeps pointing downwards, and varus or inward pointing of the heels. There is also supination in the subtalar joint and adduction of the forefoot. The joint

Fig. 8.35 Severe bilateral clubbed feet. The varus deformity is so severe that the feet are pulled upwards as well as inwards, making this a talipes calcaneovarus.

movements are limited, and the muscles that affect the joint are wasted. The calf muscle is smaller. These result in the foot having a bean-shaped appearance.

Flat feet

(Pes planus)

The foot has a longitudinal and a transverse arch. The patient has a flat foot if the longitudinal arch flattens to the extent that the medial border of the foot rests on the ground. It is usually associated with a mild valgus deformity of the hindfoot, which results in pronation of the forefoot and subsequent loss of the medial arch (Fig. 8.36).

All children are flat-footed when they start walking, but the arch develops as they grow more active. The infantile pattern may persist into adult life, and the deformity may become fixed by secondary contractures or excessive laxity in the joints.

When assessing for flat feet, it is important to check for symmetry in the arches of both feet. **Ask the patient to go onto tip toe**. With normal feet, the heel moves inwards or into varus. **Tarsal coalition**, in which there is an abnormal congenital connection in the bones, is a possibility in the younger patient if the heel does not move. In older patients, it may be the result of loss of function and stretching of the tibialis posterior tendon, which holds up the arch.

Lateral view

Normal	Equinus	Cacaneous

Superior view

Normal	Varus	Valgus

Fig. 8.34 Deformities of the foot.

Fig. 8.36 Flat feet (pes planus). The medial border of the foot rests on the ground. There is also mild genu valgum (knock knees).

Contrary to popular opinion, **flat feet rarely cause trouble in adult life** as the body weight is spread over a large flat area. The fastest runners often have flat feet!

High-arch foot

(Pes cavus)

This is the opposite of a flat foot; the longitudinal arch is accentuated (Fig. 8.37). Pes cavus occurs secondary to muscle imbalance. A specific cause is usually not found, but **it is important to carry out a full neurological examination** as peripheral neuropathies, especially Charcot–Marie–Tooth disease, spina bifida and poliomyelitis, can all present with pes cavus. Asymmetry with a unilateral high-arch foot is a 'red flag' suggesting significant underlying neurological problems.

The high arch is clearly visible and easy to diagnose (Fig. 8.38). The **toes are always 'clawed'** (hyperextension of the metatarsophalangeal joints and flexion of the interphalangeal joints) and the patient **cannot straighten their toes**.

Fig. 8.37 A high-arched foot (pes cavus).

Fig. 8.38 A unilateral high-arch (cavus) left foot.

Extension of the metatarsophalangeal joints combined with a high arch makes the ball of the foot more prominent and lifts the tips of the toes off the ground so that they do not participate in weight-bearing. As a consequence, **callosities develop** on the ball of the foot beneath the heads of the metatarsal bones and on the dorsal aspect of the toes where they rub against the shoes.

Unlike the flat foot, the high-arched foot **frequently causes pain and discomfort**.

Hallux valgus

(Bunion)

A valgus deformity at the metatarsophalangeal joint of the great toe is a common abnormality (Fig. 8.39). It can be congenital or acquired, with the latter more common in females because of poorly fitting

Fig. 8.39 Bilateral hallux valgus.

footwear. The bunion is the name given to the bursa that forms over the medial aspect of the prominent head of the first metatarsal. It often swells up. The local sensory nerve can get stretched by the bunion and squashed between the bunion and the shoe. The patient has difficulty finding comfortable shoes as the bunion is painful when rubbed or touched. The fluctuant subcutaneous swelling or bursa is easy to feel and distinguish from the underlying bony prominence.

Osteoarthritis develops as a result of prolonged abnormal stresses in the first metatarsophalangeal joint. This causes pain in the joint during movement and weight-bearing.

Clinical examination should start with inspection of the arch as hallux valgus is more common in patients with flat feet. There may also be lesser toe abnormalities. Look for evidence of abnormal loading in the sole of the foot with callus formation under the lesser metatarsals heads.

Check for tenderness over the actual bunion. Check the range of movement in the joint and whether the deformity is passively correctable.

Hallux rigidus

(Arthritis of the first metatarsophalangeal joint)
The first metatarsophalangeal joint is a joint that is commonly affected by osteoarthritis even when it is in normal alignment. This can cause **pain** and a **progressive reduction of joint movement**.

Clinical examination may reveal a bony prominence on the top of the joint, produced by the underlying bony osteophytes. These osteophytes block free motion, so dorsiflexion and plantar flexion of the great toe is significantly reduced.

Gouty arthritis

This has been discussed in Chapter 6, but is mentioned here as it is an important cause of arthritis in the first metatarsophalangeal joint.

History

Severe acute pain, redness and swelling usually develop in the first metatarsophalangeal joint. The ankles and knees and other toes can also be affected, most commonly in a middle-aged or elderly male.

Examination

The joint is red, swollen and exquisitely tender. Septic arthritis must be considered, but the absence of systemic symptoms combined with the presence of tophi and a raised serum urate confirm the diagnosis.

Mallet and hammer toes

In a mallet toe, the contracture is at the level of the distal interphalangeal joint, and in a hammer toe it is at the level of the proximal interphalangeal joint.

Patients often **present with pain** and **notice the deformity** There may be hard skin over the affected joint (Fig. 8.40), which can also be painful.

Clinical assessment involves checking for other associated conditions such as a bunion, which can cause the hammer toe, or hard skin on the sole of the foot. It is not always easy to say if it is a mallet toe, hammer toe or both. Sometimes it is just easier

Fig. 8.40 A row of hammer toes. The tips of some of the toes are off the ground, and there are callosities over the flexed proximal interphalangeal joints. The distal interphalangeal joints of the second and third toes are only slightly hyperextended.

to call it what you see, i.e. a flexion deformity of the lesser toe.

Claw toes and the neurological foot

There is usually a neurological basis to a claw toe. In a claw toe, there is extension of the joint at the level of the metatarsophalangeal joint, with flexion at the interphalangeal and distal interphalangeal joints. Check for a high arch or cavus foot as a claw toe is often associated with this deformity (see above). Look for symmetry in the arch. The great toe may also be clawed. Note whether there are any calluses on the tops of the toes, and assess the correctability of the joints. If they cannot be passively corrected, this affects treatment options (see *Investigation and Management*, Chapter 9).

Morton's neuroma

This is a neuroma of a digital nerve caused by repetitive trauma or tight-fitting shoes. It usually causes **pain on weight-bearing** over the ball of the foot (metatarsalgia).

Externally, there may be no visible signs of this condition. Squeezing the third web space between your middle and ring fingers can recreate the pain. Lateral compression at the same time makes the pain worse as you are now compressing the enlarged digital nerve between your fingers and the metatarsal neck. This is painful, and a soft click can sometimes be heard, the so-called **Mulder's click**.

Bunionette

This is a prominence on the outer aspect of the foot – a bunion of the fifth toe – just like a bunion of the great toe. There may be hard skin or an inflamed bursa over it. The foot is wider, and finding comfortable shoes is more difficult.

Osteoarthritis of the ankle

History

This is less common than osteoarthritis of the hip or knee, and unlike hip arthritis, it is usually post-traumatic, as a consequence of either previous sprains or fractures. It therefore often develops in younger patients with a history of major injury.

It causes **pain and swelling** and can **seriously limit walking**.

Examination

There may be **visible malalignment** of the joint. When the patient stands, the heel may be in valgus or varus, with the whole ankle joint tilted. The joint can be bulky as a consequence of joint swelling and new bone formation.

The most striking abnormality is a reduction in dorsal and plantar flexion of the ankle when compared with the normal side. Sometimes there is no movement at all, and the ankle may be in equinus and held in plantar flexion.

Rheumatoid arthritis of the foot and ankle

This has been already covered in Chapter 6 and discussed with the upper limb, where it commonly affects the joints of the hand (see Chapter 7). It is, however, nearly as common in the joints of the foot and ankle. It starts as a synovitis in the metatarsophalangeal, tarsal and ankle joints, and also involves the tendons.

History

It presents with pain swelling and deformity in the foot, which interferes with mobility.

Examination

There is often swelling of the ankle and the small joints of the foot. Ankle movements, especially inversion and eversion, are reduced, and the ankle eventually develops a severe valgus deformity. The forefoot often has a hallux valgus deformity of the great toe. Lesser toes develop multiple hammer or claw type deformities and there may be dislocation of the lesser metatarsophalangeal joints. This is caused by stretching of the capsule, which is damaged by the inflammatory process.

It is essential to examine the plantar aspect of the foot where the metatarsal heads are more prominent following subluxation of the fat pad. (This is a common exam case.)

Achilles tendinitis

This occurs in runners and hikers, and is caused by local inflammation of the paratenon, or degeneration within the actual tendon.

It is important to delineate whether the pain is in the middle of the Achilles tendon (non-insertional tendinitis) or is present where the tendon joins the bone (insertional tendinitis).

CHAPTER 8 | LOWER LIMB SYMPTOMS AND SIGNS

History

It typically causes **pain in the tendon**, which is experienced during activity.

Non-insertional tendinitis is associated with a tendon that is very tender to pinch and may be thicker as a consequence of repeated small tears in the tendon healing up with bunched up scar tissue. It is essential to assess whether the tendon is in continuity. Also compare its thickness with that of the normal side.

Insertional tendinitis often presents with an enlargement at the back of the heel from a bony prominence (a **Haglund bump**) or from calcium build-up in the tendon itself (Fig. 8.41).

Fig. 8.41 A Haglund bump.

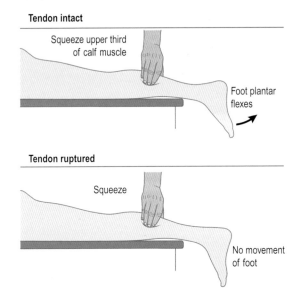

(a) Place the patient prone with the feet hanging freely over the end of the couch. Squeeze the calf muscles. If the Achilles tendon is intact, the foot will plantar flex.

(b) This patient has reruptured his Achilles tendon. Note the position of the ankle before the calf is squeezed.

(c) The ankle remains in the same position despite firm squeezing of the calf muscle. The calf tendon complex is not in continuity.

Fig. 8.42 THE SQUEEZE TEST FOR ACHILLES TENDON DYSFUNCTION

Achilles tendon rupture

It is important not to miss this diagnose as the consequences of loss of function from a missed tear are severe (see *Investigation and Management*, Chapter 9).

History

Patients typically feel a **searing pain** or **hear a loud pop or bang** as they push off. Typical activities in which this happens are tennis, badminton, squash and football. The pop is often so loud that others can hear it. They often think that they have been kicked or 'shot' in the leg.

Examination

There is usually **bruising and tenderness** at the site of the rupture. Surprisingly, it **may not be painful**, but the patient will **limp** and **step high** to clear the foot. The patient should be examined prone on the couch. A **palpable gap** can be felt in the tendon, and the foot has an abnormal lie being more dorsiflexed because of a lack of the downward pull from the calf musculature.

Squeezing the calf muscles normally causes plantar flexion of the ankle, but a **calf squeeze test** does not produce plantar flexion of the ankle if the Achilles tendon is ruptured. This is very easy to see when this is compared with the normal side (Fig. 8.42).

Plantar fasciitis

This is caused by inflammation of the plantar fascia.

History

This is the most common disorder of the foot.

Pain is experienced in the heel. The condition can be brought on by a change of footwear, walking barefoot or high-impact exercise, or it can just arise without an obvious cause. The complaint is of **start-up pain**, which is pain that is experienced first thing in the morning or when getting up having been static for a long time at a desk. After a few minutes, the pain gets a little better. The foot often again becomes sore at the end of the day.

Examination

Check for the alignment of the heel as the condition is more common in high-arched feet. There may be point tenderness where the plantar fascia inserts onto the medial third of the heel. Ankle dorsiflexion

is often reduced because of associated calf tightness. The great toe may be stiff. Thickened nodules appear on the plantar surface of the foot and may attach to the skin (Fig. 8.43).

Fig. 8.43 Plantar fibromatosis of the feet. There are bilateral thick nodules in the plantar fascia but no flexion deformities of the toes.

Plantar fibromatosis
Ledderhose's disease

This condition is very similar in aetiology to the more common Dupuytren's disease of the hand.

Callosities and corns

Continual pressure and friction on small areas of the skin of the foot caused by poor-fitting shoes or skeletal deformities stimulate thickening of the skin. A patch of thickened hyperkeratotic skin is called a **callosity**. It is often called **a corn** if it is pushed into the skin so that it appears to have a deep central core. These can also be painful when squeezed, making the differential diagnosis from a plantar wart difficult.

Frieberg's disease

This is an osteochondritis of the second and sometimes third metatarsal head. It is most often seen in young females and presents with **metatarsalgia**. The enlarged bone may be palpable as a lump in the forefoot, and is tender on movement or pressure.

FRACTURES OF THE LOWER LIMB

PROXIMAL FEMORAL FRACTURES

Proximal femoral fractures can occur about the femoral neck or distal to the intertrochanteric line.

There are four principal fracture patterns about the femoral neck:

- intracapsular: subcapital and transcervical;
- extracapsular: intertrochanteric and basal (between the trochanters).

Intracapsular fractures have the greatest risk of avascular necrosis and non-union. These fractures may be described as incomplete, complete or slightly or significantly displaced, according to the **Garden classification** (Fig. 8.44). Displaced fractures carry the worst prognosis.

Mechanism of injury This is usually a simple fall on to the greater trochanter, a direct blow in a road traffic injury or fall from a height. The latter is often associated with other injuries.

Elderly patients with extracapsular or intracapsular injuries may have reduced bone density as a result of osteoporosis. These fractures occur more commonly in females.

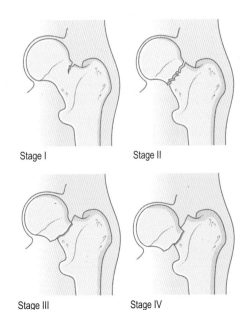

Stage I   Stage II

Stage III   Stage IV

Fig. 8.44 Garden's classification of fracture.

Occasionally, the patient may have a pathological fracture from osteomalacia, Paget's disease or bony metastases.

History

After a minor fall or accident, an elderly patient complains of persistent pain in the hip, often radiating to the thigh. Standing and walking are impossible if the fracture is unimpacted and displaced. The patient may still, however, be able to weight-bear if the fracture is impacted. In younger patients with normal bones, the injury will be more violent. Such injuries are more common in males.

Examination

In patients with femoral neck fractures, the limb is usually shortened, adducted and externally rotated. The presence or absence of external rotation varies depending on the level of the fracture and the amount of displacement.

The joint may be tender over the femoral neck anteriorly, and hip movements, particularly flexion and internal rotation, are very painful. The thigh may be swollen.

General complications are shown in Revision panel 8.4.

Revision panel 8.4

General complications of proximal femoral fractures

Venous thromboembolism: deep vein thrombosis or pulmonary embolus

Fat embolus

Adult respiratory distress syndrome

Pneumonia

Blisters or pressure sores

Local complications include:

    Infection
    Avascular necrosis of the femoral head
    Heterotopic ossification
    Malunion
    Non-union
    Osteoarthritis of the hip joint

DISLOCATIONS OF THE HIP

These are usually the result of road traffic accidents, where force is transmitted up the femoral shaft. They can also result from falls from a height. The most common is a posterior dislocation, but anterior and central dislocations can also occur.

Posterior dislocation

This often occurs when a vehicle passenger or driver is thrown forwards and hits their bent knee against a rigid structure, such as the dashboard. The femoral head is forced backwards, often fracturing the posterior acetabulum.

History

Pain in the hip is severe, the limb is shortened, and patients cannot weight-bear or walk.

Examination

The limb is shortened, internally rotated, adducted and flexed. All movements of the hip are restricted and painful. The greater trochanter may appear prominent, and the buttock appears swollen.

There may be an associated femoral shaft fracture, which may mask the signs of the hip dislocation (see below).

Complications

There may be other associated fractures of the femoral head, neck and shaft, and these must not be missed if a an attempt is to be made to reduce the dislocation. Sciatic nerve injury (see Chapter 3) complicates over 10 per cent of dislocations, although fortunately most recover. Avascular necrosis of the femoral head is common, appearing within 12 months of the injury in 10 per cent of cases. Heterotopic ossification can also occur.

Osteoarthritis is a late complication.

Anterior dislocation

The history is similar, but the limb lies abducted, externally rotated and slightly flexed.

The femoral head is usually seen and felt bulging anteriorly.

Complications

Femoral vein thrombosis, arterial injury and femoral nerve damage are associated complications.

Central dislocation

This occurs when a fall or blow on the greater trochanter drives the femoral head through the acetabular floor, causing a pelvic fracture (see Chapter 9).

FRACTURES OF THE FEMORAL SHAFT

These are usually caused by high-energy injuries such as road accidents, and are most common in young male adults. In elderly individuals, a pathological fracture must always be considered, especially if the force involved seems insignificant. Fractures can also occur around the prosthesis of hip and knee replacements in this age group. Open fractures occur when the skin is breached by the external force or by the sharpened bone ends.

History

There is severe thigh pain and an inability to weight-bear.

Examination

The thigh is very swollen, and all movements are painful. The leg is often shortened, abducted and externally rotated. There may be significant blood loss into the torn thigh muscles, and there may be signs of hypovolaemic shock.

Complications

Complications are shown in the Revision panel 8.5.

Revision panel 8.5
Complication of fractures of the femoral shaft

Neurovascular injury

Infection

Fat embolus

Venous thromboembolism

Joint stiffness

Delayed union

Mal union

Non-union

SUPRACONDYLAR FRACTURES OF THE FEMUR

These follow falls in elderly osteoporotic females and direct violence in young males involved in high-speed car accidents. A previous knee arthroplasty is also a risk factor.

The fracture can be extra- or intracapsular, and may involve one or both condyles.

History

The knee is painful, and the patient notices swelling and deformity in and around the knee.

Examination

The knee is tender and swollen, and all movements are painful and restricted. Weight-bearing is usually impossible. The distal pulses must be carefully palpated as injuries to the popliteal artery are common (see Chapter 10).

FRACTURES OF THE PATELLA

These are caused either by direct violence, where the knee strikes a hard surface or is hit by an object, or by indirect violence, where there is a sudden muscular contraction. This latter mechanism may also cause a rupture of the quadriceps tendon or avulsion of the tibial tubercle.

The fracture may be transverse, vertical, oblique, comminuted and either displaced or undisplaced. A patellar fracture needs to be differentiated from a congenitally bipartite patella.

History

The front of the knee is painful and swollen, and weight-bearing is painful.

Examination

There is local tenderness, bruising and abrasions over the knee cap, and there may be evidence of a haemarthrosis of the joint. Knee extension is usually painful and may be impossible. The ability to extend the knee does not rule out a fracture, as the surrounding soft tissues including the retinaculum may be intact. A palpable fracture gap resulting from displacement of the patella may be noted.

DISLOCATION OF THE PATELLA

The patella is normally pulled laterally as the quadriceps contracts because the normal knee is in slight valgus. The risk of patellar dislocation increases in subjects with:

- severe genu valgum;
- ligamentous laxity;
- an underdeveloped lateral femoral condyle;
- a shallow intercondylar groove;
- a small or high patella.

The dislocation occurs when there is sudden severe contraction of the quadriceps with the knee joint in a valgus position and externally rotated, such as when a rugby player executes a jink or side-step. It can also follow a direct hit to the medial side of the patella.

Recurrent dislocation happens in patients with the congenital anomalies listed above. The injury may be trivial because the medial capsule has been torn at the time of the first dislocation. Bilateral dislocations can occur.

History

Knee pain comes on suddenly while running or twisting. The joint is stuck in flexion, invariably causing the patient to fall to the ground. The patient may volunteer that 'the knee has gone out of joint'.

Age Patients are mostly young, usually in their teens and twenties.

Sex Sporadic, recurrent and bilateral dislocations are all more common in females.

Examination

Immediately after the dislocation, the medial femoral condyle appears prominent because the patella has shifted laterally, where it can usually be felt. The patella often returns spontaneously to its normal position, and the joint becomes swollen with a haemarthrosis.

In patients with recurrent dislocation, there may be signs of generalized joint laxity. The patella often seems small or lies in a high position.

Patellar apprehension test The patient resists vigorously if the patella is pushed laterally with the knee in slight flexion.

DISLOCATION OF THE KNEE

Posterior displacement of the femur occurs as the result of a force severe enough to tear both cruciate ligaments and one or both lateral ligaments. Road traffic accidents are the most common cause.

History

The knee is extremely painful, swollen, deformed and unable to move or weight-bear.

Examination

The knee joint is very swollen, bruised and deformed. There is often a loss of the anterior bulge of the knee, with the femoral condyles being easily palpable in the upper part of the popliteal fossa.

Complications

The popliteal vessels and nerves are often damaged by the injury, with the popliteal artery sometimes being torn or divided. Common peroneal nerve palsies, fractures of the tibial spines and meniscal injuries can also all occur.

PROXIMAL FRACTURES OF THE TIBIA AND FIBULA

These usually occur in adults and can be extra-articular fractures, fractures of the articular surface or fractures of one or both condyles. Most are confined to the tibia and often involve the tibial plateau.

These fractures can be caused by a car striking a pedestrian on the side of the knee (a direct blow) or by a fall from height, when the tibial condyles are split by a femoral condyle. When a severe valgus stress is applied to the knee (as in skiing), it may cause a fracture of the lateral tibial condyle that may be associated with a fracture of the fibular neck and damage to the medial collateral ligament.

History

This is usually of knee pain, swelling, deformity and an inability to stand or walk.

Examination

There may be blood in the knee joint (haemarthrosis), with a tender doughy swelling, bruising and overlying skin abrasions. A varus or valgus deformity indicates the side of the fracture. There may also be tenderness over the fracture or any damaged ligament.

Complications

These include peroneal nerve damage, compartment syndrome, residual joint deformity and osteoarthritis of the knee.

FRACTURES OF THE SHAFTS OF THE TIBIA AND FIBULA

Fracture of the tibia is common because it lies subcutaneously and is thus very exposed. This increases the risk of associated skin damage, leading to an open fracture.

The mechanisms of injury include twisting in football or skiing injuries (spiral fractures of both tibia and fibula), angulation (transverse, comminuted or oblique fractures) or direct blows in road accidents.

History

This is of pain, deformity and an inability to weight-bear or walk.

Examination

Bruising, local tenderness and deformity are all present. The skin, nerves and pulses must all be very carefully examined.

Complications

Compartment syndrome and vascular injuries (veins and arteries) are common associations of these fractures. Malunion and delayed union can also occur.

FRACTURES OF AND AROUND THE ANKLE

These are common injuries in children, skiers, footballers and rugby players, and are often associated with sprains and dislocations.

They are usually caused by the ankle twisting and the talus rotating within the tibiofibular mortise, resulting in fractures of one or both malleoli.

CHAPTER 8 | LOWER LIMB SYMPTOMS AND SIGNS

Inversion, lateral rotation and abduction cause the lateral (fibular) malleolus and also sometimes the medial malleolus to fracture obliquely. An equal and opposite twist causes a fracture of the medial (tibial) malleolus and sometimes the lateral malleolus.

The posterior end of the tibia may occasionally be sheared off by the tibia moving rapidly forward over the talus.

The classification of ankle fractures is largely determined by the level of the fibular fracture. Distal to the syndesmosis is type A, level with the syndesmosis is type B, and above the syndesmosis is type C (the **Weber classification**) (Fig. 8.45). The **Lauge–Hansen** classification is based on the position of the foot at the time of injury and the direction of the applied causal load.

Occasionally, a fall from height causes a pilon (hammer) fracture, in which the articular surface of the tibia or the upper end of the talus becomes comminuted.

Fig. 8.45 The Weber classification of fractures around the ankle.

History

Pain and inability to weight-bear follow an ankle twist.

Examination

The ankle is swollen and very tender. Deformity suggests that there is a fracture or dislocation. Tenderness is maximal over the fracture sites at the ankle. However, tenderness may also be felt higher up the fibula because of a further fracture (**Maisonneuve fracture**).

Complications

These include instability, stiffness, malunion and late osteoarthritis.

ANKLE DISLOCATION

This is usually associated with an ankle fracture.

FRACTURES OF THE TALUS AND CALCANEUM

These fractures are often associated with other foot injuries or fractures, and the whole of the foot, its nerves and its blood vessels must always be carefully examined.

Fractures of these bones are caused by falls from a height (e.g. painters, scaffolders and window cleaners) or severe road accidents, where the foot is on the brake at the time of impact. Fractures of the spine, pelvis or hip are often associated.

Calcaneal fractures are more common than talar fractures.

As the talus articulates in three joints – the ankle joint (tibia/fibula), the subtalar joint (calcaneus) and the talonavicular joint (navicular bone) – injuries can have significant long-term implications.

History

The history of the accident may be suggestive, and the ankle and foot are usually painful and swollen. Weight-bearing is painful and often impossible.

Examination

The foot is usually very swollen and bruised and may be deformed, with the heel appearing broad and squat (Fig. 8.46). Movements at the subtalar joint are impossible. The relevant bone is tender.

Complications

These include avascular necrosis in up to 50 per cent of severe cases and osteoarthritis. There may be an associated talar or subtalar dislocation, but marked swelling often masks the deformity. Skin necrosis may occur over the displaced talus, hence the need for early reduction.

(a)

(b)

Fig. 8.46 HEEL DEFORMITIES CAUSED BY CALCANEAL FRACTURES WITH ASSOCIATED FRACTURE BLISTERS

MID-TARSAL FRACTURES

Fractures of other individual tarsal bones are rare, and when they occur are often associated with a combination of other fractures and dislocations in the foot.

History

There is usually a history of severe blunt trauma to the foot, which is swollen, bruised and painful.

Examination

A deformity is often present that makes the foot appear club-like or twisted and swollen.

METATARSAL FRACTURES

These are caused by a direct blow or a twisting force, and are common in footballers and rugby players whose boots are trodden on while their momentum is maintained. They are also a common site for stress fractures in army recruits and professional sportsmen.

The metatarsal bones can also dislocate. A fracture at the base of the second metatarsal associated with dislocation is known as a **Lisfranc fracture**.

History

There is pain and swelling in the forefoot.

Examination

Localized tenderness over the fracture may be the only sign as the fractures are usually undisplaced. There may be marked swelling. Compartment syndrome may occur.

FRACTURED TOES

These are caused by stamping or heavy objects falling on the toes.

Pain, swelling, deformity and local tenderness are suggestive, and fractures may be associated with subluxations and dislocations.

FRACTURED SESAMOID BONES

These can be fractured directly, by traction or by stress. Pain is experienced over the bone and is reproduced by digital pressure or hyperextending the great toe.

CHAPTER 8 | LOWER LIMB SYMPTOMS AND SIGNS

The spine and pelvis

Common spinal complaints include:

- mechanical type neck or low back pain;
- pain in the neck with radiation to the arm;
- back pain with radiation to the leg;
- cauda equina syndrome;
- spinal cord compression.

There are a number of well-defined clinical syndromes produced by prolapsed discs in the cervical and lumbar spine.

Pain is the dominant symptom (brachalgia, sciatica) and is often severe and of sudden onset. With chronic neck or back pain, always ask about **night pain**, as this is associated with metastatic disease. **Fever** may indicate an epidural abscess, seen most commonly in those with diabetes and intravenous drug abusers.

Any **interscapular pain** waking the patient at night is likely to be caused by metastatic destruction of a vertebral body until proved otherwise.

In a patient with cancer and intractable back pain, ask about any **disturbance of bladder or bowel control**, and perform a neurological examination of the lower limbs.

Clinical assessment of the spine is the same as for any other joint or series of joints, namely a careful history, followed by an examination based on the principles of 'look–feel–move'.

The spine is considered in two sections: the cervical spine and the thoraco-lumbar-sacral spine.

THE CERVICAL SPINE

EXAMINATION OF THE CERVICAL SPINE

The patient must be undressed appropriately with both shoulders exposed.

Inspection

The head should be held in a neutral position with preservation of the natural lordosis, the normal range being between 20° and 30°. Is there anterior, posterior or lateral flexion? Is the head tilted in position to try to relieve the pain of acute disc prolapse? Can the patient look straight ahead, or does he or she look down to the ground, as for instance in ankylosing spondylitis?

Look for asymmetry, particularly of the sternocleidomastoid muscles, the clavicles and the supraclavicular fossae. Is there a visible mass or scars indicating previous surgery?

Palpation

Feel posteriorly from the occiput to the upper thoracic spine, looking for areas of tenderness or any deformity such as a 'step' indicating spondylolisthesis. Note that the most prominent spinous process is T1 and not C7, although C7 is known as the vertebra prominens.

Palpate the trapezius region, the shoulders, the clavicles and then the posterior and anterior triangles of the neck, looking for tenderness and masses such as a cervical rib. Assess the thyroid, larynx and supraclavicular fossae.

Range of movement

Test actively, asking the patient to move their head, and then passively, in which you hold the head gently and move the cervical spine. Try to differentiate between active movement limited by pain and passive movement limited less by pain than by intrinsic stiffness of the cervical column, most commonly caused by degenerative spondyolytic changes. The normal range of movement is shown in Table 9.1.

Table 9.1   The normal range of movement of the cervical spine

Direction of movement	Range of movement
Flexion/extension	120°
Axial rotation	160°
Lateral flexion	60–70°

Specific signs

Spurling's sign (Fig. 9.1)

The head is extended and rotated towards the side of the patient's symptoms, with simultaneous gentle downward compression of the head. The test is positive if the patient's pain is reproduced and radiates down the arm.

A positive Spurling's sign indicates cervical radiculopathy, commonly due to acute intervertebral disc prolapse or, in older patients, intravertebral osteophytes causing nerve root compression in the exit foramen.

Fig. 9.1 Spurling's sign.

L'Hermitte's sign

On sudden flexion or hyperextension of the neck, an electric shock sensation passes down into the upper and lower limbs. The patient may mention this in the history. The sign may be positive in patients with severe spinal cord compression from degenerative stenosis, or central large disc herniation causing spinal cord compression.

Other systems

In all patients presenting with what are thought to be symptoms arising from the cervical spine, an examination of the shoulders and a full neurological examination of the upper and lower limbs must be carried out (see Chapter 3).

COMMON CONDITIONS OF THE CERVICAL SPINE

Cervical axial mechanical type neck pain

This is the most common symptom arising from the cervical spine.

Age It occurs in adults, more commonly over the age of 45 years.

Site The pain is sited in the midline, radiating into the shoulders and down into the interscapular region of the thoracic spine, but not into the arms (Fig. 9.2). There are no associated neurological symptoms.

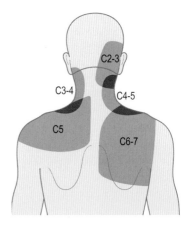

Fig. 9.2 This illustrates the sites where pain is perceived from the cervical spine. The commonest origin for pain is the C5/6 and C6/7 levels with the pain felt across the shoulders and in the interscapular region, significantly below the cervical spine.

Precipitating factors A history of minor trauma is common but not invariably present.

Pain The pain is variable in intensity, and waxes and wanes with time. There is rarely pain at night, but patients may complain of difficulty in getting to sleep, after which they sleep satisfactorily.

Stiffness This is usually worse in the morning, improves on movement, but may be exacerbated by being in one position for prolonged periods of time, such as when leaning forward working at a computer.

The symptoms are usually self-limiting and are significantly improved with an active physiotherapy programme. Investigations are only warranted in cases when the pain is failing to resolve or when there are associated neurological symptoms and signs suggestive of more significant pathology (see *Investigation and Management*, Chapter 10).

Whiplash injury

This is a combination of a hyperextension and a hyperflexion injury of the cervical spine, usually as a consequence of being hit from behind in a motor vehicle accident.

Symptoms Patients may present immediately or 2–3 days later with neck pain, neck stiffness, occipital headaches and occasionally neurological symptoms in the upper limbs. Approximately 25 per cent of patients develop chronic pain that lasts for longer than 2 years, severe in a one-third of cases.

Examination There are no significant abnormal signs except some stiffness.

Differential diagnosis Significant injury to bones or joints needs to be excluded by appropriate investigations.

Medicolegal implications As the diagnosis is based on the history and there are no significant physical signs or abnormal investigations, many claims for compensation for this condition may unfortunately be fraudulent.

Acute cervical intervertebral disc prolapse

Age and sex This is most common in the fourth decade, and slightly more common in males than females (1.4 to 1).

Level It most commonly occurs at the C5/6 disc level followed by C6/7 and then C4/5.

Symptoms There is acute neck pain, either generalized and diffuse in a mesodermal distribution,

or with localized and specific pain in a nerve root distribution.

Radiculopathy and *myelopathy* are defined in Revision panel 9.1. There are usually no precipitating factors. Diffuse neck pain and stiffness is followed by more specific pain in a radicular pattern down one arm, sometimes into the hand. This may be severe and be associated with sensory loss and muscle weakness with decreased or absent motor reflexes. There may also be significant night pain preventing sleep.

Rarely, there is associated myelopathy, although this must be excluded by a careful examination.

Natural history The vast majority of cases resolve within 3 months, and only 1–2 per cent require surgical treatment.

See also Chapter 3.

Revision panel 9.1

Definition of radiculopathy and myelopathy

Radiculopathy: an extradural compression of a nerve resulting in some degree of pain, paralysis, sensory loss and motor reflex changes, in the distribution of a spinal nerve

Myelopathy: a dysfunction of the spinal cord *itself*

Spondylitic myelopathy: an *extrinsic* compression of the spinal cord producing the symptoms and signs of an upper motor neuron lesion of the spinal cord

---

Cervical spondylosis and spondylitic cervical myelopathy

Cervical spondylosis

Definition Cervical spondylosis is the term used to describe degeneration of the intervertebral discs with degenerative osteoarthritis of the facet and intravertebral joints.

Age and sex It is most common in patients aged over 50 years, although the spine begins to 'age' from the late teens, equally in males and females.

Level It is most common at the C5/6 disc level, followed by C6/7 and then C4/5.

Symptoms There is midline neck pain exacerbated by movement, with diffuse radiation to the shoulder, the area between the shoulder blades and the upper arms. There is associated neck stiffness, which may interfere with driving.

CHAPTER 9 | THE SPINE AND PELVIS

Night pain is not usually a major feature, although patients may complain that they find it difficult to get comfortable in order to go to sleep. They may also wake in the morning with increased neck pain and stiffness. This improves once they get up and mobilize.

Natural history The condition is usually self-limiting, although some patients have episodic periods of neck pain, lasting from a few weeks to a few months, and continuing for years. A few develop significant chronic neck pain.

As the degenerative process proceeds, radiculopathy may develop caused by stenosis of the exit foramina caused by a combination of uncovertebral osteophytes, disc prolapse and ligamentum flavum and facet joint hypertrophy.

Spondylitic cervical myelopathy

Progressive spondylitic pathology can lead to central spinal canal stenosis and the development of a myelopathy (see Revision panel 9.1) as the spinal cord is compressed. This can be either *dynamic*, when cord compression occurs only on movement, or there may be instability of the cervical spinal column, causing compression of and damage to the spinal cord, termed *myelomalacia*. There may not be neck pain, but stiffness is a common feature.

History

Patients complain of clumsiness and dysaesthaesia (abnormal sensation) of the hands, with a loss of fine motor function. They cannot do up buttons satisfactorily, write neatly or use a keyboard.

There may be a disturbance of gait, with a sense of unsteadiness. They feel a need to look at their feet on walking, with a loss of walking distance as the legs tire easily. This is caused by loss of proprioception followed by loss of motor function. The degree of myelopathy may be graded using the Nurick classification (Table 9.2).

Natural history Those with mild symptoms and signs do not always progress and some improve, but patients with severe symptoms usually deteriorate and require surgery.

Thoracic outlet syndrome: cervical rib syndrome

Cause The cause may be a cervical rib, an associated fibrous band or hypertrophy of the scalenus anterior

Table 9.2 Nurick's classification of cervical myelopathy

Grade 0	Root signs and symptoms, no cord involvement
Grade 1	Signs of cord involvement, normal gait
Grade 2	Mild gait involvement, able to be employed
Grade 3	Gait abnormality prevents employment
Grade 4	Able to ambulate but with assistance (walk!)
Grade 5	Chair bound or bedridden

muscle compressing the subclavian artery and/or the brachial plexus, especially the T1 nerve root.

Cervical ribs occur in about 0.4 per cent of the population (70 per cent being bilateral), but only 60 per cent are symptomatic.

Symptoms There is pain and numbness of the arm and hand, with weakness of grip, especially on prolonged carrying of heavy bags. It is made worse on abduction of the shoulder.

Vascular symptoms (axillary vein thrombosis, Raynaud's phenomenon, subclavian aneurysm) are also common (see Chapter 10), and presentation is occasionally with a lump in the neck caused by the cervical rib.

Signs There may be a palpable cervical rib in the supraclavicular fossa (see Chapter 12), decreased vascular supply to the hand, or signs of T1 nerve root compression (see Chapter 3).

Adson's test (Fig. 9.3) The patient extends and turns the neck towards the affected side while abducting and extending the shoulder with the elbow in extension. This results after a few minutes in a loss of the radial pulse and an exacerbation of the patient's symptoms. Returning the neck and shoulder to the neutral position restores the pulse and relieves the symptoms.

Allen's test (Fig. 9.4) This is similar to Adson's test, but the patient turns the neck away from the affected side while abducting and externally rotating the shoulder.

Adson's and Allen's tests are unreliable, with both false-positive and false-negative results.

disease characterized by inflammation and destruction of the synovial joints. There may be atlanto-axial subluxation, vertical subluxation of the second cervical vertebra with cranial settling, basilar invagination and sub-axial subluxation.

Symptoms Patients present with progressive neck pain and stiffness. In advanced disease, cervical myelopathy (see above) may develop, but with modern treatment this is rare.

    Ranawat's classification (Table 9.3) classifies the degree of disability.

Table 9.3   Ranawat's classification of cervical myelopathy in rheumatoid arthritis

Grade 1	Neck pain, no neurological deficit
Grade 2	Subjective weakness, dysaesthesia, hyper-reflexia
Grade 3A	Objective weakness and long tract signs, ambulatory
Grade 3B	Objective weakness and long tract signs, non-ambulatory

Fig. 9.3 Adson's test for thoracic outlet syndrome.

THE THORACO-LUMBAR-SACRAL SPINE

EXAMINATION OF THE THORACO-LUMBAR-SACRAL SPINE

The patient must be adequately undressed with exposure of the whole spine and lower limbs.

Inspection

View the whole spine from behind, looking for scars, any cutaneous stigmata of underlying spinal dysraphism such as a hairy naevus, a sinus or a sacral dimple indicating any underlying spinal dysraphism, e.g. spina bifida. Look for any café-au-lait spots indicating neurofibromatosis.

Fig. 9.4 Allen's test for thoracic outlet syndrome.

Rheumatoid arthritis of the cervical spine

The cervical spine is the region most commonly affected by this chronic, systemic autoimmune

Alignment

Is there a scoliosis or kyphosis (Fig. 9.5)? Minor deformities are not immediately obvious. Look from the side with the patient's hips and knees in full extension to assess the sagittal plane and the presence of a kyphosis. Check the position of the shoulders. Are the scapulae and the loin creases symmetrical? Is the pelvis level?

Adam's forward bending test The patient is asked to lean forward with their arms hanging down in front of them in a relaxed and comfortable position. This will reveal more clearly any scoliosis or kyphosis (Fig. 9.6).

(a)

Fig. 9.5 Inspection of the spine. This illustrates quite marked thoracic kyphosis in a patient with ankylosing spondylitis, with characteristic compensatory hyperextension of the neck to allow a forward horizontal gaze.

(b)

Fig. 9.6 ADAM'S FORWARD BENDING TEST (a, b) This illustrates the rib hump that is characteristic of a right thoracic scoliosis.

Range of movement

The bulk of forward flexion and extension on bending forwards and backwards is at the hips, so methods are needed to differentiate this from true spinal flexion and extension.

For thoracic flexion, hold a tape measure with the ends on the spines of T1 and L1, and note the increased length when the patient bends forwards from the standing into the fully flexed position. This is normally around 8 cm. A similar measurement from L1 to S1 should show an increase of 8–10 cm. Less than 3 cm indicates significant pathology.

Schober's test (Fig. 9.7) Marks are made 10 cm above and 5 cm below the line that connects the two posterior superior iliac spines. On maximum forward bending, the distance should increase by 8–10 cm. Less than 3 cm indicates significant pathology.

Fig. **9.7** Schober's test.

Lateral flexion Ask the patient to run their hand down the lateral aspect of the thigh as far as they are able. The normal is approximately 30° of lateral flexion.

Rotation Rotation should be tested in the sitting position. The maximum range of thoracic and lumbar rotation is approximately 40°, largely occurring in the thoracic spine, with only 5° coming from the lumbar spine.

Chest expansion Place a tape measure under the axillae. Expansion should be at least 6 cm; less than 2.5 cm is abnormal. A common cause for loss of expansion is ankylosing spondylitis.

Gait

At this stage, while the patient is still standing, it is convenient to assess the gait. Look for an *antalgic gait* in which the stance phase of gait is shortened relative to the swing phase. This indicates pain on weight-bearing.

Look for any neurological deficit, such as muscle wasting or a foot drop. Observation of heel and

toe walking may reveal a subtle weakness of tibialis anterior (L4), extensor hallucis longus (L5) or triceps surae (S1/2).

Palpation and percussion

Feel from T1 to the sacrum, looking for tenderness of the spine itself and the paravertebral muscles. Is there continuity of the spinous processes and the interspinous and supraspinous ligaments, or is there a step indicating a spondylolisthesis?

Pain on percussion suggests spinal column sepsis.

Lower limb tension signs

These are tests for radiculopathies of the lumbar and S1 nerve roots, the most common causes of which are an acute disc prolapse causing compression of an individual nerve, or degenerative changes causing nerve root compression.

Sciatic stretch (Lasègue's) test (Fig. 9.8) With the patient lying supine, the leg is lifted until prevented by pain in a radicular distribution, that is exacerbated by dorsiflexing the ankle. If the leg can be raised above 50°, the test loses its specificity as the cause may be tight hamstring muscles.

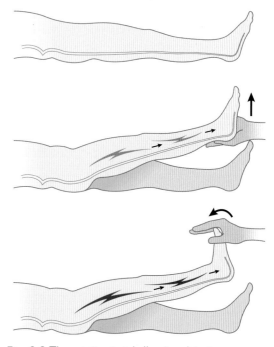

Fig. **9.8** The sciatic stretch (Lasègue) test.

If the pain is relieved by flexing the knee, it is known as the *bowstring sign*, which suggests nerve root irritation at the L4, L5 or S1 level, caused by lower lumbar disc prolapse.

Frajersztajn's sign Raising the leg on the asymptomatic side reproduces the radicular pain on the affected side. This may indicate central disc prolapse, characteristically at the L4/5 level.

Femoral stretch test (Fig. 9.9) The patient lies prone, and the knee is flexed and the hip extended. This tenses the femoral nerve. If radicular pain is produced down the front of the thigh in the L2–L4 distribution, there is likely to be an upper lumbar radiculopathy.

Fig. 9.9 The femoral stretch test.

Hip and leg length

Leg length discrepancy is the most common cause of a functional scoliosis with a tilted pelvis, present only when the patient stands. It is corrected when the patient sits, and is confirmed by measuring the leg lengths.

Hip examination is essential. Pain arising from the hip may mimic pain from the spine and vice versa. An L4/5 spondylolisthesis may present with pain referred into the groin, very similar to that of osteoarthritis of the hip. This is easily detected on examination of the hip. With a spondylolisthesis, there will be a painless full range of movement of the hip.

Neurological examination

A detailed neurological examination of the upper and lower limbs must be performed to look for myelopathy, radiculopathy or peripheral neuropathy. Inspection reveals asymmetry or muscle wasting. Tone is assessed, followed by testing sensation for light touch, pinprick, vibration and proprioception,

and then assessment of motor function. Finally, the reflexes are tested.

Myelopathy and radiculopathy are defined in Revision panel 9.1. The dermatomes are shown in Fig. 3.36 and the myotomes in Fig. 9.10.

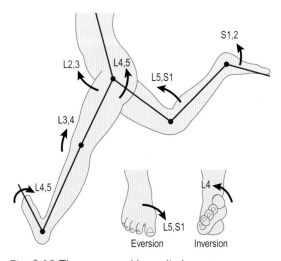

Fig. 9.10 The upper and lower limb myotomes.

Myelopathy

There is an upper motor neuron deficit caused by spinal cord dysfunction usually caused by direct compression associated with a compromise of cord perfusion. There is hypertonic (spastic) paresis, with sensory loss, hyper-reflexia and upgoing plantar reflexes (*Babinski's sign*). The level of spinal cord injury leading to a myelopathy is defined as the most caudal level with normal function.

Radiculopathy

There will be a lower motor neuron deficit caused by damage to an individual nerve root or neural plexus, leading to a hypotonic (flaccid) paresis with sensory loss, impaired or absent reflexes and absent plantar reflexes.

Rectal examination

If a cauda equina syndrome is suspected, a rectal examination is mandatory to assess the function of the S2, S3 and S4 nerve roots, which control bladder, bowel and sexual function. There are four components:

1. Assessment of perianal light touch sensation.
2. Assessment of perianal pinprick sensation and the anal wink reflex. In response to the pinprick, the anal sphincter contracts and the patient feels the pinprick. Both are absent in cauda equina syndrome.
3. Anal sphincter digital examination to assess resting anal tone and voluntary anal contraction. In cauda equina syndrome, the resting anal tone is decreased or absent, with decreased or absent voluntary contraction.
4. Assessment of the bulbo-cavernosus reflex (Fig. 9.11). In the catheterized patient, a sharp tug on the urinary catheter produces contraction of the anal sphincter detected by an examining finger within the anus. This reflex is absent in cauda equina syndrome. It is also absent in spinal shock, and its return indicates resolution of the condition.

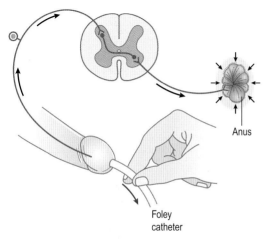

Fig. 9.11 The bulbo-cavernosus reflex.

Abdominal and vascular examinations

These are mandatory to exclude intra-abdominal pathology as a cause for back pain, and arterial ischaemia as a cause of lower limb pain (see Chapters 10 and 15).

Note that examination of the spine is not usually part of a routine physical examination, but if it is not carried out properly, much significant pathology can be missed.

COMMON CONDITIONS OF THE THORACO-LUMBAR-SACRAL SPINE

Back pain

Each year, one-half of the UK population have an episode of back pain, and one-tenth of the population seek medical advice. There are three important groups:

- Simple back pain.
- Radicular pain.
- Potentially serious pathology.

The Clinical Standards Advisory Group for Back Pain has produced a set of criteria for the identification of patients presenting with low back pain who may have serious pathology. These are called the 'red flag signs' and are listed in Revision panel 9.2.

> ### Revision panel 9.2
> #### Red flag signs for low back pain
> Age – below 20 years or above 50 years
> A history of significant trauma
> Thoracic pain
> Non-mechanical pain, namely a constant pain not related to movement and sometimes worse at night
> A past medical history of cancer, steroid use, intravenous drug abuse or HIV infection
> Being systemically unwell
> A history of weight loss
> Lumbar flexion less than 5 cm
> Neurological deficit
> Structural spinal deformity

CHAPTER 9 | THE SPINE AND PELVIS

Low back pain

Definition This is pain lasting for more than 24 hours, located between the lowest ribs and the inferior gluteal fold, and arising from the spine. It does not radiate into the legs, and there are no neurological symptoms or signs.

Age The patient is usually between 20 and 55 years old.

Character It is mechanical in nature, namely in that it varies with activity and time. In other words, it 'comes and goes'.

Causes The causes are complex and myriad, but the most common factor is degeneration. Other causes of the pain (listed in Revision panel 9.3), must however, be excluded.

Revision panel 9.3

Causes of low back pain

Spondylogenic

Degenerative:
> Disc
> Facet joint
> Vertebral bodies

Tumour:
> Benign
> Malignant – primary or secondary

Sepsis:
> Pyogenic
> Tuberculosis
> Fungal
> Yeast

Metabolic:
> Osteoporosis
> Paget's disease

Neurogenic

Nerve root (radicular):
> Disc
> Stenosis – central, posterolateral, foraminal

Cauda equina syndrome – massive prolapsed intervertebral disc causing compression of the cauda equina

Viscogenic

Renal

Retroperitoneal, e.g. pancreatic

Bowel

Vascular

Abdominal aortic aneurysm

Acute prolapsed intervertebral disc

Incidence Symptomatic lumbar intervertebral disc herniation affects 2 per cent of the population at some time. Of these, 1 in 20 require surgery.

Symptoms There is back pain lasting for some weeks that then lessens in severity and is replaced by leg pain radiating to below the knee. This is often described as *sciatica*, which is a radicular pain in the L4, L5 or S1 distribution, sometimes with associated neurological symptoms.

The pain may be very severe, exacerbated by sitting, standing and coughing, with shooting pain down the leg. It is relieved to a degree by changing position and walking, but walking too far can further exacerbate the symptoms.

Specific enquiries Ask if there is any perineal sensory loss (*saddle anaesthesia*) or loss of normal bladder and bowel control. This may indicate cauda equina syndrome, and must always be asked about.

Symptomatic thoracic disc herniation

This is a rare condition, affecting only one person per million per year. Symptoms include thoracic pain, burning sensations, and numbness and paraesthesia in the trunk and down the legs. There may be a full scale myelopathy due to spinal cord compression (see above).

Cauda equina syndrome

Definition This is compression of the cauda equina leading to compromise of the nerve supply to the sphincters of the bladder and bowel.

Cause The cause is commonly a massive central disc herniation.

Symptoms There is usually severe pain radiating down to the perineum, although pain is not invariably present. This is followed by an inability to pass urine and impaired faecal continence.

Signs There is perineal sensory loss, a palpable bladder due to painless urinary retention, laxity and weakness of the anal sphincter and absence of the bulbo-cavernosus reflex.

Unless treated rapidly, the urinary and anal sphincters will not recover. Cauda equina syndrome is therefore a surgical emergency.

Degenerative spinal stenosis presenting with neurogenic claudication

Degenerative changes within the lumbar spine lead to narrowing of the spinal canal, termed spinal stenosis. This may lead to neurogenic claudication.

Age Patients are usually over the age of 50 years.
Symptoms There is usually low back pain and stiffness. On walking, the pain radiates down into the legs, and may be associated with numbness and paraesthesia in the feet. Sometimes there is actual weakness of the feet, with a tendency to trip.

Neurological examination is usually normal except for the absence of the ankle jerks.

Relieving factors The pain may be eased to a degree by leaning forwards. The cross-sectional area of the spinal canal is increased in flexion, so the stenosis is lessened, which reduces the symptoms. Patients may say that pushing a supermarket trolley is helpful as it allows them to lean forwards with support.

Differentiation from vascular claudication The pain is relieved by resting or sitting down in both conditions. In neurogenic claudication, the symptoms recede slowly over 5–10 minutes before the patient can continue walking, and this is further improved by leaning forwards or squatting. In vascular intermittent claudication, the recovery time is much less: 1–2 minutes. The ankle–brachial pressure index is invariably reduced in vascular claudication (see Chapter 10), but it should be remembered that the two conditions can coexist.

Spinal deformity – scoliosis and kyphosis

Scoliosis

Scoliosis is a lateral curvature of the spine. It may be structural or functional.

A *structural scoliosis* is a fixed deformity of the spine associated with a rotational deformity of the vertebral bodies. The curvature may have some flexibility, but it cannot be corrected by a change in position (Fig. 9.12).

(a) Showing bend to right.

(b) Showing scoliosis with spine deviating in mid-thoracic region, to the right.

Fig. 9.12 INSPECTION OF THE ALIGNMENT OF THE SPINE

CHAPTER 9 | THE SPINE AND PELVIS

Fig. 9.13 A patient with functional scoliosis.

A *functional scoliosis* (Fig. 9.13) is a curvature of the spine that is not associated with any rotational abnormality of the vertebral body. It is more accurately described as a tilt or list of the spine and is corrected by sitting or lying down. The most common cause is a discrepancy in leg length.

Functional scoliosis may also occur when there is a painful lesion within the spine, such as an acute prolapsed intervertebral disc or osteoid osteoma that causes the spine to be held at an angle. If the source of pain is not removed, the scoliosis may become fixed and structural.

The many causes of structural scoliosis are listed in Revision panel 9.4.

Scoliosis may be congenital, idiopathic or neuromuscular. The congenital variety may be associated with structural abnormalities of the vertebrae such as hemivertebrae or a failure of segmentation under the influence of the homeobox genes. Associated abnormalities of the genitourinary

system or heart are common. Early onset idiopathic scoliosis is more common in males, while late onset (adolescent) idiopathic scoliosis is significantly more common in females.

Revision panel 9.4
Causes of structural scoliosis

Idiopathic
Early onset under 5 years old
Late onset over 5 years old

Congenital
A failure of either formation or segmentation of the vertebral body, or a combination of the two

Neuromuscular
Neuropathic
Upper motor neuron:
  Cerebral palsy
  Spinal cerebellar atrophy, e.g. Friedrich's ataxia
Lower motor neuron:
  Poliomyelitis
  Spinal muscular atrophy
  Myelomeningocele – spina bifida
Myopathic
  Arthrogryposis
  Muscular dystrophy, e.g. Duchenne

Neurofibromatosis

Mesenchymal disorders
Marfan's syndrome
Ehlers–Danlos syndrome

Trauma
Post-traumatic deformities

Osteochondrodystrophies
Achondroplasia
Mucopolysaccharidoses, e.g. Morquio's syndrome

Spinal column sepsis

Tumours
Osteoid osteoma
Histiocytosis X

Metabolic
Rickets
Osteogenesis imperfecta
Homocystinuria

Kyphosis

In the normal spine, there is lordosis in the cervical and lumbar spines, and kyphosis in the thoracic spine. A plumb line from the odontoid peg passes through the bodies of C7 and L1, and the posterior junction of the L5 and S1 vertebral bodies (Fig. 9.14). The normal thoracic kyphosis is between 20° and 45°, and increases marginally with age to 55°, measured from T4 to T12. The lumbar lordosis is between 40° and 60°, measured from T12 to S1.

The most common sagittal plane deformity is an increase in thoracic kyphosis and a loss of lumbar lordosis. This causes increasing back pain with a positive sagittal balance (anterior position of the head in relation to the pelvis as the body tilts forward) and fatigue on walking.

Severe kyphosis can lead to significant spinal cord compromise and the development of a progressive neurological deficit. Monitoring is essential.

Fig. 9.14 The normal sagittal alignment of the spine.

Symptoms Patients complain principally of their appearance. Other symptoms are back pain, a sensation of leaning forward, difficulty looking forwards, a sense of abdominal constriction and the need to use a stick to assist in holding themselves upright when standing or walking.

The most common causes of kyphosis in young people are Scheuermann's disease (osteochondritis of the spine), ankylosing spondylitis and trauma. In the older age groups, degenerative changes and osteoporotic wedge compression fractures are more common (Revision panel 9.5).

A localized kyphosis with a prominent angle is termed a *kyphus*.

Revision panel 9.5

Causes of spinal kyphosis

Traumatic
Compression fractures

Iatrogenic
Postsurgical laminectomy
Postirradiation

Inflammatory disorders
Rheumatoid arthritis
Ankylosing spondylitis

Infectious
Pyogenic
Tuberculosis

Scheuermann's kyphosis

Degenerative conditions
Osteoarthritis
Osteoporotic wedge compression fractures
Paget's disease

Congenital
Failure of formation or segmentation, or a combination of the two

Neoplastic
Primary tumours
Metastatic tumours
Multiple myeloma

Skeletal dysplasias
Achondrodysplasia
Pseudoachondrodysplasia

Osteoporosis/osteomalacia

These conditions commonly affect the spine. Osteoporosis typically occurs in elderly postmenopausal women and is symptomless until a pathological fracture occurs. A kyphosis or kyphus may be present. Osteomalacia affects those with a calcium and phosphate deficiency, usually caused by a vitamin D deficiency, and should be considered as a cause of kyphosis, especially in the Asian population.

Tumours of the spine

These may be benign, primary malignant or metastatic secondary malignancies.

Symptoms The most common presenting feature is pain that may be associated with a deformity. It is non-mechanical, constant and progressive. It is usually present at night, and there may be a radicular component to the pain if a nerve root is being compressed, or an overt myelopathy if there is spinal cord compression. Weight loss suggests a malignant tumour.

If there is associated instability of the spinal column, for example in the case of a pathological fracture, the pain will be exacerbated by movement to the extent that the patient is unable to move at all. On taking the history, look out for 'red flag' symptoms.

Signs There may be localized tenderness, and kyphosis or a kyphus secondary to vertebral collapse. Neurological examination is essential.

Benign tumours of the spine

- *Haemangiomas* are the most common hamartoma in the spine, and consist of dilated vascular channels.
- *Osteochondromas* are benign cartilaginous tumours arising from enchondral ossification.
- *Osteoid osteomas and osteoblastomas* arise in the pedicles of vertebrae and cause night pain.
- *Aneurysmal bone cysts* are rare and produce expansile osteolytic lesions.
- *Eosinophilic granulomas* occur in children.
- *Giant cell tumours* arise in vertebral bodies and are painful. They may become malignant.

Primary malignant tumours of the spine

These are rare, and usually arise in the vertebral bodies:

- *Myelomas* are myeloproliferative lesions of plasma cells.
- *Chordomas* arise from notochord remnants.
- *Sarcomas* can be osteosarcomas, chondrosarcomas or Ewing's sarcomas.

Secondary malignant tumours of the spine

These are far more common than primary tumours, and are usually metastases from primary tumours of the:

- Breast.
- Bronchus.
- Kidney.
- Prostate.
- Thyroid.
- Gastrointestinal tract.

The main symptoms are spinal pain, which is often present at night, radicular pain, neurological weakness of the limbs or bladder, and weight loss with anorexia and fatigue. The signs are tenderness and kyphosis or kyphus, with or without neurological signs. Any patient with a history of cancer with back or spinal pain needs to be fully assessed and will require imaging of the spine.

Spinal column sepsis

This may be *pyogenic* (staphylococci, *Pseudomonas*, *Escherichia coli*, *Klebsiella*, *Proteus*, *Salmonella*) or *non-pyogenic* (tuberculosis and occasional fungal infection). Ninety per cent of infections are in the thoraco-lumbar spine. The infection tends to arise in disc spaces in children and end-plates in adults, in both cases spreading to the adjacent discs and vertebrae. An epidural abscess may follow.

Tuberculosis is increasing in incidence throughout the world. Airborne spread leads to lung infection, which spreads to the bones via the bloodstream. There is granuloma formation followed by caseation.

Symptoms The presenting features of spinal column sepsis are pain that is also present at night, associated with stiffness and often neurological symptoms. There is usually but not always, constitutional upset.

Spinal tuberculosis is notoriously indolent, and there is on average a delay of 6–9 months from presentation to diagnosis.

Risk factors Specific enquiry must be made about the conditions listed in Revision panel 9.6.

Spondylolisthesis and spondylolysis

Spondylolisthesis

This is a forward slip of one vertebra in relation to the vertebra below. The causes are listed in Table 9.4.

Symptoms and signs Eighty per cent of cases are symptomless. Some patients suffer from chronic low back pain and notice tightening of the hamstring muscles. It is rare to develop radiculopathy or cauda equina syndrome.

On palpation, a step in the spinous processes at the appropriate level may be detectable, although this is an unreliable sign.

Spondylolysis

A spondylolysis is a break in the pars interarticularis, usually of the L5 vertebral body without a forward slip. The most common cause is a stress fracture of the L5 pars interarticularis.

Table 9.4   Classification of spondylolisthesis

Type	Name	Cause	Vertebral level	Age
I	Congenital or dysplastic	Dysplasia of the lumbar/sacral posterior arch and facet joints	Usually L5 on S1	8–10 years
II	Isthmic (spondylolytic)	A defect of the pars interarticularis: Stress fracture Elongation of the pars Traumatic fracture of the pars (rare)	L5	8–15 years
III	Degenerative	Degenerative changes of the facet joints and disc	L4 on L5 (90%)	Over 60 years
IV	Traumatic	A fracture of the posterior elements, excluding the pars interarticularis	Any level	Any
V	Pathological	Disturbance of the posterior elements and posterior tension band that allows the vertebra to slip forwards; this can be caused by tumour, sepsis or metabolic conditions such as Paget's disease	Any level	Any
VI	Iatrogenic, after surgery	Disruption of the posterior elements due to surgical removal of the laminar, pedicles and/or facet joints	Any level	Any

Age There is a bimodal age presentation of symptoms.

The younger age group (8–15 years) presents with back pain made worse by exercise. There may be a *spondylolitic crisis*, namely acute severe low back pain with severe hamstring spasms and tightness. Acute gluteal muscle spasms give the appearance of an inverted heart shape to the buttocks. There is difficulty in walking, with a semi-crouch-type gait with the hip and knees flexed. There may be neurological symptoms and signs, predominately in the L5 nerve root distribution.

Those in middle age present with back pain and L5 radicular pain due to facet and disc degeneration, which causes foraminal stenosis of the L5 nerve roots.

Coccydynia

This simply means pain in the coccyx.

Symptoms There is pain in the tail bone, usually with a history of slipping on a floor or stairs and landing heavily on the buttocks. The pain is worse on sitting, but is only rarely felt at night. There is no disturbance of bladder or bowel function, although opening of the bowels may be uncomfortable when they need to sit on the lavatory. There are no neurological symptoms.

Natural history The condition is self-limiting but can take up to 2 years to resolve fully.

Conditions of the sacroiliac joints

Pain arising from the sacroiliac joints can be hard to differentiate from pain arising from the lower lumbar spine and lumbar-sacral junction. The common causes of pain are:

- seronegative arthropathy, principally ankylosing spondylitis;
- sepsis, including tuberculosis;
- trauma: the sacroiliac joint is the strongest in the body, and if there is disruption, there is usually a related fracture of the pelvis.

Spina bifida and meningomyelocele

This condition is a consequence of failure of fusion of the vertebral arches with or without a defect in the neural tube, usually at a lower lumbar level.

Spina bifida occulta is a simple failure of fusion of the posterior elements and is entirely benign occurring most commonly at the L5 or S1 level. A meningomyelocele is when there is herniation of the neural structures through the posterior elements of the spine; this may be associated with neurological deficits of the lower limb and of bladder and bowel function. Cutaneous appearances vary from a simple hair-filled pit to a more obvious cystic swelling with meninges bulging through the defect, or cerebrospinal fluid leaking through neural material on the surface.

A full neurological examination is essential. There is often an accompanying hydrocephalus, so look for a bulging fontanelle or excessive head circumference.

FRACTURES OF THE SPINE AND PELVIS

A *stable* spinal fracture is not displaced by normal muscle action. *Unstable* fractures without immediate spinal cord damage can subsequently displace and cause cord damage leading to paresis or paralysis. Inadequate management of an unstable fracture without cord damage can therefore result in permanent and preventable cord damage. Hence, diagnosis and management go hand in hand.

Instability depends on the sites and extent of the damage to the vertebral bodies, the posterior arches and the stabilizing intervertebral ligaments. It occurs in the 10 per cent of fractures in which both ligaments and bones are damaged.

The most common causes of spinal fractures are high-energy injuries sustained from road traffic accidents and sports and leisure activities. These result in either axial compression, or a combination of forces on the vertebral column, resulting in failure and fracture.

Spinal fractures may also be from penetrating trauma, such as from a knife or bullet.

Pathological fractures of the vertebrae are also common. Consider this possibility if the injury was disproportionately slight, or the patient has a malignancy known to metastasize to bone.

First aid If there is the remotest possibility of a spinal fracture, the spine must be immobilized until careful clinical and radiological assessment has shown no evidence of a fracture or displacement (see Chapter 5 and *Investigation and Management*, Chapter 10).

History

Every patient with blunt injuries to the head and neck, especially if they are unconscious, should be suspected of having a spinal injury. High-speed road traffic accidents, falls from a height and crushing injuries are risk factors. Neck or back pain and the presence of neurological symptoms must also arouse suspicion of a spinal injury.

Examination

The neck must be stabilized and not moved as per the ATLS protocol. Inspect and palpate for tenderness, bogginess, bruising, entry wounds and deformity. There may be a prominent spinal process, or an increased space between the spinous processes. All spinal movements may be limited.

The patient should then be log-rolled (see Chapter 5), and the thoraco-lumbar spine inspected and palpated as above.

Always conduct a full neurological examination including a rectal examination (see Chapter 3).

FRACTURES OF THE CERVICAL SPINE

These are less common than fractures of the thoraco-lumbar spine. Many are associated with severe, immediately fatal head injuries.

Fracture of C1

(Jefferson's fracture)
This is a burst fracture of the ring of the atlas usually caused by a fall on the head; it accounts for 10 per cent of all cervical fractures (Fig. 9.15). This is best seen on an axial CT scan, demonstrating the fractures through the ring of the axis (C1). If there is greater than 7 mm displacement of the C1 lateral masses then the fracture is unstable because of rupture of the transverse ligament. There are no specific signs, and the diagnosis is made by X-ray. Neurological problems are rare.

Fracture of the C2 pedicles

(Hangman's fracture)
This was the means of death in judicial hanging when both the pedicles of the axis were fractured and the C1/2 disc torn by a hyperextension/distraction force (Fig. 9.16). Nowadays it is usually caused by the chin hitting the dashboard in a road traffic injury, which causes a traumatic spondylolisthesis of C2 on C3, combined with an avulsion fracture of the anterior lower body of C3.

The fracture is unstable and neurological damage can cause death.

(a) AP view. If the distance A + B is >7 mm, the fracture is unstable.

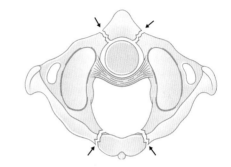

(b) Axial view (fractures arrowed).

Fig. 9.15 JEFFERSON'S FRACTURE

Fig. 9.16 Hangman's fracture (arrows).

Atlanto-axial dislocation

This often fatal injury follows hyperextension, distraction and rotation of the cranio-cervical junction. A patient who survives may be seen supporting their head in their hands.

CHAPTER 9 | THE SPINE AND PELVIS

Fracture of the odontoid process

This is the most common fracture of the cervical spine (17 per cent), and usually results from a direct blow on the occiput during a fall or in a road traffic accident (Fig. 9.17) There is hyperflexion in a young road traffic victim, or hyperextension in an elderly patient with osteoporosis from a fall on the face. There is cord damage in 25 per cent of cases.

There are no specific symptoms or signs and the diagnosis is made on X-ray (see *Investigation and Management*, Chapter 10).

Fig. 9.17 Fracture of the odontoid process (arrow).

Wedge compression fractures

These follow hyperflexion with compression. The anterior bodies of the mid and lower cervical vertebra are crushed (Fig. 9.18). The fracture is stable, and cord damage is rare.

Fig. 9.18 Wedge compression fractures (arrow).

Burst fractures

The vertebra is crushed in all directions, often as a result of diving into shallow water and landing on the head, with resulting violent axial compression. These fractures are often associated with permanent cord damage.

Comminuted fractures of the vertebral body

(Flexion compression fractures)

There is severe compression with or without hyperflexion, often the result of a dive. The vertebral body is comminuted and unstable, with one or more bone fragments (the teardrops) forced into the cord, with the posterior portion of the body forced into the spinal canal, which may lead to neurological damage (Fig. 9.19).

Fig. 9.19 Stage IV flexion compression (arrow).

Fracture/dislocation and subluxation

There is a pure flexion or flexion-rotation injury that either tears the posterior spinal ligaments of the lower cervical spine (subluxation) or causes the articular facets to ride forwards over the facets below. There may also be associated fractures of one or both articular masses, with posterior ligamentous tears. This fracture/dislocation renders the spine unstable (Fig. 9.20).

A step may be felt on palpation of the cervical spinous processes as one vertebra is displaced forwards over another.

Fig. 9.20 Fracture/dislocation of the cervical spine with bilateral facet dislocation. There is a high incidence of neurological injury associated with this injury pattern that may be progressive if the facets are not reduced as expeditiously as possible.

Hyperextension avulsion fractures

Avulsion fraction of the anterior inferior corner of the vertebral body is caused by hyperextension injury (Fig. 9.21). This is not associated with any neurological deficit, is stable and is managed conservatively. This fracture is also confusingly known as a teardrop fracture.

Fig. 9.21 This is a stable fracture. The teardrop is the anterior portion of the vertebral body (arrow).

Avulsion injury of the spinous process of C7

(Clay shoveller's fracture)
Severe muscular contraction of the posterior spinal muscles pulls off the spinous process. There is localized tenderness (Fig. 9.22).

Fig. 9.22 Avulsion injury of the spinous process of C7 (clay shoveller's fracture) (arrow).

FRACTURES OF THE THORACO-LUMBAR SPINE

Except for the specialized fractures of C1and C2 described above, the various types of fracture described in the cervical spine can also occur in the thoraco-lumbar region.

In the thoracic spine, wedge compression and fracture dislocations from hyperflexion are usually stabilized by the rib cage. There is often underlying osteoporosis, and multiple fractures may lead to kyphosis (see above). The spinal canal is narrow in this region, increasing the likelihood of cord damage, which is usually complete.

Fractures of the lower two thoracic and the upper lumbar vertebrae are more common, because this is the relatively mobile area between the fixed zones of the thorax and the sacrum and pelvis. A fall from a height producing axial compression and hyperflexion of this region is a common cause.

The strength of the spine at this level is in three columns: anterior, middle and posterior (Fig. 9.23). Fractures of the middle column and at least one other should be considered unstable.

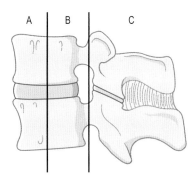

Fig. 9.23 Lumbar spinal columns.

CHAPTER 9 | THE SPINE AND PELVIS

There are four main types of fracture:

- Compression.
- Burst/hyperflexion.
- Distraction (seat belt).
- Fracture/dislocation.

Wedge compression fractures

These are the most common type, the result of axial compression and hyperflexion. They are stable unless a lot of vertebral height has been lost, which is indicated by severe tenderness and a palpable gap between the vertebral spines.

Burst fractures

These fractures are due to axial compression that squashes the vertebral body. The pedicles are splayed and the laminae are fractured, with bone fragments and disc material driven into the spinal canal. A significant loss of vertebral height combined with a kyphosis indicates instability.

Flexion/distraction fractures

(Seat belt injuries)

These are fractures through the spinous processes into the pedicles and the posterior part of the vertebral bodies. They occur in high-velocity road accidents when a seat belt is worn. Neurological injuries are unusual, but the fracture is unstable and is often associated with abdominal injuries (see Chapter 5).

Fracture/dislocations

These are caused by flexion, compression, rotation and distraction, and rarely by hyperextension. One or both facet joints are subluxed or dislocated, and there are associated fractures of the vertebral body or disruption of the intervertebral disc. Associated spinal cord injury is common, especially if both facet joints are dislocated (90 per cent complete paraplegia), and the spine is always unstable.

Fractures of a transverse process are caused by muscle avulsion.

FRACTURES OF THE SACRUM AND COCCYX

These bones may be fractured by a fall on or a direct blow. Pain, local tenderness, bruising and abnormal mobility are all indicative of a fracture.

Fractures of the sacrum are often associated with fractures of the pelvis (see below).

The Denis classification (Fig. 9.24) divides the sacrum into three zones:

1. fractures lateral to the neural foramina;
2. fractures passing through the foramina;
3. fractures medial to the foramen and involving the spinal canal.

The likelihood of neurological damage is greater in Zone 2 (30 per cent) and Zone 3 (50 per cent). A full neurological examination is essential, including an assessment of anal sphincter tone and the bulbo-cavernosus reflex (see Chapter 3).

Fig. 9.24 The Denis classification of sacral zones.

PELVIC FRACTURES

Pelvic fractures are often associated with other major injuries (see Chapter 5) but may be isolated, as when for example a simple fall in an elderly patient causes a fracture of the pubis or iliac crest without any instability of the pelvic ring.

High-velocity road accidents or falls from a height usually cause major pelvic bone disruptions, and are often associated with other life-threatening injuries of the head, brain, abdomen and chest. In addition, local injuries to the bladder and urethra, bowel and blood vessels are also life-threatening, and effective resuscitation is essential if a successful outcome is to be achieved (see Chapter 5).

The pelvis is a strong bony ring (Fig. 9.25) that carries weight from the spine to the lower limbs. A break in one part of the ring is invariably accompanied by a break elsewhere. They may be classified as stable where the sacroiliac complex is intact, partially unstable or completely unstable.

Fig. 9.25 The pelvic bony ring.

Initial assessment Look for other system injuries and hypovolaemic shock. Then assess the degree of pelvic stability and any local organ or soft tissue damage.

Resuscitation precedes any assessment of the pelvic injury.

History

Local pain is suggestive, but a fractured pelvis must be considered in all patients who have been subjected to high-energy trauma, especially if there are signs of unexplained hypovolaemic shock and they are unconscious.

Examination

There may be no overt signs of injury, but skin abrasions, local tenderness over the pubic symphysis, iliac crest or sacrum and the presence of crepitus are all highly suggestive of a pelvic fracture. Leg length discrepancy and malrotation in the absence of lower limb fractures are also important signs.

A bimanual assessment of transverse stability should then be carried out by compressing and distracting the iliac wings (Fig. 9.26). This must be done gently to avoid causing further bleeding. An experienced surgeon may be able to assess vertical and acetabular stability by pulling on the leg while palpating the pelvis.

Rectal and vaginal examinations should be performed to assess the presence of associated injuries and the presence of an occult open fracture.

Neurological examination of the lower limb (see Chapter 3) should exclude a spinal injury. The peripheral pulses should also be checked (see Chapter 10).

Urethral and bladder injuries should be looked for before catheterization in all displaced anterior ring injuries (see Chapter 17).

If there is pain in the hip and lateral bruising, and the leg is in an abnormal position, there may be an acetabular fracture. Neurovascular assessment must then be carried out as sciatic, femoral and obturator nerve injuries may be associated.

Fig. 9.26 Bimanual assessment of pelvic stability.

The arteries, veins and lymphatics

Examination of the arteries, veins and lymphatics requires special techniques, which are described before detailed descriptions of the history and clinical features of the individual conditions.

THE ARTERIES

CLINICAL ASSESSMENT OF THE ARTERIAL CIRCULATION OF THE LOWER LIMB

Always examine the patient in a warm room. A routine for assessment is listed in Revision panel 10.1.

Inspection

Colour

The first, most notable, feature of an ischaemic limb is its colour. The skin may be as white as marble or show varying degrees of redness or blueness, which becomes more obvious in the lower parts of the leg and the toes. Excessive deoxygenation of the blood in the skin capillaries sometimes gives the foot a purple–blue cyanosed appearance, but the blue fades to white within a few seconds when the patient lies down. Dark skin of ethnic origin masks these subtle colour changes, making the diagnosis of mild and moderate arterial insufficiency more difficult.

In acutely ischaemic legs, blue streaks around white patches produce a mottled discolouration. When the cyanotic areas become fixed, the ischaemia is irreversible.

Gangrene turns the skin a permanent blue–black colour, which is usually first seen in the toes (see page 328).

Vascular angle

The vascular angle, which is also called Buerger's angle, is the angle to which the leg has to be raised before it becomes white. In a limb with a normal circulation, the toes stay pink even when the limb is raised by 90°. In an ischaemic leg, elevation to 15° or 30° for 30–60 seconds may cause pallor (Fig. 10.1). A vascular angle of less than 20° indicates severe ischaemia. This test is useful as a comparator. When both limbs are raised together, the ischaemic foot goes white, while the normal foot remains pink.

After elevating the legs, patients should be asked to sit up and dangle their feet over the side of the couch. A normal leg and foot will remain a healthy pink colour, whereas an ischaemic leg will slowly turn from white (after elevation) to pink and then take on a suffused purple–red colour (Fig. 10.2). The latter is caused by deoxygenated blood filling the dilated capillaries. This is indicative of severe ischaemia.

Venous filling

In a warm room, the veins of a normal foot are dilated and full of blood, even when the patient is lying horizontally. In an ischaemic foot, the veins collapse and sink below the skin surface to look like pale blue gutters. This appearance is called guttering of the veins (Fig. 10.3).

(a) The limb becomes pallid on elevation.

(b) A pale ischaemic right leg.

Fig. 10.1

Fig. 10.2 A limb showing the red/purple changes of chronic ischaemia.

Fig. 10.3 Left limb shows pallor of left great toe, following digital compression.

Pressure areas

Inspect all areas subjected to pressure or trauma during walking or bed rest very carefully, because these are the first sites to show evidence of trophic changes, ulceration and gangrene. It is important to look at the bottom, back and lateral surfaces of the heel, and the ball of the foot. It is also important to look at the skin over the malleoli. The skin over the head of the fifth metatarsal must be carefully inspected, as must the tips of the toes, as well as between the toes, where the pressure of one toenail against the side of the adjacent toe can cause ulceration (Fig. 10.4).

Pressure necrosis is manifest by thickening of the skin, a purple or blue discolouration, blistering, ulceration or patches of black, dead, gangrenous skin.

Fig. 10.4 An ischaemic ulcer developing between the toes where one toe is pressing on the other.

Revision panel 10.1

Routine for assessing the arterial circulation

Inspection

Colour when:
Horizontal
Elevated (vascular angle)
Dependent
Venous filling

Look at the pressure areas and between the digits

Palpation

Skin temperature

Capillary refilling time

Palpate the pulses

Auscultation

Listen for bruits

Measure the blood pressure and index

Many textbooks state that loss of hair on the skin of the lower leg, foot and toes is a sign of ischaemia. This is a very unreliable sign and does not need to be recorded.

Palpation

Temperature

The skin temperature can only be assessed reliably if both lower limbs have been exposed to the same ambient temperature for a full 5 minutes. Uncover the limbs and perform some other part of the physical examination to allow the skin temperature to adjust to the temperature of the surrounding air. Most clinicians prefer to use the backs of their fingers to assess temperature. The cool, dry backs of the fingers are ideal temperature sensors.

The whole limb should be assessed to discover which parts are warm or cold, and the level at which these changes occur. A blue or even red foot can be very cold.

Capillary refilling

Press on the pulp of a toe or finger for two seconds, and then observe the time taken for the blanched area to turn pink after you have stopped pressing. This gives a crude indication of the rate of blood flow in the capillaries and the pressure within them.

Feel all the pulses

Pulses are most easily felt where an artery is superficial and crosses a bone. In the neck, shoulder and upper limbs, the carotid, subclavian, brachial and both wrist arteries are close to the skin and easy to palpate.

The femoral pulse in the groin lies half way between the symphysis pubis (in the midline) and the anterior superior iliac spine (the mid-inguinal point) (Fig. 10.5a). The artery is so superficial that it can usually be felt, even when it is pulseless.

The dorsalis pedis artery runs from a point on the anterior surface of the ankle joint, midway between the malleoli, towards the cleft between the first and second metatarsal bones (Fig. 10.5b). In 10 per cent of subjects, the anterior tibial artery is absent and replaced by a branch of the peroneal artery.

The posterior tibial artery lies one-third of the way along a line between the tip of the medial malleolus and the point of the heel, but is easier to feel 2.5 cm higher up, where it lies just behind the medial malleolus (Fig. 10.5c).

It is often helpful to feel the dorsalis pedis and posterior tibial pulses in both limbs simultaneously. Stand at the end of the bed or couch and feel the dorsalis pedis artery of each foot, simultaneously, by placing the pulps of all the fingers of each hand along the line of the artery, with your thumbs beneath the arch of the foot. From this position, the hands can be rotated over the foot until the pulps of the fingers lie in the groove between the Achilles tendon and the medial malleolus. The pulps of the fingers can then be pulled up against the back of the tibia, trapping the posterior tibial artery against the bone.

The popliteal pulse is difficult to feel because it does not cross a prominent bone and is not superficial. There are three ways to feel it, and all three may have to be tried before deciding that the pulse is present or absent:

- The most convenient technique for feeling the popliteal pulse is to extend the patient's knee fully and place both hands around the top of the calf, with the thumbs placed on the tibial tuberosity and the tips of the fingers of each hand touching behind the knee, over the lower part of the popliteal fossa. The pulps of all the fingers are then pulled forwards against the posterior part of the tibial condyle, trapping the popliteal artery between them and the posterior surface of the tibia (Fig. 10.5d and 10.5e).

(a) Palpating the femoral pulse at the mid-inguinal point, halfway between anterior superior iliac spine and pubic symphysis. Normally more than one finger is used.

The pulsating artery can be felt in the midline (provided the fingers are held still). If in doubt, count any pulse you feel against the rate detected by a second examiner feeling the radial or superficial temporal pulse to check for synchronization.

- Flexing the knee to 135° loosens the deep fascia and may make the lower half of the artery easier to feel. The vessel is, however, moved further from the surface by bending the knee, and this may make palpation of the upper half of the artery more difficult as it sinks into the large fat pad between the femoral condyles.
- It is sometimes worth turning the patient into the prone position and feeling along the course of the artery with the fingertips of both hands.

(b) Palpating the popliteal pulse with the knee extended.

(c) The position of the fingers when feeling the popliteal pulse with the knee fully extended.

(d) Simultaneous palpation of the dorsalis pedis pulses.

(e) Simultaneous palpation of the posterior tibial pulses.

Fig. 10.5 PALPATION OF THE PERIPHERAL PULSES

Remember that:

- when a popliteal pulse is very easy to feel, the artery may be aneurysmal;
- the popliteal pulse should be palpable if the foot pulses are easy to feel and there are no adductor canal or femoral artery bruits.

Test the muscles and nerves

Severe ischaemia causes a loss of muscle and nerve function, ultimately producing an immobile, numb limb.

Auscultation

Use your stethoscope to listen along the course of all the major arteries, especially if the pulses are weak. It is an important part of the routine examination to listen to the arteries in the neck, the abdomen, the groin and the thigh (Fig. 10.6). Always remember to listen over the adductor canal.

Bruits are caused by turbulent flow beyond a stenosis, or an irregularity in the artery wall. Do not press too hard over a superficial artery with the bell of your stethoscope, as pressure can distort the flow and cause a bruit. Bruits may change in volume and character if there are changes in blood flow.

Before finishing the physical examination of the lower limb, you should always measure the blood pressure in both arms to exclude significant subclavian or innominate artery disease.

Pressure measurement with the Doppler flow detector

Small hand-held Doppler ultrasound instruments can be used in the clinic to detect blood flow. The sound waves generated by the device are focused into a beam and directed towards the vessel to be examined by placing the probe over the surface of the vessel, after removing any air between the probe and the skin with a coupling jelly. Moving red cells alter the frequency of the reflected ultrasound according to the Doppler principle.

The chosen vessels, usually the dorsalis pedis, posterior tibial or peroneal arteries at the ankle, are located by placing the Doppler probe over their known anatomical course, and listening for regular changes in the sound generated by the pulsatile flow. A sphygmomanometer cuff previously placed around the ankle is then inflated until the noise created by the flow ceases (Fig. 10.7). The pressure at which this occurs is the systolic blood pressure. This can be measured in all three ankle vessels.

The **pressure index** is the ratio between the pressure measured by this technique and the

Fig. 10.6 The common sites to hear bruits over the arteries of the lower limbs.

Fig. 10.7 The technique for measuring the Doppler pressure index, which is the pressure at which the cuff needs to be inflated to abolish the noise of the arterial flow.

pressure in the brachial artery. It is normally unity or 1.1; i.e. both foot and brachial artery pressures should be almost identical. Ratios above 1.0 indicate stiff, calcified limb vessels (often diabetic arteries), which cannot be squashed by the external pressure applied by the sphygmomanometer cuff. Ratios below 1 indicate occlusive disease upstream of the foot vessels.

The Doppler ultrasound flow detector is a very useful tool because it can detect pulsatile flow when the pulse is impalpable to the fingers. The pressure index provides a rough indicator of disease severity. A more accurate assessment of the severity of the disease can be obtained by measuring the pressure before and after exercise.

SYMPTOMS PRODUCED BY ACUTE ARTERIAL INSUFFICIENCY OF THE LIMBS

Severe limb pain of sudden onset

This occurs when the arterial blood supply of a limb is suddenly interrupted, with no time for collaterals to form. It is much more common in the lower limbs. The pain comes from ischaemic muscles and nerves, which develop irreversible changes within a few hours.

The *symptoms* are easy to remember, as each begins with P (Revision panel 10.2):

- Pain, usually very severe and of sudden onset.
- Paraesthesiae ('pins and needles') and numbness, which develop over a few hours and eventually progress to
- Paralysis.

The *three principal physical signs* also begin with P:

- Pallor.
- Pulselessness, and the limb feels
- Perishingly cold to the touch.

The limb looks white and feels cold. These findings can be compared with the appearance of the other side if the symptoms are unilateral. The capillary circulation is poor, with a prolonged refilling time after digital compression. The veins are empty, and the limb may become blue and develop a blotchy, blue–white appearance.

The femoral pulse may be present if the arterial occlusion is at the division of the common femoral artery into the superficial and profunda femoris arteries, or is situated more distally. Similarly, in the upper limb, the subclavian and axillary pulses may be palpable, whereas the distal pulses, for example the brachial, wrist and ankle pulses, are not.

Muscle tenderness, a bad prognostic sign, especially in the muscles of the anterior and posterior calf compartments, should be sought by gently pressing the bellies of these muscles.

A full neurological examination should concentrate on power, sensation and reflexes (see Chapter 3).

The Doppler ultrasound probe should be used to confirm the absence of pulsatile blood flow in the peripheral arteries. If any pulsatile flow is detected, it is likely to be severely diminished in height and intensity.

The leg will become mottled and marbled if the ischaemia persists. The muscles will eventually become hard, and the skin will begin to blister and develop gangrene, which usually starts in the toes before spreading proximally. The causes of acute limb ischaemia are shown in Revision panel 10.3.

Revision panel 10.2

The symptoms and signs of acute ischaemia

Pain

Paraesthesia and numbness

Paralysis

Pallor

Pulseless

Perishing cold

Revision panel 10.3

Causes of acute arterial ischaemia

An arterial embolus

Thrombosis on an atheromatous plaque

Thrombosis of an aneurysm (usually popliteal)

Arterial dissection (usually aortic)

Traumatic disruption

External compression, e.g. a cervical rib or popliteal entrapment

Examination

Examine the heart and general circulation with care to ascertain the cause of a sudden arterial occlusion, such as the following.

An arterial embolus is suspected if the patient is fibrillating, has had a recent heart attack, or is known to have heart valve disease. Patients may never have had any symptoms of arterial ischaemia, for example intermittent claudication, before the embolus occurs.

An acute arterial thrombosis is suspected if the patient has already experienced symptoms of chronic arterial ischaemia, such as intermittent claudication or even rest pain (see below).

A thrombosed aneurysm is suspected if other arteries, such as the popliteal artery of the opposite limb, are found to be dilated.

An aortic dissection is suspected if the patient presents with severe chest and/or back pain. Other pulses, such as the left subclavian artery, may be absent.

A traumatic arterial disruption is suspected if there is a clear history of injury or vascular intervention.

A cervical rib is suspected if there is a palpable supraclavicular swelling (see Chapters 9 and 12). Patients with cervical ribs may have experienced neurological symptoms in the arm and hand for many years. (Special investigations are required to diagnose the other causes of subclavian artery compression.)

Also exclude two of the major non-arterial causes of an acute limb pain of sudden onset – acute venous thrombosis (see page 356), and spinal cord compression or infarction (see Chapters 3 and 9).

SYMPTOMS OF CHRONIC ARTERIAL INSUFFICIENCY OF THE LOWER LIMB

Intermittent claudication

Strictly speaking, *intermittent claudication* means intermittent limping (Latin *claudicare*, to limp, a word derived from the disability of the Emperor Claudius). This term is used to describe a cramp-like pain in a muscle that appears during exercise. It is caused by an inadequate blood flow to the muscles. The pain stops the patient using the muscle and, if the affected muscle is in the leg, causes them to limp and then stop walking.

History

Age The majority of patients presenting with intermittent claudication are males, over the age of 50 years, and with smoking-related atherosclerotic disease of the lower limb vessels. Claudication can also develop in young adults with Buerger's disease, or after an arterial embolism or the traumatic occlusion of a major artery.

Sex Claudication is more common in males than in females. In males, it may be associated with impotence if the occlusive disease is at the aortic bifurcation.

Pain The pain of intermittent claudication is quite specific and must fulfil three criteria:

- The patient must experience the pain in a muscle, usually the calf.
- The pain should only develop when the muscle is exercised.
- The pain must disappear when the exercise stops.

Walking distance Limitation of walking is the principal complaint. Patients find that they can only walk a limited distance before an ache begins in the muscles of the leg, which then becomes a cramp, and eventually stops them walking any further. The distance covered by the time walking has to stop is called the claudication distance. This should be recorded. The patient should if necessary be observed walking to see when the pain develops.

They should also be asked how long they have to wait until the pain goes away, and whether they can then walk the same distance again. Some patients complain of an ache or cramp that does not stop them walking and that fades away if they force themselves to continue walking. Others find they can prevent the pain developing by walking slowly.

The severity of the pain and the time taken for it to begin and cease vary from patient to patient. Any muscle can be affected. The calf muscles are most often affected, but a claudication pain can arise in the thigh, buttock or foot muscles, and in the muscles of the upper limb and forearm.

Patients may also describe numbness and paraesthesiae in the skin of the foot at the time that the muscle pain begins. This is the result of blood being shunted from the skin to the muscle.

Pains that begin when at rest or immediately the patient stands up, and pains that occur in tissues

CHAPTER 10 | THE ARTERIES, VEINS AND LYMPHATICS

other than muscles and that do not abate with rest, are not claudication pains.

Onset and progression The pain of claudication usually begins insidiously. The walking distance gradually shortens over a few months before becoming static. In one-third or more of affected patients, the walking distance then increases, with spontaneous remission of the symptoms as the collateral circulation develops.

It is always important to ask about '**rest pain**' in a patient with claudication, as this symptom signifies the onset of critical limb ischaemia (see below). Patients with rest pain may have had intermittent claudication in the affected limb for many years .

Examination

Examination of the legs

Inspection The appearance of the limb on inspection is often remarkably normal, although if the condition is severe, there may be some blanching on elevation of the legs (see Fig. 10.1).

Palpation The foot and leg may be cold. The pulse immediately above the affected group of muscles is likely to be weak or absent. Thus, if claudication is experienced in the calf, the popliteal pulse is usually impalpable, but the femoral pulse is likely to be present. The femoral pulse is likely to be absent if the pain is felt in the thigh muscles. Thus, the level of the symptoms and signs often indicates the level of disease. It is possible to have claudication in the calf with palpable ankle pulses, but careful examination often reveals a bruit in the thigh, and if the pulses are re-examined after exercise, they may no longer be palpable.

The Doppler pressures are invariably reduced and fall still further with exercise.

Auscultation The common sites to find bruits in association with intermittent claudication are over the aortic bifurcation, the iliac and common femoral arteries, and the superficial femoral artery at the adductor hiatus.

Examination of the motor and skeletal systems

This should be normal.

Differential diagnosis

Other causes of a claudication-like pain include osteoarthritis of the hip and knee, spinal stenosis, prolapsed intervertebral disc and venous claudication.

The hip and knee should always be carefully examined, as should the spine, especially if all the pulses are palpable (see Chapter 6).

Venous claudication should be considered if the limb is swollen, or if there is lipodermatosclerosis of the gaiter skin (see page 346).

Rest pain

'Rest pain' is a term used to describe the continuous, unremitting pain caused by severe ischaemia. In contrast to the pain of intermittent claudication, which only appears during exercise, this pain is present at rest throughout the day and night.

History

Age Most patients with arterial disease severe enough to cause rest pain are 60 or more years old, but Buerger's disease and trauma can cause rest pain in young males.

Symptoms Patients complain of a continuous, severe aching pain that stops them sleeping. Rest pain is usually experienced in the most distal part of the limb, namely the toes and forefoot. If any gangrene is present, the patient feels the pain at the junction of the living and dead tissues.

Rest pain is often relieved by putting the leg below the level of the heart, so patients hang their legs over the side of the bed or prefer to sleep sitting in a chair. The painful part is very sensitive. Movement or pressure exacerbates the pain. The patient often sits in bed with the knee bent, holding the foot still to try to relieve the pain. Strong analgesic drugs are the only means of providing relief. Rest pain is unremitting and gets steadily worse.

Systematic questions It is important to enquire about symptoms suggestive of pre-existing arterial disease in the affected limb, such as claudication, and any symptoms that indicate the presence of atherosclerosis elsewhere. Chest pains, a previous myocardial infarction, fainting, weakness, paraesthesiae in the upper limbs, episodes of blurred vision and stroke are all important indications of serious vascular disease elsewhere.

Family history Arterial disease is often familial, so it is important to ascertain the cause of death of parents and siblings, and whether they had any symptoms of vascular disease.

Risk factors These include cigarette smoking, hypertension, diabetes and hypercholesterolaemia.

Examination

General appearance

Patients with rest pain usually look drawn and haggard because of continuous pain and sleepless nights. They are often unwilling to lie flat on a couch with the leg horizontal for more than a short period because elevation of the leg exacerbates the pain.

An arcus senilis (see Chapter 1) is not diagnostic of vascular disease but may be present. Xanthelesmata and xanthomata, which are cholesterol deposits around the eye and in the subcutaneous tissues, are indicative of hypercholesterolaemia (see Fig. 1.22). Pallor suggesting anaemia or a rubicund appearance suggesting polycythaemia (rubra vera) is worth noting, as both these conditions can predispose to claudication and rest pain (see Chapter 1).

General examination

The whole cardiovascular system must be examined with care. The blood pressure must be measured in both arms and recorded, the heart examined, the major arteries auscultated and the abdominal aorta felt in case it is dilated and aneurysmal (see below).

Inspection

When dependent, a painful ischaemic foot is a deep reddish-purple colour. The tips of the toes may be grey or white if they are completely bloodless. There may be black patches of gangrene on the toes or the heel (Fig. 10.8).

When horizontal, the foot rapidly becomes pale or marble white, and the veins empty, becoming guttered. Further elevation of the leg increases the pallor. If the foot is not white when horizontal, it will certainly become so when elevated to 20°.

It is possible to have severely ischaemic toes and a good circulation in the rest of the foot. In these circumstances, the description above applies only to the toes. The pain is unlikely to be an ischaemic pain if the whole foot is painful but stays pink above an angle of 20°. The foot may be swollen and blue if the patient has been sitting with the leg dependent to ease the pain.

(a) Black areas of clearly defined (demarcated) gangrene (dry and uninfected).

(b) Gangrene caused by frostbite.

(c) Gangrene caused by trenchfoot.

Fig. 10.8 GANGRENE

CHAPTER 10 | THE ARTERIES, VEINS AND LYMPHATICS

The pressure areas on the heel and the skin between the toes may be gangrenous, ulcerated or infected (Fig. 10.9). Ischaemic changes often develop at the site of the nail beds.

Fig. 10.9 Pressure necrosis of the heel.

Palpation

The skin temperature from mid-calf downwards is usually reduced, even when the foot is dependent and congested. Capillary refilling is retarded.

In general, rest pain is caused by a combination of large and small vessel disease, so it is common to find that the popliteal and femoral pulses are absent. Small vessel disease should be suspected if these pulses are palpable. The likely cause is then diabetes or Buerger's disease.

Auscultation

Bruits may be heard over the iliac and femoral arteries (see Fig. 10.6).

Other signs

There may be muscle wasting caused by disuse, and if the patient has been sitting holding the ischaemic foot for many weeks, there may be a fixed flexion deformity of the knee and hip joint.

Examination of the nervous system is important because a severe, constant pain in the lower limb may be caused by a neurological abnormality (see Chapter 3). The nervous system may be abnormal in individuals with diabetes, but these patients rarely have very severe rest pain as the diabetes destroys the limb's pain sensation.

Gout may cause severe pain in the foot, with redness and tenderness (see Chapter 8).

Very occasionally, an abscess or foreign body needs to be excluded.

Chronic ischaemia can occur in the upper limb, but is far less common.

Pregangrene and gangrene

This is also far more common in the lower limb, because upper limb vessels have less atherosclerosis and a better collateral circulation.

Pregangrene

This term is used by clinicians to describe the changes which indicate that a tissue's blood supply is so precarious that it will soon be insufficient to keep the tissue alive.

The principal symptom of pregangrene is rest pain, which is described in detail above.

The principal signs are pallor of the tissues when elevated, congestion when dependent, guttering of the veins, thick and scaling skin, and wasting of the pulps of the toes or fingers. The limb is cold and has poor capillary refilling. Ischaemic tissue is tender. Any further reduction in the blood supply will result in tissue death, or gangrene (see below). These symptoms must therefore be treated with the utmost urgency.

Gangrene

Gangrene is the term used to describe dead tissue. Dead tissue is brown, dark blue or black, and gradually contracts into a crinkled, withered, hard mass (Fig. 10.10). These changes can happen if a patch of skin, a toe or the whole of the lower limb becomes ischaemic. The nerves in the dead part die, and therefore gangrenous tissues are not painful.

Fig. 10.10 A blue ischaemic toe caused by emboli from a femoral artery stenosis.

The junction between the living and dead tissue gradually becomes distinct, provided there is adequate venous drainage and the proximal blood supply remains intact. This junction is known as the *line of demarcation*. The dead tissue may eventually separate and fall off. The living tissue on the proximal side of the line of demarcation is usually ischaemic, so is often constantly painful (rest pain) and tender. If the gangrene is the result of local trauma and the surrounding tissues are normal, they are not usually painful.

Gangrene usually develops in the extremities of the limbs – the tips of the toes and fingers – and in areas of skin subjected to pressure. The dead tissue does not become shrivelled if its venous drainage is impaired or if it becomes infected. In these circumstances, the gangrene becomes soft and boggy, and the line of demarcation often becomes purulent.

A hard, shrunken, non-infected patch of gangrene with a clear line of demarcation is called dry gangrene. A soft, swollen, infected patch of gangrene without a clear margin is called wet gangrene (Fig. 10.11). However, it is better to use the terms 'infected' and 'non-infected' rather than wet and dry. This difference is important because sometimes, as in those with diabetes, the gangrene is actually secondary to the infection and not the ischaemia.

Diabetic gangrene is often associated with gas in the tissues (tissue crepitus) and a foul smell.

Venous gangrene, which may complicate a massive deep vein thrombosis and phlegmasia caerulia dolens, usually affects all the toes (Fig. 10.12).

Fig. 10.12 Venous gangrene in a patient with a massive venous thrombosis, which has presented with very symmetrical gangrene of all the toes combined with foot swelling.

Ischaemic ulceration

An ischaemic ulcer is the aftermath of gangrene. By definition, it is caused by an inadequate blood supply.

History

Ischaemic ulcers are common in the elderly, who often also have symptoms of coronary or cerebral vascular disease. Patients sometimes remember a minor precipitating injury.

Symptoms Ischaemic ulcers, except those associated with a neurological abnormality, are very painful. They cause rest pain.

They do not bleed, but they discharge a thin serous exudate, which can become purulent. They are usually indolent, and often get slowly deeper and larger. Ischaemic ulcers may occasionally penetrate into joints, making movements very painful. The causes of ischaemic ulcers are (Revision panels 10.4, 10.5):

- large artery obliteration: atherosclerosis and embolism;
- small artery obliteration: Buerger's disease, atheroembolism, diabetes, scleroderma and physical agents such as prolonged local pressure, radiation, trauma and electrical burns.

Systematic questions and past history The patient may give a history of prior claudication or symptoms of generalized vascular disease such as chest pain.

Fig. 10.11 Wet gangrene with no clear line of demarcation.

CHAPTER 10 | THE ARTERIES, VEINS AND LYMPHATICS

Revision panel 10.4

The causes of ischaemic ulceration

Large artery obliteration

Atherosclerosis

Embolism

Small artery obliteration

Scleroderma

Buerger's disease

Embolism

Diabetes

Physical agents:
   Pressure necrosis
   Radiation
   Trauma
   Electric burns

Fig. 10.13 A typical ischaemic ulcer with pale granulations in the base of a gently sloping ulcer edge surrounded by normal skin.

Revision panel 10.5

The causes of chronic ulceration

Infection

Repeated trauma

Ischaemia

Oedema

Denervation

Localized destructive disease (tuberculosis, carcinoma)

Examination

Site Ischaemic ulcers are found at the tips of the toes or fingers, and over the pressure points.

Size Ischaemic ulcers vary in size from small, deep lesions a few millimetres across, to large, flat ulcers 10 cm or more wide on the lower leg (Fig. 10.13).

Shape The ulcers are most often elliptical.

Tenderness The ulcer and the surrounding tissues are often very tender. Removing a dressing can cause an exacerbation of the pain that lasts for several hours.

Temperature The surrounding tissues are usually cold because they are ischaemic. Adjacent, warm, healthy tissue suggests another cause for the ulceration.

Edge The edge of an ischaemic ulcer is either punched out if there is no attempt at healing by the surrounding tissues, or sloping if the ulcer is beginning to heal (see Chapter 1). The skin at the edge of the ulcer is usually a blue–grey colour. There is no lipodermatosclerosis in the surrounding skin unless venous disease coexists.

Base The base of the ulcer usually contains grey–yellow slough covering flat, pale, granulation tissue.

Depth Ischaemic ulcers are often very deep. They may penetrate down to and through deep fascia, tendon, bone and even an underlying joint.

Discharge This may be clear fluid, serum or pus.

Relations The base may be stuck to, or be part of, any underlying structure. It is quite common to see bare bone, ligaments and tendons exposed in the base of an ischaemic ulcer.

Lymph drainage Infection in an ischaemic ulcer usually remains confined to the ulcer, so the local lymph glands are not normally enlarged.

State of the local tissues Surrounding tissues may show signs of ischaemia – pallor, coldness and atrophy.

Distal pulses These are invariably absent.

Doppler pressures The Doppler pressure index is invariably reduced.

Neurological examination If the ulcer is caused by a neuropathy (see below), there may be a loss of superficial and deep sensation, weakness of movement and a loss of reflexes (see Chapter 3).

General examination There may be evidence of vascular disease elsewhere. The urine should be tested for sugar.

Neuropathic ulceration

Tissue ischaemia is usually painful. Pain is the mechanism by which the body appreciates that any part of the skin is becoming deprived of blood. The feet and buttocks become painful after prolonged standing or sitting, encouraging movement to remove the pressure from the painful part. When pain sensation is lost, this warning is lost, and any compressed tissue may become permanently damaged.

Neuropathic ulcers are therefore only indirectly caused by local ischaemia. The main cause is lack of sensation in the tissues, allowing unrecognized trauma to occur.

Neuropathic ulcers are deep, penetrating ulcers that occur over pressure points (Fig. 10.14), but the surrounding tissues are healthy and may have a good circulation. The diagnostic features are as follows:

- The ulcers are painless.
- The surrounding tissues are unable to appreciate pain.
- The surrounding tissues may have a normal blood supply.

These ulcers can easily be mistaken for ischaemic ulcers, which is why a neurological examination is always important. The causes of neuropathic ulceration (Revision panel 10.6) are:

- peripheral nerve lesions: diabetes, nerve injuries or leprosy;
- spinal cord lesions: spina bifida, tabes dorsalis and syringomyelia (see Chapters 3 and 9).

Fig. 10.14 A neuropathic ulcer that is deep and painless over a pressure area in a non-sensate limb.

All these conditions may, however, occur in patients with vascular disease, so true ischaemic and neuropathic ulcers may occur together, and the combined effect of both diseases may be synergistic.

Careful examination of the arterial and neurological systems is required to identify the major cause.

Pulsatile swellings

(Aneurysms)

An aneurysm is a localized dilatation of an artery. The majority of aneurysms are caused by degeneration of the arterial wall, often with associated atherosclerosis, but some are caused by a primary weakness in the connective tissues of the arterial wall.

The causes of aneurysms are shown in Revision panel 10.7.

Revision panel 10.6

The causes of neuropathic ulceration (ulcers secondary to a loss of sensation)

Peripheral nerve lesions

Diabetes

Nerve injuries

Leprosy

Spinal cord lesions

Spina bifida

Tabes dorsalis

Syringomyelia

CHAPTER 10 | THE ARTERIES, VEINS AND LYMPHATICS

Revision panel 10.7

The causes of aneurysms

Congenital

A localized weakness:

  Berry aneurysm
  Marfan's syndrome
  Ehlers–Danlos syndrome
  Arterial dilatation associated with a congenital
      arteriovenous fistula

Acquired aneurysm

Trauma

Direct injury

Infection:

  Bacterial arteritis (mycotic)
  Syphilis
  Acquired immunodeficiency syndrome

Atherosclerotic

False aneurysms

Trauma

Post arterial surgery

In a true aneurysm, all the layers of the arterial wall (intima, media and adventitia) are involved. In a false aneurysm, the arterial wall is breached, and the wall of the aneurysm consists of blood clot and compressed surrounding normal tissues.

Although an aneurysm can develop in any artery, most occur in the abdominal aorta and the femoral and popliteal arteries.

Berry aneurysms (see Chapter 3) arise in a weakened area of the circle of Willis. They are often associated with hypertension, and are responsible for many subarachnoid haemorrhages at any age. It is debatable whether they are truly congenital, but the weakness responsible for their development may possibly be inherited.

Syphilitic aneurysms of the thoracic aorta were once common, but are now extremely rare.

History

Age Aneurysms are rare before the age of 50 years. Thereafter, their frequency increases with age.

Sex Males are affected six times more often than females.

Other causative factors A family history, cigarette smoking and hypertension are well-recognized risk factors.

Symptoms Many aneurysms cause no symptoms during life and are discovered by chance during a routine physical examination or by a screening programme.

The most common presenting symptom is dull, aching pain. With abdominal aneurysms, this is usually experienced over the swelling in the centre of the abdomen, but the pain often radiates to the back and may be experienced only in this site. The abdominal pain is caused by stretching of the artery, and the back pain by erosion of the lumbar vertebrae.

Some patients with abdominal aneurysms present with sciatica or loin pain as a consequence of local pressure on the nerves.

Acute pain occurs if the vessel suddenly stretches or begins to tear. This becomes a very severe pain if the aneurysm ruptures and a large haematoma forms (see Chapter 15). The patient may collapse from the accompanying hypotensive shock or suddenly die.

A few thin patients notice a pulsatile mass. This is a common presentation for femoral aneurysms, but is rare for abdominal aneurysms.

Occasionally, patients notice their abdomen pulsating when they lie in the bath or in bed.

Severe ischaemia of the lower limb follows the thrombosis of an aneurysm. This is a rare event in aortic and femoral aneurysms, but is a common presentation of popliteal aneurysms.

Less severe ischaemia may be caused by emboli originating in the aneurysm. One of the best examples of this complication is the multiple small emboli that may block the digital arteries of a patient with a subclavian aneurysm.

Peripheral emboli in the lower limb may cause intermittent claudication or rest pain.

The aorta, femoral and popliteal arteries are closely related to the inferior vena cava and the femoral and popliteal veins, respectively. Dilatation of an artery may block its adjacent vein by direct pressure, or cause it to thrombose. Patients may then present with a swollen, blue, painful limb.

Very occasionally, aneurysms rupture into an adjacent vein. The resulting acute arteriovenous fistula may cause severe cardiac embarrassment. The tissues distal to the fistula become cyanosed, the neck veins are elevated, and there is usually a loud machinery murmur over the aneurysm.

Systematic questions and past history Coronary or cerebral vascular disease can coexist.

(a) The bimanual technique used for palpating an abdominal aortic aneurysm. Assess the width of the abdominal aorta by placing your hands on either side of the pulse in the epigastrium.

Fig. 10.15 ABDOMINAL AORTIC ANEURYSM

(b) The position of an aneurysm of the abdominal aorta. If there is a gap between the top of the aneurysm and the costal margin, the aneurysm probably begins below the origin of the renal arteries. The femoral pulses are usually palpable.

Examination

Abdominal aneurysms

The abdominal aorta divides into the iliac arteries at about the level of the umbilicus. Consequently, most abdominal aneurysms are felt in the upper umbilical and epigastric regions (Fig. 10.15). Iliac artery aneurysms present as a pulsating mass in the iliac fossa or hypogastrium.

Aneurysms produce an expansile pulsation. In order to feel the expansion, both hands must be placed on either side of the mass to confirm that the hands are pushed apart as well as being pushed upwards (Fig. 10.15a). Many lumps in the upper abdomen transmit aortic pulsation and may be misdiagnosed as aneurysms. Real difficulty may occasionally be encountered if the aorta is encased by pathologically enlarged lymph glands.

Aneurysms feel firm and smooth, and can sometimes be moved a little from side to side. The presence of tenderness implies that there is inflammatory change, or that the wall of the aneurysm is stretching and likely to rupture.

The pulses at the groins and in the legs are usually present, and the vessels often slightly dilated. All pulses must be carefully palpated and their presence or absence documented, as aneurysmal and occlusive disease may coexist in some patients (Fig. 10.16).

The signs and symptoms of a ruptured aneurysm are described in Chapter 15. When an aneurysm

(c) A large central/upper abdominal expansile pulsatile mass indicative of an abdominal aortic aneurysm.

ruptures, it becomes very painful and tender. The patient may collapse with signs of hypovolaemia – pallor, tachycardia and hypotension. An expanding retroperitonal haematoma may be felt as a large mass in the abdomen spreading down into the iliac fossa or posteriorly into the loins.

Femoral aneurysms

These usually arise in the common femoral artery, and produce a bulge just below the inguinal ligament (Fig. 10.17). They have an expansile pulsation. A mass of enlarged lymph glands may transmit pulsation and can be misdiagnosed as an aneurysm (see the

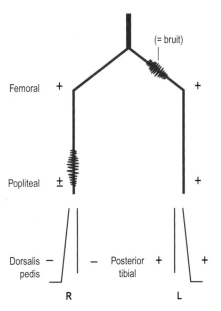

Fig. 10.16 Record the pulses and bruits on a simple diagram.

should always be excluded in patients presenting with an idiopathic calf vein thrombosis. Unfortunately, popliteal aneurysms often thrombose before they are noticed, and present with acute ischaemia of the lower limb (see above).

The diagnosis is confirmed by finding an expansile pulsation in the popliteal fossa (Fig. 10.18). The pulse is easy to feel. The examiner's fingers are pushed apart and away by the pulse, which can often be felt on both sides of the popliteal fossa. A popliteal aneurysm should always be suspected when a popliteal pulse is easy to feel. A bruit may be present above or over an enlarged segment of the vessel.

A thrombosed popliteal aneurysm is smooth and solid, and does not pulsate or fluctuate. It can be moved slightly from side to side, but never moves up and down. It may be confused with a Baker's cyst or semimembranosus bursa (see Chapter 8), but its size does not change when the knee is flexed, and it occupies the whole length of the midline of the popliteal fossa.

Fig. 10.17 A femoral aneurysm seen as a widened vertical pulsatile mass in the left groin.

differential diagnosis of a groin lump, Revision Panel 14.4). The other pulses in the leg must be documented, as there is often an associated popliteal aneurysm. Femoral and popliteal aneurysms are often bilateral, but do not necessarily develop or present at the same time (see below).

Popliteal aneurysms

Aneurysms of the popliteal artery are occasionally noticed by patients if they bulge out of the popliteal fossa. They may be found by chance in patients presenting with claudication. Popliteal aneurysms

Fig. 10.18 A popliteal aneurysm.

The ankle pulses will not be palpable. The legs should be examined for signs of venous obstruction, as this is a common complication of popliteal aneurysms (see below).

False aneurysms

A false aneurysm is a large haematoma whose centre contains fluid blood and connects with the lumen of the blood vessel. The most common cause is a therapeutic or diagnostic vascular puncture or a stab wound. Following the arterial puncture, a haematoma forms outside the artery. At first, thrombus plugs the defect, but pulsatile blood pressure gradually pushes out the haemostatic plug from the defect in the artery wall and excavates the haematoma to form a cavity connected to the vessel.

The symptoms, signs and complications of false aneurysms are exactly the same as those of a true aneurysm except for the following:

- There is a history of trauma or iatrogenic intervention, followed by
- The sudden appearance of a pulsatile swelling.
- False aneurysms tend to occur at unusual sites, for example the wrist or ankle, although iatrogenic false aneurysms are now most common in the groin.

False aneurysms also occur when a surgical graft separates from the native vessel. A pulsatile mass beneath an incision in the groin at the site of a previous vascular anastomosis is most likely to be a false aneurysm.

HAEMORRHAGE

A major vascular disruption, which may be the result of a penetrating, blunt or hyperextension injury, is likely to result in severe haemorrhage. The bleeding may be concealed, as when, for example, a serrated or spiculated end of a fractured long bone pierces an artery or a ruptured aneurysm bleeds into the tissues or a body cavity, or may be revealed, as when an aneurysm erupts through the skin or a congenital vascular malformation bleeds onto the skin surface.

Concealed haemorrhage from an arterial injury is suspected if a large swelling rapidly develops in association with signs of hypovolaemia, i.e. pallor, sweating, venoconstriction, tachycardia and eventually hypotension. The pulses distal to the injury will not be palpable if the artery has been transected, when the limb may show signs of acute ischaemia (the six Ps, see above).

In patients presenting with visible (revealed) haemorrhage, the diagnosis is straightforward. There is usually a jet of bright red, high-pressure, pulsatile blood coming out of an obvious cutaneous defect or wound. (Venous bleeding, in contrast, is dark red and wells up out of the wound.) The pulses distal to the injury may be absent if the artery has been transected. Direct pressure or proximal arterial compression over a bony point should arrest the bleeding until definitive treatment can be administered.

When the bleeding is coming from the site of a penetrating wound, it is important to assess local nerve and muscle, as other vital structures may be damaged. This may be difficult because the arrest of the haemorrhage must take precedence.

Artery, vein, nerve and muscle injuries commonly coexist.

When the haemorrhage occurs into a body cavity or is deeply seated, there may be no signs of swelling and the symptoms of hypovolaemia predominate. Haemorrhage into the peritoneum or retroperitoneum often causes pain as well as collapse, and may be associated with bruising around the umbilicus or flank (see Chapter 15).

TRANSIENT AND PERMANENT NEUROLOGICAL WEAKNESS, PARALYSIS AND BLINDNESS

Transient cerebral ischaemia

A transient ischaemic attack (TIA) is defined as a brief episode of neurological dysfunction (i.e. paralysis, paraesthesiae or speech loss) resulting from focal temporary cerebral ischemia not associated with permanent cerebral infarction. The classical definition of a TIA stipulated that symptoms must recover completely within 24 hours, but this time limit has been removed as it is now considered arbitrary.

Persistent cerebral ischaemia causes a stroke. This is a sudden episode of prolonged cerebral malfunction caused by cerebral infarction or haemorrhage, both caused by vascular disease, which usually takes the form of a prolonged weakness or paralysis of one-half of the body (a hemiplegia) (Fig. 10.19) and sometimes an associated sensory or speech defect,

Fig. 10.19 A patient who is hemiplegic with a facial weakness (upper motor; see Chapter 3) that is indicative of a cerebral infarct from a cerebral vascular accident.

which may predominate (see Chapter 3). The malfunction does not begin to recover for several days, and may never recover completely. Ischaemia of the midbrain that damages the vital centres in this area may cause coma and cardiovascular and respiratory instability.

It is important to remember that the right side of the brain controls the left side of the body, and vice versa.

The speech area (*Broca's area*) is invariably in the left temporoparietal area in right-handed people, although it can be in the right hemisphere in left-handed patients.

Strokes are more commonly caused by infarction than by cerebral haemorrhage, and are usually embolic or thrombotic, although an arterial wall dissection can occlude an artery's lumen.

Stroke caused by cerebral haemorrhage produces identical cerebral symptoms, but is more common in females and is associated with hypertension.

Both types of stroke usually cause upper motor neuron signs, with reduced power, spastic tone and brisk reflexes in the limbs, associated with an upgoing plantar reflex (*Babinksi's sign*). A cerebral haemorrhage can only be differentiated from an infarct with certainty by computed tomography scanning, and not by the history or physical signs.

Transient ischaemic attacks

These are caused by emboli or hypoperfusion (TIAs).

The emboli that cause TIAs come from the carotid arteries, heart valves and the great vessels. Platelet clumps and cholesterol crystals originally attached to ulcerated plaques break off and are swept up into the retinal or cerebral vessels (Fig. 10.20). Retinal emboli cause transient loss of vision, known as amaurosis fugax (fleeting blindness), which seems to the patient like a curtain coming across the visual

(a) A retinal platelet embolus arising from a carotid plaque presenting as amaurosis fugax.

(b) A retinal infarct. The pale area is the infarct.

Fig. 10.20 RETINAL INFARCT

field or a grey veil blocking out all or part of the vision in one eye.

Anyone presenting with a brief episode of weakness, paraesthesia or loss of sensation in one-half of the body that lasts a few minutes or several hours and then recovers completely must be suspected of having a TIA.

There are usually no physical signs by the time the patient presents, but evidence of previous ischaemic episodes – facial weakness, expressive dysphagia, upper motor neuron lesions and cholesterol emboli in the retinal vessels or areas of retinal infarction – should be sought.

The detection of a **carotid bruit** over the carotid artery just below the angle of the jaw indicates the presence of at least some stenosis in the region of the carotid bifurcation.

A severe internal carotid artery stenosis can, however, be present without any bruit, and a loud bruit can be caused by a stenosis of the external carotid artery.

Arrhythmias and cardiac murmurs suggest a cardiac source for the emboli. A low pulse pressure and an ejection systolic murmur suggest the presence of aortic valve disease, while an irregularly irregular or very slow pulse suggests a possible cause of Stokes–Adams attacks (see Chapter 2 page 56).

Transient hypoperfusion

Whereas emboli are common, hypoperfusion is rare because autoregulation usually ensures adequate cerebral perfusion, unless there is a very severe reduction in carotid blood pressure and flow. Episodes of hypoperfusion usually occur with much greater frequency than embolic attacks, often several times a day or week, and can be brought on by exercise or vasodilatation. They may cause 'global brain ischaemia', and present with dizziness and collapse rather than motor cortical symptoms.

Differential diagnosis

The differential diagnosis of a TIA is shown in Revision panel 10.8.

A history from a bystander or relative may be very helpful in making the diagnosis.

Any history of aura, twitching, tongue-biting or incontinence is indicative of *grand mal epilepsy*, whereas *petit mal* causes patients to lose touch temporarily with their surroundings (see Chapter 3).

Revision panel 10.8
The differential diagnosis of a TIA
Embolism from carotid artery atherosclerosis
Grand or petit mal epilepsy
Stokes–Adams attacks from a tight aortic stenosis
Arrhythmias
Vasovagal attacks
Hypoglycaemia
Migraine
Vertebrobasilar disease
Subdural haematoma
A space-occupying lesion in the brain

Hypoglycaemic attacks

These occur during periods of food abstinence, especially at night. Patients often describe hunger, malaise and vague abdominal pain, which is accompanied by trembling, dizziness and blurred vision. They may also notice incoordination, slurred speech, diplopia and drowsiness. The blood and urinary sugar is low during an attack, the symptoms of which can be instantly relieved by glucose.

Migraine

These attacks are usually heralded by severe unilateral headache, often situated over one eye and associated with photophobia and vomiting, and occasionally transient blindness. There are no physical signs, and the diagnosis relies entirely on the history. Sometimes there is a preceding 'aura' before the migraine begins.

Vertebrobasilar insufficiency

It can sometimes be quite difficult to separate TIAs from vertebrobasilar insufficiency, but the symptoms of the latter are often precipitated by neck movements or looking up. Neurological signs may indicate pathology in the hindbrain or cerebellum. Bruits may be heard over the origin of the vertebral artery.

Subclavian steal syndrome

This syndrome occurs when the first part of the subclavian artery is blocked and blood flows down the vertebral artery, because, during arm exercise, the vertebral artery acts as a collateral vessel to supply

Fig. 10.21 The flow of blood up the carotid artery and down the vertebral artery in a patient with subclavian steal syndrome, which results from a block in the first part of the subclavian artery (shown). Use of the left arm increases the flow to the limb at the expense of flow to the hindbrain, causing faintness.

— Blocked left subclavian artery

the arm (Fig. 10.21). This steals blood away from the hindbrain, and gives rise to hindbrain and cerebellar symptoms. Patients present with transient motor or sensory symptoms, and even loss of consciousness, after arm exercise. The presence of a weak brachial and radial pulse, reduced blood pressure in the affected arm, and a bruit over the subclavian artery should suggest the diagnosis of subclavian steal syndrome.

Other intracranial disease

Patients with a subdural haematoma may experience fluctuations in their level of consciousness, and will almost always develop some localizing neurological signs before eventually developing signs of raised intracranial pressure (see Chapter 3). This is also true of cerebral tumours and metastases, which can initially cause diagnostic confusion until the patient eventually develops signs of fixed and expanding defects.

Multiple sclerosis, acute glaucoma, retinal tears and temporal arteritis can cause transient blindness. Multiple sclerosis can cause considerable diagnostic confusion, but multiple lesions occurring in time and space eventually indicate the likely diagnosis.

Completed strokes

A full neurological examination is essential in all patients who present with a completed stroke, in order to exclude a vascular cause as well as a neurological dysfunction caused by space-occupying lesions, abscesses, haematomas and multiple sclerosis (see Chapter 3).

The blood pressure and heart must be carefully assessed (see Chapter 2). The superficial temporal arteries should be palpated. The carotid bifurcation and lower neck should be auscultated for bruits. A stethoscope placed over the closed eye can occasionally detect intracerebral bruits in patients with a stenosis in the carotid siphon.

COLD, BLUE DIGITS, HANDS AND FEET

Intermittent colour changes of the skin of the periphery of the limbs suggest the presence of vasospasm or recurrent minor episodes of arterial occlusion, and must be excluded before the diagnosis of vasospastic disease is accepted.

To do this, the supraclavicular fossa must be inspected and palpated for a fullness or occasionally a bony lump caused by a cervical rib or a dilated subclavian artery. The subclavian, axillary, brachial, radial and ulnar pulses must all be palpated and auscultated. The blood pressure should be measured in both arms, and Doppler pressures must be measured in the radial, ulnar and brachial pulses. Abnormalities detected by these examinations may require special tests such as plain radiographs, Duplex scanning and arteriography.

Patients not found to have a physical obstruction of their blood vessels are likely to be suffering from excessive vasospasm of the small vessels in their hands in response to cold and emotional stimuli. Some conditions can be diagnosed by the physical appearances they produce, but their aetiology is still largely conjectural, and there is a considerable overlap between each condition.

Raynaud's phenomenon

This is the best known vasospastic disorder. The term is used to describe a series of colour changes in the skin of the hands or feet following exposure

Revision panel 10.9

The causes of Raynaud's phenomenon

Atherosclerosis and Buerger's disease

Platelet emboli from:

Subclavian aneurysm (secondary to cervical rib)

Atherosclerotic stenosis of the subclavian artery

Collagen disease:

Scleroderma

Systemic lupus erythematosus

Rheumatoid arthritis

Vibrating tools

Irritation of nerves:

Cervical spondylosis

Cervical rib

Spinal cord disease

Old poliomyelitis

Repeated immersion in cold water

Working in a cold environment

Previous frostbite

Blood abnormalities:

Cold agglutinins

Cryoglobulins

Polycythaemia

Drugs:

Ergot

General diseases:

Hypothyroidism

Diabetes

Malnutrition

(a) Raynaud's phenomenon.

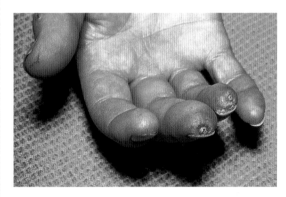

(b) Ischaemic ulceration of the fingertips. This usually indicates permanent, rather than spastic, occlusion of the digital vessels.

Fig. 10.22 VASOSPASTIC DIGITAL CHANGES

to cold (Fig. 10.22a). The condition can be most distressing in cold climates, especially in winter:

- The skin first turns white, and becomes cold and numb.
- It next turns blue, but remains cold and numb.
- Finally, it turns red, hot and painful.

Many attacks are brought on by cold or emotion, and many do not pass through all the classic colour changes (Revision panel 10.9).

History

Sex Ninety per cent of those affected are female, and many are cigarette smokers. It affects 5–20 per cent of the population.

Past history It is worthwhile asking patients if they have a history of frostbite, have ever worked in a cold storage environment or have regularly used vibrating tools.

Joint problems, rashes and swallowing difficulty indicate the likelihood of scleroderma or another collagen vascular disease.

Examination

Those conditions which, in addition to the colour changes, cause permanent damage to the digital arteries, such as scleroderma, vibration injury and blood abnormalities, gradually cause atrophy of the pulps of the fingers, poor nail growth and ulceration of the fingertips. The fingers waste, especially the pulps, and become thin, stiff and pointed if the digital arteries become occluded. The hand is cold and the joints may be stiff. Sometimes there are small, painful, ischaemic ulcers on the fingertips, which are slow to heal, or small scars at the site of the resolution of previous patches of ischaemia. Both are very painful and tender. The patient may eventually develop rest pain and gangrene of the fingertips. Repeated infections around the nails (paronychia) are common.

CHAPTER 10 | THE ARTERIES, VEINS AND LYMPHATICS

Many patients eventually develop the signs of scleroderma, evidence that the phenomenon is a secondary abnormality, not a primary disease.

When the cause of the colour changes is solely vasospasm, the hands look normal between attacks, making the diagnosis of the underlying cause far more difficult. The symptoms are often secondary to other conditions, and the diagnosis of idiopathic Raynaud's disease is only made when these have been excluded.

The common causes are the collagen vascular diseases, especially scleroderma, the excessive use of vibrating tools and cold exposure. Patients with scleroderma, systemic lupus erythematosus and rheumatoid arthritis may show the characteristic changes in their skin and face (see Chapter 1).

Fig. 10.23 Hands demonstrating the red/blue colour changes of acrocyanosis.

Primary Raynaud's disease

When all the other causes of Raynaud's phenomenon have been excluded, a diagnosis of primary Raynaud's disease is upheld. This condition is quite common in teenage females. It is mild, familial and often associated with chilblains. It often disappears in the late twenties, but a few females have symptoms all their life, and occasionally the disease becomes very severe.

If the symptoms start in adult females, often around the menopause, they are likely to be the first sign of scleroderma.

It is always worthwhile measuring the Doppler pressures at the wrist, especially if the pulses are impalpable. The digital vessels may also be insonated with the Doppler flow detector, and in patients with collagen diseases, pulses in these may well be absent near the tips of the fingers.

Some doctors use a cold exposure test – dipping the hands in cold water and re-mapping and re-measuring the Doppler digital pressures in the fingers – to reproduce the symptoms and confirm the existence of a cold sensitivity.

Acrocyanosis

This is a condition, usually affecting females, in which the hands and feet are persistently blue and cold (Fig. 10.23). The colour of the skin does not vary with the environmental temperature as it does in Raynaud's phenomenon, but the blueness may come and go. The hands may be pink and normal

between attacks, or cold with sweaty palms. As the attack subsides, the hands may become warm, sweaty and painful. The fingers are susceptible to chilblains. The diagnosis is based solely on the colour, temperature and appearance of the hands.

Erythrocyanosis crurum puellarum frigidum

This condition affects the posterior and medial aspects of the lower legs of young (15–25 years old) females in response to cold. The legs are often fat and hairless.

The affected areas become red/blue (erythrocyanotic) and swollen. Dusky reddish purple blotches appear and may feel cold to the touch. The swollen area is tender and may progress to chilblains and superficial ulceration (Fig. 10.24). When the chilblains break down and ulcerate, they must be differentiated from other forms of leg ulcer.

ERYTHROMELALGIA

This is a condition in which the patient complains of burning red extremities. These symptoms may be exacerbated by the pressure of bedclothes against the skin. The condition is much more common in females. It appears to result from the release of vasodilator neurochemicals, with 5-hydroxytryptamine accumulating in the tissues. It must be differentiated from gout, Buerger's disease,

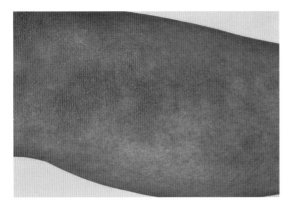

Fig. 10.24 Erythrocyanosis crurum puellarum frigidum (erythrocyanosis frigida), seen as painful, red, cold areas of induration (chilblains).

systemic lupus erythematosus, rheumatoid arthritis and peripheral neuritis.

Examination of the extremities confirms that they are red, and patients complain that dependency causes an increase in the pain.

LARGE LIMBS

Local gigantism, multiple arteriovenous fistulas and Klippel–Trenaunay syndrome all cause a limb to grow larger and thicker than its fellow.

The presence of multiple arteriovenous fistulas throughout a single limb is known as Parkes Weber syndrome (Fig. 10.25). This is a congenital abnormality. The limb, as well as being enlarged, feels hot. The subcutaneous veins are often dilated. There may be palpable thrills and audible machinery murmurs over the major sites of fistulation.

A tourniquet inflated around the root of the limb should cause slowing of the pulse (the *Branham–Nicoladoni sign*). This is a consequence of reducing the venous return by abolishing the shunt. The differential diagnoses are the other causes of limb hypertrophy mentioned above. Rarely, patients with a swollen, lymphoedematous limb are misdiagnosed as having a hypertrophic limb.

SURGICALLY CORRECTABLE CAUSES OF HYPERTENSION

Patients with *high blood pressure* rarely present as surgical outpatients, but renal artery stenosis

(a)

(b)

Fig. 10.25 PARKES WEBER SYNDROME
(a, b) Limbs with Parkes Weber syndrome, in which the multiple arteriovenous fistulas cause limb enlargement and vascular dilatation. A machinery murmur can often be heard over the limb.

CHAPTER 10 | THE ARTERIES, VEINS AND LYMPHATICS

Fig. 10.26 The retinal appearances of a patient with severe hypertension. Haemorrhages and exudates are visible.

retinal haemorrhage (Fig. 10.26), adrenal tumours and coarctation of the aorta are important, surgically correctable causes of hypertension. Renal function must be assessed, and the abdomen should be auscultated for bruits in all atherosclerotic patients who are found to be hypertensive.

A 'moon' face, abdominal striae and a 'buffalo' hump (see Chapter 1) are indicative of Cushing's syndrome, while the presence of neurofibromas suggests the possibility of a phaeochromocytoma (see Chapter 4).

Coarctation of the aorta is a rare but important cause of hypertension (in the upper limbs), and is discussed in Chapter 2.

INTESTINAL ISCHAEMIA

Ischaemia of the bowel may have an acute or chronic onset.

Acute obstruction of the superior mesenteric artery by an embolus or by thrombosis causes acute abdominal pain, peritonitis and shock (see Chapter 15).

Chronic atherosclerotic occlusion or stenosis of the coeliac or mesenteric vessels can cause intestinal angina – abdominal pain that develops 30–60 minutes after eating – causing fear of eating, and weight loss.

A reduced blood flow in the arteries of the colon, particularly the splenic flexure, can cause ischaemic colitis with diarrhoea and sometimes rectal bleeding.

The only physical sign in the chronic syndromes may be the presence of an abdominal bruit.

THE VEINS

CLINICAL ASSESSMENT OF THE VENOUS CIRCULATION OF THE LOWER LIMB

Anatomy and physiology

The veins of the lower limb are divided into the superficial and deep systems, separated by the deep fascia of the leg. At certain points, veins pass through the deep fascia to provide a communication between the two systems (Fig. 10.27). The valves in these communicating veins usually only allow blood to pass from the superficial into the deep system. The deep veins have many valves to ensure that blood only flows upwards against the force of gravity towards the heart.

In the erect position, the venous return is heavily dependent on the calf muscle pump. Large venous sinusoids within the soleus muscle are compressed during contraction of the calf muscles, for example during walking. This forces blood out of the calf veins into the popliteal veins, and on towards the heart. During calf muscle relaxation, the intramuscular veins open, but blood is prevented from refluxing back into them from the proximal deep veins by the valves in the popliteal veins. The negative pressure in the deep veins then sucks blood in from the superficial system through the communicating veins to reduce the superficial venous pressure, incrementally, with each calf muscle contraction.

The superficial veins all eventually join either the great (long) or the lesser (short) saphenous system. These two major subcutaneous veins end where they communicate with the femoral and popliteal veins, respectively (Fig. 10.27). The two superficial systems are also joined to the deep veins by a number of other communicating (perforating) veins, the most important of which are in the calf.

The tributaries of the saphenous veins become varicose because they, unlike the saphenous trunks, do not contain a strong coat of smooth muscle in their wall. They lie in a more superficial position and are not bound down to the deep fascia.

The deep veins accompany the arteries of the lower leg and join to form the popliteal vein, which also receives blood from the calf muscle sinusoids.

Deep vein thrombosis usually starts in the soleal sinusoids and venae commitantes, before extending up into the popliteal vein, the femoral vein, the iliac veins and even into the vena cava.

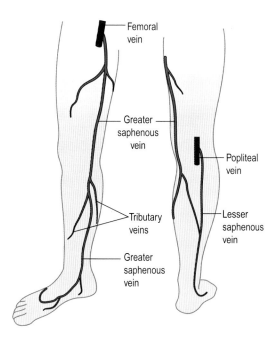

Fig. 10.27 A line diagram of the superficial, deep and communicating veins of the lower limb.

Symptoms of lower limb venous disease

Most patients with venous disorders complain of:

- **'unsightly veins'** in their lower limbs;
- pain or discomfort when standing;
- minor ankle swelling.

They may also complain of skin changes (lipodermatosclerosis, eczema, pigmentation and ulceration) in the skin of the gaiter region.

Superficial veins may occasionally bleed or thrombose.

Superficial vein thrombosis causes painful lumps or cords.

Deep vein thrombosis presents with calf pain and leg swelling (Fig. 10.28) or, if it is complicated by a pulmonary embolism, with pleuritic chest pain, haemoptysis and dyspnoea.

Examination of the veins of the lower limb (Revision panel 10.10)

Inspection

The lower limbs need to be fully exposed with the patient standing erect on a low stool in a warm, well-lit examination room. Many patients with venous

Fig. 10.28 Superficial thrombophlebitis in the greater saphenous vein, shown as dark area, which is palpable as 'lumps'.

> ### Revision panel 10.10
> #### Routine for assessing the venous circulation
> Ask the patient to stand up
>
> Inspection:
>
> Site, tortuosity and size of visible veins
> Effect of elevation and dependency
> Ankle oedema
> Skin colour, especially above the medial ankle
>
> Palpation:
>
> Palpate the trunks of the long and short saphenous veins
> Palpate the sapheno-popliteal junction
> Feel the texture of the skin and subcutaneous tissues
>
> Percussion:
>
> Percussion wave conduction upwards or downwards
>
> Auscultation:
>
> Listen for bruits over prominent varices
> Tourniquet tests
> Doppler ultrasound

CHAPTER 10 | THE ARTERIES, VEINS AND LYMPHATICS

(a)

(b)

Fig. 10.29 TWO SAPHENA VARICES
(a) Left, (b) right. A saphena varix is a bluish swelling over and below the saphenous termination, which collapses and disappears when the patient lies flat.

(a) Blue.

(b) Red.

Fig. 10.30 SPIDER VEINS
(a, b) 'Spider veins' are dilatations of the intracutaneous veins.

disorders have visible, dilated and tortuous subcutaneous veins, which are described as '**varicose veins**'.

Both limbs must be examined from all aspects. The site and course of all the varicosities should be recorded on anterior and posterior outline drawings of the lower limb.

A blue-tinged bulge in the groin, which disappears on lying down, is likely to be a **saphena varix** (Fig. 10.29). This is a dilation of the termination of the long saphenous vein or one of its major tributaries.

Some varicose veins are large and prominent, whereas others are minute and intradermal. The latter may cause a blue patch, which can arise from a single feeding vein. Intradermal veins are called **spider veins** or **venous stars** (Fig. 10.30). Slightly larger intermediate veins are often called **reticular veins**.

Large, prominent, distended veins on the medial side of the lower calf have been called '**ankle blow-outs**' if they lie in close proximity to the site of incompetent calf communicating veins (Fig. 10.31).

(a)

(b)

Fig. 10.31 ANKLE 'BLOW-OUTS'
(a, b) Dilatations of the surface veins over or close by incompetent ankle perforating (communicating) veins.

Fig. 10.32 An example of an 'ankle flare' or corona phlebectatica, in which there is a considerable dilatation of the intracutaneous veins below the ankle in limbs with venous hypertension.

The network of small dilated venules that develops beneath the lateral and/or medial malleolus of limbs with severe venous hypertension is called an **ankle flare** or **corona phlebectatica** (Fig. 10.32).

Distended veins crossing the groins and extending up over the abdominal wall are collateral veins, and indicate the presence of a deep venous obstruction. Cross-pubic collateral veins may be visible if one iliac system is obstructed (Fig. 10.33).

The skin of the lower medial third of the leg, the gaiter region, must be carefully inspected. Venous hypertension caused by venous outflow obstruction or severe reflux may cause an area of skin pigmentation, tenderness and subcutaneous induration, called **lipodermatosclerosis**, and eventually **eczema and ulceration** (Fig. 10.34).

Palpation

The examiner's dominant hand should be gently run over the course of the main veins and their tributaries because dilated veins can sometimes be more easily felt than seen, especially in fat legs. Veins in the lower leg may lie in a gutter of indurated subcutaneous fat. Dilated long and short saphenous veins are usually easy to feel.

The termination of a distended short saphenous vein is easier to feel if the patient is asked to bend the knees slightly to relax the deep fascia covering the popliteal fossa.

CHAPTER 10 | THE ARTERIES, VEINS AND LYMPHATICS

(a)

(b)

Fig. 10 33 LARGE CROSS-PUBIC COLLATERAL VEINS
(a, b) These large veins have opened up to bypass a block in the iliac veins of one limb.

Carefully palpate the sapheno-femoral junction (2.5 cm below and lateral to the pubic tubercle) and the sapheno-popliteal junction, which has a variable position in the popliteal fossa (high or low). The patient should be asked to cough while the dilated veins are palpated to see if there is any impulse or thrill (a cough impulse), indicating that the valves at their junctions with the deep veins are incompetent, and the back flow is turbulent.

Palpate the skin of the calf to define any areas of induration and tenderness (**lipodermatosclerosis**).

Percussion

The distended, dilated trunks of the long and short saphenous systems transmit a percussion wave in an orthograde direction whether or not the valves are competent. The more distended the vein, the better the wave is transmitted. The valves must be incompetent if a percussion wave is transmitted retrogradely, i.e. downwards while the patient is standing.

Percussion can also be used to help to define the terminations of the long and short saphenous veins by placing the fingers of one hand gently over the upper end of the dilated saphenous trunk and percussing the vein below it, using the middle finger of the other hand to 'flick' distended varicosities further down the leg. The process can then be repeated in reverse, with the upper end of the vein being 'flicked' and the lower hand detecting a downward percussion wave, to check the competence of the valves.

Auscultation

Listen with your stethoscope over any large clusters of veins, especially if they remain distended when the patient lies down and the limb is elevated. A machinery murmur over such veins indicates that they are secondary to an **arteriovenous fistula**.

Tourniquet tests

Many clinicians have abandoned tourniquet tests as a means of assessing varicose veins in favour of more sophisticated investigations such as duplex ultrasound, but these tests are simple to perform and, if correctly carried out, can provide useful information on the major sites of communicating vein incompetence.

The patient should lie on a couch that has a small foot stool attached to it, onto which the patient

(a) A red weepy skin rash (venous eczema) developing in a limb with venous hypertension.

(c)

(b, c) An indurated, pigmented, inflamed plaque of ankle skin (which develops in the area covered by old fashioned gaiters) that is associated with venous hypertension and is now known as lipodermatosclerosis.

(b)

Fig. 10.34 VENOUS ECZEMA, LIPODERMATOSCLEROSIS AND ULCERATION

(d) A venous ulcer. This occurs in the gaiter region of the ankle skin, surrounded by lipodermatosclerosis. The ulcer edge is sloping.

CHAPTER 10 | THE ARTERIES, VEINS AND LYMPHATICS

can rapidly stand. The limb to be examined is then elevated – often by placing it on the examiner's shoulder – to empty the veins, a process that can be expedited by stroking the blood within the veins towards the heart.

A tourniquet made from a long length of 1 cm diameter soft rubber tubing is then pulled tight around the upper thigh and held in place by strong artery forceps (Spencer Wells). The rubber tubing must press firmly into the subcutaneous tissues of the thigh to ensure that the subcutaneous veins are completely occluded (Fig. 10.35). *The Velcro tourniquets used by many junior doctors for venesection do not apply enough pressure, but the soft tubing on a stethoscope is an effective alternative if rubber tubing is not available, provided it is long enough.*

Leg horizontal, superficial veins empty

The patient stands up

An incompetent communicating vein below the tourniquet fills the superficial veins below the tourniquet

An incompetent communicating vein above the tourniquet fills the superficial veins above the tourniquet

By moving the tourniquet up and down the leg it is possible to determine the level of the incompetent communicating veins.

Fig. 10.35 The principles of the tourniquet test.

The patient is then asked to stand up quickly, and the legs are observed for 10–15 seconds. If the sapheno-femoral junction is the only site of superficial to deep valvular incompetence, the veins above the tourniquet will rapidly fill, but those below it will remain collapsed (Fig. 10.36b). This can be confirmed by suddenly releasing the tourniquet and watching the veins below the site of the tourniquet rapidly distend from above, as blood regurgitates down the long saphenous vein. There must be other sites of superficial to deep incompetence below the level of the tourniquet if the veins below the tourniquet fill immediately the patient stands up.

This test can be repeated with the tourniquet moved progressively down the whole length of the leg to try to define all the sites of superficial to deep vein incompetence, but it is easier and simpler to apply it once below the knee to exclude short saphenous incompetence.

(b) Tourniquet controlling veins.

(a) Before tourniquet applied.

Fig. 10.36 TOURNIQUET TESTS

(c) Veins distending after release of tourniquet.

CHAPTER 10 | THE ARTERIES, VEINS AND LYMPHATICS

Tourniquet tests are often difficult to interpret in patients with recurrent varicose veins, and the value of applying multiple tourniquets in an effort to locate the precise level of calf communicating veins has never been scientifically verified.

A modification of the tourniquet test is to empty the limb as described above and apply direct digital pressure over the upper end of the long saphenous vein while the patient stands up to see if this prevents retrograde filling. This is called the *Trendelenburg (tourniquet) test.*

Venous hypertension caused by proximal vein obstruction or the presence of an arteriovenous fistula should be suspected if the varicose veins fail to collapse on elevation. This can be confirmed by asking the patient to stand up after placing a tourniquet just below the knee, to cut off long and short saphenous reflux, and then to stand repeatedly on tip toes. This exercise empties a normal superficial venous system by sucking the blood in the surface varicosities into the deep veins, through competent perforating veins. A failure to achieve superficial vein emptying indicates deep vein obstruction or reflux through incompetent valves in the deep or communicating veins. This is called *Perthes' walking test.*

Doppler flow detector studies

The simple directional Doppler ultrasound flow probe described on page 323 can also be used to assess venous reflux. The patient is asked to stand up, and the ultrasound probe is placed over the termination of the long and then the short saphenous veins using coupling jelly. The direction of venous blood flow, augmented by rapid intermittent manual compression of the calf or any prominent varicosities in the lower limb, is then assessed.

A uniphasic signal on squeezing, with no sound on relaxation, indicates competent valves with forward flow (Fig. 10.37a). A biphasic signal, with prolonged retrograde flow on releasing the compression, indicates reflux and valvular incompetence (Fig. 10.37b).

Retrograde flow can also be confirmed by asking the patient to perform the Valsalva manoeuvre. This consists of taking a deep breath, pinching off the nose, closing the mouth and attempting a forced

(a) Uniphasic Doppler signal (forward flow only).

(b) Biphasic Doppler signal (forward and retrograde flow).

Fig. 10.37 DOPPLER SIGNALS

expiration. This causes venous flow to reverse if the valves are incompetent.

The Doppler ultrasound flow detector can also be used in association with the tourniquet test to demonstrate retrograde flow in the saphenous trunks when the tourniquet is released.

The simple hand-held Doppler flow detector cannot detect retrograde flow in either the deep or calf perforating veins with any accuracy. The detection of deep vein flow abnormalities requires more sophisticated duplex scans.

LOWER LIMB VENOUS DISEASE

Varicose veins

A varicose vein is a dilated, tortuous vein (Fig. 10.38). The cause of 'primary' varicose veins is unknown, but the erect stance and abnormalities in the components and structure of the vein wall may be important factors.

'Secondary' varicose veins may be the result of a proximal venous obstruction, destruction of the valves by thrombosis or an increase in flow and pressure caused by an arteriovenous fistula (Revision panel 10.11).

Varicosities do not cause symptoms, apart from unsightliness. Symptoms are caused by the physiological malfunction that follows the valvular incompetence and retrograde flow.

(a)

(b)

Fig. 10.38 VARICOSE VEINS
(a, b) Varicose veins are, by definition, dilated and tortuous, and usually have incompetent valves. They occur on both the medial (a) and the lateral (b) side of the leg.

Consequently, many patients have massive varicose veins but no symptoms, while others have severe symptoms with very few visible varicose

veins. To add to the confusion, many patients with normal veins have symptoms similar to those caused by venous disease.

History

Age Varicose veins affect all age groups, but are more common in older people. In children, they are usually caused by a congenital vascular abnormality.

Sex Ten times more females than males attend hospital with venous complaints, but surveys in the community have shown there is little difference in the incidence of varicose veins between the sexes.

Ethnic groups Varicose veins are said to be less common in Africa and the Far East than in Europe and North America.

Occupation Many patients with symptomatic varicose veins have occupations that involve standing for prolonged periods. It is doubtful whether standing, by itself, causes varicose veins, but it certainly exacerbates the leg symptoms.

CHAPTER 10 | THE ARTERIES, VEINS AND LYMPHATICS

Symptoms Many patients with varicose veins have no symptoms. The disfiguring effect of the veins is often the principal complaint.

The next most common complaint is pain. This is usually a dull ache felt in the calf and lower leg that gets worse throughout the day, especially when the patient is standing up for prolonged periods. It is relieved by lying down for 15 or 30 minutes, or by wearing compression hosiery. The pain is often experienced in the dilated varicosities.

Night cramps and itching are also common complaints.

Mild swelling of the ankle by the end of the day is common, but marked ankle oedema is not, and other causes of oedema should be eliminated before accepting that it is caused by the varicose veins. Some patients present with red, painful, tender lumps caused by acute superficial thrombophlebitis (see below).

Lipodermatosclerosis, eczema and ulceration are important complications that indicate the need for treatment.

Always exclude conditions that may obstruct the iliac veins and cause secondary varicose veins, such as pregnancy and abdominal tumours.

Previous history

Most patients with varicose veins have had them for years, and many have had various forms of treatment such as operations and injections. It is important to exclude a previous deep vein thrombosis that may have accompanied previous illnesses, operations, accidents or pregnancies. All females should be asked if they had swelling of their legs or a deep vein thrombosis during pregnancy.

Family history

It is common to find that the patient's mother and sisters also have varicose veins. A definite family history is obtained in one-third to one-half of the patients who present with varicose veins.

Examination

Local examination

Inspection Look for large visible veins. Record their site, extent and size on large drawings of the front and back of the limbs. The skin of the leg should be inspected, especially the skin of the lower third of the medial side of the calf, for signs of chronic venous hypertension, lipodermatosclerosis,

pigmentation, induration and inflammation, as well as eczema and ulceration.

Palpation Assess the texture of the skin and subcutaneous tissue of the lower leg by palpation. There may be pitting oedema or thickening, redness and tenderness. These changes are caused by chronic venous hypertension and are known as **lipodermatosclerosis**, a term which indicates that there is a progressive replacement of the skin and subcutaneous fat by fibrous tissue, induration and an associated inflammation caused by the fibrin deposition that proceeds the fibrosis.

Feel for a cough impulse and thrill in the groin, and in a dilated trunk of the short saphenous vein behind the knee. This is easier if the fascia is relaxed by slightly flexing the knee.

Percussion Test whether a percussion impulse is conducted up and, more significantly, down the main superficial veins.

Auscultation Listen over any large bunch of varicosities, especially if the veins do not collapse when the patient lies down.

Tourniquet and Doppler flow detector tests The Trendelenburg and tourniquet tests must be carried out to detect the site of any incompetent superficial to deep communicating veins. Confirm the presence of reflux with the Doppler flow detector.

General examination

Because varicose veins are so common, it is tempting to omit a full general examination. Never do this. Always examine the abdomen, and make sure the patient is not pregnant.

Inspection of the abdomen may reveal dilated collateral veins crossing to the other groin, or up over the abdomen and chest to join the tributaries of the superior vena cava. The direction of flow in these veins is detected by placing two fingers on the veins, sliding one finger along the vein to empty it and then releasing the other finger and watching which way the empty segment fills (*Harvey's test*) (Fig. 10.39). This test may have to be repeated moving the fingers in either direction before the direction of blood flow can be confirmed.

A rectal or vaginal examination may be required to exclude a pelvic or abdominal cause for the varicose veins. In males, it is important to feel the testes. Massive enlargement of the abdominal lymph

(a)

(b)

Fig. 10.39 HARVEY'S TEST
(a, b) The test demonstrates that blood flows in only one direction through competent venous valves.

glands by metastases from small testicular tumours can cause inferior vena cava obstruction.

Venous ulceration

Many patients with venous ulcers do not have visible varicose veins. Approximately one-half of all venous ulcers are associated with primary varicose veins. The remainder are the result of post-thrombotic deep vein damage (see below).

History

Age Venous ulcers usually follow many years of venous disease, so the majority are seen in patients over the age of 40 years, many of whom have had recurrent ulceration for some years before seeking medical help. Post-thrombotic disease can cause ulceration in young adults, and ulcers can occur in children and teenagers with congenital venous malformations.

Sex Venous ulcers are more common in females than in males.

Symptoms Patients have often had aching pain, discomfort and tenderness of the skin (lipodermatosclerosis and pigmentation) for many months or years before an ulcer appears.

Some ulcers are painful, but many are not.

The discharge may be very smelly, leading to depression and social isolation.

An episode of trauma often initiates the breakdown of the skin, but sometimes itching and scratching may start an ulcer.

Previous history Many venous ulcers are caused by deep and communicating vein damage, so there is often a history of venous thrombosis during an illness or pregnancy. The patient may have had previous episodes of ulceration.

Cause The ulcer invariably begins after the skin of the leg has been knocked and damaged. The initial incident is sometimes remembered, but often not.

Examination

Site Venous ulcers are commonly found around the gaiter area of the lower leg, and usually begin on the medial aspect. Ulcers situated lower down on the foot or higher up on the fleshy part of the calf are rarely caused by venous disease.

Shape and size Venous ulcers can be of any shape and any size (Fig. 10.40).

Edge The edge is gently sloping and, when healing begins, pale pink as new epithelium migrates across its surface.

Base This may be covered with yellow slough but becomes covered with pink granulation tissue when the ulcer is healing. Areas of white fibrous tissue may be seen between the granulations, and there may be more white fibrous tissue than granulation tissue when the ulcer is very chronic and indolent. The base is usually fixed to the deep tissues. Tendons and the tibial periosteum may be exposed in the base of the ulcer.

Depth Venous ulcers are usually relatively shallow.

Discharge The discharge is usually seropurulent but can occasionally be bloodstained.

Surrounding tissues The surrounding tissues usually show the signs of chronic venous hypertension – induration, inflammation, pigmentation and tenderness, i.e. **lipodermatosclerosis**.

There may be old white scars (atrophie blanche) from previous ulceration, and many dilated intradermal and subcutaneous veins. Movements of the ankle joint may be limited by scar tissue, which can cause an equinus deformity of the joint. Occasionally, true cellulitis occurs.

CHAPTER 10 | THE ARTERIES, VEINS AND LYMPHATICS

(a) Venous.

(b) Arterial.

(c) Rheumatoid.

(d) Neuropathic.

(e) HIV (AIDS).

(f) Sickle cell.

(g) Systemic lupus erythematosus.

(h) Pemphigoid.

(i) Self-induced.

Fig. 10.40 MONTAGE OF DIFFERENT TYPES OF LEG ULCER

(j) Martorell's.

(k) Gout.

(l) Gumma.

(m) Osteomyelitis.

(n) Foreign body (orthopaedic screw).

(o) Pyoderma gangrenosum.

(p) Yaws.

(q) Basal cell carcinoma.

(r) Marjolin's.

Local lymph glands Ulcers are usually colonized rather than infected, so the inguinal lymph glands should not be enlarged or tender.

Remember that squamous cell carcinoma can arise in a chronic venous ulcer, particularly in a patient known to have a long-standing venous ulcer that has enlarged, become painful and malodorous, and especially if the edge of the ulcer is found to be raised or thickened. Malignant change is also suggested by finding enlarged inguinal lymph glands. Biopsy is indicated should any of these changes appear. Malignant change in a chronic venous ulcer is known as a Marjolin's ulcer (see Chapter 4) (Fig. 10.40r).

The lower limbs The whole of both lower limbs must be examined for the presence of varicose veins, competent and incompetent communicating veins and skin changes, as described above. Most patients have bilateral disease, and the majority of patients with venous ulcers have incompetent communicating veins.

It is also important to assess the arterial circulation and the nerves, to exclude an ischaemic or neuropathic cause of the ulcer (see page 331).

General examination The abdomen should be examined to exclude an abdominal cause of venous insufficiency, and the other leg should be examined for signs of venous disease.

Look for any general features of the many other causes of skin ulceration, such as ischaemia, rheumatoid arthritis, skin tumours, pyoderma gangrenosum, collagen diseases, anaemia, polycythaemia, neuropathic ulcers and sickle-cell disease (Fig. 10.40).

Deep vein thrombosis

Only a quarter of deep vein thromboses cause symptoms and signs. Many occur spontaneously, but in more than one-half there is a predisposing cause such as an operation, bed rest, thrombophilia or recent air travel.

History

Patients complain of pain and swelling in the calf or the whole leg. The onset of symptoms is sudden, and they are usually severe enough to make walking difficult. The first indication may be a pulmonary embolism, which causes symptoms such as pleuritic pain, dyspnoea, haemoptysis and collapse.

Examination

Swelling of a leg, particularly if it is unilateral, is the most significant physical sign (Fig. 10.41). The ankle may be the only site of swelling if the thrombosis is confined to the calf. Swelling of both ankles needs to be differentiated from other causes of oedema. The swelling may extend up to the groin if the iliac vein is thrombosed.

The muscles that contain the thrombosed veins may become hard and tender. A change in texture of the muscle is more significant than tenderness because, although there are many conditions that make a muscle tender, there are few that make it stiff and hard. 'Pain' on stretching the calf muscles by forced dorsiflexion is known as *Homan's sign*. This sign is a poor discriminator and should be abandoned.

The superficial veins may be dilated, and the leg may feel hot. A large, swollen limb that is made pale by severe oedema is called **phlegmasia alba dolens**.

(a) Mild.

(b) Severe.

Fig. 10.41 ANKLE OEDEMA/SWELLING CAUSED BY A DEEP VEIN THROMBOSIS

When the venous thrombosis blocks almost all the main outflow veins, the skin of the leg becomes congested and blue. This is called **phlegmasia caerulea dolens**.

Venous gangrene can develop when there is very severe venous outflow obstruction. Venous gangrene usually affects the peripheral tissues (toes or fingers).

Chest signs The neck veins may be dilated, and there may be central cyanosis and signs of right ventricular hypertrophy if the patient has had a pulmonary embolus. A fixed-split second heart sound may be heard indicative of pulmonary hypertension, and there may be a pleural rub from the infarcted lung rubbing against the pleura.

The post-thrombotic limb

The symptoms and signs that follow the damage caused by a deep vein thrombosis, obstruction and valvular incompetence may appear months or years after the thrombosis. The initiating thrombosis may have passed unrecognized, but more often it has produced clinical signs and required treatment.

The earliest symptoms are usually a slowly progressive swelling of the leg that becomes painful as the day wears on. The skin of the gaiter area initially becomes pigmented, but eventually it becomes a hard inflamed, indurated, pigmented plaque (lipodermatosclerosis). These changes may spread around the whole circumference of the gaiter area.

Varicose veins become more prominent and, if the thrombosis obstructs the venous outflow at the base of the limb, collateral veins may develop across the groins and the pubis, and the superficial veins will not empty when the patient is asked to carry out heel-raising on the spot with a mid-thigh tourniquet in place (*Perthes' walking test*).

A small group of patients develop true venous claudication. This is a severe calf and sometimes thigh pain caused by walking. It must be differentiated from intermittent claudication caused by arterial insufficiency. These patients usually have a swollen, tender limb, multiple varicose veins, collateral veins and lipodermatosclerosis, all indicating the likelihood of a previous deep vein thrombosis. The pain of venous claudication is usually accompanied by an increase in the swelling, and the pain fades very slowly.

Superficial thrombophlebitis

Deep vein thrombosis begins in normal veins, the vein wall becoming secondarily inflamed. In superficial thrombophlebitis, the inflammation of the vein wall is invariably the cause of the thrombosis.

The causes of superficial thrombophlebitis are given in Revision panel 10.12.

Revision panel 10.12
The causes of superficial thrombophlebitis
Varicose veins
Occult carcinoma:

   Bronchus
   Pancreas
   Stomach
   Lymphoma

Thromboangiitis obliterans (Buerger's disease)
Polycythaemia
Polyarteritis
Idiopathic
Iatrogenic
Intravenous injection and injuries

An occult carcinoma should be suspected when the episodes occur in the arms of patients over the age of 45 years, especially if they are transient and migrate. Thrombophlebitis migrans is, however, a rare condition.

History

Patients complain of the sudden appearance of a painful lump on their arm or leg. The pain usually subsides in 3–7 days, leaving a tender lump or subcutaneous cord that takes several weeks to disperse. There may be a preceding injury such as a venepuncture or, if the vein is varicose, a direct injury.

Examination

The swelling is in the subcutaneous tissues. It has an elongated, cord-like shape and may be several centimetres long, running along the long axis of the limb (see Fig. 10.28). The lump is tender. The overlying skin is at first red and inflamed, before becoming pigmented and brown. Enlargement of the local lymph glands is rare, and other tissues in the limb are normal, unless the condition is secondary to varicose veins.

The whole patient must be examined for an occult carcinoma, even if they have varicose veins.

Axillary vein thrombosis

Thrombosis of the axillary/subclavian vein may follow excessive use of the limb, especially above the head, or compression of the vein by musculoskeletal abnormalities such as a cervical rib.

History

The patient complains of a sudden discomfort and swelling of the arm. The arm, forearm and hand swell up, and there is discomfort on the medial side of the upper arm and in the axilla. The arm may feel hot, and if it becomes very swollen, movements may become restricted. The patient may give a history of unusual activity in the preceding 24 hours, such as painting a ceiling.

Examination

The whole arm is swollen, congested and blue, and the surface veins are usually distended. When the hand is raised above the level of the heart, the veins at the back of the hand do not collapse. The axillary vein may be palpable and tender. Distended cutaneous veins develop across the anterior chest wall and over the scapula to provide collateral drainage. The supraclavicular fossa must be carefully palpated to exclude a causative mass such as a cervical rib, a subclavian aneurysm or lymph glands enlarged by secondary malignant disease.

Congenital vein abnormalities

Klippel–Trenaunay syndrome

This is a rare syndrome in which dilated veins develop early in life, often on the outer side of the leg, the leg being longer than the normal leg and covered in cutaneous angiomas (port wine stains) (Fig. 10.42a).

Venous angiomas

These are localized hamartomatous overgrowths of small to middle-sized veins (Fig. 10.42b). They mostly occur in the subcutaneous tissues and skin. They have a blue discolouration, and become distended when dependent, collapse on elevation and are compressible.

(a) A limb with Klippel–Trenaunay syndrome that demonstrates hypertrophy, persistent vestigial veins and a capillary naevus.

(b) A large venous angioma of the hand.

Fig. 10.42 CONGENITAL VEIN ABNORMALITIES

THE LYMPHATICS

Primary abnormalities of the lymphatic vessels are rare. Disease in the lymph glands that interrupts the flow of lymph is common.

CONDITIONS AFFECTING THE LYMPH GLANDS

Lymphangitis

When bacterial infection spreads through the tissues, the bacteria get into the lymphatics and pass along in the lymph to the draining lymph glands. Inflamed lymphatics close to the skin are visible as thin, tender, red streaks on the skin (Fig. 10.42). Lymphangitis is most often seen as a complication of infection starting in the hands or feet.

History

The patient complains of a throbbing pain at the site of the primary infection, tenderness along the red streaks and tenderness in the groin or axilla.

Examination

Inspection of the limb reveals the red, tender lymphatics. The overlying skin may be slightly oedematous. The axillary or inguinal lymph glands are usually swollen and tender.

The site of the primary infection is often not obvious. It may be a small crack between the toes or alongside a fingernail.

If a lymph gland in an oedematous limb with poor lymphatic drainage becomes infected, the infection quickly spreads throughout the oedematous tissues – cellulitis.

Lymphoedema

Lymphoedema is the accumulation of lymph in the interstitial spaces as a consequence of defective lymphatic drainage. The oedema fluid is rich in protein, in contrast to the oedema of heart and kidney failure, which has a low protein content.

The causes of lymphoedema are given in Revision panel 10.13.

The most common cause of lymphoedema is from disease in the lymph glands. Primary lymphoedema is only diagnosed when all the causes of secondary lymphoedema have been eliminated, or there is a clear family history of the condition.

Revision panel 10.13
The causes of lymphoedema

Primary
Congenital genetic disorders causing dilatation, incompetence, aplasia or obliteration of the lymphatics

Secondary
Neoplastic infiltration of the lymph glands:
   Secondary carcinoma
   Lymphomas (Hodgkin's, non-Hodgkin's)

Infection
Filariasis
Lymphogranuloma inguinale
Tuberculosis
Recurrent non-specific infection

Iatrogenic
Surgical excision of the lymph glands
Irradiation of lymph glands

History

Age Primary lymphoedema may present at birth, in young adults or, much less often, in middle age. Secondary lymphoedema presents in middle and old age, and is common after treatment for cancer.

Family history Many forms of primary lymphoedema are familial, and abnormal genes have now been discovered in several of them.

Sex Females are affected three times more often than males. Even secondary lymphoedema is more common in females, because tumours of the uterus and ovary metastasize to the iliac lymph glands, and carcinoma of the breast spreads to the axillary lymph glands.

Geography Filariasis – infestation with the parasite *Wuchereria bancrofti*, which is found in tropical and subtropical countries – is a common cause of lymphoedema (elephantiasis).

Symptoms The patient notices a slowly progressive swelling of the limb or genitalia (Figs 10.43 and 10.44). Primary lymphoedema most often affects the lower limb, often beginning after a sprained ankle or another form of trivial injury. The swelling takes many years to develop, and is often bilateral.

Fig. 10.43 Lymphoedema of the right leg.

Fig. 10.44 Genital oedema.

increased weight, which may produce a mechanical disability.

Patients with lymphoedema often develop severe episodes of acute cellulitis, which may be accompanied by septicaemia. Acute cellulitis is often preceded by a prodromal period of sweating, rigors and malaise, which is then followed by the development of pain, tenderness, redness and swelling in the limb. The infection often gets in through cracks between the toes caused by athlete's foot (tinea pedis). Vesicles may appear on the skin and leak a clear, colourless fluid.

Examination

The swollen limb

Lymphoedema has no special characteristics. It is often said that lymphoedema does not pit – this is incorrect. All oedema pits. The longer the lymphoedema has been present, the denser the accompanying fibrosis, and the firmer and more 'doughy' the oedema; nevertheless, lymphoedema always pits if you press hard enough and long enough.

Lymphoedema of the lower limb affects the toes much more often than other forms of oedema. If it has

Fig. 10.45 Secondary lymphoedema. The patient's right arm lymphoedema was caused by infiltration of the axillary lymph glands by metastases from a carcinoma in the right breast. Some carcinomas of the breast present in this way.

In contrast, the swelling of secondary lymphoedema (Fig. 10.45) may appear in a few weeks and may progress rapidly.

The swelling is not painful. There is no discomfort in the swollen limb apart from that caused by the been present for years, the toes are squashed together and become square in cross-section. This hardly ever occurs with other types of oedema. *Stemmer's sign* is an inability to pinch the skin together on the dorsal surface of the second toe (Fig. 10.46). This indicates the presence of lymphoedema, and is a consequence of secondary thickening and hyperkeratosis of the skin. Skin nodules sometimes grow outwards, looking like warts.

Lymphoedema is usually diagnosed when other general causes of oedema (cardiac, renal, hypoproteinaemia) and other local causes (venous obstruction, multiple arteriovenous fistulas, local gigantism and excessive fat deposition – lipodystrophy) have been excluded. It is therefore essential to examine the whole patient, especially the heart, the abdomen and the veins of the limb, once the presence of oedema has been confirmed.

Fig. 10.46 Stemmer's sign: an inability to pinch the skin together on the dorsum of the toes.

The lymph glands

The lymph glands are often slightly thickened and enlarged in patients with primary lymphoedema. They are usually enlarged and hard if they are infiltrated with primary or secondary tumour.

All the areas that drain to any palpable glands must be carefully examined.

General examination

A full examination of the patient must be carried out to look for any possible causes for secondary lymphoedema.

Oedema after breast surgery

Swelling of the arm is a common complication of any form of axillary lymph node surgery, particularly axillary clearance, and also of axillary radiotherapy. It is not seen after simple mastectomy.

In the first days or weeks after treatment, remember the possibility of an axillary vein thrombosis.

Late swelling may be caused by recurrent carcinoma, especially if there is any enlargement of the axillary lymph glands.

Lymphatic reflux

A relatively small number of patients have dilated ectatic incompetent lymphatics that allow lymph and chyle (which is the milky lymph draining from the intestine) to reflux back into the skin, or drain into large cavities such as the peritoneum, pleura or intestine. Patients with lymphatic reflux can develop leaky vesicles on their skin, ascites and pleural effusions, and may even pass chyle in their urine (chyluria). These conditions are rare.

Lymphangiomas

These are rare malformations with distinct clinical features that are easy to recognize.

History

A patient or, in the case of a child, the parents, first notice a small soft subcutaneous swelling. There are sometimes associated small vesicles on the surface of the skin, which may weep clear fluid. These abnormalities may be present at birth or appear later in life. The subcutaneous swellings slowly enlarge, and the vesicles increase in number, but neither are usually painful.

Examination

The skin over the subcutaneous cysts usually contain many small vesicles (Fig. 10.47). Lymphangiomas tend to occur at the junction of the leg, arm or neck with the trunk.

The subcutaneous swellings cannot be compressed or emptied. They are often indistinct and multiple. They fluctuate and transilluminate if they are of a reasonable size, and have the same signs as a cystic hygroma (see Chapter 12).

Regional lymphadenopathy is described in the various sections of the book, but as lymphoedema is so often secondary to lymph gland disease, you should refresh your knowledge of the causes of lymph gland enlargement by studying Revision panel 10.14.

Fig. 10.47 Lymphangioma circumscriptum.

Revision panel 10.14
The causes of lymphadenopathy

Infection:

    Non-specific
    Glandular fever
    Tuberculosis
    Toxoplasmosis
    Syphilis
    Cat-scratch fever – Bartonella (Rochalimaea) henselae
    Filariasis

Lymphogranuloma (inguinale)

Metastatic tumour

Primary reticuloses

Sarcoidosis

The mouth, tongue and lips

Always inspect the mouth with a good light and a spatula, and most importantly palpate the tissues. More can be revealed in the soft tissues with a finger than an eye.

- Inspect the external appearance of the lips.
- Retract the lips to see the buccal mucosa.
- Push the cheek outwards to see the buccal side of the gum.
- Push the tongue away from the inside of the gum and the floor of the mouth.
- Push the tongue to one side to see the lateral aspect of its posterior third.
- Depress the tongue to look at the fauces, tonsils and pharynx.

Always remember to wear gloves and to palpate the structures in the floor of the mouth bimanually.

CONGENITAL OROFACIAL ABNORMALITIES

Cleft lip and palate, and facial cleft

The face, jaw and palate are formed by the fusion of the frontonasal (nose, philtrum of the upper lip, premaxilla), maxillary (cheek, upper lip, upper jaw, palate) and mandibular (lower jaw, lip) processes.

Failure of these processes to meet and fuse produces a group of congenital abnormalities: cleft lip, cleft palate and facial clefts.

Partial failure of fusion produces a unilateral cleft lip and palate, which may be partial (Figs 11.1 and 11.2). Complete failure of fusion causes a bilateral

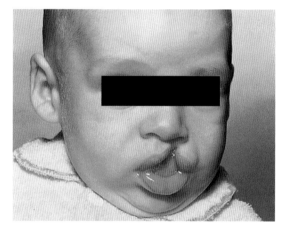

Fig. 11.1 A child with a simple cleft lip.

(a) A partial cleft of the hard and soft palates

(b) A partial cleft of the soft palates

Fig. 11.2 THE VARIETIES OF PARTIAL CLEFT PALATE

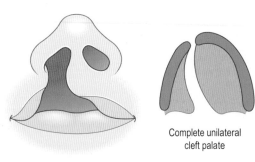

Unilateral cleft palate

Complete unilateral cleft palate

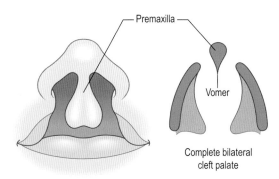

Premaxilla

Vomer

Complete bilateral cleft palate

Bilateral cleft palate

Fig. 11.3 Schematic presentation of combined cleft lip and palate.

(a) Bilateral cleft lip.

(b) Combined cleft lip and palate. Note the way in which the premaxilla protrudes.

Fig. 11.4 COMBINED CLEFT LIP AND CLEFT PALATE

cleft lip, a cleft palate and a protuberant premaxilla (Figs 11.3, 11.4). The diagnosis is apparent from inspection of the lip and palate.

The symptoms of cleft lip and palate, apart from the disfigurement, are an inability to suckle, interference with speech (particularly the formation of consonants such as D, T and G) and distortion of the dental arch.

Congenital vascular malformation (see also Chapters 4 and 10)

These comprise a heterogeneous group of dysplasias that involve the arterial, capillary, venous or lymphatic vessels or any combination of these. They are present at birth and may increase in size.

Haemangiomas usually present shortly after birth and tend to involute with age. Simple vascular malformations are divided into low flow (capillary, venous, lymphatic) and high flow (arterial, arteriovenous) (Fig. 11.5).

Complex malformations may be regional or diffuse and are usually part of a syndrome (von Hippel–Lindau, Sturge–Weber or Maffucci) (Fig. 11.6).

Age Vascular malformations can be congenital (hamartomas) or acquired (haemangiomas).

Symptoms These malformations usually only cause cosmetic problems, but they can thrombose, causing pain, or bleed.

Site They occur any where in the head and neck as well as on the lips, tongue or buccal mucosa (Fig. 11.7).

Size Haemangiomas often are small (0.5–1 cm in diameter), but they are extensive in Sturge–Weber syndrome.

Colour They are usually deep red or blue-purple. Those with a predominant venous component (low flow) blanch on pressure.

Shape They are irregular in shape.

Surface Lesions are smooth or lobulated.

Composition The malformations are soft, spongy and occasionally fluctuant if large. They may be pulsatile if they are high flow.

Relations They are very occasionally discrete and encapsulated, but the vessels usually merge with the local soft tissues. They are not adherent to the underlying tissues.

(a) Front view of an arteriovenous malformation of the upper lip.

Fig. 11.7 Venous malformation of the lip (formerly termed haemangioma).

(b) Profile view of the above arteriovenous malformation.

Fig. 11.5 VASCULAR LESION

Fig. 11.6 Sturge–Weber syndrome.

Local tissues The local tissues should be normal, but may be inflamed and tender if thrombosis has occurred.

Lymph drainage No regional lymph node enlargement is seen.

Lymphangioma

These may be isolated but can also be associated with a congenital vascular malformation when it is a 'mixed lesion'.

History

Age Lymphangiomas are hamartomas of the lymphatic system and may enlarge with age. They may be huge (as with a cystic hygroma) and cause airway embarrassment in infancy.

Symptoms Small lymphangiomas are usually symptomless and can suddenly appear in adolescence, usually associated with inflammation in the head and neck.

Examination

Site They mainly arise in the floor of the mouth, on the tongue and in the submandibular triangle (Figs 11.8, 11.9).

Size In childhood or adolescence, they present with cystic lesions of moderate size (10–15 cm³).

Colour They often have the same colour as the skin or mucous membrane under which they have developed. The cystic component in the neck will transilluminate.

CHAPTER 11 | THE MOUTH TOUNGE AND LIPS

Fig. 11.8 Extensive congenital lymphangioma of the cheek and floor of mouth.

Fig. 11.9 Isolated lymphangioma of the tongue.

Shape They are spherical or multilobulated.
Surface In the mouth, the small cystic lesions give a granular or 'frogspawn' appearance.
Composition They are soft–spongy on palpation.
Relations Rarely, there is a well-defined border; more commonly, they merge into the local structures. They usually lie in the submucosal level but may extend to the deep layers, causing obstructive problems (e.g. at the base of tongue).
Local tissues Local tissues are normal.
Lymph drainage There is no associated lymphadenopathy.

THE LIPS, BUCCAL MUCOSA AND TONGUE

Begin by inspecting the external appearance of the lips, looking for any discolouration, pigmentation (such as that of Addison's disease or Peutz–Jegher syndrome; Fig. 11.10) or telangiectasia (Rendu–Osler–Weber syndrome; Fig. 11.11). Then look for any swellings or irregularities of the buccal mucosa lining the inside of the mouth.

Fig. 11.10 The pigmentation of the lips seen in Peutz–Jegher syndrome.

Fig. 11.11 Telangiectasia in a patient with Rendu–Osler–Weber syndrome.

Mucous retention/ extravasation cysts

The mucosal lining of the lips, oral cavity and pharynx is studded with minor salivary glands whose purpose is to keep it moist. These minor salivary gland differ from their major salivary counterparts (the parotid and submandibular glands; see Chapter 12) in that they are continual secretors and more importantly can secrete against a significant pressure gradient. So if they are traumatized, for example by biting of the lower lip (a favoured site of presentation), they will continue to secrete into the adjacent tissues. Saliva generates a connective tissue reaction that walls in the fluid (forming an extravasation cyst).

The typical pattern of presentation is for the swelling to enlarge before bursting and deflating. Then once the tear has healed, the cyst reinflates. Saliva has antibacterial properties, and infection is rare.

History

Age Cysts can occur at any age. There is usually a history of previous inadvertent trauma (e.g. self-biting) in the area.
Symptoms They are usually symptomless but are repeatedly traumatized.

Examination

Site Cysts are most common on the lower lip and in the buccal mucous membrane at the level of occlusion of the teeth (Fig. 11.12).
Colour The colour varies according to the size of the cyst and the thickness of the overlying epithelium. Cysts appear pale pink when small, but as they get larger they develop a blue colour. The epithelium may be thickened and white and the cyst partly deflated if it has been traumatized.
Shape The cysts are spherical.
Size They range from 0.5 to 2 cm in diameter.
Surface They are smooth, but may be ulcerated if the cyst has ruptured.
Composition Their composition varies from soft to tense.
Local tissues The surrounding tissues should be normal, but they may be inflamed if they rupture.
Lymph drainage The local lymph glands should not be enlarged.

Fibroepithelial polyp

This is the result of connective tissue hypertrophy induced by some form of trauma.

History

Age These polyps occur at any age, usually in association with a history of minor repeated trauma/irritation. Similar lesions may be present in elderly persons with ill-fitting dentures (fibrous hyperplasia).
Symptoms The patient complains of a lump on the inner side of the lip or cheek. It slowly increases in size and is not painful unless it is caught between the teeth during mastication.

Examination

Site Polyps are most common on the lower lip but can also be found in the buccal mucosa, and less commonly on the side of the tongue where the teeth occlude. Rather firmer and sometimes ulcerated polyps are sometimes present in the upper, or more commonly the lower, sulcus of elderly individuals with poor-fitting dentures. The diagnosis is supported by replacing the denture, which may help to distinguish the lesion from a cancer.
Colour The colour is that of the normal pink mucosa.
Shape Polyps are spherical or oval shaped and can be pedunculated or broad based (Fig. 11.13).
Size They are 0.5–2 cm in size.
Surface Polyps are usually smooth.
Composition They are soft to firm. They are never fluctuant.
Relations Polyps are mobile and not fixed to the underlying tissues.
Local tissues The local tissues should be normal.
Lymph drainage The local lymph glands should not be enlarged.

Fig. 11.12 Mucocele.

Fig. 11.13 A fibroepithelial polyp with a broad base.

CHAPTER 11 | THE MOUTH TONGUE AND LIPS

Papilloma

Papillomas are small, pink, frond-like excrescences on a stalk that protrude from the mucosal surface. Some papillomas (*condyloma acuminata*) are related to human papillomavirus (HPV) infections. More than 100 HPVs have been described, and HPV-16 has been implicated in the pathogenesis of oropharyngeal carcinoma.

History

Age Papillomas can occur at any age.
Symptoms They are not painful but they grow slowly, causing local irritation.

Examination

Site A proportion of these lesions are usually sexually transmitted and are normally sited on the tip of the tongue or soft palate.
Colour The colour varies according to the state of the overlying epithelium. They may be pink, or may be pale or white if they are keratinized.
Shape They are typically exophytic and cauliflower-like.
Size They vary in size from 1 to 2 mm.
Surface Papillomas have an irregular granular surface similar to the much large finger wart. They are occasionally spiky.
Composition They are soft and fleshy lesions that are often friable.
Relations Papillomas are pedunculated in shape, arising from a narrow, stalk-like base. They are not attached to underlying structures.
Local tissues The local tissues are normal.
Lymph drainage The local lymph glands should not be enlarged.

Stomatitis

Stomatitis is a general term used to describe an inflammation of the lining of the mouth, which can include the surface of the tongue. It can have a variety of clinical appearances and has many causes (see Revision panel 11.1).

History

Stomatitis occurs in all age groups and equally in both sexes.

Symptoms The patient complains of soreness in the mouth. The mouth may feel dry.

Revision panel 11.1

The causes of stomatitis

Local trauma
Poorly fitting dentures
Sharp teeth
Excessive smoking
Radiotherapy

Local infection
Herpes
Monilia
Vincent's angina
Glandular fever
Foot and mouth disease

General conditions
Stevens–Johnson syndrome
Behçet's syndrome
Aphthous ulceration

Vitamin deficiencies
Vitamin C (scurvy)
Vitamin B and C (coeliac disease, pellagra, pernicious anaemia, kwashiorkor)

Blood diseases
Acute leukaemia
Agranulocytosis
Aplastic anaemia
Purpura

Immunosuppression
Acquired immunodeficiency syndrome (AIDS)
Chemotherapy

Drugs
Phenytoin
Lead, mercury and bismuth poisoning

Debility
Tuberculosis
Carcinomatosis

Movements of the tongue and cheeks are painful, and individual ulcers if present are very painful. The mucosa is fiery red, and the tongue may lose its papillae and become smooth. Mastication may be difficult.

Stomatitis can arise from a local or systemic condition, such as a blood dyscrasia or liver failure. In such circumstances, glossitis and oral manifestations are accompanied by signs and symptoms of the parent condition. It is important to obtain full medical history as stomatitis, and especially oral ulcers, may be a manifestation of an underlying metabolic disorder or be drug induced (nicorandil, antibiotics, chemotherapy).

Examination

The physical appearances vary according to the cause.

Aphthous stomatitis

The cause is unknown but is thought to be an inappropriate and excessive immune response to a minor stimulus.

The result is a superficial, well-defined ulcer normally situated on the buccal mucosa (Fig. 11.14) but never on the attached mucosa around the teeth or palate (this signifies primary herpes).

There are three types:

- *Normal* (groups of 3–4 ulcers cycling every 2–3 weeks).
- *Major aphthae* (one or two ulcers, which are much larger and deeper). These last for weeks or months before they heal, leaving a scar.
- *Herpetiform stomatitis*, which consists of tiny ulcers all over the mouth.

Recurrent aphthous ulcers are common in otherwise healthy young people, particularly at times of stress. They tend to disappear with age.

Behçet's syndrome should be considered if the mouth ulcers are accompanied by systemic symptoms and genital ulcers.

Candidiasis

This is the result of monilial overgrowth (of *Candida albicans*) and has four forms in the mouth:

- *Acute monilial stomatitis* (thrush). Infection of the alimentary tract is common in children and in people with debilitating disease. It is well recognized as a complication of any antibiotic therapy that changes the balance of the bacteria in the alimentary canal. It is characterized by a discreet white plaques that can be wiped from the mucosa, leaving a red or bleeding (pseudomembranous) surface (Fig. 11.15)
- *Erythematous* (atrophic).
- *Hyperplastic* (Fig. 11.16).
- *Angular cheilitis*.

(a) Monilial glossitis. The colonies of monilia on the tongue and mucous membranes look like patches of cream-coloured paint.

Fig. 11.14 Multiple aphthous ulcers of the buccal mucosa. Largest ulcer is arrowed.

(b) Monilial stomatitis affecting the palate.

Fig. 11.15 STOMATITIS

CHAPTER 11 | THE MOUTH TOUNGE AND LIPS

Fig. 11.16 Hyperplastic candidiasis of the palate.

Acute ulcerative stomatitis

(Vincent's angina)

This is caused by an infection (*Borrelia vincentii*) and is often known as Vincent's angina.

The appearance is dramatic. The attached gingiva around the teeth is bright red, and the pathognomonic feature is necrosis of the interdental papillae. Another important feature is a characteristic smell that pervades the room. The condition may be secondary to very poor oral hygiene or ushered in by a period of immunosuppression.

The cervical lymph glands are enlarged and tender.

The patient feels ill and has a fever and loss of appetite.

Gangrenous stomatitis

(Cancrum oris)

The last reported case of gangrenous stomatitis in Europe was at the end of the Second World War. Now it is largely confined to a latitude range that includes dry barren sub-Saharan Africa.

The cause is poor nutrition, coupled with poor personal hygiene and immunosuppression (viral infection, measles, human immunodeficiency virus [HIV]).

It normally commences as a small ulcer in the cheek that quickly extends with obvious signs of infection (redness, oedema, pain and loss of function). Necrosis soon follows. The dead tissue eventually separates, and with this the contours of the mouth and face are destroyed. The disease is so destructive that only 10 per cent of children survive.

Angular stomatitis

(Perlèche)

This term describes red, inflamed fissures present at the corners of the mouth (Fig. 11.17). It is common in the elderly, particularly those using old worn dentures. The creases get soiled with saliva, and the moist environment encourages maceration of the epithelium and superinfection with commensal organisms (staphylococci and *Candida*).

Angular stomatitis may be a manifestation of iron or vitamin deficiency, especially when accompanied by glossitis and oral ulcers.

Fig. 11.17 Angular stomatitis.

Syphylis

This disease was much more important in the pre-antibiotic era, when it was recognized as the 'great mimic' and could masquerade as other diseases. Everything changed with antibiotics, and the disease, with its signs and symptoms, has now been all but eradicated in Western countries. However, it shows a limited resurgence in isolated promiscuous environments

Chancres of primary syphilis can occur on the tongue or lips (Fig. 11.18). For a full description, see Chapters 3 and 18.

Mucous patches and snail-track ulcers are part of the skin abnormalities that develop with secondary syphilis (see Chapter 4). These patches or ulcers can arise in the mouth.

Gummas can arise in the tongue or hard palate as painless masses that may ulcerate.

Fig. 11.18 Primary chancre of the lower lip.

(a) Leukoplakia of the buccal mucosa.

Leukoplakia (white patch)

The term 'leukoplakia' refers to any oral white patch (Fig. 11.19a) and covers a broad spectrum of pathology. Leukoplakia can be idiopathic, viral (HPV, Epstein–Barr virus) or fungal (*Candida*), or may be related to tobacco or alcohol, when it represents a premalignant condition.

It is estimated that 2 per cent of the population have a white patch in their mouth, but in only 2 per cent of this population is the condition premalignant. The challenge is to distinguish premalignant lesions from the rest. Lifestyle factors (alcohol and tobacco use in all its forms – chewing, snuff, pan), the site of the lesion (the salivary gutters) and its appearance (erythroleukoplakia – red and white) point to the premalignant form of leukoplakia (Fig. 11.19b). White patches are usually asymptomatic.

Site Leukoplakia may present in any area of the oral mucosa. High-risk regions for malignant transformation are the ventrolateral surface of the tongue and the soft palate.
Colour The lesions are (by definition) white, but there might be an erythematous component (erythroplakia).
Size The plaques vary in size and may occupy large areas of the oral mucosa.
Shape and surface Leukoplakia can be homogenous (uniform) or heterogenous (verrucous, nodular or speckled).
Local tissues The local tissues should be normal.
Lymph drainage The local lymph glands should not be enlarged, and pathological lymphadenopathy suggests a carcinoma.

(b) Leukoplakia of the ventral surface of tongue (sublingual keratosis). This condition is considered premalignant.

Fig. 11.19 ORAL LEUKOPLAKIA

Lichen planus

This is an idiopathic, immune-related condition of unknown origin. The mucosa starts to thin and absorbs water, becoming white in appearance. The tissues are friable so are vulnerable to trauma, and small superficial ulcers are a common feature of the condition. It has a premalignant potential in less than 3 per cent of cases.

A lichenoid reaction mimics the condition, having a similar appearance, but the patch will be in contact with a large dental filling that is responsible for the changes in the mucosa.

Symptoms Patients often complain of a burning sensation with spicy or acidic foods, although many are symptomless.
Site It mostly occurs in the buccal mucosa bilaterally, but may appear on the tongue or the gingiva (*desquamative gingivitis*).

Colour The mouth lesions are typically white but may have an erythematous component in erosive forms.

Size They vary in size and may occupy the whole extent of the buccal mucosa.

Shape and surface Six clinical types have been described:

- *Reticular:* a network of white raised striae (Fig. 11.20a).
- *Papular:* white papules of variable size.
- *Plaque-type:* white patches like leukoplakia.
- *Erosive:* mucosal atrophic areas (potentially premalignant) (Fig. 11.20b).
- *Ulcerative:* painful erosions or irregular ulcers (potentially premalignant).
- *Bullous:* rare.

Local tissues The surrounding tissues should be normal, but there may be associated inflammation.

Lymph drainage The local lymph glands should not be enlarged.

Submucous fibrosis

Oral submucous fibrosis is associated with betel nut and pan chewing. This disorder is limited to the communities that are in, or originate from, the Far East that practise this habit. Alkaloids leach out of the plant and cause a band of dense fibrosis to accumulate just below the mucosa. It affects the buccal mucosa, and if the soft palate is involved a degree of rhinolalia (a nasal quality to the voice) can occur. It is easy to diagnose the submucosal thickening by oral palpation, and it is almost always symmetrical. It causes oral dysaesthesia and a progressive restriction of mouth opening. The affected sites appear shiny pale or white with atrophic mucosa (Fig. 11.21). Submucous fibrosis should be considered to be a premalignant condition.

(a) Reticular type.

(b) Erosive lichen planus presenting as erythroleukoplakia. The biopsy demonstrated areas of dysplasia.

Fig. 11.20 LICHEN PLANUS

Fig. 11.21 Submucous fibrosis.

Carcinoma of the lip

In the current age, in which smoking clay pipes has long ceased (Fig. 11.22), the main cause of lip cancer is actinic radiation. It is for this reason that it is all but restricted to the lower lip, which catches the sunlight (Fig. 11.23).

History

Age Most of the patients with carcinoma of the lip are over the age of 60 years and have an occupation or hobby that exposes them to sunlight.

Sex Males are affected more often than females.

Occupation It is particularly common in males with outdoor occupations such as fishermen, builders and farmers. It is sometimes called 'countryman's lip'.

Fig. 11.22 Carcinoma of the lip in a habitual pipe smoker. The lesion developed where he used to rest his pipe.

Fig. 11.24 A small, early carcinoma that has just ulcerated.

Fig. 11.23 Solar keratosis on the lower lip – a premalignant change.

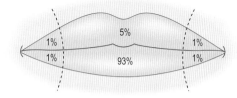

Fig. 11.25 The distribution of carcinoma of the lips.

Ethnic group In sun-bleached countries, people with dark skin are less susceptible to melanoma (see Chapter 4) but not necessarily squamous cell cancer. They are therefore not exempt from diseases induced by sunlight.

Geography It is more common in countries such as South Africa and Australia with a tropical or semi-tropical climate, where the target population is white Caucasians with a fair complexion such as those of Celtic origin.

Symptoms The lesion at first mimics a 'cold sore' on the lip (Fig. 11.24). A relapsing ulcer of the lip with actinic changes signifies an area of mucosa that is not maturing correctly and is, with minimal trauma, prone to ulceration. The relapsing nature gives false reassurance as it is eventually (perhaps after 18 or 24 months) realized that it is clearly a non-healing indurated ulcer of neoplastic origin.

Examination

Site The lower lip is affected over ten times more often than the upper lip. Carcinoma in the angle of the lips is uncommon (Fig. 11.25).

Colour The skin over the lump or round the ulcer may show evidence of a premalignant condition: blistering, thickening and pigmentation, or white boggy patches.

Shape The cancer starts as a small non-healing crack in the mucosa, which ultimately ulcerates in its centre and develops the typical everted edge of a carcinoma (Fig. 11.26).

Edge Once the lump has ulcerated, the edges proliferate and evert. They are red and, at their junction with the base of the ulcer, bleed easily.

Base The base is covered with a thin, soft, friable, grey–yellow slough which is a mixture of dying tissue and inflammatory exudate. It is thin because the ulcer is repeatedly rubbed by the tongue.

Fig. 11.26 An ulcerated carcinoma of the lower lip.

CHAPTER 11 | THE MOUTH TOUNGE AND LIPS

Depth The ulcer is initially shallow but can erode deep into the lip, destroying the epithelium and the underlying muscle (Fig. 11.27).

Fig. 11.27 A large proliferating and infiltrating carcinoma distorting the whole upper lip.

Discharge The discharge is thin, watery and slightly blood stained. It is usually infected but rarely purulent.

Relations The lump is invariably fixed to the subcutaneous structures of the lip but can be moved, with the lip, separately from the jaw. Only very advanced lesions are fixed to the gum and jaw.

Lymph drainage Lip cancer has a relatively good prognosis compared with mouth cancer, primarily because metastasis to the cervical lymph nodes occurs only late in the disease.

The lymph glands are firm and discrete if they contain metastases. When the enlargement is caused by secondary infection, the nodes are usually mildly tender.

Surrounding tissues Away from the ulcer, the rest of the lip is usually normal or mildly affected by the predisposing causes of cancer already mentioned.

General examination Distant metastases are rare.

Carcinoma of the tongue

Carcinoma of the tongue, like all squamous cell cancers of the upper aerodigestive tract, invades the local tissues and then spreads to the regional lymph nodes in the neck. Distant blood-borne metastases are a late event.

History

Age Patients are usually over the age of 50 years, with the peak incidence between 60 and 70 years.

Sex Males were affected more than females when smoking and heavy alcohol consumption was the preserve of males. Now there are almost as many females affected as males, and this is more evident in the younger age groups where other aetiological factors such as HPV may play a part in tumour induction.

Symptoms The most common complaint is of a painful ulcer, but in 20 per cent of patients the ulcer is painless and late diagnosis tends to be the result.

It is useful from a diagnostic perspective to break the tongue in the anterior two-thirds and the posterior third. In tissue untainted by previous surgery or radiotherapy, cancers situated on the anterior tongue always break the surface and appear as an ulcer. In contrast, some of those that occur on the posterior tongue burrow down beneath the lymphoid tissue and are invisible to the eye. They can be palpated but not seen, and again this is a source of diagnostic delay.

Cancer symptoms progress inexorably, and clinicians should be alert to this fact.

Referred pain to the ear is a cardinal symptom that should never be overlooked in a high-risk patient (of appropriate age and alcohol and tobacco consumption) complaining of oral discomfort. It is important to remember that most of the tongue is hidden from view.

Small tongue ulcers less than 1 cm in diameter are easily overlooked because of a protective reflex – when the mouth is examined, the patient automatically retracts the tongue.

If the tumour has spread extensively and invaded the musculature, it may cause immobility of the tongue (ankyloglossia) and difficulty with speech (dysarthria).

Tumours on the base of the tongue may alter the quality of the voice, the patient developing a 'hot potato' speech.

Alternatively, the patient may present with a lump in the neck (enlarged lymph gland) before noticing any abnormality of the tongue.

Previous history The history helps to identify some high-risk patients. The major factors that are linked to mouth cancer are excessive alcohol and tobacco consumption, but the aetiological picture is not as clear cut as previously thought. There is an increasing group of young (20–30-year-old) individuals without classical risk factors who develop mouth cancer possibly related to prior infection with HPV, as do patients with lichen planus and those receiving transplants.

Examination

Site Tongue cancer is most common on the edge and the lateral border of the tongue (Fig. 11.28).

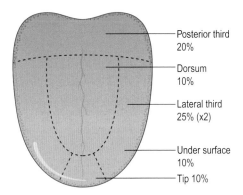

Fig. 11.28 The distribution of carcinoma of the tongue.

Colour The epithelium and papillae over a deep-seated tumour look normal, but if the carcinoma is near the surface, the epithelium loses its papillae and looks smooth, shiny and stretched. Ulcers are usually covered with a transparent, yellow–grey slough.

Shape, size and composition Cancer of the tongue may present in four forms:

- An ulcer (predominately).
- A nodule.
- A papilliferous or warty nodule.
- A fissure in an area of induration.

A carcinomatous lump is hard and indurated. Often, more can be learned with a finger than a mirror, and it is always prudent to palpate the oral tissues.

A carcinomatous ulcer of the tongue usually has the typical features of a carcinoma: a florid, friable, bleeding, everted edge, a sloughing yellow–grey base, a thin serous discharge and induration of the surrounding tissues (Fig. 11.29a).

The papilliferous or verrucous carcinoma looks like any other papilloma in that it is covered with an excess of proliferating filiform epithelium, which is usually paler than the surrounding pink epithelium, although the base is broad and firm, and the area of tongue from which it arises is indurated. It may be of any size but rarely juts out far from the tongue because of the restriction of the mouth (Fig. 11.29b).

A fissure in an area of carcinomatous induration is a rare form of tongue cancer. The fissure may be a cleft in the tongue that has deepened and lost its epithelium, or a deep linear ulcer.

(a) A large ulcer with an everted edge on the side of the tongue.

(b) An ulcerated nodule on the side of the tongue.

(c) Not all nodules are primary lesions. This one was a metastasis from a carcinoma of the bronchus.

Fig. 11.29 CARCINOMA OF THE TONGUE

Relations It is very important to examine the floor of the mouth, gums, jaw, tonsils and fauces because a carcinoma can spread into any of these structures, and once it has done so its treatment becomes much more difficult.

Tumours on the side or undersurface of the tongue are more likely to spread into the floor of the mouth than are carcinomas on the dorsum.

Spread to the floor of the mouth causes thickening of the tissues and reduces the mobility of the tongue. Infiltration of the gum and jaw fixes the tumour to

CHAPTER 11 | THE MOUTH TOUNGE AND LIPS

the bone, and the jaw itself may be swollen. Tumours of the posterior third of the tongue spread into the tonsil and the pillars of the fauces.

Lymph drainage

- The lymph from the tip of the tongue drains to the submental glands and then to either or both jugular lymph chains.
- The lymph from the rest of the anterior two-thirds drains to the glands on the same side of the neck, usually the middle and upper deep cervical glands.
- Lymph from the posterior third drains into the ring of lymph tissues around the oropharynx and into the upper deep cervical lymph glands.

More than half of the patients who present with a cancer of the tongue have palpable cervical lymph glands, but in some cases the enlargement is caused by secondary infection rather than tumour.

Local tissues Involvement of the lingual nerve causes a pain that is referred to the ear, probably through its connections with the auriculotemporal nerve.

Infiltration of the mandible causes pain and swelling of the jaw.

The surface of the tongue around the cancer may be affected by leukoplakia, and there may be other primary tumours (field changes).

Differential diagnosis The causes of ulcers on the tongue are given in Revision panel 11.2.

Revision panel 11.2

The causes of ulceration of the tongue

Aphthous ulcer

Trauma (dental)

Medication induced (nicorandil)

Non-specific glossitis

Median rhomboid glossitis

Chancre

Gumma

Tuberculosis

Carcinoma

OTHER CONDITIONS OF THE TONGUE

Macroglossia

Macroglossia is a large tongue. The causes of macroglossia are:

- multiple haemangiomas;
- lymphangiomas;
- plexiform neurofibromatosis;
- amyloid infiltration;
- infiltrating carcinoma;
- muscle hypertrophy (in cretinism);
- endocrine disorders such as acromegaly.

Tongue-tie

A congenitally shortened frenulum (Fig. 11.30) can lead to a degree of tongue-tie. This rarely causes any significant impairment of speech, but if it is severe and remains uncorrected into late infancy, it can interfere with speech.

Fig. 11.30 Tongue-tie: a congenitally short frenulum. This rarely causes any significant impairment of speech.

Median rhomboid glossitis

Median rhomboid glossitis is associated with candidiasis. Smoking, denture-wearing and conditions that cause immunosuppression are predisposing factors. It does not usually cause any symptoms, but is usually noticed by the patient.

It occurs in the midline of the dorsum of the tongue, anterior to the sulcus terminalis. It has a rhomboidal shape. The mucosa may be eroded or raised, and the colour varies from red to white and yellow or combinations of these (Fig. 11.31). There might be a nodular component, and in the past the condition was mistaken for cancer. Cancers in the midline of the tongue are rare.

Fig. 11.32 A right hypoglossal nerve palsy. When this patient was asked to protrude his tongue, it could be seen to be wasted on the right and deviated to the right.

Fig. 11.31 Median rhomboid glossitis.

Wasting of the tongue

Paralysis of the XIIth cranial nerve (the hypoglossal nerve) causes disuse atrophy of one side of the tongue. This leads to the generation of a fatty lump where the muscle has atrophied. When the patient is asked to 'put out your tongue', the tongue deviates towards the paralysed side (Fig. 11.32). The cause of the hypoglossal nerve neuropathy must be elucidated (see Chapter 3).

Mucosal neuromas (neurofibroma)

These may be solitary or, in conjunction with the uncommon condition of multiple endocrine neoplasia type 2b (see Chapter 12), multiple mucosal neuromas can be seen, particularly on the tongue (Fig. 11.33).

Fig. 11.33 Solitary tongue plexiform Schwannoma.

THE PALATE

The varieties of congenital cleft palate were described earlier in the chapter.

Exostosis

(Torus palatinus)

This is a completely benign bone lump in the midline of the hard palate. Another favoured site is along the lingual plate of the mandible. Its grows slowly and is usually spherical or oval shaped (Fig. 11.34). The overlying mucosa has a normal appearance, but if the lump is large the mucosa is stretched over the bone surface and tears easily. The exposed dense bone can be very painful and slow to heal. A torus palatinus may interfere with the fitting of a denture.

Fig. 11.34 An exostosis is recognizable by its midline cleft and is known as a torus palatinus.

Perforation of the palate

(Oro-antral/oro-nasal fistula)

A perforation in the palate can be acquired if disease or trauma destroys the bones of the palate (Fig. 11.35).

It can be caused by:

- iatrogenic injury when removing an upper molar tooth;
- tumours of the maxillary antrum bursting through the palate into the mouth;
- Wegener's granulomatosis: a rare vasculitis causing necrotizing granulomatous inflammation;
- surgical excision of the palate to approach the maxillary antrum.

Fig. 11.35 Large perforation of the palate. The nasal septum and turbinate bones are clearly visible.

Necrotizing sialometaplasia

Necrotizing sialometaplasia is a benign, inflammatory condition that mostly affects the minor palatal salivary glands. It usually occurs in young male smokers. It presents as irregular ulcers in the area of the junction between the hard and soft palates (Fig. 11.36). It is almost indistinguishable from a cancer except by biopsy. The condition is self-limiting.

Fig. 11.36 Necrotizing sialometaplasia. The clinical picture mimics carcinoma.

Tumours of the palate

The mucous membrane covering the hard palate is identical to that of the rest of the buccal mucosa. Cancers similar to those of the lips and buccal mucosa are not uncommon.

The hard palate also contains many minor salivary glands. A *pleomorphic salivary adenoma* (mixed salivary tumour – see Chapter 12) is a common cause of a lump at the junction of the hard and soft palate.

Approximately 40 per cent of minor salivary gland tumours are malignant (adenocarcinoma, mucoepidermoid carcinoma, adenocystic carcinoma), and the risk increases from the soft palate down to the floor of the mouth. Almost all tumours of the sublingual gland are malignant.

The patient's sole complaint is of a lump on the palate that grows slowly but steadily If it is not treated, it can fill the arch of the palate and make speech and eating difficult.

On examination, the lump feels smooth and hard (Fig. 11.37).

The overlying mucous membrane is not attached to it, and if the lump is small it can be moved over the underlying palate. As the tumour grows, it becomes less mobile and more difficult to distinguish from a tumour growing in or above the palate. Other rare tumours can occur in the palate (Fig. 11.37c).

THE TONSILS

Tonsillitis

This is a condition familiar to all because almost everyone has had it. It causes a sore throat and pain on swallowing.

On examination, the tonsils are seen to be enlarged and red, with pus exuding from their crypts. The surrounding pillars of the fauces, soft palate and oropharynx are also red and tender, and may be covered with small yellow-based ulcers.

Bilateral enlargement of the tonsils, together with the above signs, is diagnostic of tonsillitis.

Unilateral enlargement of a tonsil, even if it is red and tender, is not always caused by infection and may be a tonsillar cancer or lymphoma. Remember the other causes described below.

Carcinoma of the tonsil

Carcinoma of the tonsil occurs in the elderly. The enlarging tonsil and deep infiltration by the tumour cells may cause severe pain in the throat, which is referred to the ear.

The surface of the growth eventually ulcerates to form a deep indolent ulcer (Fig. 11.38), rarely with everted edges, which bleeds and causes severe dysphagia and a pungent fetor oris. The cervical lymph glands often become involved early in the disease process.

(a) A pleomorphic adenoma of a minor salivary gland on the palate.

(b) A carcinoma on the side of the palate.

(c) A malignant melanoma of the hard palate. This is a rare condition, but is included as a reminder that malignant melanoma can arise at the mucocutaneous junctions, i.e. around the mouth and anus.

Fig. 11.37 TUMOURS OF THE PALATE

Fig. 11.38 Carcinoma of the right tonsil.

CHAPTER 11 | THE MOUTH TOUNGE AND LIPS

Lymphoma of the tonsil

Lymphoma of the tonsil occurs in late-middle and old age. In contrast to carcinoma, it causes a painless swelling. The patient's only complaints are a sensation of a lump in the back of the mouth and throat and some times mild dysphagia.

Gross swelling may interfere with speech and make the patient's words indistinct.

Bilateral enlargement of the cervical lymph glands is a common feature as this is a systemic disease.

Both carcinomatous and lymphomatous tonsils can look infected, but acute tonsillitis in the elderly is not common, so be on your guard and search for an underlying cause.

Peritonsillar abscess

(Quinsy)

This is an abscess, lateral to the tonsil, that pushes the tonsil towards the midline and makes it look enlarged. It is a very painful condition. Opening the mouth and swallowing saliva is particularly painful.

The diagnosis rests on observing a red bulge in the anterior pillar of the fauces, tender cervical lymph glands, fever and tachycardia. It is very difficult to distinguish from a submasseteric abscess arising from a third molar tooth except that in the former the patient can open their mouth, whereas the latter causes profound trismus, as the masseter muscle goes into spasm.

THE FLOOR OF THE MOUTH

Exostosis

(Torus mandibularis)

A torus mandibularis is a completely benign bony lump in the medial aspect of the mandibular alveolus in the premolar region. They are typically symmetrical and may grow slowly. They are usually spherical but may be multilobulated, and the overlying mucosa should be normal. They may interfere with the fitting of a denture.

Ranula

A ranula is a mucus extravasation cyst that arises from the sublingual gland. The sublingual gland has a head that is fixed to the floor of mouth by the duct of Ranvier and a tail that lies beneath the mucosa and is drained by a single duct. The head is formed by a concrescence of independent minor salivary gland units (see mucous retention cysts earlier in the chapter).

Ranula is the Latin for a small frog. It is said that the swelling was given this name by Hippocrates because he thought it looked like the inflated belly of a frog.

History

Age Ranulas appear most often in children and young adults.

Sex Both sexes are equally affected.

Symptoms The patient complains of a swelling in the floor of the mouth that has grown gradually over a few weeks.

Some ranulas fluctuate in size, and when large they may burst and discharge the saliva into the mouth, but once the tear has sealed they fill again. They can interfere with eating or speech.

Examination

Position The swelling lies in the floor of the mouth, between the symphysis menti and the tongue, just to one side of the midline.

Colour The lump has a characteristic semi-transparent blue appearance. The colour and the site are the diagnostic features (Fig. 11.39).

Tenderness The swelling is not tender. Saliva has bacteriocidal properties, and these cysts do not get infected.

Shape Ranulas form spherical cysts, but only the top half is visible.

Fig. 11.39 A ranula: a tense, translucent, spherical swelling just below the mucosa of the floor of the mouth.

Size They vary from 1 to 20 cm in diameter.

Surface Their surface is smooth, but their edge is difficult to feel because they lie deep within the arch of the mandible.

Composition The swelling is soft and usually fluctuant and transilluminates, but it cannot be compressed or reduced.

Relations The overlying mucosa is not fixed to the wall of the cyst, and the cyst is not fixed to the tongue or the jaw.

The swelling is usually closely related to the duct of the submandibular salivary gland (Wharton's duct) and the lingual nerve.

Ranulas occasionally extend through the mylohyoid muscle into the neck. This variety is called a plunging ranula. These cysts mimic a developmental lymphangioma. The diagnosis is clinched by needle aspiration and the finding of sticky yellow fluid that has a high amylase count.

Lymph drainage The cervical lymph glands should not be enlarged.

Local tissues These should all be normal.

Sublingual dermoid cyst

When the face and neck are formed by fusion of the facial processes, a piece of epidermis may get trapped deep in the midline just behind the jaw and later form a sublingual dermoid cyst.

Such cysts are in the midline, but they may be above or below the mylohyoid muscle (see Chapter 12, page 405).

History

Age The swelling is usually noticed when the patient is between the ages of 10 and 25 years.

Sex Both sexes are equally affected.

Symptoms The patient complains of a swelling under the tongue or just below the point of the chin. It is generally symptomless. It can be differentiated from other lesions by needle aspiration, but these cysts can become infected.

Examination

Position The lump is easily visible, either in the centre of the floor of the mouth between the tongue and the point of the jaw, or bulging down below the chin, looking like a double chin (Fig. 11.40).

(a) Front view of a sublingual dermoid cyst giving the impression of a 'double chin'.

(b) Intraoral view showing bulging of the anterior floor of the mouth and displacement of the tongue posteriorly.

Fig. 11.40 A SUBLINGUAL DERMOID CYST

Colour The mucous membrane of the mouth and the skin beneath the chin overlying the lump are normal.

Tenderness Sublingual dermoid cysts are not tender.

Shape The cyst is clearly spherical, even though its whole surface cannot be felt.

Size By the time these cysts are noticed, they are 2–5 cm across.

Surface The surface is smooth.

Edge The edge is clearly defined.

Composition The lump feels firm, but bimanual palpation reveals that it fluctuates.

These cysts do not usually transilluminate as their contents are often opaque. They cannot be compressed or reduced.

Relations Sublingual dermoid cysts can be felt bimanually, with one finger in the mouth and one beneath the chin.

When the tongue is lifted up, the supramylohyoid variety bulges into the mouth. The submylohyoid variety bulges out below the chin if the tongue is pushed against the roof of the mouth with the teeth clenched. Neither variety is attached to the surrounding structures.

Local tissues The nearby tissues should all be normal.
Lymph drainage The local lymph glands should not be enlarged.

Stone in Wharton's duct

Stones and infection in the submandibular gland and duct are common (see Chapter 12). A stone may migrate to the punctum, where it is both visible and palpable. If the stone lies in the mid-portion of the duct, it sits under the sublingual gland and may be obscured from view or palpation. The submandibular gland is usually swollen and tender (Fig. 11.41).

Fig. 11.41 A swollen (obstructed) submandibular gland as a result of a calculus.

THE GUMS

Fibroma
(Fibrous epulis)
An epulis is a swelling that arises from the alveolar margin of the jaw. The most common variety is the fibrous epulis. This is a fibroma that arises from the gingival tissues, forming a firm nodule at the junction of the gum and tooth. It may be polypoid in shape (Fig. 11.42).

Fig. 11.42 A fibrous epulis.

Granuloma
(Granulomatous epulis)
This is a pyogenic granuloma arising from the mucosa of the gum (Fig. 11.43). It is usually associated with gingivitis or local infection.

Fig. 11.43 A pyogenic granuloma or granulomatous epulis.

Dental cyst

A developmental (odontogenic) or inflammatory (radicular) cyst may cause alveolar bone expansion and present as a hard lump in the gingival area (Fig. 11.44).

Bone tumour

A variety of giant cell 'tumours' (peripheral giant cell) can extend out of the bone and have a appearance similar to that of a pyogenic granuloma (a friable gingival lump) (Fig. 11.45). They are distinguished by biopsy.

Fig. 11.44 A small developmental odontogenic cyst (keratocyst) between two viable teeth.

Fig. 11.46 An alveolar mucosa carcinoma.

involved tooth as this leads to tooth extraction. The inevitable result is that the patient returns a month later with a more advanced cancer in an unhealed tooth socket.

THE JAW

Swellings of the jaw

Swelling of the whole jaw may be caused by infection, a cyst or a tumour. These are classified in Revision panel 11.3.

Alveolar (dental) abscess

The most common cause of swelling of the jaw is a dental or alveolar abscess. This is an abscess that forms at the base of the root of a decaying tooth and tracks outwards, through the external surface of the mandible or maxilla, to form an abscess beneath the cheek or jaw.

History

Age An alveolar abscess can develop at any age.
Symptoms A constant dull ache in the jaw, which gets gradually worse and becomes throbbing in nature.
Previous history The patient may know that they have bad teeth, having had toothache and avoided dental care.

Examination

Position Most alveolar abscesses point to the labial (outer) side of the jaw. Those in the lower jaw also

Fig. 11.45 A giant cell epulis.

Carcinoma

Carcinoma of the gum presents as a granular area that later develops a rolled edge. In its early stages of development, it can mimic a chronically infected periodontal pocket. It is painful and progresses inexorably over time (Fig. 11.46). The pitfall is to think that it is a granuloma related to a periodontally

Revision panel 11.3

The causes of swelling of the jaw

Infections

Alveolar (dental) abscess

Acute osteomyelitis

Actinomycosis

Cysts

Inflammatory odontogenic cysts

Developmental odontogenic cysts

Other non-odontogenic cysts and cystic tumours

Neoplasms

Benign

Fibrous dysplasia

Giant cell granuloma

Odontogenic tumours

Locally invasive

Ameloblastoma

Malignant

Osteosarcoma

Malignant lymphoma (Burkitt's tumour)

Secondary tumours (by direct invasion or bloodstream spread)

Fig. 11.47 A dental abscess arising from a lower carious tooth spreading to the submental and submandibular regions.

point downwards to the inferior margin of the mandible.

Colour The overlying skin or mucosa is reddened by hyperaemia.

Shape The abscess takes the form of a flattened hemisphere, but its edges merge into the surrounding tissues, so it does not have a clear-cut shape or edge. The swelling is hot and acutely tender (Fig. 11.47).

Surface The surface is indistinct.

Composition It is difficult to assess the composition of the swelling because it is so tender.

The deep part of the mass feels firm, but the overlying tissues may be soft and boggy with oedematous fluid. Large abscesses may fluctuate.

Relations The mass is clearly fixed to, and feels as if it is part of, the underlying bone.

Lymph drainage The upper cervical lymph glands are usually enlarged and tender.

Local tissues The arteries and nerves of the face, jaw and tongue should be normal. There may be visible evidence of neglect of the teeth, such as caries and gingivitis, and there may be unerupted teeth. If the abscess is allowed to point and discharge, it may become a chronic discharging sinus.

Odontogenic cyst

These cysts arise from odontogenic epithelium left behind in the mandible as the tooth buds develop and leave their position to erupt into the mouth. The epithelial remnants can be stimulated to coalese and form a cyst (inflammatory or developmental).

An inflammatory cyst (radicular) is attached to the root of an erupted but decayed and non-vital tooth (Fig. 11.48a). These cysts are common and can be up to 2–3 cm in diameter.

Clinical examination can get no further than detecting that the swelling is in the bone. Sometimes the bone is so thin that it 'crackles' when touched, like a broken eggshell (Fig. 11.48b and 11.48c).

Developmental cysts (Fig. 11.49a) that arise in relation to the crown of an unerupted tooth (most being third molar or canine) are dentigerous cysts. Keratocysts are more aggressive, tend to be larger and do not normally reside around the crown of the tooth. The distinction is made by biopsy.

These cysts can enlarge, cause swelling of the jaw (Fig. 11.49b) and produce tooth mobility. Resorption of a root is normally associated with keratocysts, dentigerous cysts or ameloblastomas.

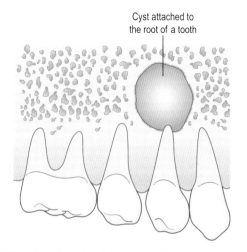

(a) The site of origin of a dental radicular cyst (inflammatory).

(b) A large dental cyst expanding the maxilla and bulging into the vestibular sulcus.

(c) Because the bone was so thin, it crackled when palpated.

Fig. 11.48 ODONTOGENIC CYSTS

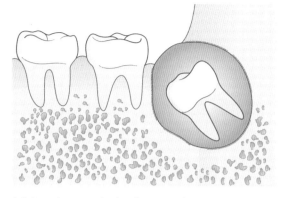

(a) An odontogenic developmental cyst.

(b) A dentigerous cyst causing swelling at the angle of the mandible.

Fig. 11.49 DEVELOPMENTAL CYSTS

Tumours of the jaw

Many types of benign and malignant tumours of the jaw are listed in Revision panel 11.3. They all present as a bony swelling that grows steadily and usually painlessly.

Four neoplastic causes of swelling of the jaw deserve special mention.

Carcinoma of the antrum

These are much more common than primary bone tumours, and when they invade downwards into the maxilla they cause swelling of the upper jaw and palate. They are silent tumours and normally present at a late stage of development.

Ameloblastoma

This tumour arises from the ameloblast that is responsible for forming the crown of a tooth. Characteristically, it is a painless tumour that causes progressive swelling of the jaw (Fig. 11.50). It is locally invasive. If it is found to have extended into soft tissue, it may have become malignant. The tumour may be solid or cystic, and a definitive diagnosis requires a biopsy.

Fig. 11.50 A maxillary ameloblastoma causing buccal and palatal bulging.

Osteosarcoma

Osteosarcomas can occur in both the upper and the lower jaw. They are rare and present as a mass that is diagnosed by biopsy (Fig. 11.51).

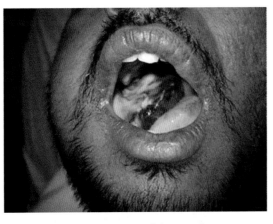

Fig. 11.51 A large sarcoma of the maxilla.

Malignant lymphoma

Burkitt's lymphoma is a malignant tumour of B-lymphocytes associated with Epstein–Barr virus infection. In its endemic form, it affects children below the age of 12 years and occurs in those areas of sub-Saharan Africa that have a warm, wet climate and endemic malaria.

Lymphomas present with progressive, painless swelling of the jaw that distorts the face, may displace the eye and partially occludes the mouth (Fig. 11.52).

Lymphomatous tissue may also be present elsewhere, causing abdominal and skeletal symptoms.

Fig. 11.52 A lymphoma arising from the upper jaw.

12 The neck

HISTORY AND EXAMINATION OF SWELLINGS IN THE NECK

The majority of surgical conditions that arise in the neck present as a swelling. Taking the history and performing the physical examination should follow the standard pattern, but there are some important features that deserve special attention.

The history of swellings in the neck

The most common cause of a swelling in the neck is an enlarged lymph gland, and the most common causes of such enlargement are infection and secondary tumour deposits.

Systemic illness

Symptoms such as general malaise, fever and rigors and contact with people with infectious diseases may indicate an infective cause of the swelling.

Loss of appetite, loss of weight and pulmonary, alimentary or skeletal symptoms may suggest a malignant cause.

Irritation of the skin associated with enlarged cervical lymph glands is often seen with lymphoma.

Head and neck symptoms

The patient should be asked about pain in the mouth, discomfort on eating, sore throats or ulceration, nasal discharge, pain or blockage of the airway, pain in the throat or neck, dysphagia, odynophagia, changes in voice and difficulty with breathing. Enquiries should be made for any lumps or ulcers on the skin of the head and face, and for whether they have changed in size, shape or consistency, or have begun to bleed.

The skin, mouth, nose, larynx and pharynx are common sites for neoplasms, and although head and neck cancers commonly present with metastases in the lymph glands, they are not usually associated with symptoms of distant metastases such as general malaise and loss of weight.

The examination of swellings in the neck

Site

It is essential to define the site of a lump in the neck.

The neck is divided into two triangles (Fig. 12.1). The *anterior triangle* is bounded by the anterior border of the sternomastoid muscle, the lower edge of the jaw and the midline. In clinical practice, the structures deep to the sternomastoid muscle are considered to be inside the anterior triangle.

The upper part of the anterior triangle, below the jaw but above the digastric muscle, is sometimes called the digastric or submandibular triangle.

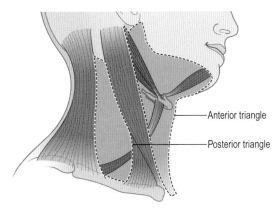

Fig. 12.1 The anatomical triangles of the neck.

The *posterior triangle* is bounded by the posterior border of the sternomastoid muscle, the anterior edge of the trapezius muscle and the clavicle.

To define the triangles, it is necessary to get the patient to tense their neck muscles:

- The sternomastoid muscle is made to contract by putting your hand under the patient's chin and asking them to push their head down against the resistance of your hand. This tightens both sternomastoid muscles.
- The trapezius muscle is made to contract by asking the patient to shrug (elevate) their shoulders against resistance.

Relation to muscles

Lumps in the neck should always be felt with the muscles initially relaxed and then with them contracted. If the lump is deep to a muscle, it will become impalpable when the muscle contracts.

Relation to the trachea

Swellings that are fixed to the trachea will move when the trachea moves. The trachea is pulled upwards during swallowing. Assess the relationship to the trachea of every lump in the neck by watching to see if it moves with the trachea during swallowing.

Relation to the hyoid bone

The hyoid bone moves only slightly during swallowing, but ascends when the tongue is protruded. Ask the patient to open their mouth. When the jaw is still, ask them to protrude their tongue. If the swelling in the neck moves as the tongue protrudes, it must be fixed to the hyoid bone.

CERVICAL LYMPHADENOPATHY AND OTHER NECK SWELLINGS

Causes of cervical lymph gland enlargement

Enlargement of the cervical lymph glands is the most common cause of a swelling in the neck (Revision panel 12.1). Even when only one gland is palpable, the adjacent glands are invariably diseased.

The four main causes of cervical lymph gland enlargement are:

- *infection* – non-specific tonsillitis, glandular fever, toxoplasmosis, tuberculosis, cat-scratch fever;
- *metastatic tumour* from the head, neck, chest and abdomen;
- *primary reticuloses* – lymphoma, lymphosarcoma, reticulosarcoma;
- *sarcoidosis*.

The diagnosis of lymphadenopathy caused by systemic illnesses such as glandular fever, toxoplasmosis and sarcoidosis depends on finding lymphadenopathy elsewhere, on other evidence of the underlying disease and on special blood tests.

Revision panel 12.1
Causes of cervical lymphadenopathy

Infection

Non-specific

Glandular fever

Tuberculosis

Syphilis

Toxoplasmosis

Cat-scratch fever (*Rochalimaea henselae*)

Metastatic tumour

From the head, neck, chest and abdomen

Primary reticuloses

Lymphoma

Lymphosarcoma

Reticulosarcoma

Sarcoidosis

Non-specific cervical inflammatory lymphadenopathy

Non-specific reactive lymphoid hyperplasia can follow any inflammatory process or be associated with skin conditions, particularly of the scalp, when it is termed *dermatopathic lymphadenopathy*. However, non-specific inflammatory lymphadenopathy commonly follows recurrent bouts of tonsillitis, especially if the attacks have been treated inadequately. The upper deep cervical glands are most often affected (Fig. 12.2).

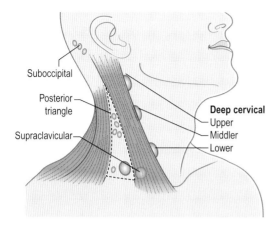

Fig. 12.2 The anatomy of the cervical lymph glands.

In a healthy child, small normal lymph glands are often palpable, especially in the posterior triangle.

History

Age When the lymphadenopathy is associated with tonsillitis, the majority of patients are below the age of 10 years. Other reactive conditions can occur at any age.

Symptoms The common presenting symptom is a painful lump just below the angle of the jaw.

The severity of the pain may vary. It is usually more a discomfort, which becomes acute when the patient has a sore throat.

The lump may be large enough to be visible or felt by the child's parent when washing their neck.

The child may snore at night, have difficulty in breathing, have nasal speech because of tonsillar and adenoid hyperplasia or suffer from recurrent chest infections.

Cause The child or parents frequently recognize the relationship between the appearance of the lump and an episode of tonsillitis.

Systemic effects When the lump is tender, the patient often feels ill, has a sore throat and pyrexia and does not want to eat.

Recurrent severe episodes can cause loss of weight and slow the rate of growth and body maturation.

Social history Recurrent sore throats and upper respiratory tract infections are more common in malnurtured children in substandard, cold, damp houses.

Examination

Position Lymph from the tonsils drains to the upper deep cervical lymph glands. The gland just below and deep to the angle of the mandible is often called the tonsillar gland (Fig. 12.3). This gland and those just below it are likely to be enlarged.

Tenderness If the infection is active, the enlarged glands will be tender.

Shape and size The tonsillar gland is usually spherical and approximately 1–2 cm in diameter. It is rarely bigger than this. The glands below it are usually smaller, even when inflamed.

Composition and relations Each gland is firm in consistency, solid, discrete, tender and not very mobile.

Local tissues The tonsils are likely to be enlarged and hyperaemic. Pus may be seen exuding from the surface crypts.

The glands on the other side of the neck are often just as large but may not have been noticed by the parents.

General examination Look for the presence of enlarged lymph glands elsewhere. None should be enlarged.

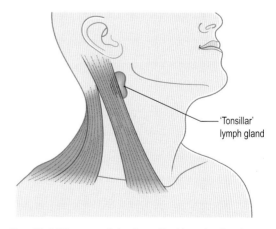

Fig. 12.3 The site of the 'tonsillar' lymph gland.

Recurrent chest infections may have damaged the lungs – assess the patient for any evidence of lobar collapse, bronchiectasis and lung abscess.

Tuberculous cervical lymphadenitis and abscess

The human tubercle bacillus can enter the body via the tonsils, and from there move to the cervical lymph glands. The upper deep cervical glands are most often affected. There is no generalized infection, so there is little systemic disturbance of health. Infection with bovine tuberculosis ceased in the UK when the control and testing of dairy cattle was introduced.

History

Age and ethnic groups Tuberculous lymphadenitis is common in children, young adults and the elderly. In the UK, the incidence in the young has diminished since the introduction of *Bacille Calmette–Guérin (BCG)* vaccination, mass radiography screening and the discovery of effective antituberculosis antibiotics, but the prevalence of cervical lymph gland enlargement caused by anonymous mycobacteria is increasing. In the UK, tuberculous lymphadenitis is found most often in young immigrant adults (Fig. 12.4).

Fig. 12.4 A tuberculous cervical lymph gland in a young immigrant adult.

Symptoms The patient complains of a lump in the neck. This appears gradually with or without pain.

The pain can be intense if the glands grow rapidly and necrose.

Systemic symptoms are unusual in the young, but the elderly sometimes have anorexia and slight weight loss.

If the glands break down into an abscess, the swelling increases in size, becomes more painful, and the patient notices discolouration of the overlying skin.

When the glands are very painful, neck movements and swallowing may be uncomfortable.

Previous history Elderly patients often have a history of swollen neck glands when young – sometimes treated at that time by surgical excision.
Immunization Enquire for vaccination with BCG.
Family history Check for a family history of tuberculosis.
Social history Tuberculosis is more common in the poor and socially underprivileged.

Examination

The signs of tuberculous lymphadenitis

Position The upper and middle deep cervical glands are most often involved (Fig. 12.5).
Temperature The mass of glands does *not* feel hot.
Tenderness The glands are often slightly tender, but pain is not a prominent feature.
Colour If there is no abscess present, the overlying skin should look normal.
Shape, size and consistency In the early stages, the glands are firm, discrete and between 1 and 2 cm in diameter.

As caseation increases and the glands necrose, the infection spreads beyond the capsule of the glands. This makes the lumps enlarge and coalesce.

A typical patch of tuberculous lymphadenitis is an indistinct, firm mass of glands that occupies the upper half of the deep cervical lymph chain, partly beneath and partly in front of the sternomastoid muscle.

The glands are commonly matted together, but there may be some discrete glands above or below the matted mass.

Fig. 12.5 Enlargement of the upper deep cervical lymph glands caused by tuberculosis.

Local tissues Other cervical lymph glands may be palpable. The tonsils and the other tissues in the neck should be normal.

The signs of a tuberculous abscess

When an infected lymph gland caseates and turns into pus, it becomes an abscess. The natural tendency of an abscess is to weaken the overlying tissues until it bursts through them to reach and burst through the skin. This is known as *pointing*. At the stage when a tuberculous abscess has burst through the deep cervical fascia into the subcutaneous tissues, it has two compartments, one on either side of the deep fascia, connected by a small central track. This is called a *collar-stud abscess* (Fig. 12.6).

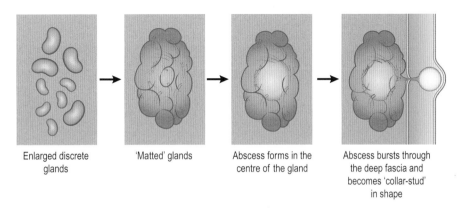

Enlarged discrete glands → 'Matted' glands → Abscess forms in the centre of the gland → Abscess bursts through the deep fascia and becomes 'collar-stud' in shape

Fig. 12.6 The development of a tuberculous 'collar-stud' abscess.

Position Because a tuberculous abscess forms in tuberculous lymph glands, it is most often found in the upper half of the neck (Fig. 12.7).

Colour When the pus reaches the subcutaneous tissues, the overlying skin turns reddish-purple.

Temperature The skin temperature is normal because the process of caseation and pus formation is slow and does not stimulate excessive hyperaemia – hence the name cold abscess.

Tenderness The mass is tender, sometimes exquisitely so if the abscess is tense.

Shape The deep part of the abscess tends to be sausage shaped, with its long axis parallel to the front edge of the sternomastoid muscle. The superficial pocket of the abscess is usually lower than the deep part.

Size Most tuberculous abscesses are 3–5 cm across, but they can be much larger.

Surface The surface is irregular and indistinct.

Edge The edges are moderately well defined if the abscess is tense, but if the pocket of pus is lax there will not be a definite edge.

Composition The abscess feels firm and rubbery, and it will fluctuate if sufficient pus is present. This latter sign cannot be elicited if the abscess is small and lies deep to the sternomastoid muscle.

The subcutaneous part of a collar-stud abscess should be clearly fluctuant, but it is not usually possible to reduce the superficial pocket of pus into the deep pocket.

Relations The original abscess is deep to the deep fascia, partly under the sternomastoid muscle, and fixed to surrounding structures. The superficial part of a collar-stud abscess is immediately below the skin and becomes more prominent when the sternomastoid muscle is contracted. If spontaneous discharge occurs, a chronic sinus may form. Tuberculous sinuses are characterized by minimal erythema and lack of pain, unless secondarily infected (Fig. 12.8).

The other lymph glands in the neck near the abscess may be enlarged.

General examination In tuberculous lymphadenitis, there are often no systemic abnormalities, but when a tuberculous abscess develops, there may be tachycardia, pyrexia, anorexia and general malaise.

There may be signs of tuberculosis in the lungs, in other lymph glands and in the urinary tract.

(a)

(b)

Fig. 12.7 A LARGE TUBERCULOUS 'COLLAR-STUD' ABSCESS

Fig. 12.8 A chronic tuberculous sinus that has become secondarily infected.

Carcinomatous lymph glands

Malignant metastatic deposits in the cervical lymph glands are the most common cause of cervical lymphadenopathy in adults.

The primary tumour is most often in the buccal cavity (tongue, lips and mucous membrane) and larynx, but every possible primary site must be examined when cervical glands are enlarged by secondary deposits, including the skin (Fig. 12.9).

History

Age Most head and neck cancers occur in patients over the age of 50 years. Most patients presenting with metastatic deposits in their cervical lymph glands are between 55 and 65 years.

The exception is papillary carcinoma of the thyroid, which occurs in children and young adults.

Sex Most of the head and neck cancers, other than those of the thyroid, are more common in males than females.

Local symptoms The patient complains of a painless lump in the neck.

It is uncommon for carcinomatous glands to be tender or to become so large that they interfere with neck movements before being noticed.

The lump tends to grow slowly, and further lumps may appear.

General symptoms The patient may have symptoms from the primary lesion in the head or neck, such as a sore tongue, a hoarse voice or a separate lump in the neck such as in the thyroid or salivary glands. If the primary is in the chest, they may have a cough or haemoptysis; if it is in the abdomen, they may have dyspepsia or abdominal pain.

Generally speaking, head and neck cancers do not cause anorexia and weight loss, whereas cancers in the lungs and intra-abdominal organs do.

Examination

Site The site of the affected glands gives a crude indication of the site of the primary. Lesions above the hyoid bone drain to the upper deep cervical glands. The larynx and thyroid drain to the middle and lower deep cervical glands. An enlarged supraclavicular lymph gland commonly indicates intra-abdominal or thoracic disease. When enlarged by metastases, this gland is called *Virchow's gland*; its presence is *Troisier's sign*.

Colour The overlying skin is a normal colour unless the mass is so large that it stretches or infiltrates the skin, which makes it pale or blotchy red (Fig. 12.10).

Temperature The skin temperature will be normal unless the tumour is very vascular.

Tenderness Glands containing secondary deposits are usually not tender.

Fig. 12.9 This patient presented with hard, enlarged lymph glands in the neck. The primary lesion was the insignificant mole above his right eyebrow.

Fig. 12.10 Secondary malignant deposits in the skin of the neck.

Shape and size Glands containing metastases vary in size and shape. Both features depend upon the amount of tumour within them and its rate of growth. At first the glands are smooth, discrete and vary in size. As they grow, they may coalesce into one large mass.

Composition Glands containing tumour are hard, often stony hard. Rarely, a very vascular tumour deposit will be soft, pulsatile and compressible.

Relations The glands are tethered to the surrounding structures, so they can usually be moved in a transverse direction but not vertically.

Their relation to the sternomastoid muscle varies according to the group to which they belong. Secondary cancer is more common in the glands of the anterior than the posterior triangle. These glands lie deep to the anterior edge of the sternomastoid.

If the tumour spreads beyond the capsule of the glands, the mass becomes completely fixed.

Local tissues The overlying skin and muscle may be infiltrated with tumour, in which case the tumour must be distinguished from secondary deposits actually lying in the skin.

Lymph drainage Other lymph glands on the pathway between the primary lesion and the noted gland may be enlarged.

General examination Examine all the sites that might contain the primary lesion (Fig. 12.11; Revision panel 12.2), in particular:

- the skin of the scalp, the ear and the external auditory meatus;
- the lips, tongue, buccal mucous membrane and tonsils;
- the nose, maxillary antra and nasopharynx;
- the thyroid gland;
- the salivary glands;
- the skin of the upper limb;
- the breasts;
- the lungs;
- the stomach, pancreas, ovaries and testes.

The symptoms and signs of malignant disease originating in these organs are discussed in the appropriate chapters. Some aspects of this examination require special instruments, for example a head or laryngeal mirror and light.

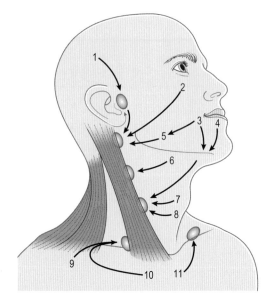

Fig. 12.11 Sites of primary neoplasms that metastasize to the cervical lymph glands.

Revision panel 12.2

Sites of primary neoplasms that metastasize to cervical lymph glands

1 Scalp
  Parotid gland
  Upper face
  Ear
2 Maxillary antrum and other air sinuses
  Nasal cavity and nasopharynx
3 Tongue
  Buccal mucosa
  Floor of mouth
  Mandible
4 Lips
5 Tonsil
  Base of tongue
  Oropharynx
6 Submandibular gland
  Skin of neck
7 Larynx and laryngopharynx
8 Thyroid
  Upper oesophagus
9 Upper limb and both sides of the chest wall
10 Breast
11 Lungs, stomach and all the viscera

Primary neoplasms of the lymph glands

(Reticuloses, lymphoma)

The most common primary tumour of lymphoid tissue is malignant lymphoma. There are many histological varieties, but they are often loosely divided into Hodgkin's and non-Hodgkin's lymphoma.

History

Age The reticuloses are common in children and young adults.

Sex Males are affected more often than females.

Symptoms The most common presenting symptom is a painless lump in the neck, which is noticed by chance and grows slowly.

Malaise, weight loss and pallor are common symptoms.

Itching of the skin (pruritus) is an unexplained but distinctive complaint.

There may be fever with rigors, occurring in a periodic fashion (*Pel–Ebstein fever*).

Lymphomatous infiltration of the skeleton may cause pains in the bones, and there may be abdominal pain after drinking alcohol.

If there are large masses of lymph glands in the mediastinum, they may occlude the superior vena cava, causing venous congestion in the neck and the development of collateral veins across the chest wall.

Large masses in the abdomen can obstruct the inferior vena cava and cause oedema of both legs.

Examination

Site Any of the cervical lymph glands can be affected, often with bilateral involvement (Fig. 12.12, Revision panel 12.3). Lymphoma is one of the few conditions, apart from infection, that may cause lymphadenopathy in the posterior triangle.

Tenderness The glands are not tender.

Shape, size and surface The lymph glands in Hodgkin's disease are usually ovoid, smooth and discrete.

It is possible to define individual glands even when they become large. This is the opposite of tuberculosis, in which the lymph glands become matted and indistinct.

Fig. 12.12 Bilateral cervical lymphadenopathy caused by Hodgkin's lymphoma.

Revision panel 12.3

Plan of examination for source of secondary cervical lymphadenopathy

(Start at the top and work downwards)

Examine the *skin* of the scalp, face, ears and neck

Look in the *nose*

Look in the *mouth* at the tongue, gums, mucosa and tonsils

Palpate the parotid, submandibular and thyroid glands

Examine the arms and the chest wall – including the breast

Examine the abdomen and genitalia

Transilluminate the air sinuses

Examine the nasopharynx and larynx with mirrors

Consistency Glands infiltrated by lymphoma are solid and rubbery in consistency.

Relations Although tethered to nearby structures, these glands can usually be moved from side to side and rarely become completely fixed.

Local tissues The surrounding tissues should be normal.

General examination Other groups of lymph glands may be enlarged. The liver and spleen may be palpable. The patient is often anaemic and may be jaundiced.

CHAPTER 12 | THE NECK

Spread to the skin produces elevated, reddened, scaly patches of skin known as mycosis fungoides (Fig. 12.13).

Fig. 12.13 Cutaneous deposits of lymphoma.

Branchial cyst

A branchial cyst is a remnant of a branchial cleft, usually the second cleft, and often appears from beneath the upper third of the sternomastoid muscle (Fig. 12.14). It is lined with squamous epithelium, but there are often patches of lymphoid tissue in the wall that are connected with the other lymph tissue in the neck and can become infected.

History

Age Although these cysts are present at birth, they may not distend and cause symptoms until adult life. The majority present between the ages of 15 and 25 years, but they can present in childhood (Fig. 12.15), while a number can appear later when patients are in their forties and fifties.

Sex Males and females are equally affected.

Symptoms The common presenting complaint is a painless swelling in the upper lateral part of the neck.

The lump may be painful when it first appears, and later attacks of pain may be associated with an increase in size, usually caused by infection in the lymphoid tissue in the cyst wall (Fig. 12.16).

A severe throbbing pain, exacerbated by moving the neck and opening the mouth, develops if the contents of the cyst become infected and purulent.

General effects These cysts have no systemic effects and are not associated with any other congenital abnormality.

Fig. 12.15 A branchial cyst presenting in childhood.

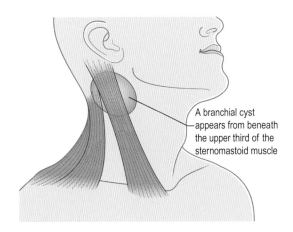

A branchial cyst appears from beneath the upper third of the sternomastoid muscle

Fig. 12.14 The site of a branchial cyst.

Fig. 12.16 A large branchial cyst that had become painful. This commonly follows recurrent bouts of tonsillitis, especially if the infection has been inadequately treated.

Examination

Position A branchial cyst lies behind the anterior edge of the upper third of the sternomastoid muscle and bulges forwards (Fig. 12.17). Rarely, the cyst can bulge backwards behind the muscle.

Fig. 12.17 A branchial cyst that presented in adult life. The back of the swelling is clearly deep to the sternomastoid muscle.

Colour and tenderness The overlying skin may be reddened and the lump may be tender if the cyst is inflamed.

Shape The cyst is usually ovoid, with its long axis running forwards and downwards.

Size Most branchial cysts are between 5 and 10 cm long.

Surface Their surface is smooth and the edge distinct.

Composition The consistency varies with the tension of the cyst. Most cysts are tense, but a lax cyst feels soft. They are dull to percussion.

The lump fluctuates, but this sign is not always easy to elicit, especially if the cyst is small and the sternomastoid muscle thick.

The lump is usually opaque because it contains desquamated epithelial cells that make its contents thick and white. Sometimes the fluid is golden yellow and shimmers with fat globules and cholesterol crystals secreted by the sebaceous glands in the epithelial lining. Such cysts may transilluminate.

The cyst cannot be reduced or compressed.

Relations The bulk of the mass lies deep to the upper part of the sternomastoid muscle. It is not very mobile because it is closely tethered to the surrounding structures.

Lymph drainage The local deep cervical lymph glands should not be enlarged. If they are palpable, the diagnosis should be reconsidered in favour of an inflammatory process such as a tuberculous abscess rather than a branchial cyst. Other cystic lesions that are often presumed to be branchial cysts are secondary cystic lymph gland deposits from a papillary carcinoma of the thyroid.

Local tissues The local tissues should be normal.

If the cyst has turned into an abscess, the surrounding tissues will be oedematous and the skin hot and red.

Branchial fistula (or sinus)

This is a rare congenital abnormality. It is the remnant of a branchial cleft, usually the second cleft, which has not closed off.

The patient complains of a small dimple in the skin at the junction of the middle and the lower third of the anterior edge of the sternomastoid muscle (Fig. 12.18) that discharges clear mucus, and sometimes becomes swollen and painful and discharges pus.

When the whole branchial cleft stays patent, the fistula connects the skin with the oropharynx, just behind the tonsil. In most cases, the upper end is obliterated and the track should really be called a branchial sinus.

Swallowing accentuates the openings on the skin.

Fig. 12.18 A branchial fistula opening at the lower edge of sternomastoid muscle.

Carotid body tumour

This is a rare tumour of the chemoreceptor tissue in the carotid body. It is therefore a chemodectoma. It is usually benign but can become quite large and occasionally is malignant.

History

Age Chemodectomas commonly appear in patients between the ages of 40 and 60 years.

Symptoms The common presentation is a painless, slowly growing lump. The patient may notice that the lump pulsates, and may suffer from symptoms of transient cerebral ischaemia (blackouts, transient paralysis or paraesthesia). These symptoms are unusual because the increasing compression of the carotid artery by the tumour is a very slow process.

Development The lump grows so slowly that many patients ignore it for many years.

Multiplicity Carotid body tumours may be bilateral.

Examination

Always be especially gentle when palpating a lump close to the bifurcation of the carotid artery. Pressure in this area can induce a vasovagal attack.

Position The carotid bifurcation is at, or just below, the level of the hyoid bone. Carotid body tumours are therefore found in the upper part of the anterior triangle of the neck, level with the hyoid bone and beneath the anterior edge of the sternomastoid muscle (Fig. 12.19).

Tenderness, colour and temperature These tumours are not tender or hot, and the overlying skin should be normal.

Shape The lump is initially spherical but, as it grows, it becomes irregular in shape, often narrower at its lower end, where it is situated in the bifurcation of the common carotid artery.

Size Carotid body tumours may vary from 2–3 cm to 10 cm in diameter.

Composition The majority of these tumours are solid and hard. They are dull to percussion and do not fluctuate, and can be mistaken for an enlarged lymph gland (Fig. 12.20). They are often called *potato tumours* because of their consistency and shape (Fig. 12.21).

Fig. 12.20 A carotid body tumour. Note that the visible mass is lower than that of a branchial cyst (see Fig. 12.17) but indistinguishable on inspection from an enlarged cervical lymph gland. Most carotid body tumours are initially mistaken for enlarged lymph glands.

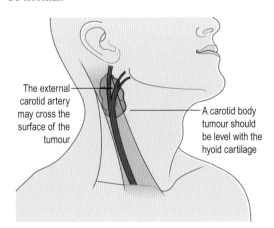

The external carotid artery may cross the surface of the tumour

A carotid body tumour should be level with the hyoid cartilage

Fig. 12.19 The site of a carotid body tumour.

Fig. 12.21 A very large, firm, bosselated carotid body tumour – hence the name 'potato tumour'.

Fig. 12.22 A carotid artery aneurysm.

Sometimes these tumours pulsate. This is either a transmitted pulsation from the adjacent carotid artery, a palpable external carotid artery running over the superficial aspect of the lump, or a true expansile pulsation from a soft or very vascular tumour or an aneurysm (Fig. 12.22).

It is surprising that, in spite of their vascularity, most of these tumours are hard. Those which are soft and very vascular not only have an expansile pulsation, but can also be compressed and may exhibit a bruit.

Relations The lump is deep to the cervical fascia and beneath the anterior edge of the sternomastoid muscle.

The common carotid artery can be felt below the mass, and the external carotid artery may pass over its superficial surface. Without this close relationship to the arteries, this tumour is indistinguishable from an enlarged lymph gland.

Because of their intimate relationship with the carotid arteries, these tumours can be moved from side to side but not up and down.

Cystic hygroma

(Lymph cyst, lymphocele, lymphangioma)
A cystic hygroma is a congenital collection of lymphatic sacs that contain clear, colourless lymph. They are probably derived from clusters of lymph channels that failed, during intrauterine development, to connect with and become normal lymphatic pathways. Lymph cysts commonly occur near the root of the arm and the leg (i.e. in the anatomical junctions between the limbs and head and the trunk).

(a)

(b)

Fig. 12.23 CYSTIC HYGROMA
(a, b) Two examples of cystic hygroma: in a very young child – the common age of presentation – and in a young adult.

History

Age The majority of cystic hygromas present at birth or within the first few years of life (Fig. 12.23), but they occasionally stay empty until infection or trauma in adult life causes them to fill up and become visible. Occasionally, large lymphoceles can be seen in elderly patients (Fig. 12.24).

Fig. 12.24 A large lymphocele in an elderly female.

Symptoms The only symptom is the complaint about the lump, but the parents of an affected child are usually more concerned about the disfigurement caused by the cyst.

Family history This condition is not familial.

Examination

Position Cystic hygromas are commonly found around the base of the neck (Fig. 12.25), usually in the posterior triangle, but they can be very big and occupy the whole of the subcutaneous tissue of one side of the neck.

Temperature and tenderness They are not hot or tender, and the overlying skin is normal.

Shape A cystic hygroma is a mixture of soft unilocular and multilocular cysts, so the whole mass looks lobulated and flattened.

Size Small cysts are a few centimetres across. Large cysts can extend over the whole of one side of the neck.

Surface If the cysts are close to the skin, it may be possible to feel a distinct surface. Deep cysts feel smooth, but because they are lax, their edges are often indistinct.

Composition Cystic hygromas are soft and dull to percussion. They fluctuate easily, but their distinctive physical sign is a **brilliant translucence**.

Large cysts will conduct a fluid thrill, and in some multilocular swellings the fluid in one loculus can be compressed into another.

They cannot be reduced.

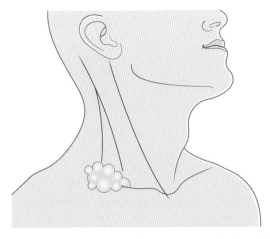

Fig. 12.25 The cystic hygroma is commonly found in the subcutaneous tissue at the base of the posterior triangle. It is brilliantly translucent.

Relations Cystic hygromas develop in the subcutaneous tissues. They are thus superficial to the neck muscles and close to the skin but are rarely fixed to the skin. However, a cyst in the posterior triangle may extend deeply beneath the sternomastoid muscle into the retropharyngeal space.

Lymph glands The local lymph glands should not be enlarged and, as the lymph drainage of the tissues around the cyst is normal, there is no lymphoedema. If there is associated lymphadenopathy, the diagnosis should be reconsidered, as cystic nodal metastases of papillary thyroid carcinoma can present as large, painless cystic swellings in the neck.

Local tissues The local tissues are normal.

Pharyngeal pouch

A pharyngeal pouch is a 'pulsion' diverticulum of the pharynx through the gap between the horizontal fibres of the cricopharyngeus muscle below and the lowermost oblique fibres of the inferior constrictor muscle above. If swallowing is uncoordinated so that the cricopharyngeus does not relax, the weak unsupported area just above these fibres (known as *Killian's dehiscence*) bulges out (Fig. 12.26). The bulge eventually grows into a sac, which hangs down and presses against the side of the oesophagus.

History

Age Pharyngeal pouches appear in middle and old age.

Sex They are more common in males than in females.

Symptoms Patients often have a long history of halitosis and recurrent sore throats before noticing the common presenting symptom of regurgitation of froth and food. The regurgitated food is undigested and comes up into the mouth at any time. There is no bile or acid taste to it.

Regurgitation at night causes bouts of coughing and choking, and if pieces of food are inhaled a lung abscess may develop.

As the pouch grows, it presses on the oesophagus and causes dysphagia. Patients can sometimes swallow their first few mouthfuls of food (until the pouch is full), but thereafter have difficulty in swallowing.

By the time these symptoms become severe, the patient may have noticed a swelling in the neck, and find that pressure on the swelling causes gurgling sounds and regurgitation. The swelling changes in size and often disappears.

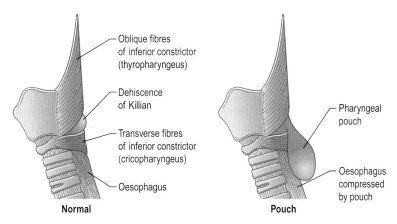

Fig. 12.26 The anatomy of a pharyngeal pouch.

If the dysphagia continues, the patient may become malnourished and lose weight.

Examination

Position In most patients, there is no palpable swelling, but when a swelling caused by a pharyngeal pouch is apparent, it appears behind the sternomastoid muscle, below the level of the thyroid cartilage (Fig. 12.27).

Shape Its shape is indistinct because only part of its surface is palpable. It feels like a bulging deep structure.

Size Most pouches cause a swelling of only 5–10 cm diameter. The pouch is not palpable when it is smaller, so many patients have symptoms but no abnormal physical signs.

Surface and edge When palpable, the surface is smooth, but the edge is not definable.

Composition The lump is soft and sometimes indentable. It is dull to percussion and does not fluctuate or transilluminate.

It can be compressed and sometimes emptied. Compression may cause a gurgling sound and be associated with regurgitation. Although the mass may disappear with compression, not to return until the patient eats again, it cannot be said to have been 'reduced' according to the usual meaning of the word.

Relations A pharyngeal pouch lies deep to the deep fascia, behind the sternomastoid muscle, and is fixed deeply. Its origin from a structure behind the trachea can be appreciated during palpation, but the neck of the pouch and its attachment to the oesophagus cannot be felt.

It cannot be moved about in the neck.

Lymph glands The cervical lymph glands should not be enlarged.

Local tissues The surrounding tissues feel normal. Indeed, when the pouch is empty, the whole neck feels normal.

General examination Pay special attention to the chest, as there may be an aspiration pneumonia, collapse of a lobe or a lung abscess.

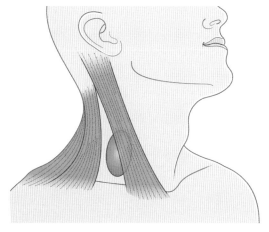

Fig. 12.27 A pharyngeal pouch rarely causes a detectable swelling. If it does, the swelling is behind the sternomastoid muscle.

CHAPTER 12 | THE NECK

Sternomastoid 'tumour'

(Ischaemic contracture of a segment of the sternomastoid muscle)

This is a swelling of the middle third of the sternomastoid muscle (Fig. 12.28). In neonates, it consists of oedema around an infarcted segment of the muscle, caused by the trauma of birth. As the patient grows, the lump disappears and the abnormal segment of muscle becomes fibrotic and contracted.

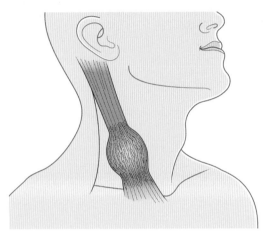

Fig. 12.28 A sternomastoid 'tumour' is an area of oedema and necrosis in the lower third of the sternomastoid muscle.

History

Age The lump is noticed at birth or in the first few weeks of life.

Symptoms The mother may notice the lump or that the child keeps their head turned to one side – torticollis (Fig. 12.29). Attempts to turn the head straight may cause pain or distress.

If the muscle is not extensively damaged, the swelling slowly subsides, the muscle spasm relaxes and the torticollis disappears. If the muscle damage becomes an area of permanent fibrosis, the twist and tilt of the head to one side becomes more noticeable as the child grows.

Examination

The lump

Position The swelling lies in the middle of the sternomastoid muscle (i.e. in the middle third of the neck on the anterolateral surface) (Fig. 12.30).

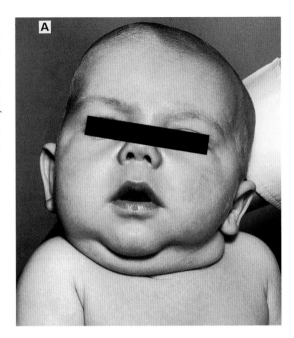

Fig. 12.29 An infantile torticollis caused by ischaemia of the sternomastoid muscle.

Fig. 12.30 A localized swollen segment of sternomastoid with a slight torticollis in an older child, caused by ischaemia and fibrosis of the muscle after birth; this is a typical sternomastoid 'tumour'.

Tenderness The lump may be tender in the first few weeks of life.

Shape and size The swelling is fusiform, with its long axis along the line of the sternomastoid muscle. It is usually 1–2 cm across.

Surface The surface is smooth.

Edge The anterior and posterior edges of the lump are distinct, but the superior and inferior edges, where the lump becomes continuous with normal muscle, are indistinct.

Composition At first the lump is firm and solid and easy to feel, but as it gradually becomes harder, it begins to shrink and may become impalpable.

Surrounding structures and local lymph glands These should be normal.

The neck

Examine the movements of the neck. As the child is too young to obey commands, watch how they move their head when lying in their cot, and then manipulate the head and neck very gently.

The sternomastoid muscles rotate and tilt the head. Contraction of the left sternomastoid turns the head towards the right, but tilts the head to the left. Both these deformities may be present. Forced movement to correct the deformity may cause pain and be resisted by the child.

Apart from the restriction of movement caused by spasm of the sternomastoid muscle, the neck movements should be normal.

The eyes

Look at the eyes and watch their movements to detect any squint. Torticollis can be a means of correcting a squint. Move the head into a vertical and central position and watch the eyes. If the torticollis is secondary to a squint and not a sternomastoid tumour, the squint will appear as the head is straightened.

The head

An uncorrected torticollis may affect the growth of the facial bones and cause facial asymmetry.

In adults, recent onset torticollis usually just represents muscle spasm (Fig. 12.31).

Fig. 12.31 An adult form of torticollis caused by muscular spasm.

Cervical rib

Although a cervical rib can cause serious neurological and vascular symptoms in the upper arm, clinical examination of the neck does not usually reveal any abnormalities. The abnormal rib is usually detected with an X-ray (Fig. 12.32). Sometimes there is a fullness at the root of the neck, but it is rarely distinct enough to justify a firm clinical diagnosis

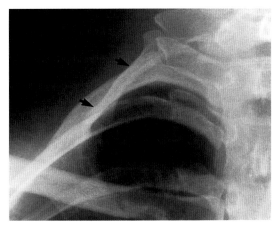

Fig. 12.32 An X-ray demonstrating a cervical rib.

of cervical rib (Fig. 12.33). It can occasionally be associated with aneurysmal change in the subclavian artery.

The common neurological symptoms caused by a cervical rib are pain in the C8 and T1 dermatomes, and wasting and weakness of the small muscles in the hand. Vascular symptoms such as Raynaud's phenomenon, trophic changes and even rest pain and gangrene may occur but are uncommon.

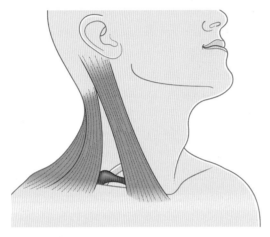

Fig. 12.33 A cervical rib rarely causes a visible swelling. It may cause a subclavian artery aneurysm.

THE SALIVARY GLANDS

Saliva is produced by the paired parotid, submandibular and sublingual glands and many other small, unnamed glands scattered beneath the buccal mucous membrane.

The most common surgical conditions affecting the salivary glands are:

- infection and calculus formation in the submandibular gland;
- tumours of the parotid gland.

Mumps is the most common medical disease; all other diseases of the salivary glands are uncommon (Revision panel 12.4).

The submandibular salivary gland

Submandibular calculi

Submandibular calculi are common because the submandibular gland lies below the opening of its duct on the floor of the mouth, and because the secretion of the submandibular gland contains a

---

Revision panel 12.4

Causes of swelling of a salivary gland

Acute infection

Viral (e.g. mumps)

Bacterial (e.g. *Staphylococcus*)

Duct obstruction

Sialectasis (chronic infection)

Tumour

Benign

Malignant

Sarcoidosis (Mikulicz's syndrome)

Sjögren's syndrome

---

considerable quantity of mucus, two factors that encourage stasis in the duct. Calculi in the parotid gland are less common.

A salivary gland calculus is composed of cellular debris, bacteria, mucus, and calcium and magnesium phosphates – a mixture similar to the 'scale' (tartar) on the teeth.

History

Age Most submandibular salivary calculi occur in young to middle-aged adults. They are rare in children.
Sex Males and females are equally afflicted.
Symptoms The main symptoms are pain and swelling beneath the jaw, caused by obstruction of Wharton's duct.

Swelling is usually the principal complaint, because it appears before, and persists after, the pain. The pain is a dull ache, which occasionally radiates to the ear or into the tongue.

Both symptoms appear, or worsen, before and during eating. The swelling begins just before eating, and the pain develops as the gland enlarges. Both symptoms last through the meal, but afterwards the pain goes away before the swelling. If the gland becomes irreparably damaged, the swelling persists between meals and the dull aching pain may also become constant.

Very rarely, the patient may notice discomfort and a swelling in the floor of the mouth caused by distension of the duct and/or the stone (Fig. 12.34). Patients may be able to relieve their symptoms by pressing on the gland, and they may notice that this

Fig. 12.34 Stone in the submandibular duct. When a stone impacts at the end of the submandibular duct, the floor of the mouth looks asymmetrical. In this patient, there is a bulge over the right submandibular duct due to an impacted stone.

action produces a foul-tasting fluid in their mouth (purulent saliva).

Development The symptoms may recur and remit for periods of a few days or weeks if the stone moves about in the duct, sometimes obstructing it, sometimes not.

If the stone passes through the orifice of the duct, the symptoms disappear.

Persistent obstruction damages the gland, making it harder and more tender.

Previous history The patient may have had similar symptoms on the other side of the face. Simultaneous bilateral calculi are uncommon.

Examination

The lump

Position The submandibular gland lies beneath the horizontal ramus of the mandible on the mylohyoid muscle (Fig. 12.35). It is 2–3 cm in front of the anterior border of the sternomastoid muscle and should not be confused with enlarged upper deep cervical lymph glands, which are deep to the sternomastoid muscle.

Colour and temperature If the gland is not infected, the overlying skin will have a normal colour and temperature (Fig. 12.36). If the gland is infected, the skin becomes red, oedematous and hot.

Superficial part

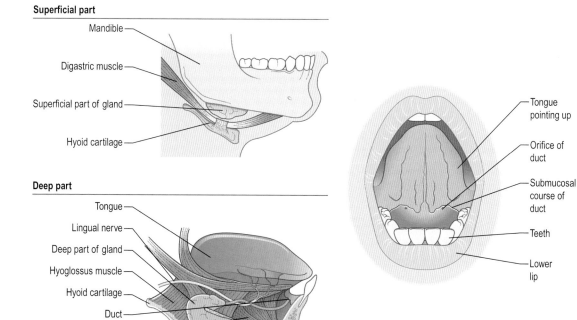

- Mandible
- Digastric muscle
- Superficial part of gland
- Hyoid cartilage

Deep part

- Tongue
- Lingual nerve
- Deep part of gland
- Hyoglossus muscle
- Hyoid cartilage
- Duct
- Glenioglossus muscle
- Mylohyoid muscle
- Jaw

- Tongue pointing up
- Orifice of duct
- Submucosal course of duct
- Teeth
- Lower lip

Fig. 12.35 The anatomy of the submandibular gland.

Fig. 12.36 A swollen right submandibular gland. Although some of the swelling seems to spread over the jaw, the upper part of the gland is actually deep to the mandible.

Tenderness The gland is tender when it is tense (before and during eating) but is not usually tender between meals, unless it is infected.

Shape The shape of the superficial part of the submandibular gland is a flattened ovoid (almond shaped).

Size If the gland is enlarged solely by obstruction of its duct, it rarely becomes more than 3–5 cm across. If it becomes infected, it may get much larger.

Surface Its surface is smooth but the lobules of the gland may make it bosselated.

Edge The anterior, posterior and inferior edges of the gland are distinct and easy to define, but the upper edge is wedged between the mandible and the mylohyoid muscle and is impalpable.

Composition A distended submandibular gland has a rubbery, hard consistency and will not fluctuate, transilluminate or reduce. It is dull to percussion and has no bruit.

Occasionally, prolonged pressure on the gland may make it a little smaller and produce a jet of saliva from the orifice of the submandibular duct.

Relations The skin is freely mobile over the swollen gland. The gland itself can be moved a little from side to side, but most movements are restricted by the tethering of the gland to the underlying muscles. When the muscles of the floor of the mouth are tensed by asking the patient to push their tongue against the roof of the mouth, the gland becomes less mobile.

It is important to ascertain the relations of the lump to the floor of the mouth and the tongue by bimanual palpation. Feel the lump between the gloved index finger of one hand inside the mouth and the fingers of the other hand on the outer surface of the lump.

It should be possible to appreciate that the lump is outside the structures that form the floor of the mouth. It should not be fixed to the mucosa of the floor of the mouth or to the tongue.

Lymph drainage Lymph from the submandibular gland drains to the middle deep cervical lymph glands, but there is also some lymphoid tissue within the gland that can contribute to its enlargement.

The local lymph glands are usually not enlarged unless the gland is infected.

Local tissues The nearby tissues, except the submandibular duct in the floor of the mouth, should be normal.

The floor of the mouth

Inspection Ask the patient to open their mouth and lift their tongue up to the roof of the mouth. This displays the orifices of the submandibular ducts on their small papillae on either side of the frenulum of the tongue.

If a stone is impacted at the end of the duct, its grey–yellow colour may be visible in the open orifice of the duct.

The presence of a stone in the duct makes that side of the floor of the mouth bulge upwards, look asymmetrical and a little reddened (see Fig. 12.34).

Press the gland gently and watch for any discharge from the orifice of the duct.

Palpation Feel along the course of the duct in the floor of the mouth for lumps and tenderness.

A stone in the duct will not feel stony hard if it is small and surrounded by inflammatory oedema. The lump caused by such a stone will feel soft with a hard centre.

General examination Examine all the salivary glands in case the symptoms are due to a systemic disease such as Sjögren's syndrome (see page 414) and not just a stone.

Submandibular sialadenitis

Infection of a submandibular gland invariably occurs secondary to the presence of a stone in its duct or the damage done by a stone that has passed through the duct. The infecting organism is usually *Staphylococcus*.

The symptoms are identical to those caused by a stone except that when the gland is infected the pain is severe, throbbing and continuous.

The physical signs of the lump in the neck are similar to those of the obstructed gland described above, with the addition of heat and tenderness. An infected gland may become quite big (5 × 10 cm). If the duct system becomes dilated (*sialectasis*), pus may pool in the gland and the whole structure turn into a multilocular abscess, which may then point externally onto the skin.

Submandibular salivary gland tumours

The tumours that often occur in the parotid gland – pleomorphic adenoma, cylindroma and carcinoma – may occur in the submandibular gland, but they are rare.

The physical features of pleomorphic adenoma and carcinoma in the submandibular gland are identical to the features of these tumours when they occur in the parotid gland, apart from the site.

A pleomorphic adenoma forms a painless, slow-growing, non-tender, hard, well-defined, spherical mass within the gland. Carcinoma causes an indistinct, warm, slightly tender, rapidly growing, painful mass. Numbness of the anterior two-thirds of the tongue indicates infiltration of the lingual nerve and is diagnostic of carcinoma.

It may be difficult to distinguish a pleomorphic adenoma from enlargement of the lymph tissue within the gland. A long history of slow, gradual growth is the most useful distinguishing feature.

The parotid gland

Acute bacterial parotitis

The most common infection of the parotid gland is mumps (Fig. 12.37). This is an epidemic viral parotitis; when it occurs in an epidemic, with bilateral painful, swollen glands and excessive oedema that spreads down into the neck giving the child a double chin, it is easy to diagnose.

When it causes unilateral gland enlargement (Fig. 12.38), little pain and no oedema, and there are no obvious contacts with the infection, it can be much more difficult to diagnose.

Non-specific parotitis, usually a staphylococcal infection, is caused by:

Fig. 12.37 Bilateral mumps in a young female.

Fig. 12.38 Unilateral mumps. A young female with diffuse swelling of the left parotid gland caused by mumps. Much of the swelling is caused by oedema.

- poor oral hygiene;
- dehydration;
- obstruction of Stensen's duct by a stone or scar tissue.

In the days before the fluid balance of sick or postoperative patients was properly controlled and administered, fulminating parotitis, with subsequent septicaemia, was a common cause of death.

History

Age Acute parotitis is more common in the elderly and the debilitated.

CHAPTER 12 | THE NECK

Symptoms The patient complains of a sudden onset of pain and swelling in the side of the face.

The pain is continuous and throbbing, and radiates to the ear and over the side of the head.

Speaking and eating cause pain because any movement of the temporomandibular joint is painful.

The patient feels hot, sweaty and ill and may complain of shivering attacks (rigors).

Systematic questions Systematic questioning may reveal symptoms of another illness, such as a bronchial carcinoma, which has caused the debility and dehydration.

Previous history The patient may have recently undergone a major operation or suffered a severe medical illness.

Examination

The lump

Position The parotid gland lies in front of and below the lower half of the ear. It is wrapped around the vertical ramus of the mandible, with its deep portion in between this bone and the mastoid process (Fig. 12.39).

In acute parotitis, the whole gland is swollen, so the whole of the face in front of the lower half of the ear bulges outwards.

Colour and temperature The skin over the swelling is discoloured a reddish-brown, feels hot and is smooth and shiny.

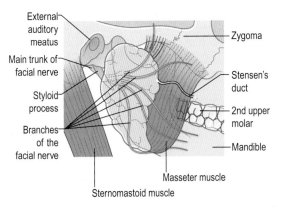

External auditory meatus
Main trunk of facial nerve
Styloid process
Branches of the facial nerve
Sternomastoid muscle
Masseter muscle
Zygoma
Stensen's duct
2nd upper molar
Mandible

Fig. 12.39 The anatomy of the parotid gland. Note that the parotid gland extends below and behind the angle of the mandible. Lumps in this part of the gland are easily mistaken for enlarged upper deep cervical lymph glands.

Tenderness The swelling is very tender.

Shape The mass has the shape of the normal parotid gland: a semi-circular anterior edge, a vertical edge just in front of the ear, and a bulge running into the gap between the mandible and the mastoid process.

Size The swollen gland may be three or four times larger than a normal gland.

Surface Its surface is smooth but difficult to define because of the oedema, inflammation and tenderness.

Composition The texture of the swelling is often described as brawny. This means that it has a firm consistency but is indentable. It is dull to percussion, not fluctuant and not compressible.

Relations If the overlying skin is red and oedematous, it will be tethered to the swelling. The swelling cannot be moved over the deep structures and becomes more prominent when the patient contracts the masseter muscles by clenching their teeth.

Lymph drainage The upper deep cervical lymph glands are usually enlarged and tender.

Local tissues Apart from the changes in the skin and the restricted movements of the temporomandibular joint, the surrounding tissues are normal. The function of the facial nerve is *not* impaired.

The mouth

Inspection The orifice of Stensen's duct is opposite the second upper molar tooth. The mouth of the duct may be patulous and the buccal mucosa over the course of the duct slightly oedematous.

Palpation Feel the mouth of the duct for any thickening or swelling.

The parotid gland cannot be palpated bimanually because it lies behind the anterior edge of the masseter muscle and the vertical ramus of the mandible.

Gentle pressure on the gland may produce a purulent discharge from the orifice of the duct.

Chronic parotitis

Chronic parotitis is usually caused by a small calculus or a fibrous stenosis blocking the drainage of Stensen's duct.

History

The patient complains of recurrent swelling of the parotid gland. The swelling is particularly noticeable before eating and is associated with an aching pain.

In severe cases, the gland becomes permanently swollen, but the pain is usually not constant.

Chronic parotitis maybe bilateral.

Examination

The whole gland is easy to feel because it is bigger and firmer than a normal gland and its edges are distinct (Fig. 12.40). It is also tender and feels rubbery hard.

If there is partial obstruction to the flow of saliva, pressure on the gland may produce a copious squirt of fluid through the orifice of the duct.

Examine all the other salivary glands to exclude a general abnormality.

Fig 12.40 Chronic parotitis. A firm, slightly tender enlargement of the whole of the parotid gland caused by recurrent infection secondary to a stone in Stensen's duct.

Pleomorphic adenoma

(Mixed parotid tumour, sialoma)

This is a true adenoma of the parotid gland. Its mixed histological appearance gave rise to its old name – mixed parotid tumour – and its currently favoured name, pleomorphic adenoma. It has also been called a sialoma.

It is a slow-growing adenoma with an incomplete capsule. The small pieces of tumour that protrude through the defects in its capsule limit its treatment by enucleation and allow its rapid extension if it turns malignant. After many years of slow, benign growth, a small proportion of adenomas can become locally invasive.

History

Age These tumours appear in early and middle adult life.
Sex They occur more often in males than in females.
Symptoms The patient complains of a painless swelling on the side of their face that has been present for months or years and is slowly growing.

The lump may be more prominent when the mouth is open or when eating. The latter symptom can cause confusion, so it is important to find out whether the lump just becomes more prominent because of contraction of the masseter muscle or actually increases in size.

Examination

Position The majority of parotid adenomas begin in the portion of the gland that lies over the junction of the vertical and horizontal rami of the mandible, just anterior and superior to the angle of the jaw.
Colour and temperature The temperature and colour of the overlying skin are normal.
Tenderness The lump is not tender.
Shape Most pleomorphic adenomas are spherical when they are small, but as they grow they become flat on their deep surface and slightly pointed superficially. They may become lobulated when very large (Fig. 12.41).
Size These tumours can vary from pea-sized nodules to large, almost pendulous, masses 20 cm across (Fig. 12.42).
Surface Their surface is smooth, sometimes bosselated, and occasionally crossed by deep furrows.

The surface of any deep extension between the mandible and the mastoid process is impalpable.

Edge The edge is quite distinct and easy to feel.
Composition The tumour mass has a rubbery, hard consistency, is dull to percussion, not fluctuant or translucent, and not compressible.
Relations The overlying skin and the ear are not attached to the lump.

Small tumours can be moved about over the deep structures, but large tumours are less mobile.

Lymph drainage The cervical lymph glands should not be enlarged.

CHAPTER 12 | THE NECK

(a)

(b)

Fig. 12.41 A PLEOMORPHIC ADENOMA
(a, b) These photographs show the typical site, the healthy overlying skin, the absence of facial nerve involvement and the lobulation that develops as the tumour grows.

Fig. 12.42 A very large, almost pendulous, pleomorphic adenoma of the parotid gland.

Local tissues Apart from any distortion caused by the mass, the local tissues should be normal. In particular, the facial nerve should function normally. Paralysis of any facial muscles indicates infiltration of the nerve, which means that the lump is a carcinoma, not a benign adenoma.

Examine the inside of the mouth

A pleomorphic adenoma in the deep part of the parotid gland will push the tonsil and the pillar of the fauces towards the midline.

Differential diagnosis

Other parotid tumours, such as acinic cell tumours (Fig. 12.43), can be difficult to differentiate simply on examination. Furthermore a preauricular lymph gland, enlarged by secondary infection or metastases, can also present as a firm, smooth swelling just in front of the tragus and be indistinguishable from a pleomorphic adenoma if it is not tender. The most distinctive physical sign of an enlarged preauricular lymph gland is its mobility. Most tumours in the parotid gland can only be moved a short distance because they are tethered to the gland; the

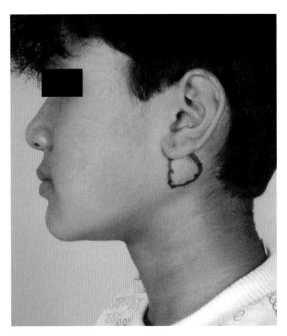

Fig. 12.43 An acinic cell tumour of the parotid gland, which is difficult to differentiate from a pleomorphic adenoma on simple clinical examination.

preauricular lymph gland lies outside the capsule of the parotid gland and is usually very mobile.

Adenolymphoma
(Warthin's tumour)

This is a cystic tumour that contains epithelial and lymphoid tissues. The epithelial element is believed to originate from embryonic parotid ducts that have become separated from the main duct system of the gland. The lymphoid element comes from normal lymph tissue associated with the developing gland.

The tumour arises on the surface of, or just beneath, the capsule of the parotid gland.

History

Age Adenolymphomas appear in middle and old age.
Sex They are more common in males than in females.
Ethnic group They do not occur in black people.
Symptoms The patient complains of a slow-growing, painless swelling over the angle of the jaw. The swelling may be bilateral.

Examination

Position An adenolymphoma usually develops in the lower part of the parotid gland, level with the lower border of the mandible (Fig. 12.44). This is slightly lower than the common site of origin of the pleomorphic adenoma.
Temperature and colour The overlying skin looks and feels normal.
Tenderness The lump is not tender.
Shape Adenolymphomas are spherical or hemispherical.
Size They are usually 1–3 cm in diameter.
Surface The surface is smooth and well defined.
Edge Its edge is distinct and sometimes makes the lump seem separate from the parotid gland.
Composition Adenolymphomas have a soft consistency, are dull to percussion and not translucent, and often fluctuate.
Relations The lump can usually be moved a little in all directions and is not attached to the skin.
Lymph drainage The cervical lymph glands should not be enlarged.
Local tissues The adjacent tissues are all normal.

Fig. 12.44 Warthin's tumour. An adenolymphoma of the parotid gland. This photograph shows the typical site of an adenolymphoma – just over the angle of the jaw. Although it looks similar to the pleomorphic adenoma shown in Fig. 12.41, it had a soft consistency.

CHAPTER 12 | THE NECK

Carcinoma of the parotid gland

Carcinoma of the parotid gland is uncommon but not rare. It can arise *de novo* or in a long-standing pleomorphic adenoma.

History

Age The patient is usually over the age of 50 years.
Sex Males and females are equally affected.
Symptoms The common complaint is of a rapidly enlarging swelling on the side of the face. The swelling is persistently painful, especially during movements of the jaw. The pain may radiate to the ear and over the side of the face (Fig. 12.45). The patient may give a history of a preceding painless lump that has been present for many years.

The patient may also complain of asymmetry of the mouth (Fig. 12.46) and difficulty in closing the eyes due to facial nerve involvement. Occasionally, the patient may require a lateral tarsorrhaphy (Fig 12.47) to protect the cornea from exposure and ulceration.

Examination

Position The swelling is in the site of the parotid gland.
Colour If the overlying skin is infiltrated by the tumour, it may be reddish-blue.
Temperature The skin and the mass are hyperaemic and hot.
Tenderness The mass is not very tender, an important difference from acute parotitis, which also presents as a hot swelling.
Shape The tumour may be of any shape. It is basically a flattened hemisphere, but as it spreads in different directions, its shape becomes irregular.
Size Its size increases inexorably.
Surface The surface is smooth but irregular.
Edge The edge is often indistinct.
Composition The mass has a firm, sometimes hard consistency, is dull to percussion but is not fluctuant or translucent. Although it may be very vascular, it does not have an audible bruit.
Relations Carcinoma of the parotid becomes fixed to the deep structures early in its growth and may also become fixed to, and infiltrate, the skin.

The thickening of the tissues around the temporomandibular joint may restrict jaw movements.

Fig. 12.45 Carcinoma of the parotid gland. This patient complained of a painful swelling in front of his ear. The swelling was hot and the overlying skin reddened. Although the swelling was not very large, there was some weakness of the muscles of facial expression.

Fig. 12.46 Asymmetry of the mouth due to facial nerve palsy.

Fig. 12.47 Lateral tarsorrhaphy to protect the cornea from ulceration after facial nerve palsy.

Lymph drainage The cervical lymph glands are likely to be enlarged and hard.

Local tissues If the facial nerve is infiltrated by tumour, the patient will be unable to use the muscles of facial expression. The signs may vary from mild weakness of the lower lip when baring the teeth to a complete VIIth cranial nerve palsy.

If the tumour has infiltrated into the mandible, the jaw will be swollen and tender.

General examination There may be evidence of disseminated blood-borne metastases.

Differential diagnosis Not all swellings in the parotid or submandibular region are caused by salivary gland pathology. Lymph nodes in these areas can mimic salivary gland enlargement (Figs 12.48 and 12.49) while primary skin lesions in these areas may potentially be misdiagnosed (Fig. 12.50).

Autoimmune disease

There are two syndromes of slow, progressive, but relatively painless enlargement of the salivary glands in which biopsy reveals that the swelling is caused by replacement of the glandular tissue by lymphoid tissue. Both conditions are believed to be autoimmune diseases.

Mikulicz's syndrome

Mikulicz's syndrome is:

- enlargement of the salivary glands: usually both the parotid and both submandibular glands enlarge, but the syndrome can begin and remain in one gland for quite a long time;

Fig. 12.49 Preauricular lymphadenopathy. Preauricular lymphadenopathy is a condition that is commonly mistaken for parotid gland enlargement. However, this woman's preauricular swelling was caused by a secondary deposit of carcinoma in the ascending ramus of the mandible.

Fig. 12.48 The submandibular swelling in this woman was a lymph gland enlarged by secondary deposits from a carcinoma of the tongue, and not a lesion of the submandibular gland.

Fig. 12.50 This ulcerating lesion over the parotid gland was initially diagnosed as a parotid carcinoma. However, there was no facial weakness and the lesion was actually in the skin. A biopsy revealed that it was a squamous cell carcinoma of the skin.

CHAPTER 12 | THE NECK

- enlargement of the lachrymal glands: this causes a bulge at the outer end of the upper eyelids and narrowing of the palpebral fissures;
- a dry mouth, which may be the presenting symptom: the patient is not thirsty.

It may be associated with lymphoma, leukaemia, sarcoidosis and tuberculosis.

Sjögren's syndrome

Sjögren's syndrome exhibits all the above characteristics, although the degree of salivary gland enlargement is often not so gross, plus:

- dry eyes;
- generalized arthritis.

Thyroglossal cyst

The thyroid gland develops from the lower portion of the thyroglossal duct, which begins at the foramen caecum at the base of the tongue and passes down to the pyramidal lobe of the isthmus of the thyroid gland. If a portion of this duct remains patent, it can form a thyroglossal cyst.

Theoretically, thyroglossal cysts can occur anywhere between the base of the tongue and the isthmus of the thyroid gland, but they are commonly found in two sites: between the isthmus of the thyroid gland and the hyoid bone, and just above the hyoid bone (Fig. 12.51). Thyroglossal cysts within the tongue and in the floor of the mouth are rare.

History

Age Thyroglossal cysts appear at any age, but the majority are seen in patients between 15 and 30 years old.

Sex They are more common in females than in males.

Symptoms The most common symptom is a painless lump in a prominent and noticeable part of the neck (Fig. 12.52). Pain, tenderness and an increase in size occur if the cyst becomes infected.

Duration of symptoms The lump may have been present for many years before an increase in its size causes the patient to complain.

Systemic symptoms There are no systemic symptoms.

(a) Subhyoid cyst.

(b) Pretracheal cyst.

Fig. 12.52 TWO THYROGLOSSAL CYSTS

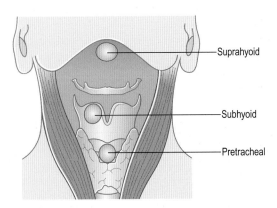

Fig. 12.51 The sites of a thyroglossal cyst.

Examination

Position Thyroglossal cysts lie close to the midline, somewhere between the chin and the second tracheal ring. In the fetus, the thyroglossal duct is in the midline, but when a cyst forms in adult life it often slips to one side of the midline, especially if it develops in front of the thyroid cartilage.

Colour, temperature and tenderness If the cyst is infected, the overlying skin will be red, hot and tender (Fig. 12.53); otherwise it is normal.

Shape and surface Thyroglossal cysts are spherical and smooth, with a clearly-defined edge.

Size They vary from 0.5 to 5 cm in diameter. Because a lump in the front of the neck is so noticeable, patients often complain of these cysts when they are very small.

Composition Thyroglossal cysts have a firm or hard consistency, depending upon the tension within the cyst. Some cysts are too tense and others too small to fluctuate, but the majority of thyroglossal cysts are between these extremes and fluctuate with ease. Some cysts transilluminate but many do not, either because the contents have become thickened by desquamated epithelial cells or the debris of past infection, or because they are too small.

Relations Thyroglossal cysts are tethered by the remnant of the thyroglossal duct. This means that they can be moved sideways but not up and down.

The thyroglossal duct is always closely related to the hyoid bone. When the hyoid bone moves, the cyst also moves.

The hyoid bone moves upwards when the tongue is protruded. First, ask the patient to open their mouth and keep the lower jaw still; next, hold the cyst with your thumb and forefinger, and then ask the patient to protrude their tongue. If the cyst is fixed to the hyoid bone, you will feel it tugged upwards as the tongue goes out. This is a difficult sign to elicit so it is easier to feel the tugging sensation than to actually see the movement. Although this test is diagnostic, the absence of movement does not exclude the diagnosis. Indeed, this sign is absent from many cysts that are below the level of the thyroid cartilage.

Lymph glands The local lymph glands should not be enlarged unless there is secondary infection of the cyst.

Local tissues Whenever there is an abnormality of thyroid gland development, examine the base of the tongue for ectopic (lingual) thyroid tissue. A lingual thyroid looks like a flattened strawberry sitting on the base of the tongue.

SYMPTOMS OF THYROID DISEASE

The thyroid gland can cause two groups of symptoms and signs: those connected with the swelling in the neck, and those related to the endocrine activity of the gland. In order to appreciate fully the symptoms and signs that may be produced by diseases of the thyroid, a clear understanding of the physiology of the gland is essential. The history and examination should be directed towards detecting both the local and general symptoms and signs that may be produced, either by any physical abnormality in the configuration of the thyroid or by any pathophysiological abnormality of its endocrine activity.

Neck symptoms

A lump in the neck

The majority of thyroid swellings grow slowly and painlessly. Quite often, the patient will come across a swelling coincidentally when washing, or a member of their family or a close friend will point

Fig. 12.53 An infected thyroglossal cyst.

CHAPTER 12 | THE NECK

it out to them. Other swellings may have been there for some years before the patient suddenly decides to seek advice concerning their nature and management. In a few patients, a lump will appear suddenly and may be painful, or a long-standing lump may enlarge quickly (Revision panel 12.5).

A rapid change in the size of part of the gland, or of an existing lump, may be caused by haemorrhage into a necrotic nodule, a fast-growing carcinoma or subacute thyroiditis. The sudden enlargement of a lump caused by haemorrhage is usually painful, whereas a fast-growing anaplastic carcinoma is not usually painful until it invades nearby structures.

A special feature of papillary and follicular carcinomas of the thyroid gland is their very slow growth. They may exist as a lump in the neck for many years before metastasizing. Thus, the length of time that a lump has been present is no indication of its underlying nature.

Discomfort during swallowing

Large swellings may give the patient a tugging sensation in the neck when they swallow. This is not true dysphagia. Thyroid swellings rarely obstruct the oesophagus because the oesophagus is a muscular tube that is easily stretched and pushed aside. However, because the thyroid has to be pulled upwards with the trachea in the first stage of deglutition, an enlarged gland can make swallowing uncomfortable, or even difficult.

Dyspnoea

Deviation or compression of the trachea by a mass in the thyroid may cause difficulty in breathing. This symptom is often worse when the neck is flexed laterally or forwards and when the patient lies down

---

Revision panel 12.5

A scheme for the diagnosis of swellings in the neck (deep to the deep fascia)

1 Is there one or more than one lump?
2 Where is the lump?
3 Is it solid or cystic?
4 Does it move with swallowing?

Multiple lumps are invariably *lymph glands*

A single lump

In the anterior triangle that does not move with swallowing

Solid:
    Lymph gland
    Carotid body tumour
Cystic:
    Cold abscess
    Branchial cyst

In the posterior triangle that does not move with swallowing

Solid:
    Lymph gland
Cystic:
    Cystic hygroma
    Pharyngeal pouch
    Occasionally a secondary deposit of a
        papillary thyroid carcinoma
Pulsatile:
    Subclavian aneurysm

In the anterior triangle that moves with swallowing

Solid:
    Thyroid gland
    Thyroid isthmus lymph gland
Cystic:
    Thyroglossal cyst

Revision panel 12.6

Physiology of the thyroid gland

Changes in hormone activity can be assessed by:

Clinical examination
Measuring circulating tri-iodothyronine (T3) and thyroxine (T4) levels
Measuring the rate and quantity of radioactive iodine taken up by the gland

Hormone secretion can be suppressed by:

Iodine, which inhibits hormone release
Potassium perchlorate, which interferes with iodine trapping
Carbimazole and propylthiouracil, which inhibit the iodination of tyrosine and the coupling of tyrosines to make thyronines
Destroying the gland surgically or with radiotherapy

supine. The whistling sound of air rushing through a narrowed trachea is called stridor.

Pain

Pain is not a common feature of thyroid swellings. Acute and subacute *thyroiditis* can present with a painful gland, and Hashimoto's disease often causes an uncomfortable ache in the neck.

Anaplastic carcinoma can cause local pain and pain referred to the ear if it infiltrates surrounding structures.

Hoarseness

A change in the quality of the voice of a patient with a lump in the neck is a very significant symptom because it is probably caused by a paralysis of one of the recurrent laryngeal nerves, which means that the lump is likely to be malignant and infiltrating the nerve.

Symptoms and signs of endocrine dysfunction

Every patient with any thyroid disorder should be carefully questioned and examined for any symptoms or signs of endocrine dysfunction (Fig. 12.54).

Symptoms and signs of hyperthyroidism/thyrotoxicosis (see also pages 426–429)

Nervous system Symptoms include nervousness, irritability, insomnia and nervous instability, and examination may reveal a tremor of the hands. Occasionally, a full-blown thyrotoxic psychosis may be apparent.

Cardiovascular system Symptoms include palpitations, breathlessness on exertion, swelling of the ankles and chest pain, which may be manifest as tachycardia, atrial fibrillation, dyspnoea and peripheral swelling.

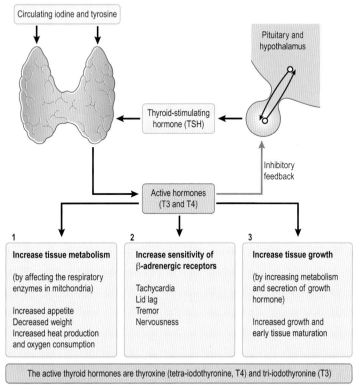

Fig. 12.54 The physiology of the thyroid gland (Revision panel 12.6).

Metabolic and alimentary systems There is an increase in appetite but loss of weight, and sometimes a change of bowel habit, usually diarrhoea. Proximal muscle myopathies may occur with wasting and weakness. The patient has a preference for cold weather, and often complains of excessive sweating and an intolerance of hot weather. Some women have a change of menstruation, usually amenorrhoea.

Symptoms and signs of hypothyroidism/myxoedema (see also pages 429–430)

There is an increase in weight, with deposition of fat across the back of the neck and shoulders. Symptoms also include: slow thought, speech and action; intolerance of cold weather; loss of hair, especially the outer third of the eyebrows; muscle fatigue; a dry skin and 'peaches and cream' complexion; and constipation.

EXAMINATION OF THE THYROID GLAND

Concentrate upon both the nature of any gland enlargement or abnormal configuration, as well as any change in endocrine activity. It is best to assess both aspects in a combined approach rather than try to assess each separately.

Look at the whole patient

First confirm that the swelling in the neck is in the thyroid gland by watching to see if it moves when the patient swallows. Then look at the whole patient.

Are they sitting still and composed, or fidgeting about, constantly moving their fingers and looking nervous and agitated, or are they slow and ponderous in their movements?

Are they thin or fat? What is the distribution of any wasting or fattening? Patients with thyrotoxicosis have a generalized loss of weight, especially about the face, but may also have localized wasting of their hands, face and shoulder muscles.

Are they under-clothed and sweaty, or wrapped up in a large number of jumpers but still cold?

Look at the hands

- Feel the pulse. Tachycardia suggests thyrotoxicosis (hyperthyroidism); bradycardia suggests myxoedema (hypothyroidism). In middle-aged and elderly patients, thyrotoxicosis may cause atrial fibrillation – in fact, it may be the only sign of this in elderly patients.
- Are the palms moist and sweaty?
- Is there a tremor? Test for a tremor by asking the patient to hold their arms out in front of them, with the elbows and wrists straight, and fingers straight and separated. Thyrotoxicosis causes a fine, fast tremor. If in doubt, hold out your own hand beside the patient's for comparison. A fine tremor may be accentuated by placing a sheet of paper over the fingers.

Examine the eyes

Eye symptoms

Patients who suffer from thyrotoxicosis may complain of staring or protruding eyes and difficulty closing their eyelids (*exophthalmos*), double vision caused by muscle weakness (*ophthalmoplegia*) and swelling of the conjunctiva (*chemosis*). They may get pain in the eye if the cornea ulcerates. (See Revision panel 12.7.)

There are four important underlying changes that can occur in the eyes of patients with hyperthyroidism that produce the above effects (Figs 12.55 and 12.56). Each one may be unilateral or bilateral.

Lid retraction and lid lag

This sign is caused by overactivity of the involuntary (smooth muscle) part of the levator palpebrae superioris muscle. If the upper eyelid is higher than normal and the lower lid is in its correct position, the patient has lid retraction. Do not be deceived into thinking this abnormality is caused by exophthalmos.

When the upper lid does not keep pace with the eyeball as it follows a finger moving from above downwards, the patient has lid lag.

Exophthalmos

If the eyeball is pushed forwards by an increase in retro-orbital fat, oedema and cellular infiltration,

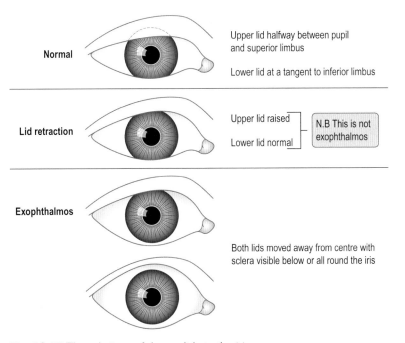

Normal — Upper lid halfway between pupil and superior limbus

Lower lid at a tangent to inferior limbus

Lid retraction — Upper lid raised / Lower lid normal — N.B This is not exophthalmos

Exophthalmos

Both lids moved away from centre with sclera visible below or all round the iris

Fig. 12.55 The relations of the eyelids to the iris.

(a) Exophthalmos.

(b) Unilateral lid retraction.

(c) Exophthalmos and lid retraction.

(d) Severe lid retraction but no exophthalmos.

Fig. 12.56 SOME EYE SIGNS ASSOCIATED WITH THYROTOXICOSIS

CHAPTER 12 | THE NECK

(e) Exophthalmos but no lid retraction.

(f) Wasting and loss of hair (and exophthalmos).

(g) Chemosis. The conjunctiva is hyperaemic and bulging over the eyelid. There is exophthalmos, lid retraction and periorbital oedema.

(h) This patient had gross chemosis and exophthalmos but the eye was pulsating. The cause of these abnormalities was a carotid artery–cavernous sinus fistula.

Fig. 12.56 SOME EYE SIGNS ASSOCIATED WITH THYROTOXICOSIS (continued)

the normal relationship of the eyelids to the iris is changed. The sclera becomes visible below the lower edge of the iris (the inferior limbus).

Because the eyes are pushed forwards, the patient can look up without wrinkling the forehead, but they will have difficulty converging. In severe exophthalmos, the patient cannot close their eyelids and may develop corneal ulceration.

Ophthalmoplegia

Although exophthalmos stretches the eye muscles, it does not usually affect their function. The cause of the weakness of the ocular muscles

(ophthalmoplegia) associated with severe exophthalmos is oedema and cellular infiltration of the muscles themselves and of the oculomotor nerves. The muscles most often affected are the superior and lateral rectus and inferior oblique muscles. Paralysis of these muscles prevents the patient looking upwards and outwards.

Chemosis

Chemosis is oedema of the conjunctiva. The normal conjunctiva is smooth and invisible. A thickened, crinkled, oedematous and slightly opaque conjunctiva is easy to recognize.

Chemosis is caused by the obstruction of normal venous and lymphatic drainage of the conjunctiva by the increased retro-orbital pressure.

Inspect the neck (Fig. 12.57, Revision panel 12.8)

After checking that the lump is in the anatomical site of the thyroid gland, ask the patient to swallow. The patient may need a sip of water to help deglutition. All thyroid swellings ascend during swallowing.

Observe the general contours and surface of the swelling. The skin can be puckered, tethered and pulled up by swallowing if the patient has an advanced thyroid carcinoma that has infiltrated into the skin, but this is a late manifestation of anaplastic carcinoma and very uncommon.

Ask the patient to open their mouth and then to put out their tongue. If the lump moves up as the tongue comes out, it must be attached to the hyoid bone, and is likely to be a thyroglossal cyst.

The neck veins will be distended if there is a mass obstructing the thoracic inlet.

Look at the position of the thyroid cartilage. Is it in the centre of the neck or deviated to one side?

Palpate the neck from the front

The most important part of palpation is done from behind, but it is worthwhile placing your hand on any visible swelling while standing in front of the patient, to confirm your visual impression of its size, shape and surface, and to find out if it is tender.

Check the position of the trachea. This is best done by feeling with the tip of two fingers in the suprasternal notch. The trachea should be exactly central at this point. When a thyroid mass extends below the suprasternal notch and obscures the trachea, you must examine the thyroid cartilage. A mass that is displacing the trachea will tilt the thyroid cartilage laterally.

Palpate the neck from behind the patient (Fig. 12.57)

Stand behind the patient. Place your thumbs on the ligamentum nuchae and tilt the patient's head slightly forwards to relax the anterior neck muscles. Let the palmar surface of your fingers rest on each side of the neck; they will be resting on the lateral lobes of the thyroid gland. A small lobe can be made prominent and easier to feel by pressing firmly on the opposite side of the neck.

Ask the patient to swallow while you are palpating the gland to confirm that any swelling moves with swallowing and is actually part of the thyroid. This manoeuvre also lifts up lumps that are lying behind the sternum into the reach of your fingers. With a retrosternal extension of the thyroid, it is important to assess whether you can feel the lower border of the gland on swallowing or whether there is still a significant extension lying behind the sternum.

At the end of palpation, you should know the following facts about the gland and/or the lump: tenderness, shape, size, surface and consistency.

A normal thyroid gland is not palpable.

Palpate the whole of the neck for any cervical and supraclavicular lymphadenopathy.

CHAPTER 12 | THE NECK

(a) Look at the eyes and the neck and ask the patient to swallow.

(b) Palpate the neck from behind, with the thumbs pushing the head forwards to flex the neck slightly.

(c) Palpate both lobes and the isthmus with the fingers flat.

(d) If one lobe is difficult to feel, make it more prominent by pressing firmly on the opposite side.

(e) Feel the trachea.

(f) Percuss the lower limit of the gland.

(g) Listen over the gland for a systolic bruit.

Fig. 12.57 EXAMINATION OF THE THYROID GLAND

Percussion

Percussion is used to define the lower extent of a swelling that extends below the suprasternal notch by percussing along the clavicles and over the sternum and upper chest wall. This can be done when standing in front of or behind the patient. However, this does not always provide a reliable assessment of the extent of a retrosternal goitre. Percussion of the lump in the neck itself is rarely helpful.

Auscultation

Listen over the swelling. Thyrotoxic and vascular glands and lumps may have a systolic bruit.

General examination

Pay particular attention to the cardiovascular and nervous systems for any evidence of hyperthyroidism or hypothyroidism, the signs and symptoms of which are described on pages 426–430.

DIFFERENT FORMS OF GOITRE (FIG. 12.58)

Simple hyperplastic goitre

Simple enlargement of the thyroid gland is invariably caused by excess stimulation with thyroid-stimulating hormone (TSH), the production of which is stimulated by low levels of circulating thyroid hormone. Relative iodine deficiency is the most common pathological cause for a low level of

(a) A large colloid goitre. The patient was euthyroid.

(b) A large central solitary nodule.

(c) A nodular goitre extending below the sternum and causing venous obstruction. Distended veins are visible above the right clavicle. The patient was euthyroid.

(d) Beware! Not all lumps in the neck are thyroid swellings. This mass was soft and did not move with swallowing. It was a lipoma. Never make a spot diagnosis; examine every lump carefully and thoroughly.

Fig. 12.58 VARIOUS GOITRES

thyroid hormone production. Physiological states that require increased activity of the thyroid gland, such as puberty and pregnancy, are also associated with enlargement of the gland.

The term 'colloid goitre' is used to describe the late stage of diffuse hyperplasia, when all the acini are distended with colloid that has not been released because the stimulation by TSH has dropped off.

History

Age In areas where goitre is endemic (i.e. prevalent in the local population), hyperplastic goitres appear in childhood.

Sporadic physiological hyperplastic goitres appear at puberty, during pregnancy and during severe illnesses and emotional disturbances, so they are commonly seen in puberty and young adult life.

Sex Hyperplastic goitres are five times more common in females than in males.

Geography Endemic goitre is common in places where the drinking water has a low iodine content, such as the habitable valleys of the Alps, Andes, Himalayas and Rocky Mountains, and the lowland areas a long way from the sea that depend upon water from mountain ranges, such as the Nile Valley, Congo Delta and Great Lakes of the USA. The rain that falls on the mountains has a normal iodine content, but the iodine is filtered out by the time it reaches the springs and streams of the highland valleys.

Diet Some vegetables contain chemicals that are goitrogens (i.e. they interfere with hormone synthesis). An excess dietary intake of the brassica family of foods (e.g. cabbage, sprouts and kale) can cause a goitre.

Local symptoms The principal complaint is of a swelling in the neck. This appears slowly and without pain.

If it becomes large – especially if it remains as a colloid goitre after the initial stimulus has gone – it can cause pressure symptoms such as dyspnoea, venous engorgement and mild discomfort during swallowing.

General symptoms Diffuse hyperplastic goitres are not usually associated with clinically significant hyperfunction or hypofunction of the gland.

Long-standing colloid goitres often become nodular goitres and occasionally secondary thyrotoxicosis (*Plummer's syndrome*), or secondary hypothyroidism may develop.

Examination

Position The swelling occupies the anatomical site of the thyroid gland.

Tenderness It is not tender.

Shape The swelling usually follows the configuration of the gland and can be seen to have two lobes and an isthmus.

Size Physiological goitres are only two or three times larger than a normal gland, but iodine-deficiency goitres can become very large.

Surface The surface of a hyperplastic goitre is smooth. If it turns into a colloid goitre, its surface becomes bosselated and, in time, nodular.

Composition The gland feels firm and is dull to percussion. Hyperaemic physiological goitres may have a very soft systolic bruit.

Relations The gland moves upon swallowing. The other tissues in the neck should be normal.

Lymph glands The deep cervical lymph glands should not be palpable.

The eyes The eyes should be normal.

General examination The patient is usually euthyroid.

Multinodular goitre

Multinodular goitres develop spontaneously and in glands subjected to prolonged stimulation (i.e. hyperplastic glands). They can therefore be endemic (in iodine-deficient areas) or sporadic (occurring haphazardly).

A nodular goitre results from a disorganized response of the gland to stimulation, and contains areas of both hyperplasia and hypoplasia.

The cut surface of a nodular goitre reveals nodules with haemorrhagic, necrotic centres, separated by normal tissue. The normal tissue contains normal active follicles; the nodules contain both hyperactive and degenerate, involuting, follicles.

When the nodules are hyperplastic, the patient may develop secondary thyrotoxicosis.

In long-standing nodular goitres, most of the nodules are inactive and the quantity of normally active follicles may be so reduced that thyroid hormone production is inadequate and hypothyroidism may develop.

History

Age In endemic areas, nodular goitres appear in early adult life (15–30 years). Sporadic nodular goitres appear later, between the ages of 25 and 40 years.

Sex Nodular goitres are six times more common in females than in males.

Geography These goitres are common in areas where the drinking water is deficient in iodine (see 'Simple hyperplastic goitre').

Symptoms The most common presenting symptom is an enlarging, painless swelling in the neck, which may cause dyspnoea, discomfort when swallowing, stridor and engorged neck veins.

Sudden enlargement and pain can occur if there is haemorrhage into a necrotic nodule. Necrotic nodules are not cysts, and it is wrong to call this event a haemorrhage into a cyst.

Secondary thyrotoxicosis (Plummer's syndrome) occurs in a significant proportion (maybe as high as 25 per cent) of patients with long-standing nodular goitres. The symptoms of thyrotoxicosis are listed earlier in the chapter.

Myxoedema/hypothyroidism: as the follicular hyperplasia and its stimulation subside, the patient is left with a devastated gland that has little normal tissue. Ultimately, its endocrine secretions are inadequate and the patient has a considerable chance of becoming hypothyroid by the time they reach 60 or 70 years of age. The symptoms of myxoedema/hypothyroidism are described below.

Examination

Position The swelling is in the lower third of the neck in the anatomical site of the thyroid gland and is usually asymmetrical.

Tenderness A nodular goitre is only tender when there has been a recent haemorrhage into a nodule.

Shape and size The nodules are asymmetrical and the gland can become any shape. Nodules in the isthmus are prominent. The nodules may extend below the clavicles and the sternal notch, into the superior mediastinum.

Surface The surface of a nodular goitre is smooth but nodular. Frequently, only one nodule may be palpable, even though the rest of the gland is grossly diseased. This is termed a 'dominant nodule' and malignancy must be excluded.

Composition The consistency of the nodules varies: some feel hard, others feel soft. There is an old saying that 'Solid lumps in the thyroid feel cystic, whereas cystic lumps feel solid'. The explanation is that a nodule composed of thyroid tissue is soft, whereas a nodule full of blood and liquefied necrotic tissue becomes tense and feels hard.

The nodules do not fluctuate or transilluminate. There should be no bruit over the gland.

Relations The lump will move upwards during swallowing, indicating that it is fixed to the trachea. It should not be fixed to any other nearby structures.

Lymph drainage The cervical lymph glands should not be palpable.

Local tissues The trachea may be compressed and/or deviated, depending on the site of the nodules. Bilateral nodules will compress the trachea into a narrow slit, causing dyspnoea and stridor – especially during lateral flexion of the neck. Large unilateral nodules will push the trachea laterally.

When the trachea is pushed to one side, the 'keel' of the larynx is tilted away from the midline.

If the gland is jammed in the thoracic inlet, it may obstruct and distend the jugular veins.

Rarely, the goitre is so large that it starts to cause pressure on the overlying skin, and on occasions it may even start to ulcerate through (Fig. 12.59).

Fig. 12.59 A large goitre causing skin changes and imminent ulceration.

The eyes The eyes should be normal. It is unusual to get neurological or eye changes with secondary thyrotoxicosis associated with a nodular goitre. These systems are affected more often in primary thyrotoxicosis.

General examination There may be general signs of thyrotoxicosis – especially the cardiovascular signs or, in elderly patients with very long-standing nodular goitres, signs of hypothyroidism.

The solitary nodule

Although only one nodule may be palpable, approximately one-half of the patients who present with a solitary nodule actually have a multinodular goitre, i.e. a clinically dominant nodule in a macroscopical multinodular goitre (see Revision panel 12.9).

Revision panel 12.9

Causes of a 'solitary' nodule in the thyroid gland

A dominant nodule in a multinodular goitre

Haemorrhage into a nodule

A cyst

Adenoma

Carcinoma (papillary or follicular)

Enlargement of the whole of one lobe (usually Hashimoto's disease)

It is unusual to be able to determine the pathology of a solitary nodule by clinical examination. Thus, although the majority of solitary nodules are benign, they must all be investigated, as many well-differentiated carcinomas of the thyroid present as solitary nodules. Fine-needle aspiration to determine the cytology of the nodule has become part of the routine clinical examination in most clinics.

Thyrotoxicosis caused by a solitary toxic/autonomous adenoma is uncommon and is rarely caused by a solitary malignant nodule.

The causes of a solitary nodule in the thyroid gland are:

- a dominant nodule in a multinodular goitre;
- haemorrhage into, or necrosis of, a hyperplastic nodule;
- a cyst;
- an adenoma;
- carcinoma (papillary or follicular);
- enlargement of the whole of one lobe by thyroiditis.

THYROTOXICOSIS AND MYXOEDEMA (HYPERTHYROIDISM AND HYPOTHYROIDISM)

Thyrotoxicosis

Thyrotoxicosis is caused by an excess of circulating thyroid hormone. The gland may be diffusely hyperplastic (Graves' thyroiditis), nodular or the site of disease such as thyroiditis or an adenoma, but rarely a carcinoma.

The terms 'primary' and 'secondary' are used to describe thyrotoxicosis arising in a previously normal or previously abnormal gland, respectively. They can be confusing terms, but primary thyrotoxicosis (Graves' disease) is usually caused by a form of autoimmune thyroiditis, whereas secondary thyrotoxicosis (Plummer's syndrome) usually occurs in a long-standing multinodular goitre.

The thyroid hormones tri-iodothyronine (T3) and thyroxine (T4) have three effects:

- They increase the metabolic rate of all cells.
- They increase the sensitivity of beta-adrenergic receptors.
- They stimulate all cells to grow, but the effect on growth is only significant before natural growth has finished.

The increased tissue metabolism causes an increased appetite, a decrease in weight and an increase in heat production.

The increased adrenergic receptor sensitivity causes tachycardia, extrasystoles, atrial fibrillation, tremor, nervousness, lid retraction and lid lag.

Stimulation of growth during childhood produces early maturation and a slight increase in the rate of growth.

In myxoedema (hypothyroidism), all of these symptoms are reversed. The lack of growth stimulation in a child causes dwarfism.

History

Age Primary thyrotoxicosis occurs most often in young women, between 15 and 45 years of age. Toxic autonomous nodules can occur at any age.

Secondary thyrotoxicosis (from a nodular goitre) occurs in middle age – between 45 and 65 years.

Sex Primary thyrotoxicosis is ten times more common in females than in males.

Geography Secondary thyrotoxicosis is more common in those areas where simple hyperplastic goitre (and nodular goitre) is endemic.

Metabolic symptoms The patient complains of a ravenous appetite, but in spite of eating excessively, tends to lose weight. Patients may also find that they always feel warm and therefore like cold weather and dislike hot weather. There may be excessive sweating.

Cardiovascular symptoms The patient complains of palpitations, shortness of breath during exertion, missed and irregular heart beats (extrasystoles and atrial fibrillation) and tiredness. Cardiovascular symptoms are often the presenting symptoms of secondary thyrotoxicosis, whereas atrial fibrillation may be the only sign of thyrotoxicosis in an elderly patient.

Neurological symptoms Symptoms such as nervousness, irritability, insomnia, depression and excitement, even mania and melancholia, may be noticed by close relatives long before the patient is aware of them.

There may be hyperaesthesia, headaches, vertigo and tremors of the hands and tongue.

The patient may complain that their eyes have become more protuberant and that some eye movements are difficult.

Alimentary symptoms The changes in appetite and weight have been mentioned under metabolic symptoms. There is often a slight change in bowel habit – usually mild diarrhoea.

Genital tract symptoms Most women have a reduction in the quantity of their menses; some have amenorrhoea.

Musculoskeletal symptoms In addition to generalized weight loss, there may be specific wasting and weakness of the small muscles of the hand, shoulder and face. These muscles rarely become completely paralysed.

Cause Patients with primary thyrotoxicosis may relate the onset of their symptoms to puberty, pregnancy, an illness or a sudden emotional upset. Although it is difficult to be certain that events of this sort are the prime cause of hypersecretion of the thyroid gland, they undoubtedly exacerbate any hidden or developing abnormality. They are sometimes remembered as the three S's – sex (puberty and pregnancy), sepsis and psyche!

Examination

Signs in the neck

The thyroid gland is usually enlarged, but thyrotoxicosis can be present without any enlargement of the gland.

The enlargement may be diffuse, nodular or tender, depending on the local pathology (Fig. 12.60).

A diffusely enlarged hyperaemic gland usually has a systolic bruit audible over its lateral lobes.

Signs in the eye

Thyrotoxicosis is associated with four groups of physical signs in the eyes (see Figs 12.55 and 12.56).

Lid retraction and lid lag These are common signs. In lid retraction, the upper eyelid crosses the eye above its usual level (midway between the pupil and the superior limbus of the iris) because the autonomic part of the levator palpebrae superioris muscle is hypertonic.

Ask the patient to follow your finger as you move it slowly from above, downwards. If the upper eyelid does not keep pace with the eye, the patient has lid lag. This is also caused by the increased tone of the levator palpebrae superioris muscle.

The patient may blink less frequently than normal.

Exophthalmos Oedema of the retro-orbital tissues pushes the eye forwards. The first abnormality is the appearance of sclera below the inferior limbus, but when the condition is extreme the eye appears to be popping out and the eyelids cannot be completely closed.

(a) A small goitre, nervousness and agitation, with the start of weight loss.

Fig. 12.60 THE VARIED APPEARANCES OF THYROTOXICOSIS

(b) A nodular goitre. No eye or nervous system signs, but palpitations, breathlessness and atrial fibrillation.

Exophthalmos makes convergence difficult and allows the patient to look up without raising their eyebrows or wrinkling their forehead. Corneal ulceration may complicate severe exophthalmos.

Ophthalmoplegia Infiltration of the ocular muscles weakens the eye muscles and diminishes the eye movements. The muscles most often affected are the superior rectus and inferior oblique muscles. As these muscles normally turn the eye upwards and outwards, this is the first movement to become weak.

Chemosis This is oedema of the conjunctiva. The conjunctiva becomes thick, boggy and crinkled and may bulge over the eyelids. The eyes water excessively.

General signs

These are best described in systems.

Metabolic signs The patient looks thin and their face and hands may be particularly wasted. They may look hot and be sweating, even in a cold room.

(c) A large goitre, increasing appetite but weight loss – particularly of the face and shoulder girdle – with no eye signs.

Cardiovascular signs There is usually a tachycardia of 90 beats per minute or more at rest, which persists during sleep.

If there are extrasystoles or atrial fibrillation, the pulse will be irregular.

If there is mild heart failure, there may be râles at the bases of the lungs and oedema of the ankles.

Neurological signs The patient looks worried and nervous and moves in an agitated, jerky way. They will often twist a handkerchief between their fingers.

A fine tremor may be demonstrated when they stretch out their hands with their fingers spread. A similar tremor may be present in the protruded tongue.

Musculoskeletal signs The muscles of the hands, shoulders and face may be wasted and weak and the fingertips enlarged.

Skin In certain patients with Graves' disease, red, blotchy, raised areas may be seen over the shins. This is termed *pretibial myxoedema* and is caused by deposits of myxoid tissue within the skin (Fig. 12.61).

Myxoedema

History

Myxoedema is the clinical state that follows a severe lack of thyroid hormone (*hypothyroidism*). The term myxoedema means 'mucous swelling' and is used because when it was first described it was believed that the increase in weight and body swelling was caused by a new form of oedema.

Age Myxoedema tends to occur in middle and old age.

Sex It is more common in females than in males.

Metabolic symptoms The patient complains of tiredness and weakness, which can lead to intense physical and mental lethargy. These symptoms may come on insidiously, and therefore the patient simply ascribes their symptoms to their age or the everyday pace of life.

The patient always feels cold, and therefore likes hot weather and dislikes cold weather. They gain weight but have a poor appetite.

Cardiovascular symptoms Breathlessness and ankle swelling indicate the onset of cardiac failure.

Neurological symptoms The patient finds it difficult to think and to speak quickly and clearly.

Fig. 12.61 Pretibial myxoedema.

Hallucinations, dementia ('myxoedema madness') and, in severe cases, 'myxoedema coma' can occur.

Alimentary symptoms Progressive and obdurate constipation is common.

Genital tract symptoms Menorrhagia is common when myxoedema occurs before the menopause.

Examination

Signs in the neck

The thyroid gland may be enlarged by long-standing disease such as a nodular goitre, but in many cases the neck is normal.

Signs in the eyes

The eyes are normal but the eyelids become swollen and heavy, making the patient look sleepy and lethargic.

The hair of the outer third of the eyebrows falls out.

CHAPTER 12 | THE NECK

General signs

General appearance and metabolic signs Myxoedema produces a puffy face, a generalized, non-pitting increase in the subcutaneous tissues of the trunk and limbs, and a dulling of thought, speech and action. In a white-skinned patient with myxoedema, the complexion is said to resemble 'peaches and cream'. The skin is smooth and has a pale-yellow (the cream) colour. The cheeks are often slightly flushed and have a pink-orange tinge (the peaches) (Fig. 12.62).

The skin is dry and inelastic and does not sweat. Although it may look oedematous, it does not pit after prolonged pressure.

The patient is overweight, with excess connective tissue and fat in the supraclavicular fossae, across the back of the neck and over the shoulders.

The hair looks thin, ragged and falls out.

The hands are puffy and spade-like.

The tongue enlarges and seems to fill the mouth during speech and interferes with the articulation of words. The voice becomes deep and hoarse.

All the signs of myxoedema may develop insidiously and may not always be obvious; therefore, they must be looked for carefully if a hypothyroid state is suspected (Fig. 12.63).

Cardiovascular signs The pulse rate is slow (40–60 beats per minute) and the blood pressure is low. Both these changes may be reversed if heart failure develops.

The hands are usually cold and the fingertips blue.

Neurological signs Mental alertness and the ability to respond to questions and solve problems are noticeably retarded. Conversation is hampered by the difficulty in articulation caused by enlargement of the tongue.

All movements are slow and deliberate.

The reflexes are sluggish and their relaxation period prolonged.

Cretinism

A cretin is a child whose mental and physical development has been retarded by a lack of thyroid hormone. Nowadays this condition is rare because the hormone deficiency can be replaced.

Cretinism is likely to occur in those places where goitre is endemic. The child may have a goitre.

Fig. 12.62 The facies of myxoedema. Thinning of the hair, loss of the outer third of the eyebrows, a 'peaches and cream' complexion and thickening and heaviness of the eyelids.

Fig. 12.63 This woman has myxoedema. There is some loss of hair, especially the outer third of the eyebrows, and heaviness of the face and creamy skin, but none of these features is diagnostic. This emphasizes that early myxoedema is difficult to recognize.

The child has an underdeveloped skeleton (dwarfism) and a large protruding tongue, the eyes are wide apart, and the skull is also wide. The limbs and neck are short and the hands spade-like.

The skin is dry and there are supraclavicular pads of fat.

The abdomen is distended and protruberant, and there is often an umbilical hernia.

There is mental retardation, even imbecility.

When hypothyroidism occurs in older children, they develop a mixture of the symptoms of cretinism and myxoedema.

CARCINOMA OF THE THYROID GLAND

The thyroid gland is a very vascular organ, and secondary tumour deposits from primary lesions in the breast, stomach, colon and lung can be found at autopsy. However, these secondary deposits rarely become large and noticeable and rarely present as a thyroid swelling. The majority of the neoplasms in the thyroid gland that present as a lump in the neck are primary thyroid tumours.

There are three varieties of carcinoma of the thyroid follicles:

- papillary carcinoma;
- follicular carcinoma;
- anaplastic carcinoma.

The parafollicular (C) cells can also undergo malignant change, and this cancer is called *medullary carcinoma*.

The lymphoid tissue in the gland can also undergo malignant change to become a lymphoma, but this is not a true thyroid tissue neoplasm. Lymphoma is more common in patients with Hashimoto's disease.

Papillary carcinoma

This tumour contains a few formed follicles, but its bulk consists of hyperplastic follicular epithelium with a papilliferous configuration that sometimes produces a small quantity of colloid. This tumour spreads in the lymphatics. The cervical lymph glands may be palpable long before the primary lesion in the thyroid gland becomes palpable.

History

Age Papillary carcinoma is a tumour of children and young adults. Because it occurs in young children, the metastases in the lymph glands were once thought to be clusters of 'lateral aberrant thyroid' tissue, but they are not. They are true metastases and may often be the presenting feature. These enlarged nodes may present as large cystic swellings and mimic a branchial cyst.

Sex Females are affected three to four times more often than males.

Symptoms The common presenting symptom is a lump in the neck. The lump may be in the region of the thyroid gland or, if it is caused by secondary deposits in the lymph glands, in the anterolateral part of the neck.

Distant secondary deposits or a change in thyroid function are very uncommon.

Duration of symptoms The lump may have been present for many years before the patient seeks advice, because these tumours are slow growing and slow to spread beyond the thyroid gland and its draining lymph glands.

Cause It is important to ask for any history of radiation to the neck or mediastinum. There is a greater incidence of papillary carcinoma in children who have had their neck or chest irradiated intentionally for conditions such as asthma, tuberculosis, enlargement of the thymus, tonsillitis and acne (a form of treatment no longer practised), or unintentionally following a nuclear reactor accident.

Examination

The principal abnormality is a lump or lumps in the neck.

Position The lump may be in the region of the thyroid gland or deep to the sternomastoid muscle.

Temperature and tenderness The skin of the neck should be normal, provided there is no tumour infiltration. The lumps are usually not tender.

Shape and size The primary nodule in the thyroid gland may vary in size from a minute, impalpable nodule to a nodule 3–5 cm in diameter. When palpable, it is usually spherical, smooth and clearly defined, but its surface may be bosselated.

Lymph glands containing thyroid carcinoma metastases are ovoid or nodular, and usually smooth and clearly defined. Occasionally, they are cystic, providing a diagnostic dilemma. The thyroid gland lymph first drains to the pretracheal and paratracheal lymph glands and then to the lower deep cervical lymph glands, which lie beneath the anterior edge of the lower third of the sternomastoid muscle.

Composition The consistency of both the primary nodule and the secondary lymph glands is hard or firm. Both are dull to percussion, do not fluctuate and do not cause a bruit.

Relations The primary nodule in the thyroid gland will move upon swallowing and is not usually fixed to superficial structures.

Enlarged lymph glands move more easily in a transverse than in a vertical plane and do *not* move with swallowing. They are not usually attached to the skin.

Lymph drainage If a nodule is felt in the thyroid gland, examine all the lymph glands in the neck with care.

General examination The patient usually appears fit and well, without any of the systemic signs which suggest a disseminated neoplasm or thyroid dysfunction.

Follicular carcinoma

The cells in this well-differentiated thyroid cancer retain their normal follicular configuration. Most of the follicles contain a small amount of colloid, which implies that the cells are synthesizing hormone. This has an important bearing on treatment because the tumour cells will often take up radioactive iodine. This tumour spreads by the bloodstream.

History

Age Follicular carcinoma occurs in adults between the ages of 20 and 50 years.

Sex Females are affected more than males.

Symptoms The common presenting symptom is a lump in the neck, which may have been present for many years.

If the tumour has spread beyond the thyroid gland, the patient may complain of breathlessness, chest pain or pain or swelling in a bone, caused by lung and bone metastases, respectively. In these circumstances, the pathologist usually finds that the tumour has a thin capsule and has spread into the substance of the gland – the 'invasive' variety of follicular carcinoma.

Multiple lumps in the neck caused by metastases in lymph glands do occur, but not as frequently as with papillary carcinoma.

Systemic effects These patients are euthyroid.

Examination

The principal abnormality is a lump in the neck.

Position Follicular carcinoma usually arises in one of the lateral lobes of the thyroid gland.

Temperature and tenderness The overlying skin is not hot and the lump is not tender.

Shape and size The lump is usually spherical and smooth, with distinct edges. Even the invasive variety feels as if it has a distinct surface. Occasionally, a poorly differentiated follicular carcinoma can arise in a long-standing multinodular goitre (Fig. 12.64).

Composition The lump is firm to hard, does not fluctuate, is dull to percussion and has no bruit.

Relations The lump moves with swallowing but is not attached to overlying structures.

Lymph glands The deep cervical lymph glands may be enlarged and hard.

Local tissues The local tissues are usually normal.

General examination Examine the chest carefully for any evidence of consolidation or collapse. Pulmonary secondary deposits are quite common but may not cause any abnormal physical signs.

Metastases in the skeleton are often painful and tender. A bone near to the skin containing a metastasis may be visibly deformed, swollen and hot. Some thyroid cancer metastases are so vascular that they are soft and pulsatile and have an audible bruit.

Anaplastic carcinoma

This is the worst variety of thyroid cancer because it spreads rapidly. Most patients with this disease

Fig. 12.64 A poorly differentiated follicular carcinoma arising in a long-standing multinodular goitre.

are dead within 1 year of diagnosis. Its cells do not synthesize thyroid hormone.

History

Age Anaplastic carcinoma of the thyroid gland appears between the ages of 60 and 80 years.

Sex Females are affected more often than males.

Symptoms The common complaint is a swelling of the neck rather than 'a lump', which may be rapidly growing. The patient complains of swelling because the tumour is diffuse and infiltrating, not localized.

A dull aching pain in the neck is quite common.

Dyspnoea occurs when the tumour begins to compress the trachea, especially when the neck is flexed. It may also occur if there are multiple pulmonary metastases.

Hoarseness or a change in the quality of the voice is a diagnostic symptom because it implies infiltration of the recurrent laryngeal nerve.

Pain in the ear, caused by infiltration of the vagus nerve, is not uncommon.

There may be bone pain. Any bone can be the site of a secondary deposit, and pathological fractures can occur.

General malaise and weight loss appear when there is disseminated disease.

Duration of symptoms The symptoms of an anaplastic carcinoma often develop rapidly as this carcinoma grows quickly and is highly invasive. Local invasion and compression of the trachea can lead to death from asphyxia or precipitate a fatal pneumonia.

Examination

Position The swelling in the neck is in the region of the thyroid gland. At first this is in one lobe, but in advanced cases the whole gland may be enlarged and irregular (Fig. 12.65).

Colour The overlying skin often has a red–blue tinge because the underlying infiltration interferes with its venous drainage.

Temperature The skin temperature is normal or slightly raised.

Tenderness The mass often becomes tender as the tumour infiltrates beyond the thyroid gland.

Shape The mass in the neck has no definable shape once it has spread beyond the thyroid gland, and before this stage it is not easy to define because the surface is so indistinct.

Fig. 12.65 An anaplastic carcinoma of the thyroid.

Size The mass may become so big that it interferes with neck movements.

Surface and edge The surface is irregular and indistinct and the lump often has no palpable edge.

Composition The mass is hard and solid. It does not fluctuate, is dull to percussion and has no bruit.

Relations Provided the mass is not infiltrating the whole neck, it will move during swallowing.

It may be fixed to one or both sternomastoid muscles and the overlying skin as well as to the trachea. When the sternomastoid muscle is contracted, the movement of the lump during swallowing is limited and the skin becomes puckered. With wider extension and fixation to surrounding tissues, the mass becomes fixed.

The skin may be infiltrated with tumour, making it thick, nodular and a reddish-brown colour.

Lymph glands Although the deep cervical lymph glands are invariably involved in the disease, their enlargement may be obscured by the primary mass in the gland.

If the local lymph glands are palpable, they feel hard and fixed. At first they are smooth and discrete, but they become irregular and indistinct when the tumour begins to spread through their capsules.

CHAPTER 12 | THE NECK

Local tissues The skin of the neck may be tethered or fixed to the lump or even infiltrated with tumour.

The trachea is often compressed and deviated, causing stridor.

One vocal cord may be paralysed by infiltration of the recurrent laryngeal nerve. This may be suspected if the patient has a hoarse voice, but it must be confirmed by indirect laryngoscopy.

All the soft tissues of the neck may be fixed and hardened by infiltrating tumour.

General examination Patients often breathe with difficulty and have stridor. There may be basal pneumonia or collapse caused by pulmonary secondary deposits or the restriction of lung expansion by the narrowed trachea.

There is often wasting and anaemia.

There may be evidence of skeletal metastases – even pathological fractures.

In advanced cases, the liver may be enlarged, and secondary deposits occasionally appear in the skin.

Medullary carcinoma

This is a rare condition but can sometimes be diagnosed before operation. It is a neoplasm of the parafollicular (C) cells.

The common presentation is a firm, smooth and distinct lump in the neck, indistinguishable from any other form of thyroid solitary nodule.

The majority of patients are between the ages of 50 and 70 years when the tumour is sporadic in nature. When the condition occurs in young adults (20–30 years), often with a family history, it may be a manifestation of the *multiple endocrine neoplasia syndrome* (MEN) type 2a or 2b.

In these cases, the medullary thyroid carcinoma may be accompanied by associated conditions such as:

- phaeochromocytoma – MEN 2a;
- parathyroid tumours;

or

- phaeochromocytoma;
- neuromas of the tongue, lips and conjunctivae – MEN 2b (Fig. 12.66);
- pale brown birthmarks;
- megacolon;
- a marfanoid habitus.

Fig. 12.66 Tongue neuromas in a patient with multiple endocrine neoplasia type 2b and medullary carcinoma of the thyroid.

Symptoms that may indicate a medullary tumour, apart from a lump in the neck and the presence of the above lesions in the patient or their family, are diarrhoea and flushing. Diarrhoea occurs in one-third of the patients. The fluidity of the stool and the frequency of defaecation are both increased.

If this tumour is suspected, it is important to measure the serum calcitonin level.

THYROIDITIS

There are three varieties of thyroiditis that can be diagnosed clinically: Hashimoto's disease, de Quervain's thyroiditis and Riedel's thyroiditis.

The term 'thyroiditis' is a non-specific description of the histological changes occurring in the gland. Although the aetiology of these conditions is only partly understood, the eponyms are useful because they do not imply an aetiology but rather a clinical description.

Hashimoto's disease

This is an autoimmune thyroiditis. The body fails to recognize part of itself – in this case both the mitochondria of the thyroid cells and the thyroglobulin they produce – and sets up an immune response against its own tissues. The result is a lymphocyte and plasma cell infiltration of the gland that ultimately destroys the thyroid cells. In the first instance, the thyroid cells respond by becoming hyperplastic, causing a degree of thyrotoxicosis, but eventually and inevitably the gradual destruction of the thyroid cells causes myxoedema (hypothyroidism).

History

Age and sex Hashimoto's disease is most common in middle-aged females, especially those near the menopause, but it can occur in males and at any age.

Symptoms in the neck The patient usually complains of a swelling or lump in the neck. This lump may appear gradually or rapidly and is often painful, particularly when it appears rapidly.

The swelling, or lump, fluctuates in size, and the pain is often intermittent. The symptoms are worse when the patient is tired or run down, or has an intercurrent illness.

The voice should not alter.

Systemic effects The symptoms of mild thyrotoxicosis or myxoedema may be present.

The common course of events is for the mild symptoms of thyrotoxicosis, which appear at the onset of the disease, to die out gradually and become replaced by the opposite symptoms of myxoedema.

The majority of patients are euthyroid when they complain of the lump, having ignored or not had any symptoms of thyrotoxicosis, and not reached the myxoedematous phase.

This variability of the local and systemic effects of the disease makes the diagnosis difficult.

Family history Other members of the family may have suffered from the same or other forms of autoimmune disease, such as pernicious anaemia and autoimmune gastritis.

Examination

The main complaint is usually a lump in the neck.

Position The swelling is in the region of the thyroid gland and may be unilateral or bilateral.

Temperature In the initial acute phase − if it occurs − the overlying skin may feel warm.

Tenderness The swelling is often slightly tender.

Shape The swelling may be any shape − a solitary nodule, the whole of one lobe or the whole gland. When one lobe or more is involved, the swelling is usually lobulated.

Size Hashimoto's disease usually causes a moderate swelling of the gland, easily visible but rarely gross.

Surface The swelling has a smooth surface and the edge is distinct.

Composition The swelling has the texture of firm rubber. This texture is homogeneous, in spite of the lobulated shape, which helps to distinguish the swelling from a nodular or colloid goitre.

There is no bruit.

The composition and mild tenderness are the features that may alert you to the possibility of the diagnosis.

Relations The swelling moves with swallowing but is not fixed to any other structures.

Local tissues All the local tissues should be normal.

Lymph glands The nearby lymph glands should not be enlarged.

General examination The majority of patients are euthyroid, but some will have the signs of mild thyrotoxicosis and others of early myxoedema.

De Quervain's thyroiditis

This condition is a true subacute inflammation of the thyroid gland, often associated with mild hyperthyroidism. It may be caused by a virus infection and sometimes occurs in epidemics.

History

De Quervain's thyroiditis occurs in adults. The main complaint is of the sudden appearance of a painful swelling in the neck. The patient feels ill and may notice that they are anxious, sweaty and hungry and have palpitations.

Examination

Examination reveals a diffuse, firm, tender swelling of the whole of the thyroid gland.

There may be signs of mild thyrotoxicosis − nervousness and agitation, lid lag and tachycardia.

De Quervain's thyroiditis is self-limiting. It disappears in 1−3 months.

CHAPTER 12 | THE NECK

If only one lump is palpable it may be:

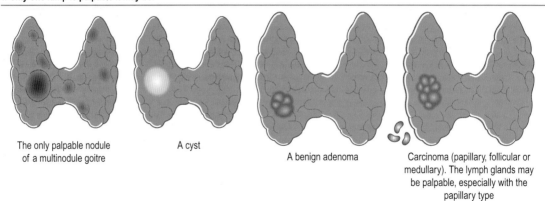

The only palpable nodule
of a multinodule goitre

A cyst

A benign adenoma

Carcinoma (papillary, follicular or
medullary). The lymph glands may
be palpable, especially with the
papillary type

If more than one lump is palpable the swelling may be:

The whole of one lobe involved by
Hashimoto's thyroiditis

A multinodular goitre

An anaplastic carcinoma especially
if the voice is hoarse and the mass
is fixed to the surrounding tissue

If diffusely enlarged it may be:

Grave's disease. Primary
thyrotoxicosis. Slight to moderate
enlargement. Soft, smooth with
a bruit

Hypoplastic (colloid) goitre.
Moderate to gross enlargement.
Bosselated. No bruit

Thyroiditis. Hashimoto's,
de Quervain's or Riedel's.
Moderate or small. Hard, tender

Multifocal carcinoma

Fig. 12.67 A SCHEME FOR THE DIAGNOSIS OF THYROID SWELLINGS

Once you have examined the patient, you should be able to draw conclusions on the nature and texture of the gland and on its endocrine activity.

The gland
1. Solitary palpable nodule
2. Multinodular goitre
3. Diffusely enlarged gland

Activity of the gland
1. Normal (euthyroid)
2. Hypersecretion (hyperthyroidism/thyrotoxicosis)
3. Hyposecretion (hypothyroidism/myxoedema)

Having established the configuration of the gland and its endocrine activity, a table of possible differential diagnoses can be drawn up (Table 12.1). This allows a degree of clarity in interpreting the presenting clinical features and in arriving at a working diagnosis.

Riedel's thyroiditis

This is a very rare condition but can be mistaken for an anaplastic carcinoma.

The gland is gradually replaced by dense fibrous tissue, which may even infiltrate beyond the gland into the nearby strap muscles.

The patient complains of a lump in the neck or, very rarely, increasing dyspnoea caused by compression of the trachea.

Examination reveals a stony hard swelling of the thyroid gland, at first of one lobe, but eventually of both lobes and the isthmus.

The lump moves with swallowing but may be fixed to the surrounding tissues, which are otherwise normal.

When both lobes are involved, the smooth, discrete surface usually excludes the diagnosis of carcinoma, but when one lobe is involved, it is impossible to make a firm clinical diagnosis.

Note A scheme for diagnosing thyroid swellings is shown in Fig. 12.67.

PARATHYROID DISEASE

Parathyroid conditions are rarely accompanied by clear physical signs. It is extremely uncommon to be able to palpate an abnormal parathyroid gland in the neck, although very rarely a large carcinoma may be felt, in itself a very rare condition. The only physical signs that may be noted in parathyroid disease relate to the functional abnormalities of the parathyroid glands.

Hypoparathyroidism

The most common cause of hypoparathyroidism is damage or removal of the glands at the time of thyroidectomy. This can result in hypocalcaemia, which can produce tingling and numbness in the face nerve irritability and a positive Chvostek's sign, which is contraction and twitching of facial muscles when the skin over the facial nerve is tapped at the angle of the jaw where the nerve leaves the parotid gland. The patient may also suffer from spontaneous carpopedal spasm. Latent tetany can be produced by placing a sphygmomanometer cuff on the arm above systolic blood pressure, when carpal spasm can occur (Fig. 12.68). This is known as Trousseau's sign.

Fig. 12.68 Trousseau's sign of hypocalcaemia.

Hyperparathyroidism

The classical clinical features of hyperparathyroidism relate to '*stones, bones and abdominal groans*'. The symptoms are attributable to both the direct effects of parathormone on the organs such as the kidneys and bones and also to the effects of the resultant hypercalcaemia.

Around 50–80 per cent of patients with primary hyperparathyroidism are said to be asymptomatic, but some will exhibit neuropsychiatric or non-specific constitutional symptoms that revert to normal after parathyroidectomy. Such non-specific symptoms can include thirst, polyuria, anorexia, weight loss and muscle weakness. Indeed, many patients will say that they feel much better after surgery without being able to specify why.

Symptomatic patients mainly present with bone changes, but few patients present with clinical bone disease or radiological evidence of bone resorption, although most will have some changes in bone density. Around 50 per cent of patients will have biochemical indications of increased bone turnover, but only 2 per cent will have radiological manifestations.

Table 12.1　Correlation between clinical state of the thyroid gland, endocrine function and pathological diagnosis

Clinical state	Hypothyroid	Euthyroid	Hyperthyroid
Diffuse enlargement	Thyroiditis	Iodine deficiency Enzyme defects Goitrogens Thyroiditis Amyloid Physiological (pregnancy, puberty)	Primary hyperthyroidism (Graves' disease)
Multinodular enlargement	Multinodular goitre with gross degeneration	Multinodular goitre Lymphoma Anaplastic carcinoma Medullary carcinoma	Secondary hyperthyroidism (Plummer's syndrome)
Solitary nodule	Coincidental nodule with myxoedema	Cyst Dominant nodule Adenoma Follicular or papillary carcinoma	Autonomous toxic nodule
No palpable goitre	Thyroiditis Primary myxoedema Post-thyroidectomy or postradioactive iodine	Normal gland	Primary hyperthyroidism Thyroxine overdose

13 The breast

More than a quarter of general surgical outpatient referrals are of females with breast symptoms, but less than 10 per cent of general surgical operations are for breast disease. Most patients require no more than reassurance, but the rapid identification of those few with malignant disease remains a challenge.

Breast cancer has the best prognosis of the common solid organ malignancies, and with constantly improving treatments up to 80 per cent of sufferers are alive and well 10 years after diagnosis. Nevertheless, public perception and constant media attention ensure that females with breast symptoms tend to be more anxious than other surgical patients.

Development and physiology of the breast

Breast development is occasionally seen in neonates as a consequence of maternal oestrogens crossing the placenta. Babies of both sexes may be affected and lactation can occur ('witches' milk'), sometimes complicated by abscess formation.

Female breast development commences shortly before the menarche. It may be asymmetrical and uncomfortable, and cause parental anxiety.

The breasts increase in size in the second half of each menstrual cycle, following ovulation. Mild pain and tenderness are common during this phase.

In pregnancy and lactation, the size and texture of the breasts change profoundly, making clinical assessment more difficult.

HISTORY AND EXAMINATION OF BREAST DISEASE

History

Age The age of the patient is a good pointer to the diagnosis. Young females rarely have cancer, but over the age of 70 years, most breast lumps turn out to be malignant.

It is essential to ask specifically about any family history of breast disease as well as the following.

Previous pregnancies How many children has the patient had? Were the children breast-fed and, if so, for how long?

Parity and breast-feeding reduce the incidence of breast cancer: a mother of five breast-fed children is less likely to have breast cancer than a nulliparous woman of the same age.

Relation of symptoms to menstruation Breast symptoms that alter with the menstrual cycle are more likely to be due to benign disease.

Medication Is the patient taking drugs containing female sex hormones? Oral contraceptives reduce the severity of cyclical change in the breasts. Hormone replacement therapy taken by menopausal and postmenopausal patients extends the age at which they are likely to suffer from benign conditions such as breast cysts.

Patient perception Patients are often fearful of the consequences of breast lumps and occasionally hide their symptoms with an impressive degree of self-delusion. One may be told, particularly by elderly patients, that a fungating cancer was only noticed last week when it has clearly been present for much, much longer. Be sympathetic – you do not know how you would react in similar circumstances.

Examination (Fig. 13.1)

Position

The patient must be undressed to the waist, resting comfortably on an examination couch with her upper body raised at 45°. This position allows good access to all areas of the breast. When a patient says that the lump can only be felt in a certain posture they should of course be examined in this position as well.

Inspection

Stand or sit directly in front of the patient, and look for the following (Revision panel 13.1).

(a) Look at the breast for asymmetry and for changes in the skin and nipple.

(b) Ask the patient to raise her hands above her head. This exaggerates asymmetry and skin tethering.

(c) Feel the breast with the flat of your fingers.

(d) Test the mobility of every lump in two directions, with the pectoralis muscles relaxed and tense. Tense the muscles by asking the patient to place her hands on her hips and press inwards.

(e) When you palpate the axilla, hold the patient's arm to relax the muscles that form the axillary folds.

(f) Compare the axillae simultaneously.

Fig. 13.1 EXAMINATION OF THE BREAST

Size There is enormous variation, with individual sensitivity at each extreme.

Symmetry It is quite normal for there to be a difference between the sides. However, any marked size difference of recent onset is likely to be caused by significant pathology.

Skin The skin may be pulled in or puckered by an underlying cancer. There may be oedema caused by obstruction of skin lymphatics by cancer cells, which is commonly referred to as *peau d'orange*, an accurate description. Other skin changes include visible tumour nodules or a malignant ulcer caused by direct invasion of the skin by a cancer.

The colour of the nipples and areolae changes with age, and there is darkening during pregnancy. The areolar skin is naturally corrugated with small nodules known as *Montgomery's tubercles*.

The nipple may be inverted. Is this bilateral, is it of recent origin or long-standing, and does it display the transverse slit pattern seen in duct ectasia? There may be evidence of fluid leaking from the nipple, or there may be eczema-like skin changes as in Paget's disease.

Duplication There may be accessory nipples along the mammary line from axilla to groin (Fig. 13.2), or visible ectopic breast tissue in the anterior axillary fold (Fig. 13.3).

Ask the patient to raise her arms slowly above her head. Skin changes may then become more apparent, particularly tethering to a carcinoma. Exposure of the underside of the breasts in an obese patient with large breasts may reveal intertrigo.

Ask the patient to press her hands against her hips to tense the pectoral muscles. This may reveal a previously invisible swelling.

Inspect the axillae, arms and supraclavicular fossae. Grossly enlarged lymph glands may be visible, and distended veins or arm lymphoedema may be obvious.

Fig. 13.2 Supernumerary nipples.

Fig. 13.3 An ectopic mass of breast tissue in the axillary tail. This is easily mistaken for a pathological abnormality.

Revision panel 13.1

Points to remember when examining the breast

History

Menarche, menopause, changes during the menstrual cycle, pregnancies, lactation, family and drug history

Examination

Expose the trunk above the waist

Inspect the breasts at rest and ask the patient to raise her arms above her head

Look at:

Size
Symmetry
Skin:
    Puckering
    Peau d'orange
    Nodules
    Discolouration
    Ulceration
Nipples and areolae
Axillae, arms and neck

Feel the normal side first

Examine the axillae and arms

Examine the supraclavicular fossae

Carry out a general examination

CHAPTER 13 | THE BREAST

Palpation

The breast should be palpated with the flat of the fingers and not with the palm of the hand.

Begin with the symptomless side or face the patient and feel both breasts simultaneously. The texture of the breast is enormously variable depending on age, parity, body mass and hormonal activity. It may be quite soft and apparently featureless, or it may be firm and fibrous, with easily palpable nodules, which are in fact normal lobules. In a menstruating woman and at the end of the second half of the menstrual cycle, the breasts may be engorged and tender.

In thin females, the lobular structure may be discernible and the breast tissue may be picked up between the fingers. In females with large breasts, gravity pulls the breast downwards and outwards, and the axillary tail may be readily palpable as a nodular ridge on each side. Sometimes the upper border of firm breast tissue is easily palpable separate from the subcutaneous fat.

Do not forget to feel the axillary tail, which lies over the anterior axillary fold. This may be very obvious in a slim woman with firm breast tissue. Occasionally, this part of the breast seems to be separate from the main breast and so presents as an apparent axillary swelling (Fig. 13.3).

Do not be discouraged by your initial difficulty in differentiating normal from abnormal breast tissue. Clinical examination remains an art, not a science.

If you find a lump, ascertain its *site*, *shape*, *size*, *surface*, *edge* and *consistency*, as with a lump in any other area of the body. This may require bimanual examination, controlling the movement of the lump with one hand and feeling the lump with the other.

Sometimes after a thorough palpation you may fail to find the swelling. If so, ask the patient to show it to you. She may then demonstrate to you a very obvious abnormality. Do not take this personally – it happens to the most experienced. Even if you still cannot feel the lump that the patient can, take the symptom seriously and arrange further investigations or a re-examination. Believe the patient and not your inexperienced fingers.

Relations to skin

There is a difference between skin fixation and skin tethering (Fig. 13.4).

When a lesion is fixed to the skin, it has spread into the skin and cannot be moved or separated from it.

A tethered lesion is one which is more deeply situated and distorts the fibrous septa (the *ligaments of Astley Cooper*) that separate the lobules of breast tissue. This puckers the skin, but the lesion remains separate from it and can be moved independently.

Most lumps can be moved anywhere within the arc depicted, without moving the skin

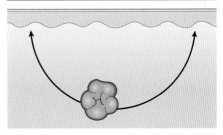

If when a lump is pulled outside the arc the skin indents, it is **tethered**

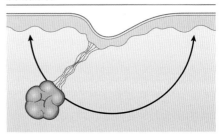

If a lump cannot be moved without moving the skin, it is **fixed**

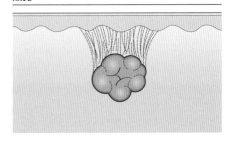

Fig. 13.4 Tethering and fixation.

Relations to the structures beneath the breast

The difference between fixation and tethering to deep structures is less obvious because the muscles beneath the breast are invisible when relaxed. If there is a deep-seated lump, ask the patient to press her hand against her hip, which tenses the pectoral muscles. If the lesion is then less mobile, it is either fixed or tethered.

The nipple

An inverted nipple may be everted by gentle squeezing the areolar edge or by asking the patient do it for you.

Nipple inversion that is easily everted is within the normal range.

If the nipple will not evert, there is likely to be underlying disease.

Unilateral inversion is more significant than bilateral inversion.

Recent-onset inversion is more worrying than long-standing nipple inversion.

If the patient complains of discharge, it may be possible to express fluid by gently pressing the areola (or the patient will again help). Observe whether any fluid comes from one or many duct orifices. Nipple discharge may be red, white, creamy yellow or watery (Revision panel 13.2).

Revision panel 13.2

The changes that can occur in the nipple

Destruction

Depression (retraction or inversion)

Discolouration

Displacement

Deviation

Discharge

Duplication

The axilla

The axilla is a difficult area to examine unless there is gross pathology. Small, firm, 'shotty' glands can commonly be felt in thin patients, but usually on both sides. In the obese, it may be virtually impossible to feel even significantly enlarged glands.

The axillary contents form a three-sided pyramid whose apex is in the narrow gap between the first rib and the axillary vessels.

Stand on the patient's right side. Take hold of her right elbow with your right hand and let her forearm rest on your right forearm. Persuade her to allow you to take the weight of her arm. The patient may try to help by holding the arm away from her side, but this tenses the muscles in the anterior and posterior axillary folds and makes palpation more difficult. Place your left hand flat against the chest wall and sweep the tips of your fingers from the top of the axilla and from side to side to feel the nodes against the chest wall.

To reach the apex of the axilla, you will have to push the tips of your fingers upwards and inwards. This may cause discomfort, so explain this to the patient, who may also be ticklish.

Next, move your left hand anteriorly over the anterior axillary fold and downwards into the axillary tail and behind the edge of the pectoralis major muscle.

To palpate the left axilla, lean across the patient, hold her left elbow with your left hand and use your right hand to feel the axilla. It may be easier to move round to her left side. With a cooperative patient who is able to relax (and is not ticklish), good access to the axillae is obtained by palpating both sides simultaneously from in front. This method is particularly useful for comparison when there are bilateral palpable but not abnormal glands.

Finally, feel the supraclavicular fossae and the neck.

General examination

A full examination includes checking the arms for any swelling or neurological or vascular abnormalities, and examination of the abdomen.

Triple assessment

In the UK, most patients with breast problems are seen in dedicated breast clinics. The diagnostic mainstay is *triple assessment*, comprising:

1   history and examination;
2   imaging by mammography and/or ultrasound scanning;
3   cytology or histology (Revision panel 13.3).

Cytological examination looks at cells obtained by aspiration of a lump with a fine needle.

Histological examination looks at tissue in biopsy specimens obtained with special core-cutting needles, often with image guidance.

Revision panel 13.3

Triple assessment of a breast lump

History and examination

Imaging by mammography and/or ultrasound scanning

Cytology by aspiration or histology by core biopsy

PRESENTATION OF BREAST DISEASE

Breast disease presents in three main ways:

- a lump, which may or may not be painful;
- pain, which may or may not be cyclical;
- nipple discharge or a change in appearance.

The most *likely* diagnoses when the patient presents with one or more of the above are listed below.

A painless lump

- Carcinoma.
- Cyst.
- Fibroadenoma.
- An area of fibroadenosis.

A painful lump

- An area of fibroadenosis.
- Cyst.
- Periductal mastitis.
- Abscess (usually postpartum or lactational).
- Occasionally a carcinoma.

Pain and tenderness but no lump

- Cyclical breast pain.
- Non-cyclical breast pain.
- Very rarely, a carcinoma.

Nipple discharge

- Duct ectasia.
- Intraduct papilloma.
- Ductal carcinoma-in-situ (DCIS).
- Associated with a cyst.

Changes in the nipple and/or areola

- Duct ectasia.
- Carcinoma.
- Paget's disease.
- Eczema.

Changes in breast size and shape

- Pregnancy.
- Carcinoma.
- Benign hypertrophy.
- Rare large tumours.

Remember that carcinoma, the only life-threatening disease of the breast, can present in almost any way, to which must be added the findings on screening mammography in asymptomatic females.

CARCINOMA OF THE FEMALE BREAST

Cancer of the breast is in females the most common cancer and the second most common cause of cancer death (after lung cancer). There are many macroscopic varieties and histological types. The amount of fibrous tissue that surrounds the cancer cells is highly variable. Sometimes most of the mass is fibrous stroma, with just a few scattered cancer cells, or the cancer may be highly cellular, vascular and rapidly growing.

The cut surface of a carcinoma is classically concave, rough, gritty and pale grey with prominent yellow and white flecks. Breast cancers are said to 'cut like an unripe pear'. The cut surface of a benign lesion bulges out to become convex, is white rather than grey, and feels smooth and rubbery, not gritty.

Cancer is the Latin word for a crab, and use of the word for malignant tumours comes from the cut surface appearance of some breast carcinomas.

In a proportion of cases, the malignant cells arising from the duct endothelium are confined to the ducts and do not invade through the epithelium. This is termed ductal carcinoma-in-situ (DCIS). It may present with nipple discharge, or as a lump in a manner similar to invasive cancer. Fine streaks of calcium deposits, known as microcalcification, are common and show clearly on mammography.

Should carcinoma cells migrate along the ducts to the nipple, they produce the skin changes known as Paget's disease.

History

Age Carcinoma of the breast is extremely rare in teenagers and unusual in the twenties. From the thirties onwards, there is a progressively increasing incidence, which peaks in the late fifties. The condition remains common into old age.

Symptoms As the breast is a surface organ, presenting symptoms relate to the primary lesion. Only rarely does it present with distant metastases.

Classically, the patient notices a painless lump, the size of which does not correlate with the length of the history. Occasionally, a prickling sensation in the breast draws attention to the swelling. The first symptom may be an axillary lump, with the primary lesion in the breast being less obvious or even impalpable.

The patient may notice skin dimpling caused by tethering.

The nipple may become retracted or destroyed.

The breast may be noticed to have changed shape or feel hard.

Backache due to bony metastases is a common symptom of advanced disseminated disease, but an uncommon mode of presentation. Occasionally, a pathological fracture may be the first sign of the disease, as may symptoms from cerebral, lung or abdominal deposits.

Curiously, systemic symptoms commonly associated with cancer, such as malaise and weight loss, are not found in patients with breast cancer. Even those with disseminated disease usually feel well in themselves (apart from bone pain) until the final stages.

Family history Two per cent of females with breast cancer have the *BRCA* gene. This declares itself before the age of 40 years, and other members of the family will have been affected, some of them with ovarian cancer as well.

Breast cancer is a common disease, so finding several sufferers in one family is not unusual. Whether there is a significantly increased risk in those with a strong family history but without the specific gene is unclear.

Parity Carcinoma of the breast is more common in nulliparous females, and less common with increasing numbers of children and with breast-feeding.

Examination (Figs 13.5 and 13.6)

A technique for examining the breast is described above.

Site Half of all breast cancers occur in the upper outer quadrant, including the axillary tail. Remember to examine the entire breast.

(a) **Displacement** and **deviation**. The left nipple is elevated (displaced) and pointing downwards and inwards, not downwards and outwards (deviation). The tumour can be seen just above the areola.

(b) **Retraction** and **displacement**. The left nipple has been pulled into the breast (retraction) and pulled upwards (displacement) by the underlying carcinoma.

(c) **Retraction** and **peau d'orange**. This carcinoma has invaded the skin and ulcerated. The skin of the lower part of the breast is oedematous and looks like the skin of an orange.

(d) **Destruction**. The right nipple and areola have been invaded and destroyed by the underlying carcinoma.

Fig. 13.5 CHANGES IN THE NIPPLE CAUSED BY AN UNDERLYING CARCINOMA

CHAPTER 13 | THE BREAST

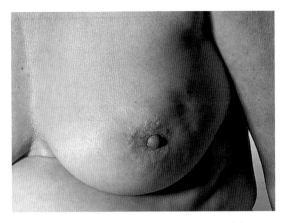

(a) Retraction, deviation and displacement of the nipple. Puckering and tethering of the skin. Visible axillary lymphadenopathy.

(b) Secondary lymphoedema of the left arm caused by metastases in the lymph glands.

(c) Fixation to the skin and the underlying muscle.

(d) Massive enlargement of the breast with secondary nodules of tumour in the skin.

(e) A fungating carcinoma with local secondary tumour nodules in the surrounding skin. The axillary lymphadenopathy is again visible as well as palpable.

Fig. 13.6 SOME DIAGNOSTIC FEATURES IN ADVANCED CARCINOMA OF THE BREAST

Tenderness Most tumours are not tender, but palpation may produce discomfort, sometimes because of the patient's fear of the consequences of the surgeon finding a lump.

Temperature Only the very rare 'inflammatory' type of breast cancer feels warm.

Shape A carcinoma of the breast may grow into any shape. The disease may also be multifocal, and it is not that unusual to find two separate primary tumours.

Surface The surface is usually indistinct, which makes it difficult to define the shape except when the lesion is small. However, a few cancers feel smooth, mimicking cysts and fibroadenomas.

Composition Carcinomas are solid, so they do not fluctuate, transilluminate or have a fluid thrill, and they usually feel firm. However, some tumours are soft, almost as soft as a lipoma, so do not attribute too much significance to consistency.

Relations to surrounding structures The terms 'fixation' and 'tethering' are defined above.

Fixation of a lump to the skin is almost diagnostic of a carcinoma. The only other condition producing skin fixation is traumatic fat necrosis (or, of course, a pointing abscess, which should be obvious).

A cancer may also attach to or infiltrate the chest wall muscle. Such a lesion will be fixed. If neglected, the tumour will invade and consume the whole breast, leaving only a large malignant ulcer on the chest wall. Such advanced lesions are still seen.

When a tumour spreads alongside the fibrous septae of the breast, it blocks the associated lymphatics. This produces oedema of the overlying skin between the many small pits that mark the openings of the hair follicles and sweat glands. The result is the orange-peel appearance known as peau d'orange.

Lymph drainage The axillary lymph glands are often palpable, depending on the build of the patient, but this may not be pathological, especially when bilateral. Involved nodes may even be visible, but conversely impalpable glands are quite commonly found on investigation to contain tumour.

Palpable lymph glands containing metastases are usually firm and discrete. As they enlarge, they may mat together and become adherent to nearby structures such as the skin, axillary vessels and nerves. Ulceration in the axilla is rare.

Glands may become fixed to the chest wall, particularly at the apex of the axilla where there is less space for gland enlargement.

Nearby tissues Extensive (but not always palpable) involvement of the axillary lymph glands may cause lymphoedema of the arm or venous thrombosis and oedema.

The other breast may contain a lump that the patient has not noticed. A second primary lesion is far more likely than a metastasis. Do not forget to examine the axilla on the non-symptomatic side, both to make a comparison and to look for separate pathology.

General examination A full general examination is essential to detect the presence of metastases, which occur commonly at the following sites:

- The skeleton – especially the lumbar spine, causing back pain and reduced spinal movements, and pathological fractures in the long bones. There may even be paraplegia from cord compression.
- The lungs – causing pleural effusions. Lung parenchymal involvement, in the form of diffuse lymphatic involvement known as *lymphangitis carcinomatosa*, may cause severe dyspnoea.
- The liver – making it palpable and causing jaundice and ascites.
- The skin – producing multiple hard nodules within the skin. These are usually in the skin of the breast containing the cancer, but may be seen in the neck, trunk and further away.
- The brain – producing any variety of neurological symptoms and signs.

Conditions mimicking breast cancer

Fat necrosis

Fat necrosis occurs in the elderly. After an injury, not necessarily noticed by the patient, there is focal necrosis of subcutaneous fat with local scarring that causes skin tethering. There may be a history of trauma or of bruising. The condition resolves spontaneously.

Mondor's disease

Mondor's disease is thrombophlebitis of the lateral thoracic vein, which produces a cord-like, linear skin puckering that can alarm both patient and clinician. It resolves spontaneously.

BENIGN BREAST TUMOURS

Fibroadenoma

A fibroadenoma is a benign neoplasm of the breast with a dominant fibrous element. The cut surface of a fibroadenoma reveals lobules of whorled, white fibrous tissue that bulge out of their capsules.

There are two histological varieties of fibroadenoma: pericanalicular, which mainly consist of fibrous tissue, and intracanalicular, which contain more glands. The former tend to be harder and more discrete. Clinically, the distinction is unimportant.

Fig. 13.7 A giant fibroadenoma of the left breast.

Most fibroadenomas present in the teens and twenties, occasionally later, but not in the elderly. They enlarge slowly and can become sizeable if left (Fig. 13.7).

History

A painless lump in the breast, usually noticed by accident. Occasionally, there is more than one lesion.

Examination

Look out for a mobile, very discrete lump.

Position It may be anywhere in the breast.
Shape and size Fibroadenomas are usually spherical or ovoid but sometimes lobulated, and may be any size.
Surface The surface is smooth, the edge definite and the consistency like firm rubber.
Mobility Fibroadenoma is the most mobile of all breast lesions and fully merits the description 'breast mouse'.

The breast swelling most like a fibroadenoma is a breast cyst, but these occur in a different age group and are not mobile.

Phyllodes tumour

This is a rare lesion, first described as *cystosarcoma phylloides* or *Brodie's sarcoma*. It is not a sarcoma but may recur locally after simple excision. It does not metastasize.

It presents in middle-aged individuals as a slow-growing, smooth swelling, rather like a large fibroadenoma, from which it can be only distinguished on histology. Overlying skin necrosis is possible (Fig. 13.8).

Fig. 13.8 A large phyllodes tumour (Brodie's tumour) causing necrosis of the overlying skin.

Intraduct papilloma

This uncommon condition is a papillary benign neoplasm arising from the duct epithelium and enlarging into the duct system. It usually presents with a bloodstained discharge from the nipple, although there may be a soft swelling near the areola.

Lipoma of the breast

Lipomas occur anywhere in the body where there is fat, which includes the breast, both subcutaneously and more deeply seated between the lobules.

Subcutaneous lipomas are just like lipomas elsewhere, and there may be others on the trunk or limbs. If more deeply seated, they may have clinical features similar to those of cysts and fibroadenomas.

BENIGN BREAST DISEASE

Most of the conditions that lead females of reproductive age to seek medical advice in relation to their breasts are not truly a pathological process, but reflect the way of life in Western civilizations, where females have relatively few children relatively late in life, and do not use their breasts for what they are designed to do, namely produce milk.

Biologically, females are able to have children at regular intervals from the menarche onwards and could be almost constantly breast-feeding until the menopause (should they survive that long!). In these circumstances, it is unlikely that so-called benign breast disease would occur, or perhaps be noticed.

The various symptom complexes seen in benign breast disease used to be termed chronic mastitis. This is inappropriate because there is no clinical or microscopic evidence of an inflammatory process, but the term is still heard. There are several other names used, such as fibroadenosis, fibrocystic disease and cystic hyperplasia. These names are derived from the histological features of breast biopsies, such as fibrosis, adenosis, microcyst formation, epithelial hyperplasia and lymphocytic infiltration. Studies of normal breasts have shown that all these changes are non-specific and are commonly present in females without breast complaints. They are the histological manifestations of the dynamic changes that occur throughout normal reproductive life during breast development, cyclical menstrual change, pregnancy and menopausal involution.

It is best when considering the manifestations of so-called benign breast disease not to apply a histopathological label to the various symptom patterns seen in clinical practice, but to use simple clinical descriptions.

Most patients' symptoms fall, with considerable overlap, into three categories:

- Lumps and nodularity.
- Pain.
- Cysts.

Lumps and nodularity

History

The symptoms of lumps and nodularity occur during the years of ovarian activity, from menarche to menopause, beginning in the early twenties and reaching a peak in the thirties. Most patients present with one or more tender lumps in the breast, the tenderness frequently drawing the patient's attention to the lump. The swelling is variable and clearly related to the menstrual cycle, usually being more obvious in the premenstrual phase and resolving when the menses begins.

Examination

Benign breast swelling can vary from a diffuse nodularity to quite discrete lesions that mimic cancer (Table 13.1; see Revision panel 13.4).

Benign nodules tend to be in the upper outer quadrants and can be quite hard, sometimes described as rubbery.

They are not fixed or tethered to skin or muscle.

Table 13.1 A comparison of the clinical features of four common breast lumps

Type of lump	Age (years)	Pain	Surface	Consistency	Axilla
Solitary cyst	40–55	Occasional	Smooth	Soft to hard	Normal
Nodularity	20–55	Often	Indistinct	Mixed	Normal
Fibroadenoma	15–55	No	Smooth and bosselated	Rubbery	Normal
Carcinoma	35+	Uncommon	Irregular	Hard	Nodes may be palpable

Comment Experience is needed to differentiate discrete lesions that might be malignant and require further investigation, from diffuse swellings that require only reassurance and perhaps re-assessment at a different phase of the menstrual cycle. Do not become discouraged, but try to see patients with obvious real pathology before attempting to interpret the more subtle physical signs of benign breast disease.

Breast pain

Breast pain falls into various patterns and may be cyclical or non-cyclical.

Cyclical breast pain

Cyclical breast pain is very common. Almost all females experience it to some degree during their reproductive life. It comes on during the second half of the cycle and is relieved, sometimes dramatically, when menstruation commences. It is unusual before the age of 30 years and resolves spontaneously in the forties.

Curiously, as it is clearly of hormonal origin, it is often unilateral. It may be felt throughout the breast, or more in the upper outer quadrants. There may be associated tenderness, sometimes to the extent that the sufferer cannot bear any pressure on the breasts at that time in the cycle, even from a brassiere. The pain is usually reduced by the use of oral contraceptives.

On examination, there may be tenderness but no discrete lump. Diffuse nodularity is common, particularly in the upper outer quadrants.

It should be emphasized that cyclical breast pain is not a symptom of cancer. Several large studies have shown that females with breast pain are no more likely to have an impalpable carcinoma than females without pain.

Non-cyclical breast pain

Non-cyclical breast pain is less common than cyclical breast pain and has many causes.

Females at the menarche sometimes experience discomfort during very early breast development.

Females in their twenties may present with a persistently painful, tender area in one breast, but this usually resolves spontaneously.

Non-cyclical breast pain without any physical signs is also seen around the menopause and again resolves on its own.

Elderly females sometimes complain of unilateral breast pain, many years after hormonal activity has ceased. Careful examination is essential, as there is very occasionally an underlying cancer, especially when the pain is described as 'prickling'.

Breast pain in the elderly is often skeletal in origin, referred from conditions such as frozen shoulder and osteoporosis of the spine.

Conversely, very large breasts may produce skeletal symptoms in the neck and shoulder region, from both abnormal posture and pressure from brassiere straps.

Tietze's syndrome

Tietze's syndrome is an uncommon condition in which pain and tenderness arise from a costochondral junction lateral to the sternum. The patient complains of pain that may be exacerbated by movement and finds what she thinks is a breast lump. Examination will demonstrate that the lump noticed by the patient is in fact behind the breast and is part of the chest wall.

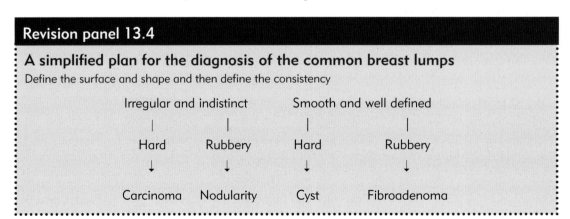

Revision panel 13.4

A simplified plan for the diagnosis of the common breast lumps

Define the surface and shape and then define the consistency

Irregular and indistinct		Smooth and well defined	
Hard	Rubbery	Hard	Rubbery
↓	↓	↓	↓
Carcinoma	Nodularity	Cyst	Fibroadenoma

Breast cyst

A breast cyst is probably the most common discrete breast swelling.

A fluid-filled cavity appears in the breast, without a demonstrable endothelial lining or a capsule. The condition is age related and occurs at times when the patient's hormone environment is changing, usually around the menopause. Cysts may be multiple and recurrent.

History

Age Breast cysts are unusual before the age of 40 years. The peak incidence is in the forties and early fifties. Hormone replacement therapy has extended the age range, and cysts are sometimes seen in females in their seventies.

Presentation Cysts often appear quite suddenly. The patient finds a large swelling that was not there the day before, and naturally assumes the worst unless she has previously had cysts. There may be associated discomfort and tenderness.

Past history Many patients have multiple cysts and will be aware that it is worth waiting for a while before consulting their doctor, as most cysts resolve.

Examination

Shape and surface A solitary cyst is smooth, spherical and of variable consistency, from soft and cystic to quite hard. The clinical diagnosis usually rests upon the smooth, spherical shape, but the swelling may be more diffuse.

Size Large breast cysts may even be visible and appear blue or green through the skin, but there will never be tethering or fixation to the skin or muscles.

Consistency It is rarely possible to elicit fluctuation or a fluid thrill or to transilluminate the lesion.

Comment The experienced clinician, having made a confident clinical diagnosis of a cyst, will proceed immediately to needle aspiration, the appropriate treatment (Fig. 13.9). The fluid obtained is variable in colour and clarity, varying from very dark green or almost black, to clear yellow. There are few more rewarding (or simpler) procedures than the aspiration of a breast cyst in a concerned woman.

Occasionally, a breast cyst communicates with the duct system and there is concomitant nipple discharge. This resolves when the cyst is aspirated.

A galactocele is a milk-containing cyst and occurs during or shortly after lactation. It presents as above

and the physical signs are similar. Aspiration produces milk, but the cyst rapidly refills and resolution must await cessation of breast-feeding.

Fig. 13.9 Aspiration of a breast cyst, a simple clinic procedure. The aspirate has the typical green colour seen with a benign cyst.

THE NIPPLE

The symptoms associated with the nipple are discharge, inversion and skin changes.

Nipple discharge

Considering that the breast is designed to produce milk, it is hardly surprising that fluid discharge is a common symptom. In many patients, no cause is ever demonstrated.

It occurs in any age group, but is most common during reproductive life. Most females who have breast-fed can express fluid on request for some time afterwards.

The fluid may be thick or thin, cloudy or clear, or bloodstained. The discharge may be unilateral or bilateral.

Endocrine causes of nipple discharge are very rare.

Significant causes of nipple discharge include DCIS, duct papilloma and, most commonly, duct ectasia.

Nipple discharge is rarely associated with invasive cancer.

Nipple inversion

Unlike nipple discharge, this condition may be associated with significant disease and always merits full assessment. The most common cause is duct ectasia, but nipple inversion is a regular presentation of breast cancer, with or without a palpable lump.

Nipple skin changes

Paget's disease of the nipple is a well-known condition, but most patients with a rash on or around the nipple have a skin and not a breast problem.

Paget's disease of the nipple (Fig. 13.10)

Paget's disease of the nipple is caused by cancer cells migrating or spreading along the duct system from a carcinoma situated deeply in the breast, which in the early stages is usually confined within the epithelium (DCIS).

The presence of carcinoma cells in the skin of the nipple produces a clinical appearance similar to that of eczema (Table 13.2). Patches of skin

Fig. 13.10 Paget's disease of the left nipple. The skin of the outer lower quadrant of the areola is red and slightly thickened. Careful palpation revealed the mass of a small underlying carcinoma.

Table 13.2   The differences between eczema and Paget's disease of the nipple

Eczema	Paget's disease
Bilateral	Unilateral
Sometimes lactating	Older females
Itches	Does not itch
Vesicles	No vesicles
Nipple intact	Nipple may be destroyed
No lumps	May be an underlying lump

first become red and then encrusted and oozy. The edges of these lesions are distinct, unlike eczema, and they do not itch, although the patient may complain of abnormal sensations and prickling. In time, the nipple is destroyed and replaced by a malignant ulcer.

In the early stages of the disease, there may be no palpable abnormality in the breast, but ultimately the in-situ carcinoma becomes invasive and a lump becomes palpable.

Never forget that proven Paget's disease of the nipple always indicates an underlying malignant process in the breast itself.

Duct ectasia

This is a common condition of unknown aetiology. As the name implies, the characteristic pathological feature is dilatation of the mammary ducts, which are full of inspissated material containing macrophages and chronic inflammatory debris. The inflammatory complications are closely related to smoking.

There are several presenting features:

- Nipple inversion, which is at first readily everted. There is a highly characteristic transverse slit appearance (Fig. 13.11). If uncomplicated and long-standing, it is usually ignored.

Fig. 13.11 The typical appearance of the nipple in duct ectasia. Note the transverse slit. The scar above the areola is the aftermath of an incision made to drain an abscess caused by periductal mastitis.

- Difficulty in breast-feeding because the infant is unable to suck the partly inverted nipple.
- Nipple discharge, of sometimes purulent material from the dilated ducts.
- Chronic low-grade infection of the periareolar area, with tender thickening around the nipple known as periductal mastitis, going on to abscess formation,. This is genuine inflammation and merits the description of mastitis (unlike the outdated expression 'chronic mastitis' mistakenly applied to the changes of benign breast disease).
- A periductal abscess may rupture (or be drained) externally and remain in communication with the duct system. This results in a mammillary fistula (Fig. 13.12). The pathogenesis is identical to that of the analogous anal fistula, and the principles of treatment are similar.

Fig. 13.12 A mammillary duct fistula. This tract connects with a mammary duct. Recurrent infection causes recurrent acute breast abscesses.

BREAST ABSCESS

Acute breast abscess

History

Acute breast abscess is associated with lactation. Bacteria may gain access to the engorged breast lobules, an excellent medium for bacterial culture, via the nipple and duct system or via the circulation.

The patient develops malaise and fever accompanied by an ache in the breast that progresses to an inexorable throbbing pain.

Examination

The infected breast displays the *signs of Celsus*, namely rubor, calor, tumour and dolor. Eventually, the abscess will point and discharge through the skin. There may be very obvious tender lymphadenopathy in the ipsilateral axilla.

Note It is safe to continue breast-feeding, even from the breast containing the abscess. Had the inflamed area communicated with the duct system, the infection would have discharged this way and the abscess would have not have formed.

When a breast abscess occurs in a female who is not lactating, there is often a predisposing risk factor such as diabetes mellitus.

Recurrent and chronic breast abscess

Recurrent and chronic breast abscess is usually associated with duct ectasia, described above.

Tuberculosis of the breast remains common in some parts of the world and is occasionally seen in the UK.

Granulomatous infections of the breast caused by atypical mycobacteria are rare but on the increase.

Both forms of infection present with a painless mass and mimic carcinoma.

PREGNANCY

Pregnancy is always associated with changes in the breast (see Revision panel 13.5).

Within a few weeks of the ovum being fertilized, the breasts become tense, heavy and slightly uncomfortable.

Revision panel 13.5

The breast changes of pregnancy

Fullness and prickling sensations

Enlargement

Distended subcutaneous veins

Increased nipple and areolar pigmentation

Circumareolar pigmentation

Hypertrophy of the subareolar sebaceous glands (Montgomery's tubercles)

A clear, expressible secretion (colostrum)

By 2 months, the breasts are enlarged and feel granular – even 'lumpy' – in texture. The subcutaneous veins dilate and become prominent, and the skin of the breasts is warm. The nipples enlarge and the areolae darken permanently. The sebaceous glands of the areola become larger, the skin over them appears stretched and pale, and they are called *Montgomery's tubercles*.

THE MALE BREAST

There are two causes of enlargement of the male breast: gynaecomastia, which is benign and common, and carcinoma, which is malignant and rare.

Gynaecomastia (Fig. 13.13)

All males have nipples and rudimentary breasts. Gynaecomastia is an abnormal development of both the ductal and stromal elements, with the following patterns of presentation:

- Transient breast enlargement in male infants due to ingestion of maternal oestrogens.
- Breast development in adolescents, presumably caused by a temporary imbalance of adrenal and testicular steroid hormones.
- Breast enlargement in middle-aged adults, usually idiopathic, but in some cases blamed on repeated minor trauma from belts and harnesses. It is usually bilateral.
- Breast enlargement in elderly males, almost invariably caused by drugs. This may be an expected part of the action of the drug, as with the use of oestrogens for prostatic carcinoma. (A similar effect occurs in younger males abusing anabolic steroids.) Gynaecomastia may also be a true side-effect of histamine antagonists, diuretics and cardiac drugs. Curiously, it tends to resolve without the offending agent having to be stopped.
- A very few cases are caused by inappropriate hormone secretion, as may occur in cirrhosis of the liver and bronchial carcinoma.

(a) Unilateral gynaecomastia in a young male.

(b) Bilateral gynaecomastia in an elderly male.

Fig. 13.13 GYNAECOMASTIA

History

The patient complains of painless, or slightly tender, enlargement of one or both breasts. Schoolboys with gynaecomastia are often teased by their (so-called) friends.

There may be a history of a recent illness.

Taking a drug history is essential.

Examination

There is sometimes a clearly palpable disc of firm breast tissue behind and attached to the areola. This is the usual form of gynaecomastia seen in younger males. Drug-induced breast enlargement tends to be more diffuse, with a fatty element. Tenderness may occur, and the axillary lymph glands will not be enlarged.

A general examination, especially of the abdomen (liver) and scrotum (testes), may yield information that indicates the likely cause.

Carcinoma of the male breast

This is an uncommon condition, usually of middle-aged and elderly males. Its symptoms and physical signs are identical to those of carcinoma of the female breast except that there is little public awareness of the condition and presentation may be late.

Because the male breast is small and not covered by a thick layer of subcutaneous fat, the disease spreads rapidly. Physical signs such as skin and muscle fixation, ulceration and axillary lymphadenopathy are often present by the time of presentation (Fig. 13.14).

Fig. 13.14 Carcinoma of the male breast. Although the mass of tumour is relatively small, it has already caused retraction of the nipple and is fixed to, and dimpling, the skin.

14 The abdominal wall, hernias and the umbilicus

The abdominal wall has a complex structure, and many of the surgical conditions affecting it are embryological in origin. It develops laterally from the vertebral column, envelops the intestinal tract, and finally fuses in the midline to form a seam-like fibrous cord, the linea alba. This is pierced at the umbilicus by the umbilical cord, which in early embryonic life contains the yolk sac and the entire mid-gut. The testes develop in the peritoneum of the posterior abdominal wall and migrate into the scrotum through the muscles just above the inguinal ligament. It is therefore hardly surprising that there are weak spots in the abdominal wall.

The abdominal wall is prone to all the lesions of skin, subcutaneous tissue, fascia and muscle described elsewhere.

To decide whether an abdominal swelling is deep to, or part of, the abdominal wall, palpate the lump with the abdominal wall relaxed and then with it tense. A lump deep to the abdominal wall becomes impalpable when the abdominal muscles contract. A lump superficial to the muscles becomes more prominent.

Contracting the abdominal muscles

If you ask a patient to lift their head and shoulders off the couch, the abdominal muscles contract – provided they do not lever themselves up with their elbows. Alternatively, lift the patient's heels and then ask the patient to hold them in that position. This tenses the rectus abdominis muscle very effectively, and any mass deep to it will become impalpable unless it is huge.

Swellings in the rectus sheath

Acute

Acute haematoma

The inferior and superior epigastric arteries lie deep to, or within, the rectus abdominis muscles. If these muscles contract suddenly and violently, the epigastric arteries or muscle fibres may be torn. The subsequent haematoma within the muscle produces pain and swelling.

Rupture of the *inferior* epigastric artery occurs during severe exercise, but also during coughing in elderly patients, especially if they are taking steroid medication. The blood is contained within the rectus sheath superiorly, but below the arcuate line (the lower edge of the posterior rectus sheath, midway between the pubis and the umbilicus) there is no posterior layer so the blood collects in the extraperitoneal space in the iliac fossa.

The patient complains of iliac fossa pain and tenderness of sudden origin, which is made worse by contracting the abdominal muscles. Examination reveals a diffuse, tender mass in the iliac fossa, deep to the abdominal wall. Skin discolouration may appear a few hours later. The condition may conceivably be confused with acute appendicitis, but there will be none of the systemic features.

Rupture of the *superior* epigastric artery follows a bout of violent coughing and causes pain and tenderness in the upper abdomen, made worse by tensing the abdominal muscles and by deep breathing. On the right-hand side, it might be confused with cholecystitis.

Chronic

Chronic haematoma

Patients occasionally present with a painless mass that examination reveals to be in the rectus sheath. The most likely cause is a chronic rectus sheath haematoma with the acute phase forgotten or not noticed. Discrete swellings are more likely to occur in the upper abdomen, confined by the fibrous intersections in the upper part of the muscle.

The swelling will be firm to hard, clearly in the abdominal wall and without a definite edge because it is deep seated.

Sarcoma

The rare desmoid tumour and other sarcomas may arise in the rectus sheath.

Lipoma

The most common swelling in the anterior abdominal wall superficial to the rectus sheath is the subcutaneous lipoma. This is clearly in the subcutaneous layer and displays the characteristic smooth surface, rounded edge and pseudo-fluctuant consistency. Solitary lipomas may be sizeable as they cause no trouble.

Dercum's syndrome is familial, and there are multiple, sometimes tender lipomas in the abdominal and chest walls and limbs. The lesions are rarely bigger than 2–3 cm.

ABDOMINAL HERNIA

A hernia is the protrusion of an organ or part of an organ through its containing wall (Revision panel 14.1). 'Rupture'/'hernia' are the common terms used for the protrusion of an intra-abdominal organ through a defect in the abdominal wall, pelvis or diaphragm.

For an organ or tissue to herniate, there must be a weakness in the retaining wall. This may be caused by a congenital abnormality, may be related to the normal anatomy, such as a place where a vessel or viscus enters or leaves the abdomen, or may be acquired as a result of trauma or disease.

This chapter deals with abdominal hernias, excluding those at the oesophageal hiatus (Fig. 14.1).

Common abdominal hernias in order of frequency in adult life are:

- inguinal;
- umbilical;
- incisional;
- femoral;
- epigastric (Revision panel 14.2).

In childhood, umbilical hernia is more common than inguinal hernia.

The common hernias

The rare hernias

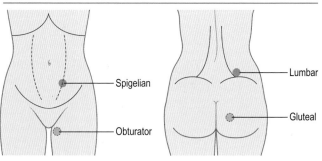

Fig. 14.1 The sites of hernias.

Rarer hernias include:

- spigelian;
- obturator;
- lumbar;
- gluteal.

You may not have a detailed knowledge of all the rare conditions, but you should be aware that hernias occur in strange places and can strangulate with the death of the patient unless treated promptly.

Hernias are common in both sexes: 9 per cent of males and 1 per cent of females develop an inguinal hernia at some time in their lives.

Although femoral hernia is found more often in females than in males, the most common hernia in females is inguinal.

Certain physical signs are common to all hernias but are not always present:

- They occur at congenital or acquired weak spots in the abdominal wall.
- Most hernias can be reduced.
- Most hernias have an expansile cough impulse.

The last two signs may be absent if the hernia has a narrow neck or the contents do not include bowel.

The diagnosis of a hernia is suggested by the site of the swelling and confirmed by the presence of reducibility and an expansile cough impulse. If these signs are absent, other causes of a lump must be considered.

Revision panel 14.1
The basic features of all hernias
They occur at a weak spot
They reduce on lying down, or with manipulation
They have an expansile cough impulse

Revision panel 14.2
The causes of abdominal hernias
Congenital anatomical defect
Alongside structures penetrating the abdominal wall
Acquired weakness from trauma or disease
Associated with raised intra-abdominal pressure

INGUINAL HERNIA

To understand inguinal hernias, it is necessary to understand the anatomy of the inguinal canal (Fig. 14.2).

Surface anatomy

The inguinal ligament runs between the anterior superior iliac spine, which is easy to see and feel, and the pubic tubercle, which is not, particularly in a fat patient. Follow the inguinal ligament downwards and medially, and you will find the tubercle 2–3 cm from the midline.

Muscles

Beneath the skin and subcutaneous tissue lies the *aponeurosis* (a flat tendon) of the external oblique muscle. The lower inwardly folded edge of this aponeurosis, which runs between the anterior superior iliac spine and pubic tubercle, is the inguinal ligament. The fibres of the aponeurosis run parallel to the inguinal ligament in the direction taken by a hand when placed in a trouser pocket, and separate above the crest of the pubis to form the external or superficial inguinal ring.

Deep to the external oblique aponeurosis are the lowermost fibres of the internal oblique muscle, arising from the lateral half of the inguinal ligament. They run medially in an arch, convex upwards, to the edge of the rectus abdominis muscle, where they join the aponeurosis of the transverse abdominal muscle to form the anterior rectus sheath. At this point, the fused aponeuroses are known as the *conjoint tendon*.

The inguinal canal

The half-moon-shaped gap beneath the arch of the internal oblique muscle is the weak spot of the inguinal region. The weak, attenuated tissue filling the gap is called the *transversalis fascia*. This area is crossed by the inferior epigastric artery as it runs upwards from the femoral artery, curving medially towards the rectus sheath.

The point where the vas deferens and testicular artery pierce the transversalis fascia is *lateral* to the inferior epigastric artery and known as the internal or deep inguinal ring. Indirect inguinal hernial sacs leave the abdomen at this point. Direct

Surface landmarks

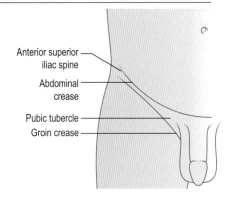

Anterior superior iliac spine

Abdominal crease

Pubic tubercle

Groin crease

The external oblique muscle

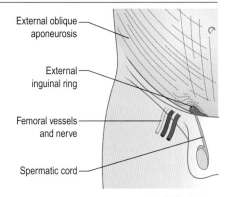

External oblique aponeurosis

External inguinal ring

Femoral vessels and nerve

Spermatic cord

The internal oblique muscle

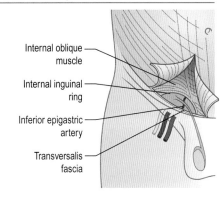

Internal oblique muscle

Internal inguinal ring

Inferior epigastric artery

Transversalis fascia

The coverings of the spermatic cord

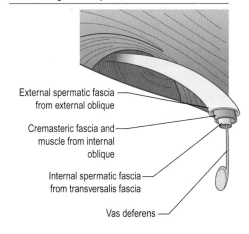

External spermatic fascia from external oblique

Cremasteric fascia and muscle from internal oblique

Internal spermatic fascia from transversalis fascia

Vas deferens

An indirect inguinal hernia

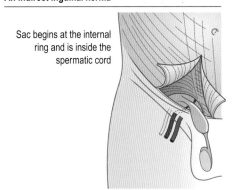

Sac begins at the internal ring and is inside the spermatic cord

A direct inguinal hernia

Sac appears medial to the inferior epigastric artery and is outside the spermatic cord

Fig. 14.2 The anatomy of the inguinal region.

inguinal hernias push through the weak area of the posterior wall *medial* to the inferior epigastric artery. Remember that the exit point of an indirect hernia is lateral to this artery and that of a direct hernia medial to it. You cannot palpate the inferior epigastric artery, but the femoral pulse, which can be felt at the mid-inguinal point (half way between the anterior superior iliac spine and the midline), will tell you where it begins. The important clinical point is that the exit point of an indirect hernia is lateral to that of a direct hernia (Revision panel 14.3).

As the vas deferens enters the inguinal canal, it takes with it a thin layer of fascia derived from the transversalis fascia, called the *internal spermatic fascia*. Further down the canal, it collects a covering of muscle fibres and fascia from the internal oblique muscle. These coverings are called the *cremaster muscle* and *cremasteric fascia*. Finally, as the vas passes through the external ring, it acquires another thin layer of fascia derived from the external oblique aponeurosis and called the *external spermatic fascia*.

Because the sac of an indirect inguinal hernia comes down obliquely alongside the vas deferens inside the spermatic cord, it has an easy path of little resistance down into the scrotum. The three fascial layers of the cord funnel the peritoneal sac towards the scrotum. By contrast, the sac of a direct inguinal hernia begins medial to the epigastric artery, outside the spermatic cord with its three external layers of tissue, so has no easy path to the scrotum, which in consequence it rarely enters.

Technique for the examination of an inguinal hernia (Fig. 14.3)

Ask the patient to stand up

It is not possible to examine or even detect an uncomplicated inguinal hernia when the patient is lying down. If you suspect the diagnosis from the history, start the examination with the patient standing. As part of any routine supine abdominal examination, conclude by asking the patient to stand up to look for hernias.

Always examine both inguinal regions.

Look at the lump from in front

Determine the exact site and shape of the lump. With practice, you may be able to distinguish an inguinal from a femoral hernia on sight.

(a) Ask the patient to stand up. When palpating the groin, stand at the patient's side.

(b) The pubic tubercle. Note that it is not low down in the crease of the groin.

(c)

(c, d) Place your examining hand flat on the groin parallel to the inguinal ligament, and your other hand on the patient's back to stop you pushing him over. You will then be able to manipulate and probably reduce the hernia.

Fig. 14.3 TECHNIQUES FOR THE EXAMINATION OF AN INGUINAL HERNIA

CHAPTER 14 | THE ABDOMINAL WALL, HERNIAS AND THE UMBILICUS

Inspection will also reveal whether the lump extends down into the scrotum, whether there are any other scrotal swellings and whether there are any swellings on the asymptomatic side.

Feel from the front

1. Examine the scrotum and its contents. It is not unusual to find an epididymal cyst or a hydrocele as well as a hernia because they are all common conditions.

2. In males, first decide whether the lump is a hernia or a true scrotal lump by seeing if you can 'get above it', namely feel its upper edge with a normal spermatic cord above. If you can, it is a scrotal swelling and not a hernia. If the lump has no upper edge because it passes into the inguinal canal, it is a hernia.

Feel from the side

Having examined the scrotal contents and decided that you cannot get above the lump, you can make a provisional diagnosis of inguinal hernia and proceed to examine the lump itself.

Stand by the side of the patient with one hand in the small of the patient's back to support him, and your examining hand on the lump with your fingers and arm roughly parallel to the inguinal ligament.

Assess the following features of the lump (discussed in detail below):

● Position.
● Temperature.
● Tenderness.
● Shape.
● Size.
● Tension.
● Composition (solid, fluid, or gaseous).
● Reducibility.

Expansile cough impulse

Compress the lump gently with your fingers; then ask the patient to turn away from you and cough. If the swelling becomes tense and expands with coughing, it has a *cough impulse*. Movement in one direction of the swelling is not a cough impulse – it has to expand or become more tense. The presence of an expansile cough impulse is diagnostic of a hernia, but its absence does not

exclude the diagnosis because the neck of the sac may be blocked or the contents may be something other than intestine.

Is the swelling reducible?

The main reason for standing at the side of the patient is to be able to place your hand in exactly the same position as the patient places his own hand when he is reducing or supporting the hernia. He puts his hand on the lump and lifts it upwards and backwards. You must do the same. You can only do this if your arm comes from a position above and behind the hernia.

First, gently compress the lower part of the swelling. As the lump gets softer, lift it up towards the external ring. It is important not to hurt the patient during this procedure as the muscles will become tense and make further efforts at reduction impossible. Once it has all passed in through this point, slide your fingers upwards and laterally towards the internal ring to see if the hernia can be controlled (kept inside) by pressure at this point.

If the hernia can be held in the reduced position by pressure over the internal ring, it is an indirect inguinal hernia. If it is above the inguinal ligament and cannot be controlled by pressure over the internal ring, it is a direct hernia.

With large hernias, it is often difficult and inappropriate to try and reduce the hernia with the patient standing up. In this case, ask the patient to lie down. In most cases, the hernia will reduce.

Finally, be very gentle with hernias that appear incarcerated. It is possible to reduce the hernia 'en masse', which means reducing the bowel together with the peritoneal sac. The hernia contents may still be incarcerated or even strangulated within the peritoneal sac.

Remove your hand and watch the hernia reappear

A reappearing indirect hernia slides obliquely downwards along the line of the inguinal canal, whereas a direct hernia will project directly forwards (Fig. 14.4).

Comment: It is not always possible, particularly in obese individuals, to differentiate between these two types of hernia. However, it is a good exercise to attempt always to do so.

(a) A left indirect inguinal hernia, moving obliquely down towards the scrotum.

(b) This is a right direct recurrent inguinal hernia. The original inguinal hernia probably developed because of the disruption and distortion of the abdominal wall caused by the previous abdominal operation. Always look for a scar in the groin. The bulge is coming out directly towards you.

Fig. 14.4 INGUINAL HERNIAS

Feel the other side

Move to the other side of the patient and examine that inguinal region. Inguinal hernias are quite often bilateral, particularly when they are direct. Even when you cannot see or feel a lump, ask the patient to cough while you are palpating the inguinal canal. There may be a small hernia that is palpable with coughing but is not visible.

Examine the abdomen

Look particularly for anything that may be raising the intra-abdominal pressure, such as a large bladder, ascites, abdominal distension or pregnancy.

With the patient lying flat, ask the patient to cough as you observe the groin. Particularly in a slim adult, you may see the contents entering the sac, which will help you to decide if the hernia is direct or indirect, as described above in the standing position. With a direct hernia, the swelling will advance directly upwards towards you. With an indirect hernia, you may be able to see oblique motion from the internal ring to the neck of the scrotum. Indirect hernias have sometimes been referred to as *oblique hernias*.

With the patient in this position, it is easier to decide whether a hernia is femoral. Femoral hernias only rarely reduce, lie below the inguinal ligament and are rather more lateral than an indirect inguinal sac extending through the external inguinal ring downwards to the same level.

Cardiovascular and respiratory assessment

Assess the cardiovascular and respiratory systems with the patient's fitness for operation in mind.

Symptoms and signs of an inguinal hernia

History

(Elective presentation)

Age Inguinal hernias may appear at any age from birth to old age.

Occupation If there is an underlying weakness, the appearance of a hernia may coincide with strenuous physical effort, or it may be first noticed at such a time. Despite the fact that hernias are no more common in manual workers than in office workers, compensation law in many countries accepts that a hernia may be an industrial injury.

Local symptoms The usual symptom is the patient finding a painless swelling. Some patients notice a dragging, aching sensation in the groin, which gets worse as the day goes on. A few present with groin pain, and the hernia is only detected by the doctor.

Other abdominal symptoms Large hernias may interfere with bowel activity and cause a change in bowel habit.

However, beware: patients with a carcinoma of the left colon, or diverticular disease, may experience progressive constipation and hence increased straining during defaecation. The increase in abdominal pressure that accompanies straining may make a coincidental hernia more prominent and lead the patient to attribute their symptoms to the hernia. Therefore, you must enquire of all patients presenting with a hernia whether their bowel action has recently changed and investigate any significant bowel symptoms in their own right before dealing with the hernia.

It is also usual to ask about other diseases that may have caused increased abdominal pressure, such as chronic bronchitis with persistent coughing, and difficulty with micturition.

History

(Emergency presentation)

Hernias, pre-existing or just discovered, may present as a surgical emergency. The patient notices that the groin swelling will not reduce or that it is painful and tender. This may be associated with the cardinal symptoms of intestinal obstruction – colicky abdominal pain, vomiting, distension and absolute constipation. The griping pain is felt not in the groin but in the midline of the abdomen, at a level that depends on which part of the intestine is involved. The hernial orifices of any patient with intestinal obstruction must always be carefully examined, as the patient may not have noticed a small lump in their groin. This is particularly so with femoral hernias.

The terms 'irreducible', 'incarcerated', 'obstructed' and 'strangulated' are used freely in the description of hernias. They must be defined carefully (Fig. 14.5).

Irreducible means simply what it states, that the contents of the hernia sac cannot be replaced into the abdomen. An irreducible hernia may be associated with three other categories of complication – incarceration, obstruction and strangulation.

Incarcerated means that contents are literally imprisoned in the sac of the hernia (usually by adhesions) but are alive and functioning normally. An incarcerated hernia is not tender.

Obstructed means that a loop of bowel is kinked or trapped within the sac of the hernia in such a way that its lumen, but not its blood supply, is obstructed. The bowel is therefore alive, and the patient has the signs and symptoms of intestinal obstruction but not of strangulation. The hernia will not be unduly tender.

Strangulation means that compression or twisting has compromised the blood supply to the contents of the sac, which are ischaemic or infarcted. The patient will be obviously unwell, and the swelling will be acutely tender. An entrapment that interferes with

the blood supply to the bowel wall will commonly obstruct the lumen as well, so most strangulated hernias containing bowel have intestinal obstruction.

However, there is a variety of strangulated hernia in which only a segment of the bowel wall is trapped and the lumen remains patent. The strangulation makes the hernia very tender, but there are no symptoms or signs of intestinal obstruction. This is called *Richter's hernia*. It occurs when the hernia has a narrow neck, so is more commonly seen with femoral than inguinal hernias.

Examination

Position An inguinal hernia will be visible in the groin in all but the obese. The anatomical landmarks and the site and line of direction of indirect and direct hernias are described above.

Colour The skin colour over an inguinal hernia should be normal. If the hernia is strangulated, the skin may be reddened. If the patient has worn a truss for many years, the skin over the external inguinal ring may be scarred and pigmented.

Temperature The temperature of the skin overlying a hernia will be the same as the surrounding skin except when the hernia is strangulated. In this event, the skin may be warm.

Tenderness A hernia may contain any viscus and, as all abdominal structures have a visceral sensory innervation, manual pressure is uncomfortable but not truly painful. By contrast, a strangulated hernia is very tender. An irreducible, non-strangulated hernia is not tender to light pressure, but any attempt at reduction by excessive pressing and squeezing can cause considerable pain.

Shape An indirect hernia moving obliquely along the inguinal canal towards the scrotum is sausage shaped, but when it extends beyond the external inguinal ring it widens out to become pear shaped. A direct hernia is usually round, like a plum in the groin.

Size Inguinal hernias vary from very small bulges that are just detectable, to large masses descending almost to knee level. The larger a hernia is, the more likely it is to be irreducible.

Comment Minor bilateral bulging of the inguinal canal in slim individuals is normal and known as *Malgaigne's bulges*. These are not true hernias.

Surface The surface will vary according to the nature of the contents but is usually smooth. In a large hernia, it is sometimes possible to palpate indentable faeces inside an incarcerated segment of colon.

Neck of sac

This tight ring of peritoneum is usually the site of any strangulation

A strangulated hernia

The blood supply of the contents of the hernia is cut off. When a loop of the gut is strangulated there will also be intestinal obstruction

A strangulated hernia

If the sac is small, a knuckle of bowel can be caught in the sac and strangled without causing intestinal obstruction. This is called a *Richter's hernia*

Maydl's hernia

When two adjacent loops of bowel are in the sac, the intervening portion in the abdomen is the first to suffer if the neck of the sac is tight, because it is the centre of the whole loop involved. Thus the strangulation piece is intra-abdominal. This is a rare variety of strangulation

Sliding hernia

If bowel which is normally extraperitoneal forms one side of the sac, it is thought to have slid down the canal pulling peritoneum with it, hence the name *hernia-en-glissade*. The sac can contain other loops of bowel, and the gut forming the wall of the sac can be strangled by the external wall ring

Incarceration

The contents are fixed in the sac because of their size and adhesions. The hernia is irreducible but the bowel is not strangulated or obstructed

Reduction-en-masse

It is possible to push a hernia back through the abdominal wall, so apparently reducing it, without actually pushing the contents out of the sac. If they were strangulated in the first position they will still be strangulated in the second. Never push hard when trying to reduce a hernia

Fig. 14.5 Some definitions.

Composition Hernias that contain gut are soft, resonant and fluctuant, and you may be able to hear bowel sounds. Peristalsis may be visible with a large scrotal hernia containing small intestine. Many hernias contain omentum, which has a rubbery feel.

Cough impulse A hernia will nearly always become larger and more tense in all directions during coughing, which is referred to as an expansile cough impulse and described above.

Reducibility This means that it is possible to return the contents of the hernia to their normal anatomical site – the abdomen.

Relations The relations of the lump will have already been defined when deciding the site and nature of the hernia.

Look carefully for any scars near the hernia. It may have been repaired in the past.

There is an increased incidence of direct right inguinal hernia in patients who have had an appendicectomy through a right iliac fossa incision because this incision weakens the adjacent muscles and occasionally divides the iliohypogastric or ilioinguinal nerves.

Revision panel 14.3

Indirect or direct inguinal hernia?

Features of an indirect inguinal hernia

Can (and often does) descend into the scrotum

Reduces upwards, then laterally and backwards

Controlled, after reduction, by pressure over the internal inguinal ring

After reduction, the bulge reappears in the middle of the inguinal region and flows medially and obliquely towards the scrotum

Found in all age groups including children

Features of a direct inguinal hernia

Does not go down into the scrotum

Reduces upwards and then straight backwards (hence the name 'direct')

Not controlled after reduction by pressure over the internal inguinal ring

After reduction, the bulge comes directly forwards

Rare in children and young adults

Special varieties of inguinal hernia

The differences between a *direct* and an *indirect* inguinal hernia are listed in Revision panel 14.3. The distinction between the two is not totally irrelevant, as well as being an excellent exercise in clinical anatomy (see Fig. 14.4). When an inguinal hernia strangulates, the usual site of constriction is the external ring. Hence a direct hernia, which does not pass through this ring, is much less likely to place the patient's life at risk by becoming strangulated. This may influence management in a poor-risk patient.

Bilateral hernias are more likely to be direct than indirect.

It is not uncommon to find both a direct and an indirect hernia in the same groin. When this occurs, the two sacs are straddled by the inferior epigastric artery and the hernia is sometimes called a *pantaloon hernia*. This is usually detected only at operation.

A *sliding hernia* occurs when a partly extraperitoneal segment of bowel (the caecum or terminal ileum on the right, or the sigmoid colon on the left) slides down into the inguinal canal, pulling a sac of peritoneum with it. The viscus involved is part of the wall of the sac. Clinical differentiation of this variety is never certain, but it is far more common on the left, and involvement of the sigmoid colon may produce disproportionate pain and even symptoms of bowel dysfunction. Sliding hernias are occasionally diagnosed during the investigation of bowel symptoms when contrast X-rays demonstrate colon on one side of a hernial sac.

Maydl's hernia (hernia-en-W; Fig. 14.5) is a rare condition in which there are two loops of bowel in the sac, with strangulation of a loop of bowel between them in the abdomen. Diagnosis is made at operation.

Recurrent hernias

Inguinal hernia is a common condition as not all of the many surgical repairs that are performed are successful.

Recurrent hernias are more likely to present with local pain. They tend to be direct and, because of the scarring from the previous surgery, are unlikely to be large. They are very rarely scrotal. The hernia may consist of extraperitoneal fat without a peritoneal sac, infiltrating itself into the defects that have arisen in the previous repair. Recognition is important because strangulation is more likely than with an untreated hernia.

Differential diagnosis

There are very few conditions that can be mistaken for an inguinal hernia provided you remember to check the scrotum, feel for a cough impulse and test reducibility (Revision panel 14.4).

Confusion may occasionally be caused by swellings which occur in the line of the spermatic cord that can pop in and out of the external ring, such as an undescended testis and a hydrocele of the cord in children. With the first, routine examination of the scrotum should reveal an absent testis. Neither has an expansile cough impulse.

Revision panel 14.4

The differential diagnosis of an inguinal hernia

Femoral hernia

Hydrocele of the cord or the canal of Nuck

Undescended testis

Lipoma of the cord

Inguinal hernia in females

In females, there is a rudimentary testicular analogue that descends through the muscles of the groin as in males. The equivalent of the spermatic cord is the round ligament, which joins the uterus just as the vas deferens joins the prostate. Hernias in females nearly always follow the round ligament and are therefore indirect. The sac passes obliquely towards the labium in the same way as it would pass towards the scrotum in the male.

There are two conditions of the groin peculiar to females:

- *Hydrocele of the canal of Nuck* is a fluid-filled distal sac of an indirect hernia. The proximal part of the sac is too narrow to admit bowel or other abdominal contents. It is analogous to the encysted hydrocele of the cord seen in children. It presents with a smooth, fluctuant swelling without a cough impulse, that will transilluminate.
- *Haematocele of the round ligament* is a curious condition in which the round ligament becomes distended with multiple small sacs containing bloodstained fluid. It presents in pregnancy with a soft, sausage-like swelling in the groin extending into the labium. This may have a weak cough impulse and when gently squeezed feels spongy and reduces in size. It is commonly confused with a hernia, but it resolves when the pregnancy is over, which hernias certainly do not.

Inguinal hernias in children

Groin hernias in male children are, for practical purposes, always indirect and are caused by failure of the processus vaginalis to obliterate after the testicle enters the scrotum. There are three clinical manifestations of this abnormality, but it is important to appreciate that the pathological process in all three is identical, namely a patent processus vaginalis. The three clinical manifestations are:

- an infantile hydrocele;
- an obvious hernia;
- an encysted hydrocele of the cord.

An *infantile hydrocele* is a fully patent processus vaginalis (i.e. one extending right down to the scrotum) that is too narrow to admit bowel but allows fluid from the peritoneal cavity to accumulate within it. The condition may present at birth or shortly afterwards as a scrotal swelling that is usually large, tense, brilliantly translucent and often bilateral. It should be possible to get above the swelling, i.e. to feel or see that its upper limit is at or below the external inguinal ring. It is rarely possible to squeeze the fluid back into the abdomen as the narrow neck of the processus acts as a non-return valve. It does not have an expansile cough impulse.

When the child cries, intra-abdominal pressure is raised and the scrotal swelling may become harder. It is important to reassure the parents that the child is not crying because the hydrocele is tense, but that the swelling is tense because the child is crying.

The usual natural history is spontaneous resolution during the first year of life as the processus slowly obliterates, but once the child begins to walk this is less likely. In ambulant children, the swelling often increases in size during the day, presumably exacerbated by gravity.

CHAPTER 14 | THE ABDOMINAL WALL, HERNIAS AND THE UMBILICUS

Fig. 14.6 A large left inguinal hernia in a child.

Fig. 14.7 This young girl's parents gave a history of an intermittent left groin swelling and pointed to the inguinal canal, but nothing was visible when she came to the clinic. Nevertheless, the history was good enough for an operation to be planned. But when on holiday in Spain, a lump appeared in the other groin, and the parents took this photograph confirming the presence of bilateral inguinal hernias.

An *inguinal hernia* in a child (Fig. 14.6) displays the physical signs listed above for an indirect inguinal hernia. The contents reduce easily, and the swelling does not transilluminate.

Children's groin hernias occasionally become irreducible, but strangulation is rare. If strangulation does occur, the gonadal vessels are more likely to be damaged than the vessels of the bowel, so testicular infarction is more common than bowel infarction.

Direct hernias do occur in children but are very rare.

Children's hernias may only appear intermittently. The swelling that the parents have definitely seen often obstinately refuses to appear in the presence of the examining doctor (Fig. 14.7). If the site of the swelling indicated by the parents is the inguinal canal, exploration is justified on the history alone, and an indirect sac is invariably found.

In females, the wall of the sac may include the ovary and Fallopian tube. In these cases, when the contents are reduced, there may remain a small mass, which is tender to touch. The child may also complain of pain in the area.

An *encysted hydrocele of the cord* is the least common variety of patent processus vaginalis; in this, a narrow-necked patent processus that does not reach the testis becomes dilated distally and filled with fluid. It presents as a discrete swelling in the spermatic cord below the external inguinal ring and above the testicle (Fig. 14.8). It transilluminates brilliantly and has no cough impulse.

Fig. 14.8 A right encysted hydrocele of the cord. It is clearly separate from the testicle. You can get above it, and there is no cough impulse in the swelling or in the groin above it.

Comment: Do not confuse the infantile with the adult hydrocele.

In children, the condition is a fluid-filled congenital inguinal hernia with a narrow sac that communicates with the peritoneal cavity on every occasion.

The adult hydrocele is an acquired condition in which fluid accumulates around the testicle, within the tunica vaginalis, in response to a local abnormality. It has no communication with the peritoneum.

FEMORAL HERNIA

Anatomy (Fig. 14.9)

A femoral hernia is a protrusion of extraperitoneal fat, a peritoneal sac and sometimes abdominal contents through the femoral canal. The anatomical margins of this canal are the inguinal ligament anteriorly, the pubic ramus and pectineus muscle posteriorly, the lacunar ligament and pubic bone medially, and the femoral vein laterally.

The femoral canal provides a space into which the femoral vein can expand. It normally contains loose areolar tissue and a lymph gland known as the *gland of Cloquet*. With bone or ligament on three sides and a major vessel on the fourth, the femoral canal cannot distend easily. A peritoneal sac coming through it therefore has a stiff, narrow neck, and any contents are at risk of strangulation.

A characteristic but not invariable feature of the sac of a femoral hernia is that it is thick walled with layers of fat and connective tissue, which when cut across look like an onion. This means that the sac remains palpable even when empty, so seems to be irreducible.

History

Age Femoral hernias are rare in children and do not become common until over the age of 50 years, with no upper age limit.

Sex Femoral hernias are much more common in females than in males. Nevertheless, do not forget that even in females the most common hernia in the groin region is the inguinal hernia, and that a male can have a femoral hernia.

Symptoms Usually, the patient discovers the swelling. The other main presentation is in the elderly, with obstruction or strangulation of a previously unnoticed hernia. Partial strangulation of the bowel wall (Richter's hernia) is likely, because of the narrow neck.

Femoral hernias are occasionally bilateral.

Examination (Fig. 14.10)

Because of the thick-walled sac, a femoral hernia can be seen and felt when the patient is lying flat. It is easier in that position to find the pubic tubercle and other related anatomical landmarks.

(a) A right femoral hernia. Note that the femoral hernia bulges into the crease of the groin.

(b) A larger femoral hernia, in an elderly female, with a wide neck stretching laterally over the femoral vein.

Fig. 14.10 FEMORAL HERNIAS

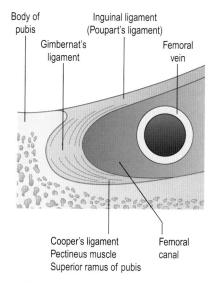

Body of pubis
Gimbernat's ligament
Inguinal ligament (Poupart's ligament)
Femoral vein
Cooper's ligament
Pectineus muscle
Superior ramus of pubis
Femoral canal

Fig. 14.9 The boundaries of the left femoral canal.

CHAPTER 14 | THE ABDOMINAL WALL, HERNIAS AND THE UMBILICUS

Position The neck of a femoral hernia, or the point at which it disappears into the abdomen, is below the inguinal ligament and lateral to the pubic tubercle (Fig. 14.11). The bulge usually appears to be directly behind the skin crease of the groin, whereas the inguinal hernia bulges out above the groin crease. With experience, this feature allows spot diagnosis.

A small hernia in a fat person is very difficult to feel, so take great care when examining this region in a patient with intestinal obstruction.

Colour The overlying skin will be of normal colour. Even if the hernia is strangulated, the sac and superficial fascia provide good camouflage.

Temperature The skin temperature is normal for the same reasons.

Tenderness Femoral hernias are not usually tender unless strangulated.

Shape and size The lump is almost spherical, and the neck cannot be defined clearly.

Most femoral hernias are small. Should they enlarge, they extend or spread upwards towards the fold of the groin because downward extension is limited by the attachment of the membranous layer of the superficial fascia (*Scarpa's fascia*) to the deep fascia of the upper thigh.

Surface The surface of the sac is usually smooth.

Composition The majority of femoral hernias feel firm because they consist of a thick-walled fatty sac. The peritoneal sac is small and is either empty or contains omentum.

Reducibility The majority of femoral hernias cannot be reduced, as most of the swelling is the sac itself.

Cough impulse Femoral hernias do not usually have a cough impulse.

Relations Diagnosis depends upon the site of the lump, hence the importance of clearly defining its relations to the surrounding structures (Revision panels 14.5, 14.6).

Local tissues Femoral hernias develop through a natural defect but are sometimes seen after the repair of an inguinal hernia. Look out for groin scars.

General examination As ever, this should be routine.

Prevascular femoral hernia (Fig. 14.12)

This is a rare variety of femoral hernia. The femoral canal expands laterally under the inguinal ligament in front of the femoral artery and vein. It has a wide neck and a flattened wide sac, which bulges downwards and laterally.

Prevascular hernias usually reduce, and have a cough impulse. They rarely strangulate. They are difficult to repair by open techniques because the femoral vessels form the posterior wall of the defect.

Fig. 14.12 A prevascular femoral hernia.

Fig. 14.11 The sites of appearance of inguinal and femoral hernia.

Inguinal hernias
Appear through the external inguinal ring, above and medial to the pubic tubercle

Femoral hernias
Appear through the femoral canal below and lateral to the pubic tubercle

Revision panel 14.5

The differential diagnosis of femoral hernia

Inguinal hernia

Enlarged lymph gland

Saphena varix

Ectopic testis

Psoas abscess (Fig. 14.13)

Psoas bursa

Lipoma

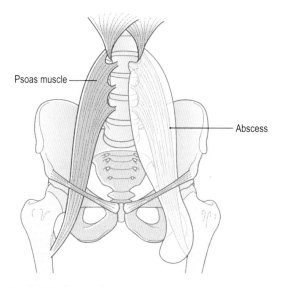

Fig. 14.13 Psoas abscess.

UMBILICAL HERNIA

All hernias that are related to the umbilicus may be called umbilical hernias. They may be congenital or acquired. All congenital umbilical hernias come through the umbilical defect itself. In adults, most umbilical hernias are acquired and come through a defect adjacent to the umbilical cicatrix, rather than through the umbilical scar itself, and should be termed paraumbilical (Fig. 14.14). In practice, the simple expression 'umbilical hernia' is used commonly for both varieties.

The normal umbilicus

Rectus abdominis muscle

Scar in linea alba tethered to the skin

Skin dimple

A congenital umbilical hernia

The umbilical scar fails to form or is weak. The abdominal contents bulge through the weak spot and evert the umbilicus

An acquired true umbilical hernia

The umbilical scar is stretched by a raised intra-abdominal pressure and the umbilicus everts

A paraumbilical hernia

The hernial orifice is at the side of the umbilical scar so the sac bulges out the umbilicus, turning it into a crescent-shaped slit

Fig. 14.14 Anatomy of an umbilical hernia.

Congenital umbilical hernia (Fig. 14.15)

In early fetal life, the whole of the mid-gut protrudes through the umbilicus. As it returns into the abdomen, the gap in the abdominal wall gradually closes, leaving a small central defect through which the umbilical vessels connect the fetus with the placenta. Should the process to obliterate the

CHAPTER 14 | THE ABDOMINAL WALL, HERNIAS AND THE UMBILICUS

(a) This baby also has a left inguinal hernia and a right hydrocele.

(b) An umbilical hernia in a 3-year-old female.

(c) A regressing congenital umbilical hernia. The defect has almost closed, and the overlying skin is collapsing inwards to become a normal umbilicus.

Fig. 14.15 CONGENITAL UMBILICAL HERNIAS

peritoneal sac fail and the defect persists, there will be a congenital umbilical hernia.

A congenital persisting protrusion of bowel through the umbilical defect without a covering of skin is called an exomphalos. This is a failure of development of the abdominal wall and not a true hernia.

History

Age Although the weakness is present at birth, the hernia may be very small and not immediately noticed.

Ethnicity Congenital umbilical hernias are more common in the Afro-Caribbean races.

Symptoms The swelling rarely causes any symptoms for the patient, but parental anxiety is common. Intestinal obstruction or irreducibility is extremely rare. A visible hernia may be embarrassing to a child when noticed by others. 'Tummy ache' in children may be attributed to the hernia, but it is unlikely that there is ever a genuine association.

Natural history The vast majority of congenital umbilical hernias resolve spontaneously during the first few years of life. It is difficult to explain how a large defect in an active child will close, but this is usual. The hernia becomes gradually smaller and then disappears. However, if there is still a defect by the age of 4 years, it is unlikely to close and operation is required.

Examination

Shape and size Congenital umbilical hernias are usually hemispherical and overlie a palpable defect in the abdominal wall. The size of the lump is variable. Very small hernias can only be found by gently palpating the umbilicus with the tip of a finger. Although the hernia may be sizeable, the palpable defect is often small.

In neonates, the remnants of the umbilical cord may be visible.

Composition Congenital umbilical hernias are soft, compressible and easy to reduce. They usually contain bowel so would be resonant to percussion, which is difficult to elicit in a small child. They reduce spontaneously when the child lies down and become tense when the child cries.

Cough impulse An expansile cough impulse is invariable.

Umbilical hernia in adults

A true umbilical hernia comes through the umbilical scar and has the umbilical skin tethered to it. It is not common in adults and is usually secondary to raised intra-abdominal pressure. The causes of an acquired umbilical hernia include pregnancy and ascites.

Paraumbilical hernia

This is the common acquired umbilical hernia. It appears through a defect adjacent to the umbilical scar (Fig. 14.16). It does not bulge into the centre of the umbilicus, and the umbilical skin is not attached to the centre of the sac.

(a) Note that the hernia is clearly coming out alongside the true umbilical scar.

(b) A large paraumbilical hernia, partially obscured by a very fat abdominal wall. Note the classical crescent shape of the umbilicus.

Fig. 14.16 PARAUMBILICAL HERNIAS

History

Age Paraumbilical hernias usually develop in middle and old age. They are more common in females than in males, and are associated with parity and obesity.

Symptoms The symptoms are swelling and discomfort. Sometimes the only symptom is pain and tenderness around the umbilicus, made worse by prolonged standing or strenuous exercise, and the doctor finds the hernia.

Strangulation of an umbilical hernia, whether or not it has been previously noticed by the patient, regularly occurs. The usual contents are extraperitoneal fat or omentum, so even though the hernial contents may be strangulated, bowel is not obstructed or damaged.

Examination

Position The main bulge of the hernia is beside the umbilicus, which is pushed to one side and stretched into a crescent shape. With a large hernia in a fat patient, there may be a crescent-shaped pit, with attachment of the skin to the umbilicus at the bottom. This pit may be too deep to clean, and in consequence there may be a foul-smelling discharge and even a collection of dried-up sebaceous secretions, an *ompholith* (see below).

Surface and edge The surface is smooth and the edge easy to define, except when the patient's abdominal wall is very fat.

Composition The lump is firm as it usually contains omentum. If it contains bowel, it is soft and resonant to percussion. It will be reducible unless the contents are adherent to the sac or the defect is very narrow.

Cough impulse Most of these hernias have an expansile cough impulse.

Relations The skin at the centre of the umbilicus is not attached to the centre of the sac as in the true umbilical hernia, but the umbilical skin is usually firmly applied to the side of the sac and may be fixed to it.

If the hernia can be reduced, the firm fibrous edge of the defect in the linea alba is easy to feel.

General examination Although abdominal distension usually causes a true umbilical hernia, it can exacerbate a paraumbilical hernia, so look for underlying causes of distension.

EPIGASTRIC HERNIA (FIG. 14.17)

An epigastric hernia is a protrusion of extraperitoneal fat, and sometimes a small peritoneal sac, through a defect in the linea alba somewhere between the xiphisternum and the umbilicus.

The patient complains of epigastric pain, which is localized exactly to the site of the hernia, but often does not notice the underlying lump.

The pain is sometimes associated with eating, so the patient calls it 'indigestion' and makes a self-diagnosis of peptic ulceration. A likely explanation for this is that the fatty hernia is 'nipped' by the linea alba on leaning forward in the sitting position adopted at the dining table. Thus, when a patient complains of epigastric discomfort, palpate the abdominal wall very carefully before concentrating on deep palpation, because all the symptoms may be caused by a small, fatty epigastric hernia.

On examination, these hernias feel firm, do not usually have a cough impulse and cannot be reduced. It is sometimes impossible to distinguish them from lipomas, only the typical position suggesting the correct diagnosis. The defect is always exactly in the midline, but the sac and hence the palpable swelling may lie to one side.

Epigastric hernia in children (Fig. 14.17)

This condition is reasonably common in childhood, sometimes associated with divarication of the rectus abdominis muscles. A small hernia may only be visible intermittently, leading to diagnostic uncertainty. As strangulation of such a sac in a child rarely, if ever, occurs, it is safe to wait until the hernia is seen before recommending surgery, unlike inguinal hernia in children, for which an operation may be indicated on the history alone.

INCISIONAL HERNIA

An abdominal incisional hernia is a hernia through a scar in the abdominal wall, caused by a previous surgical operation or injury. Scar tissue is inelastic and stretches progressively if subjected to constant stress.

History

Patients usually remember the operation or wound that caused the scar, but may not recall any complications in the original wound such as a haematoma or infection, which weakened it and made it more susceptible to the development of a hernia.

(a) A 3-year-old male with two epigastric hernias and an umbilical hernia. These small hernias can be the source of epigastric pain.

(b) A female with a large epigastric hernia, which was misdiagnosed as a lipoma and ignored for 5 years.

(c) An elderly female with an epigastric hernia. This reduced easily and caused no symptoms.

Fig. 14.17 THREE PATIENTS WITH EPIGASTRIC HERNIAS

There may be a history of factors likely to weaken the abdominal musculature, such as chronic cough, obesity or steroid therapy.

Age Incisional hernias occur at all ages but are more common in the elderly.

Symptoms The most common symptoms are a lump and pain. Intestinal obstruction and strangulation can occur.

Examination (Fig. 14.18)

Commonly, there is a lump with an expansile cough impulse, beneath an old scar. The defect in the abdominal wall may be palpable. Incisional hernias are not infrequently irreducible, the defect being plugged with adherent omentum.

If the lump does not reduce and does not have a cough impulse, it may not be a hernia, but rather a deposit of tumour, a chronic abscess or haematoma, or a foreign-body granuloma. All these lesions, except recurrent tumour, appear shortly after the initial surgery.

The first signs of incisional hernia usually appear in the first year after surgery but sometimes many years later.

Fig. 14.18 A large incisional hernia.

DIVARICATION OF THE RECTI

This is separation of the rectus abdominis muscles with extenuation of the linea alba, from the xiphisternum to umbilicus and occasionally below.

It may be seen in children in the first few years of life. It is only noticeable when the abdominal wall is tensed. Children have a relatively larger abdominal cavity than adults; even the slimmest appear somewhat 'pot-bellied'.

The condition usually improves and eventually disappears as the child grows, but occasionally it persists into adult life. There may be a coincidental umbilical hernia or an epigastric hernia.

The only clinical concern is the appearance, as strangulation is impossible with such a wide-necked bulge.

Divarication of the recti is also seen in adults, in females during and immediately after childbirth. There may be a wide separation of the muscles, with stretched overlying abdominal skin. The examiner may be able to put a hand into the abdominal cavity. (Ask permission to do this!)

As abdominal tone recovers, the defect closes, although it may become permanent after multiple pregnancies.

Although it is strictly speaking an incisional hernia, iatrogenic divarication may follow repeated surgery through a long midline incision.

Divarication is best observed with the patient lying supine. If asked to raise the head and legs together, the recti are fully tensed and the abdominal pressure rises. The thinned-out linea alba then bulges, producing a visible swelling. Patients of all ages learn the best way to produce the swelling.

RARE ABDOMINAL HERNIAS

Spigelian hernias occur at the edge of the rectus sheath, below the umbilicus and above the inguinal area. They are seen in obese patients and may be difficult to diagnose.

Obturator hernias come through the obturator foramen, and the small sac is concealed among the adductor muscles of the thigh. Only on very rare occasions will there be a palpable mass. The usual presentation is small bowel obstruction of unknown cause. The sac may compress the obturator nerve and cause pain in the medial side of the thigh.

CHAPTER 14 | THE ABDOMINAL WALL, HERNIAS AND THE UMBILICUS

Lumbar and gluteal hernias are rare. They are commonly associated with previous surgery near to the defect, such as a loin incision or an excision of the rectum. Diagnosis is difficult and often requires imaging by magnetic resonance imaging.

An *interstitial hernia* is a variety of inguinal hernia in which the sac of the hernia spreads between the muscles that form the inguinal canal, above the groin, and emerges through a defect in the internal oblique and transverse muscles rather than the external inguinal ring. It may be suspected when the sac, although clearly in the groin, appears more laterally and looks flatter than usual.

THE UMBILICUS

The most common abnormality of the umbilicus is an umbilical hernia, described above.

The important congenital abnormalities of the umbilicus are exomphalos and fistula, and the common acquired conditions (apart from hernias) are inflammation and invasion by tumour.

Exomphalos (Fig. 14.19)

This condition, present at birth, represents an intrauterine failure of the intestines to return to the abdomen, combined with a failure of the two sides of the laterally developing abdominal wall to unite to cover the embryonic defect.

All layers of the abdominal wall are deficient over the protruding intestines. Their only covering is a thin, transparent membrane formed from the remnant of the coverings of the yolk sac. Once this membrane is exposed to the air, it loses its thin, transparent appearance, becoming thicker and covered with an opaque, fibrinous exudate. Urgent surgery is required.

Umbilical fistulas

Four structures pass through the umbilicus during fetal development: the umbilical vein, the umbilical arteries, the vitello-intestinal duct and the urachus. If either of the last two tubes fails to close properly, there will be an intestinal or a urinary fistula.

A *patent vitello-intestinal duct* (Fig. 14.20) in the neonate produces an intermittent discharge of mucus and sometimes faeces from the umbilicus. It

(a) The bowel can be seen through the thin membrane.

(b) The thin membrane is covered with fibrin but has, nevertheless, ruptured. The umbilical cord is still present.

Fig. 14.19 TWO EXAMPLES OF EXOMPHALOS

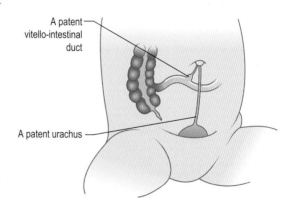

A patent vitello-intestinal duct

A patent urachus

Fig. 14.20 A patent vitello-intestinal duct or patent urachus can become an intestinal or urinary fistula, respectively.

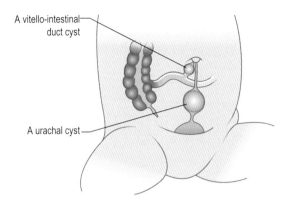

Fig. 14.21 If the vitello-intestinal duct or urachus are not completely obliterated, they may turn into cysts.

A vitello-intestinal duct cyst

A urachal cyst

is a rare abnormality. Sometimes there is visible small intestinal mucosa lining an obvious fistula, but on other occasions there may only be a small fluid leak and the condition mimics an umbilical granuloma. The duct connects to the ileum at the site of a Meckel's diverticulum.

A *patent urachus* can become a track through which urine can leak onto the external surface of the abdomen through the umbilicus. This rare condition occasionally presents in childhood, but more commonly in adult life in association with chronic retention of urine caused by disease of the prostate.

The patient complains of a watery discharge from the umbilicus.

An umbilical discharge is nearly always caused by infection in the umbilicus; nevertheless, remember the possibility of a urachal fistula, particularly if there are symptoms of urinary obstruction or a palpable bladder.

Both these embryonic tracts may partially close, leaving a patent segment that becomes a cyst (Fig. 14.21).

A *vitello-intestinal duct cyst* is a small, spherical, mobile swelling deep to the umbilicus that is tethered to the umbilicus and to the small bowel by a fibrous cord.

A *urachal cyst* is an immobile swelling below the umbilicus deep to the abdominal muscles. It may become large enough to fluctuate and have a fluid thrill. If it is still connected to the bladder, it may vary in size and be difficult to distinguish from a chronically distended bladder.

Umbilical granuloma

After the umbilical cord has been severed and tied, the proximal remnant shrivels and separates spontaneously. This leaves an area of chronic inflammation at the line of demarcation, which is quickly covered by epithelium. If the inflammatory process becomes florid, with associated infection, excess granulation tissue is formed that prevents the raw area becoming epithelialized.

The baby presents with a pouting umbilicus surmounted by a bright red, moist, friable, sometimes hemispherical mass of bleeding granulation tissue (Fig. 14.22). This condition is similar to the pyogenic granuloma seen in other parts of the skin. It usually regresses spontaneously in the first month or so of life. If the condition persists longer than this, the possibility of a patent vitello-intestinal duct or an umbilical adenoma should be considered.

Fig. 14.22 An umbilical granuloma. This is an excessive amount of granulation tissue at the point where the umbilical cord separated. These granulomas are often associated with an umbilical hernia.

Umbilical adenoma

An umbilical adenoma is a patch of intestinal epithelium left behind when the vitello-intestinal duct closes. It may produce a discharge from the depths of the umbilicus, but more often protrudes from the umbilicus and looks like a raspberry. Although it resembles an umbilical granuloma, the cause is quite different. It will not resolve spontaneously.

The mother complains that the baby has a lump at the umbilicus and a mucous discharge.

Omphalitis

Infection within the umbilicus is not uncommon in adults (Fig. 14.23). It is usually associated with inadequate hygiene and a sunken umbilicus caused by obesity, made worse by any coexisting paraumbilical hernia. The condition is similar to the intertrigo that occurs between folds of skin elsewhere associated with obesity and sweating, which become secondarily infected with skin organisms that produce an unpleasant smell.

The patient complains of umbilical discharge, pain and soreness.

On examination, the skin within and around the umbilicus is red and tender, and exuding a seropurulent discharge with a characteristic foul smell.

The whole umbilicus may feel indurated, especially if there is an ompholith or a tumour deposit.

Although simple dermatitis or skin infection is by far the most common cause of a discharge from the umbilicus, it is essential to exclude the other causes of an umbilical discharge, which are listed in Revision panel 14.7.

True omphalitis is infection of the stump of the umbilical cord following inadequate postnatal care and cleanliness.

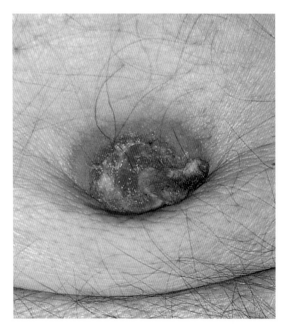

Fig. 14.23 Omphalitis. A protruding mass of infected granulation tissue caused by a large ompholith, the brown tip of which is just visible.

Revision panel 14.7
The causes of a discharge from the umbilicus

Congenital
Intestinal fistula
Patent urachus
Umbilical adenoma

Acquired
Umbilical granuloma
Dermatitis (intertrigo)
Ompholith (umbilical concretion)
Fistula (intestinal)
Secondary carcinoma
Endometriosis

Ompholith

When the sebaceous secretions that accumulate in the umbilicus are mixed with the broken hairs and fluff from clothing that become sucked into the umbilicus, the mixture can form a firm lump, worthy of the name umbilical stone or ompholith. The outside tip of the concretions dries out and may protrude like a sebaceous horn. In certain parts of the UK, there is an old wives' tale that if this stone is removed, the sufferer will bleed to death!

Routine personal hygiene will usually prevent the formation of an ompholith, but this is not always as simple as it sounds, as the umbilicus can be deep and narrow, particularly in the obese.

Small concretions are common and uncomplicated. An abscess will occasionally develop in a narrow-necked umbilicus containing an ompholith. The patient feels unwell and has a very painful, throbbing, swollen umbilicus that may be difficult to distinguish from a strangulated umbilical hernia.

Pus tracking from an intra-abdominal abscess may occasionally point at the umbilicus, the most common cause being diverticular disease.

Secondary carcinoma

(Sister Joseph's nodule)
A firm or hard nodule bulging into the umbilicus, underneath the skin or eroding through it, in a patient who is losing weight and looks unwell is likely to

be a nodule of metastatic cancer (Fig. 14.24). This presentation always indicates advanced, widespread intra-abdominal disease, and the primary tumour is usually in the abdomen.

The tumour cells reach the umbilicus via lymphatics that run in the edge of the falciform ligament alongside the obliterated umbilical vein, or by transperitoneal spread.

Nodules of secondary carcinoma may ulcerate, bleed and become infected. Rarely, the tumour deposit is in continuity with bowel and there may be an acquired intestinal fistula.

Fig. 14.24 A nodule of metastatic carcinoma bulging through the umbilicus causing a serosanguinous discharge. This is known as a Sister Joseph's nodule.

Endometrioma

If, in a female patient, the umbilicus enlarges, becomes painful and discharges blood during menstruation, it may contain a patch of ectopic endometrial tissue.

Discolouration of the umbilicus

The following physical signs are rare, but the diseases that cause them are common and serious.

A blue tinge around the umbilicus, caused by dilated, tortuous, sometimes visible, veins, is called a *caput medusae*, after Medusa, the mythical Gorgon who had small snakes on her scalp instead of hair. The dilated veins are collateral vessels that have developed to circumvent portal vein obstruction. There will be other signs of portal hypertension and liver failure.

Yellow-blue bruising around the umbilicus (*Cullen's sign*) and in the flank (*Grey Turner's sign*; see Chapter 15) may be caused by pancreatic enzymes that have tracked along the falciform ligament to the umbilicus or across the retroperitoneal space to the loin and digested the subcutaneous tissues following an attack of severe acute pancreatitis. Both appear a few days after the beginning of the acute symptoms.

Bruising at the umbilicus can also be associated with intra-abdominal bleeding, particularly when it is extraperitoneal. Causes include ruptured aortic aneurysms, ruptured ectopic pregnancy and accidental periuterine bleeding in pregnancy.

15 The abdomen

EXAMINATION OF THE ABDOMEN

The abdomen contains the stomach, duodenum, small and large bowel, liver, gallbladder, spleen, pancreas, kidneys, uterus, bladder, aorta and vena cava and, in females, the uterus, ovaries and Fallopian tubes. This relatively small cavity therefore contains a number of vital organs, all of which are susceptible to disease or malfunction. Many are inaccessible to palpation, being hidden behind the lower ribs or inside the bony pelvis (Fig. 15.1).

The close proximity of the abdominal organs to each other can make the brain incapable of distinguishing which organ is the source of a pain. Symptoms and signs will help to distinguish the likely organ and the pathology responsible for the pain.

Fig. 15.1 These drawings show the extent of the abdominal cavity. The paler lavender areas indicate the parts of the abdomen shielded from palpation by the ribs and the pelvis.

Preparation

The environment

The examination room must be warm and private if the patient is to lie undressed and relaxed. A cold couch placed in a draught or in the view of other patients makes proper examination impossible. A good light is essential, with, ideally, daylight coming obliquely from the side of the patient to emphasize the shadows. Artificial light obliterates the soft shadows that often give the first indication of asymmetry, and many neon lights falsify colours, particularly the yellows and blues.

The examination couch or bed

A hard, flat couch makes the patient lie absolutely flat and opens the gap between the pubis and the xiphisternum, but unfortunately stretches and tightens the abdominal muscles. Conversely, a soft bed lets the lumbar spine sink into a deep curve closing the gap between the pubis and the ribs. The best compromise is a hard couch with a backrest that can be raised by 15–20°. The hard couch ensures that patients retain their lumbar lordosis, opening access to the abdomen and pushing the central contents anteriorly. The elevation of the thoracic cage relaxes the anterior abdominal wall muscles.

Exposure

The full extent of the abdomen must be visible and, ideally, patients should be uncovered from nipples to knees. Many find this embarrassing and a compromise is to cover the lower abdomen with a sheet or blanket while the abdomen is being palpated. At the end of the examination, you must never forget to examine the genitalia and the hernial orifices.

Getting the patient to relax

It is not possible to feel anything within the abdomen if the patient is tense. There are several ways in which relaxation can be achieved:

- Ask the patient to rest their head on the couch or a pillow to avoid tensing the rectus abdominis muscles.
- Ask the patient to place their arms by their sides, not behind their head.
- Encourage the patient to sink their back into the couch and breathe regularly and slowly.
- Only press your hands into the abdomen during expiration as the abdominal muscles relax.

If the above manoeuvres do not work, ask the patient to flex their hips to 45° and their knees to 90° and place an extra pillow behind their head. These procedures tilt up the pelvis and reduce the access to the abdomen, but they usually relax the abdominal muscles.

The position of the examiner

The examiner's hands should be clean and warm with short nails. It is impossible to palpate deeply with long nails, and it is an insult to the patient to have dirty hands.

The whole hand should rest on the abdomen by keeping the hand and forearm horizontal, in the same plane as the front of the abdomen. To achieve this, the examiner must sit or kneel beside the bed. Do not examine the patient from a standing position by leaning forwards and dorsiflexing your wrist.

Sitting or kneeling beside the patient with your forearm level with the front of the abdomen puts your eyes about 50 cm above your hand, an ideal level for seeing any soft shadows caused by lumps and bumps (Fig. 15.2).

Fig. 15.2 When you palpate the abdomen, sit or kneel so that your forearm is horizontal and level with the anterior abdominal wall, and your eyes are 50 cm above this level. If you are higher, your wrist will be extended and you will not be able to palpate comfortably and firmly. In this illustration, the abdomen is inadequately exposed. The patient's underwear should have been removed or lowered to the level of the pubis.

The examination

This should follow the standard routine of inspection, palpation, percussion and auscultation.

Inspection

Look at the whole patient (see Chapter 1). Look for any general abnormality indicative of intra-abdominal pathology such as cachexia, pallor or jaundice.

Inspection of the abdomen from the end of the bed reveals whether there is any asymmetry or distension.

Note the position, shape and size of any bulge, any changes in its shape, and whether it moves with respiration or increases with coughing.

Observe the reaction of the patient to coughing or moving. Patients with peritonitis find movement extremely painful and consequently tend to lie very still, while patients with colic roll around with each bout of pain.

Record the presence of any scars, sinuses or fistulas.

Dilated surface veins may indicate the possibility of portal hypertension or inferior vena caval occlusion.

Palpation

Palpate gently but deliberately, firmly and with purpose. Rapid, jerky or circular movements reminiscent of kneading dough are distressing for patients and cause them to lose confidence. Keeping your hands still and feeling the intra-abdominal structures moving beneath them gives more information than rapid and thoughtless palpation.

Finish by feeling the areas that might otherwise be forgotten (see Revision panel 15.1):

- Feel the supraclavicular fossae and neck for lymph glands.
- Feel the hernial orifices at rest and when the patient coughs.
- Feel the femoral pulses.
- Examine the external genitalia.
- Look at the hands, nails and facies.

General light palpation for tenderness

This should be done by gently resting a hand on the patient's abdomen and pressing lightly. The hand should be systematically moved over the whole of the abdomen. If you are right-handed, start in the left iliac fossa and move round in an anticlockwise direction to finish in the right iliac fossa.

When a patient complains of pain, ask them to indicate its site before you begin your palpation, so that you can start over a non-tender area and move towards the tender spot. Carefully define the area of tenderness so that you can depict it as a hatched area on a drawing of the abdomen.

Assess the degree of tenderness. Palpation over an area of mild tenderness just causes pain. *Guarding*, the tightening of the patient's abdominal muscles in response to pressure, indicates severe tenderness.

The sudden withdrawal of manual pressure may cause a sharp exacerbation of the pain, which is known as *rebound* or *release tenderness*. This test may be distressing for the patient, and it is preferable to assess rebound tenderness by the patient's response to *light* percussion.

The release of pressure in a distant non-tender part of the abdomen sometimes causes pain in the tender area.

General palpation for tenderness

When no pain is elicited by systematic light palpation over the whole abdomen, repeat the process, pressing more firmly and deeply to see if there is any deep tenderness.

Palpation for masses

The whole abdomen must be carefully palpated for the presence, position, shape, size, surface, edge, consistency, fluid thrill, resonance and pulsatility of any masses.

Tender masses in the abdomen are very difficult to feel because of the protective guarding of the abdominal wall muscles. A good idea of the surface and size of a tender mass may be obtained by resting your hand gently on the tender area and pressing a little deeper during expiration and feeling the mass as it moves beneath your hand.

Rapid, hard pressure achieves nothing in these circumstances because the patient tightens their abdominal muscles.

Palpation of the normal solid viscera

The liver   To feel the liver, place your right hand transversely and flat on the right side of the abdomen at the level of the umbilicus, parallel with the right costal margin (Fig. 15.3a). Then ask the patient to take a deep breath. If the liver is grossly enlarged, its lower edge will move downwards and bump against the radial side of your index finger. If nothing abnormal is felt, repeat the process after moving your hand upwards, inch by inch, until the costal margin is reached.

The liver edge may be straight or irregular, thin and sharp, or thick and rounded. The surface may be smooth or knobbly. Palpation beginning just below the costal margin can easily miss a large liver. Gross hepatomegaly may fill the whole abdomen so, if in doubt, begin your palpation in the left iliac fossa. An enlarged liver is dull to percussion, and its upper margin should be percussed out to assess its full dimension.

(a) Palpate the *liver* by resting your fingers on the abdomen almost parallel to the right costal margin, and asking the patient to breathe in. The liver edge can be made more prominent by putting your left hand under the lower ribs and lifting them forwards.

(b) Palpate the *spleen* with your fingers lying transversely across the abdomen so that the tip of the spleen will hit the tips of your index and middle fingers when the patient breathes in. You can make the spleen more prominent by lifting the lower ribs forwards with your left hand, as you do when palpating the left kidney.

(c) Palpate the *kidneys* by pressing firmly into the lumbar region during inspiration while lifting the kidney forwards with your other hand in the loin. (The exposure is inadequate for a proper examination of the whole abdomen in these three illustrations.)

Fig. 15.3 PALPATING THE ABDOMEN

The spleen An enlarged spleen appears below the tip of the tenth rib along a line heading towards the umbilicus and, if really large, may extend into the right iliac fossa. A normal spleen is not palpable.

To feel the spleen, place the fingertips of your right hand on the right iliac fossa just below the umbilicus (Fig. 15.3b). Ask the patient to take a deep breath. If nothing abnormal is felt, move your hand in stages towards the tip of the left tenth rib. When the costal margin is reached, place your left hand around the lower left rib cage, and lift the lower ribs and the spleen forwards as the patient inspires. This manoeuvre occasionally lifts a slightly enlarged spleen far enough forward to make it palpable.

The spleen is recognized by its shape and site and, when present, the notch on its superomedial edge. It is dull to percussion as it lies immediately beneath the abdominal wall with no bowel in front of it, unlike a renal mass (see below).

The kidneys Normal kidneys are usually impalpable, except in very thin people, but both lumbar regions should always be carefully examined.

To feel the patient's right kidney, place your left hand behind the patient's right loin between the 12th rib and the iliac crest, so that you can lift the loin and kidney forwards (Fig. 15.3c). Then place your right hand on the right side of the abdomen just below the level of the anterior superior iliac spine. As the patient breathes in and out, palpate the loin between both hands. The lower pole of a normal kidney may be felt at the height of inspiration in a very thin person. When a kidney is very easy to feel, it is either enlarged or abnormally low.

To feel the left kidney, lean across the patient, place your left hand around the flank into the left loin to lift it forwards, then place your right hand on the abdomen and feel any masses between the two hands.

An enlarged kidney can be pushed back and forth between the anterior and posterior hands. This is called *balloting*. It feels like patting a ball back and forth in a pool of water. Balloting is also used to palpate a fetus in a pregnant uterus.

Percussion

The whole abdomen must be percussed, particularly over any masses. A dull area may draw your attention to a mass that was missed on palpation and indicate a more detailed and careful palpation of the area of dullness. When there is a circumscribed mass, a tap on one side while feeling the opposite side with the other hand may reveal that it conducts a *fluid thrill*. Any area of dullness should be outlined by percussion with the abdomen in two positions to see if it moves or changes shape. Free fluid (*ascites*) changes shape and moves (*shifting dullness*; see page 532).

Percussion causes pain if peritonitis is present and is a useful method for mapping out a tender area (see above).

When a part or the whole of the abdomen appears distended, the patient should be held at the hips and the abdomen shaken from side to side. Splashing sounds – a *succussion splash* – indicate that there is an intra-abdominal viscus, usually the stomach, distended with a mixture of fluid and gas.

Auscultation

Listen to the bowel sounds. Peristalsis produces gurgling noises because the bowel contains a mixture of fluid and gas. The pitch of the noise depends upon the distension of the bowel and the proportions of gas and fluid. Normal bowel sounds are low-pitched gurgles that occur every few seconds. The absence of bowel sounds indicates that peristalsis has ceased. This may be either a primary or a secondary phenomenon. If you can hear the heart and breath sounds but no bowel sounds over a 30-second period, the patient probably has a *paralytic ileus*.

Increased peristalsis increases the volume and frequency of the bowel sounds. Distension of the bowel caused by a mechanical intestinal obstruction is associated not only with increased bowel sounds, but also with a change in the character of the sounds. They become amphoric in nature with runs of high-frequency gurgles, sounding like sea water entering a large cave through a narrow entrance, often described as 'tinkling'.

Having assessed the quality of the bowel sounds, it is important to listen for any systolic vascular bruits, which indicate arterial stenosis or increased blood flow through, for example, a fistula.

Revision panel 15.1
Never forget to examine
- Supraclavicular lymph glands
- Hernia orifices
- Femoral pulses
- Genitalia
- Bowel sounds
- Anal canal and rectum

ABDOMINAL PAIN

Time spent taking a careful history is never wasted, as abdominal pain is the only symptom of many intra-abdominal diseases. The two most significant properties of an abdominal pain are its *site* and its *character* (Revision panel 15.2).

Revision panel 15.2
The features of a pain that must be elicited
- Time and nature of onset
- Site
- Character (burning, throbbing, stabbing, constricting, colicky, aching)
- Severity
- Progression
- Duration
- End
- Radiation
- Relieving factors
- Exacerbating factors
- Associated symptoms, e.g. vomiting, diarrhoea, painful micturition, missed or absent periods

The significance of the site of abdominal pain

The abdomen can be divided into three horizontal zones – upper, central and lower – by two horizontal lines. These are the transpyloric plane (a line circling the body midway between the suprasternal notch and the symphysis pubis) and the transtubercular plane (a line circling the body that passes through the

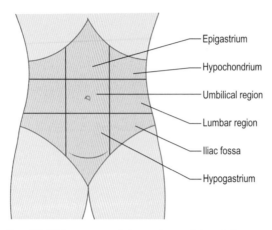

Fig. 15.4 The names of the regions of the abdomen.

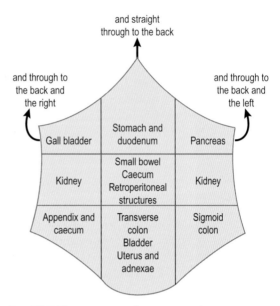

Fig. 15.5 The structures that commonly cause pain in the nine anatomical regions of the abdomen, with the pain often radiating through to the back.

two tubercles of the iliac crest) as shown in Fig. 15.4. Each of these three zones can be further vertically subdivided into three regions – central, right and left – by the two mid-clavicular lines.

The anatomical names of these nine regions are:

- the epigastrium;
- the right hypochondrium;
- the left hypochondrium;
- the umbilical region;
- the right lumbar region;
- the left lumbar region;
- the hypogastrium or suprapubic region;
- the right iliac fossa;
- the left iliac fossa.

Sometimes patients are only capable of localizing pain to the upper or lower half of the abdomen and/ or to the left or right side. Colicky pain is referred to the centre of the abdomen whatever its source, as it is a visceral sensation, whereas the pain from the parietal peritoneum is felt over the inflamed area (a somatic sensation).

Pain in the upper abdomen is most likely to arise from the biliary tree, stomach, duodenum or pancreas (Fig. 15.5). These structures produce right-sided, central and left-sided pain, respectively. The pain from these three organs radiates in different directions:

- Gallbladder pain may radiate through to the back and to the right, to reach the tip of the scapula. When felt in this area, it often seems to the patient to be a separate, independent pain.

- Ulcers in the posterior wall of the stomach or duodenum cause a pain that radiates through to the back.
- Pancreatic pain also tends to go through to the back and sometimes to the left.

Pain in the centre of the abdomen is most likely to arise from the small bowel, caecum and midline retroperitoneal structures such as the aorta. Pain from retroperitoneal structures often radiates through to the back. Pain in the lateral zones of the central region is most likely to come from the kidneys. Pain from the kidney is also felt in the loin, and may radiate down to the groin. All visceral pain may move and become localized if the inflammatory process in the viscus involves the parietal peritoneum.

Pain in the lower abdomen is most likely to come from the appendix, caecum, colon, bladder, uterus, ovaries and Fallopian tubes. Pain in the hypogastric region usually arises from the bladder, rectum, uterus and its adnexae. Pain in the right iliac fossa usually comes from the caecum and the appendix. Pain in the left iliac fossa usually comes from the sigmoid colon.

Lower abdominal pains rarely radiate, but pain from pelvic structures may be referred to the lower back or perineum.

The significance of the character of abdominal pain

It is possible to subdivide the character of the pain of the majority of the painful conditions that occur within the abdomen into two large categories: a constant pain associated with inflammation, ischaemia, infarction and neoplastic infiltration, and a colicky pain associated with obstruction of a muscular conducting tube such as the bowel or the ureter (colic).

The *constant pain* caused by inflammation, infiltration, ischaemia or infarction, whether it is the mild inflammatory response around a chronic peptic ulcer or the acute response to a perforated appendix, is made worse by any local or general movement and persists until the underlying cause subsides. Inflammation within the abdomen does not throb or burn in the same way that inflammatory pains do elsewhere.

The *colic* caused by obstruction to a muscular conducting viscus is a pain that fluctuates in severity at frequent intervals and feels griping in nature. The source of bowel colic can be suspected from the time interval between the peaks of the pain – short in the jejunum, longer in the ileum, and longer still in the colon. In biliary colic and renal colic, the peaks of pain are short, and the pain seldom goes away completely between exacerbations. Prolonged obstruction to the outflow of any hollow viscus ultimately causes it to distend. This produces a constant 'stretching' pain, which is different from the ache of inflammation but not colicky in nature. A similar pain can come from conditions that stretch the retroperitoneal tissues.

Colic can also be caused by muscular dysfunction, i.e. disorders of gastrointestinal mobility such as the irritable bowel syndrome, as opposed to true colic, which is secondary to obstruction.

The significance of radiation

Radiation of a pain signifies that other structures are becoming involved. For example, when the pain from a duodenal ulcer radiates through to the back, it indicates that the inflammation has spread beyond the duodenum into adjacent structures in the posterior abdominal wall, such as the pancreas. Radiation, therefore, not only indicates the source of the pain, but may also hint at the extent of the disease.

The significance of the rate of onset and severity

Patients with severe abdominal pain of *acute onset* are usually collectively grouped as having an 'acute abdomen'. These patients usually consult their general practitioner or seek emergency medical help once their pain has persisted for more than an hour or so. Many, however, will have had chronic symptoms over the preceding months or years caused by the condition currently causing their acute symptoms; i.e. the same condition can present acutely or chronically.

Therefore, although the rate and severity of presentation may indicate the urgency of the problem, they do not always indicate the nature of the underlying pathology.

Whatever the urgency and underlying pathology, a full history and clinical examination (as described above) must be carried out so that a working diagnosis or differential diagnosis can be made and the patient assigned to one of the following management categories:

- An acute abdomen, e.g. peritonitis, with a known or unknown underlying cause requiring urgent treatment.
- An abdominal pain of known or unknown cause requiring pain palliation pending further investigation and treatment.
- An abdominal pain with no evidence of any clinically detectable intra-abdominal pathology that can be observed and investigated later if necessary, i.e. time to wait and see.

To put it another way:

- I may or may not know the diagnosis but the problem needs urgent management.
- I understand the problem but not necessarily its cause, and have time to investigate further in order to decide what to do.
- I do not think there is anything wrong, and can wait and see whether further investigations will be required.

In almost every case, additional investigations are likely to be required to refine the diagnosis and plan treatment, but when the diagnosis is 'uncertain', careful monitoring and repeated re-examination are essential to detect any progression or resolution of the problem and ensure that important new physical signs are not missed. Acute physical signs often develop over several hours and become clear cut, often diagnostic, by the time of a later examination. In contrast, the signs of chronic conditions may take months to develop.

THE PATHOLOGY OF THE ACUTE ABDOMEN

The principal causes of acute abdominal pain are:

- inflammation of a viscus;
- perforation of a viscus;
- obstruction of a viscus;
- infarction of a viscus;
- intra-abdominal or retroperitoneal haemorrhage;
- extra-abdominal or medical causes of acute abdominal pain.

INFLAMMATION OF A VISCUS

Inflammation of a viscus results in localized pain and a condition known as *peritonitis*. The clinical features of peritonitis are as follows.

Tenderness and guarding

The tenderness is initially localized to the site of the inflammation, but can become more generalized as the condition worsens. Guarding is an excellent indication of the severity of the tenderness. If the whole abdomen is tense, there is likely to be general peritonitis.

Rebound tenderness or tenderness on percussion

This is just another way of detecting that the abdomen is very tender. It can be a valuable sign because the patient is not expecting pain when you suddenly remove your hand, so the apprehension, which can cause guarding during direct palpation, is absent. It can cause, however, considerable discomfort so should be used sparingly.

Localized pain during distant palpation

The structures in the painful area are likely to be very inflamed. When you press on a distant non-tender part of the abdomen pain can often be felt in the actual inflamed area (e.g. *Rovsing's sign* in appendicitis).

Absence of bowel sounds

The absence of bowel sounds *per se* does not indicate peritonitis, but their absence in a tender, rigid abdomen makes it highly likely that there is generalized peritonitis.

An increasing tachycardia

There is likely to be serious disease within the abdomen if the pulse rate increases gradually during 1–2 hours of observation.

Pyrexia

The temperature rises only when the peritoneal cavity becomes heavily infected. **Remember that steroids damp down the inflammatory response. Patients on corticosteroids with a severe peritonitis may have a normal temperature.**

When a peptic ulcer erodes through the wall of the stomach or duodenum at a point where it is covered only by visceral peritoneum, acid gastric juice enters the peritoneal cavity. This causes a chemical peritonitis, which later becomes infected with bacteria.

PERFORATION OF A VISCUS

A perforation in the wall of a hollow viscus allows its contents – acid, bacteria, small bowel contents, faeces, bile or urine – to enter the peritoneal cavity, where they rapidly cause a chemical or infected peritonitis. The history and physical signs may indicate the site and cause of the perforation, but whether they do or do not, it is usually necessary to perform a laparotomy to confirm the diagnosis and close the perforation. It is essential, therefore, to recognize the signs of peritonitis (see above). The pain usually begins near the site of the perforation but rapidly spreads across the whole abdomen (Revision panel 15.3).

OBSTRUCTION OF A VISCUS/ INTESTINAL OBSTRUCTION

There are many causes of intestinal obstruction (Revision panel 15.4).

Revision panel 15.3

The conditions likely to cause the perforation of a viscus

Peptic ulceration

Acute diverticulitis

Ischaemia

Gangrenous appendicitis

Trauma

Ulcerative colitis (toxic megacolon)

A perforated gallbladder

Small bowel disease (Crohn's disease, strangulation, a foreign body, typhoid)

Carcinoma of the colon

Boerhaave's syndrome

Radiation necrosis

Revision panel 15.4

Common causes of alimentary tract obstruction, by age

Neonates

Atresia (duodenum, ileum)

Meconium obstruction

Volvulus neonatorum

3 weeks

Congenital hypertrophic pyloric stenosis

6–9 months

Intussusception

Teenage

Inflammatory masses (appendicitis)

Intussusception of Meckel's diverticulum or polyp

Young adult

Hernia

Adhesions

Adult

Hernia

Adhesions

Inflammation (appendicitis, Crohn's disease)

Carcinoma

Elderly

Carcinoma

Inflammation (diverticulitis)

Sigmoid volvulus

Although it is normally possible, on the basis of the history aided by physical signs and plain abdominal radiographs, to tell whether the site of the obstruction is in the small bowel or large bowel, the clinician must always attempt to answer these three questions.

1. Is there intestinal obstruction?
2. Is the bowel strangulated?
3. Is the site of the obstruction in the small bowel or large bowel?

The signs of strangulation are the same as the signs of local peritoneal inflammation, which have been described above, namely, pain, tenderness, guarding and rebound tenderness.

The cardinal symptoms of intestinal obstruction are pain, vomiting, distension and absolute constipation (Revision panel 15.5), but the severity and time of onset of each of these symptoms depend upon the level of obstruction.

Revision panel 15.5

The cardinal symptoms of intestinal obstruction

Pain

Vomiting

Distension

Absolute constipation

Pain

The pain of intestinal obstruction is *true colic*. It occurs as a severe central griping pain interspersed with periods of little or no pain. Colic is uncommon with obstructions above the pylorus. Small bowel colic is felt in the centre of the abdomen, and large bowel colic usually in the lower third of the abdomen. Small bowel colic occurs every 2–20 minutes, depending on the level of obstruction in the small bowel. Large bowel colic occurs about every 30 minutes or more.

Vomiting

Intestinal obstruction causes frequent vomiting. The nature of the vomitus depends upon the level of the obstruction. With pyloric obstruction, the vomitus is watery and acid. High small bowel obstruction produces a greenish-blue, bile-stained vomit. Obstruction in the lower part of the small bowel is associated with a brown vomit that becomes increasingly foul-smelling as the obstruction persists. It becomes so thick, brown and foul that it is often called *faeculent vomit*. Vomiting is unusual and is usually a late symptom in patients with large bowel obstruction.

Distension

The lower the site of the obstruction, the more bowel there is available to distend. High obstructions are not associated with distension, particularly if the patient is vomiting frequently.

Obstruction of the colon causes the colon to distend around the periphery of the abdomen. The distension then extends into the small bowel if the ileocaecal valve is incompetent. If this valve remains competent, the right side of the colon, especially the caecum, can become grossly distended, causing a visible bulge in the right iliac fossa that is hyper-resonant.

Small bowel obstruction tends to cause distension in the centre of the abdomen and occasionally in a very thin patient visible peristalsis may be visible in which loops of small bowel become visible with peristaltic waves running across them during episodes of colic (Fig. 15.6).

Absolute constipation

Once an obstruction is complete and the bowel below is empty, absolute constipation develops. This means that neither faeces nor flatus is passed. This occurs early in lower large bowel obstructions and late in high small bowel obstructions.

To summarize

A high small bowel obstruction causes frequent colic and vomiting. The distension is slight and central, and absolute constipation is rare. A low large bowel obstruction causes infrequent colic, absolute constipation and peripheral abdominal distension. Vomiting is absent or occurs very late on.

The bowel sounds in a patient with mechanical obstruction are at first loud, frequent and obstructive in nature. As the bowel distends, the sounds become more resonant and high-pitched, before eventually becoming amphoteric.

Strangulated hernias and adhesions are the most common causes of small bowel obstruction, therefore, **all the hernial orifices** must be carefully examined (see Chapter 14).

Abdominal scars suggest adhesions.

Carcinoma, diverticulitis and volvulus are the most common causes of large bowel obstruction.

Rectal examination and sigmoidoscopy are essential before more detailed investigations are carried out. It is important to remember that some patients with large bowel obstruction have a *pseudo-obstruction* (*Ogilvie's syndrome*) in which large bowel peristalsis ceases as a consequence of retroperitoneal pathology.

(a) Mild distension of the abdomen.

(b) Visible peristalsis in the same patient.

Fig. 15.6 DISTENSION

INFARCTION OF A VISCUS

Table 15.1 lists the abdominal organs that may infarct and present with acute abdominal pain together with the common pathological processes responsible for infarction.

Acute pain develops when the blood supply of an organ is obstructed. When the obstructing mechanism is an external constriction or a torsion of a vascular pedicle (e.g. a volvulus), the process is gradual but the end result is the same – severe abdominal pain – as the nerve endings are damaged and die. Pain is also experienced through the somatic nerve endings of the peritoneal cavity if they are directly stimulated by the proximity of the dead organ.

Table 15.1   The intra-abdominal organs that may infarct

Organ	Mechanism
Small and large bowel	Volvulus
	Arterial thrombosis
	Arterial embolism
	Dissecting aneurysm
	Venous thrombosis
Ovary	Torsion of pedicle
Omentum/ mesentery	Strangulation of appendix epiploica
Stomach	Volvulus
Spleen/kidney/ liver	Arterial occlusion

History

The pain of infarction is usually severe and continuous and quickly develops all the hallmarks of peritonitis. The patient often finds it difficult to locate the site of the pain, which gets progressively worse if left untreated and which is aggravated by any movement and is only relieved by strong analgesics. Vomiting may accompany the pain, and most patients are severely nauseated.

Vomiting and complete dysphagia occur in the few patients who develop the rare condition of infarction of the stomach caused by a gastric volvulus.

Some patients may describe a 'classical colic' in which the pain becomes continuous and much more severe as the blood supply of an obstructed loop is compromised by the process of strangulation. Patients may know they have a hernia that has become irreducible and painful, or they may provide a history of previous abdominal surgery, indicating the possibility of adhesions as a cause of strangulation.

A history of angina, heart attacks, strokes or intermittent claudication indicates coexisting atherosclerotic disease and increases the likelihood of a mesenteric thrombosis.

Splenic infarction is common in patients with sickle-cell disease, who may also develop bowel ischaemia, as may patients with autoimmune vasculitis.

Severe chest pain preceding the abdominal pain indicates the possibility that an aortic dissection has compromised the mesenteric vessels and led to infarction.

Examination

General features Patients with abdominal infarction lie still and are often pale and sweating from the associated hypovolaemic shock. There is a tachycardia, which increases during the period of observation. An irregularly irregular pulse (atrial fibrillation) should suggest the possibility of a mesenteric embolus.

Pyrexia The temperature may be mildly elevated at first, but a high temperature only develops if treatment is delayed and bowel wall putrefaction begins to occur.

Tenderness and guarding These signs may be mild at first but become more pronounced as the condition of the bowel wall deteriorates. The abdomen also becomes more distended, and rebound or percussion tenderness can be elicited.

Bowel sounds These may be present while the infarction is beginning, but a major intra-abdominal infarct always eventually causes a paralytic ileus.

CHAPTER 15 | THE ABDOMEN

The presence of an intra-abdominal bruit (see Chapter 10) indicates the presence of atherosclerotic disease in the intra-abdominal vessels.

The hernial orifices These must be carefully examined (see Chapter 14), together with all visible incisions, and palpated for the presence of tender and irreducible lumps.

Rectal examination and sigmoidoscopy The presence of a sigmoid volvulus is usually suspected from typical appearances on plain abdominal radiographs, but sigmoidoscopy may be both diagnostic and therapeutic in this condition. Gentle pressure of the sigmoidoscope against a blind end of bowel, or the passage of a flatus tube through the sigmoidoscope, usually leads to the passage of a massive flatus with abdominal decompression and relief of pain, provided infarction has not developed.

Peripheral pulses Absence of the brachial or femoral pulses indicates the possibility of a dissecting aneurysm, especially in a patient whose pain began in the chest.

Summary Infarction of the bowel must always be considered in a patient with severe abdominal pain and few signs. **The most likely differential diagnoses are a perforated viscus causing peritonitis, severe acute pancreatitis and a ruptured abdominal aortic aneurysm.**

ABDOMINAL PAIN CAUSED BY INTRA-ABDOMINAL OR RETROPERITONEAL HAEMORRHAGE

The common conditions that cause intra-abdominal or retroperitoneal haemorrhage are a **ruptured aortic aneurysm**, a **ruptured spleen** and a **ruptured ectopic pregnancy**.

Common features of intra-abdominal haemorrhage

History

The onset of pain is always rapid, but the signs of shock and collapse may precede the pain and be the predominating symptoms.

Although patients may die from untreated hypovolaemia, the accompanying hypotension sometimes reduces the bleeding, giving a false impression of recovery, but this fortunately allows time to transfer the patient to hospital.

Examination

General appearance The patient often looks very pale and may be sweating, restless and breathless, a condition known as *air hunger*. A tachycardia is invariably present, and this is often marked if the patient is hypovolaemic. The blood pressure is maintained at first, especially in fit young adults, but eventually may fall suddenly and disastrously. The peripheral circulation is shut down so that the extremities of the limbs are pale and cold. The pupils may be dilated. The jugular venous pressure is very low and may not be visible even when the patient is lying flat.

Ruptured abdominal aortic aneurysm

History

Patients with abdominal aortic aneurysms invariably are, or have been, smokers and may have a family history of atherosclerotic aneurysms.

A previous history of angina, myocardial infarction, intermittent claudication, transient ischaemic attacks or strokes indicates the presence of generalized atherosclerosis.

Symptoms The pain from a ruptured abdominal aortic aneurysm begins in the centre of the abdomen but commonly radiates to the back and may radiate to the groin along the course of the genitofemoral nerve.

Examination

Abdomen Inspection. The abdomen is often distended. If the patient is thin, a large central pulsating mass may be visible in the epigastrium or umbilical region.

Cullen's sign and *Grey Turner's sign* – bruising around the umbilicus and in the flank, respectively – are late indicators (3–4 days) of a long-standing rupture.

Palpation. The presence of an expansile pulsatile mass may be confirmed (Fig. 15.7). It is usually tender and consists of the aneurysm and the surrounding haematoma. The upper and lower limits of the aneurysm should be defined. A clear

Fig. 15.7 Large pulsatile abdominal mass present in the centre and upper abdomen.

separation between the upper end of the aneurysm and the costal margin indicates that the aneurysm is likely to begin below the renal arteries. The finding of additional pulsatile masses in the iliac fossae suggests associated iliac aneurysms (usually in the common iliac arteries). The femoral, iliac and foot pulses must all be palpated. The presence of dilated popliteal arteries strengthens the possibility that the patient has an abdominal aneurysm. The peripheral pulses may be absent.

Large amounts of free blood in the abdomen, obesity, marked guarding and hypotension may all conspire to render a leaking aneurysm impalpable.

Severe abdominal pain and collapse with clear evidence of hypovolaemia are strongly suggestive of a leaking aneurysm in an elderly male who is known to be hypertensive and a smoker, but special investigations may be needed to confirm the diagnosis.

Auscultation. The bowel sounds may be diminished as a consequence of the irritation caused by intraperitoneal blood. Vascular bruits may be heard.

Rectal and vaginal examination Rectal examination is usually unhelpful, but occasionally an internal iliac artery aneurysm can be palpated.

Special features of other abdominal aneurysms

Aneurysms can arise in all the visceral arteries, but they are rare. Splenic artery aneurysms are the most common.

Rupture of the spleen

The spleen may be ruptured by blunt or penetrating injuries. When the spleen is ruptured by an external injury, the left lower ribs are often fractured.

Splenic haemorrhage usually causes pain in the left hypochondrium and upper abdomen. It may be associated with left shoulder tip pain if blood or a haematoma is irritating the left hemidiaphragm. Shifting dullness and flank dullness may be detected.

There will be local pain and tenderness and sharp pain on inspiration if the ribs are broken.

Very occasionally, a ruptured pathologically enlarged spleen is palpable in the right hypochondrium.

Abdominal trauma

Blunt and penetrating injuries can damage any of the intra-abdominal viscera. The spleen and liver are the most susceptible organs, and both may bleed profusely.

A history of blunt or sharp injury to the abdomen, even if trivial, provides an important clue to the diagnosis.

There may be signs of the external injury, such as cutaneous bruising or marks along the line of a seat belt, if the patient has had blunt trauma to the abdomen (see Chapter 5).

Ectopic pregnancy

When an ectopic pregnancy is the source of haemorrhage, the patient may know she is pregnant (morning sickness, amenorrhoea, breast swelling or a positive pregnancy test) and is likely to have experienced some intermittent lower abdominal pain before the sudden onset of severe pain in this area. This is usually associated with faintness and collapse, although less acute presentations are common. The lower abdominal pain becomes generalized if left untreated.

A history of any abnormality in the menstrual cycle in a female of child-bearing age coupled with the sudden onset of severe abdominal pain should suggest the possibility of an ectopic pregnancy. A previous history of pelvic inflammatory disease (see below) or fertility problems also raises suspicions of the diagnosis. If available, a rapid pregnancy test can be very helpful.

Physiological rupture of ovarian luteal cysts

These can cause minor episodes of bleeding and lower abdominal pain when they rupture at the middle of the menstrual cycle. This is called *mittleschmertz*.

Rupture of pathological ovarian cysts

Large pathological ovarian cysts can sometimes rupture and bleed profusely. Patients may collapse from the associated hypovolaemic shock or present with lower abdominal pain and then develop the signs of internal bleeding.

Rupture of liver adenomas

Liver adenomas can develop in young females taking the contraceptive pill and may rupture spontaneously. The pain is usually felt in the upper abdomen, and hypovolaemic collapse is common.

Summary

All the conditions described above present with a combination of abdominal pain and haemorrhagic shock in varying proportions (Revision panel 15.6). Their presentation needs to be distinguished from the symptoms of intra-abdominal infarction and peritonitis caused by a perforated viscus and acute pancreatitis, all of which can produce a similar clinical picture.

EXTRA-ABDOMINAL AND MEDICAL CONDITIONS CAUSING ACUTE ABDOMINAL PAIN (REVISION PANELS 15.7, 15.8)

The conditions described below are not unusual causes of abdominal pain, which emphasizes the need to conduct a full clinical examination on every patient however obvious it may seem that their problem is in the abdomen.

The chest and heart must be examined and special tests must be performed, such as chest X-ray and electrocardiography, especially when there are no or minimal signs in the abdomen.

The pain of spinal abnormalities can radiate to the abdomen, so the back should be examined carefully, especially if the pain is felt in the lumbar region.

Revision panel 15.6

The sources of intra-abdominal haemorrhage

Ruptured abdominal aortic aneurysm

Ruptured spleen

Ruptured ectopic pregnancy (tubal rupture)

Ruptured ovarian cyst

Haemorrhage from a liver adenoma

Ruptured visceral aneurysms:

    Splenic
    Hepatic
    Mesenteric

Torn mesentery

Retroperitoneal haemorrhage (over-anticoagulation)

Revision panel 15.7

Extra-abdominal and medical conditions causing acute abdominal pain

Pneumonia/pleurisy

Pulmonary infarction

Acute Coxsackie infection (Bornholm disease)

Myocardial infarction

Spinal disorders, e.g. prolapsed disc

Epigastric artery haematoma

Acute porphyria

Mesenteric adenitis

Infectious hepatitis

Curtis–Fitz-Hugh syndrome

Herpes zoster

Diabetic ketoacidosis

Syphilis (lightening pains)

Henoch–Schönlein purpura

Acquired immunodeficiency syndrome (AIDS)

Collagen disease

Sickle-cell disease

Retroperitoneal fibrosis

Non-specific abdominal pain

Munchausen's syndrome

Acute porphyria

This is associated with severe intestinal colic that is particularly precipitated by barbiturates and alcohol. The urine is often dark and turns red–purple on standing (Fig. 15.8).

Fig. 15.8 Acute porphyria. These are a series of urine samples taken from a patient with acute porphyria showing the characteristic development left to right of the red–purple pigment over time.

Mesenteric adenitis

This is associated with an upper respiratory tract infection and cervical lymphadenopathy. It can cause pain in the right iliac fossa, which may be mistaken for appendicitis. The pain is caused by swollen glands in the mesentery, so the area of tenderness may move when the patient moves from side to side.

Epigastric artery haematoma

Both superior and inferior epigastric arteries may rupture causing swelling and subsequent haematoma (Fig. 15.9).

Fig. 15.9 Swelling and haematoma caused by rupture of a superior epigastric artery.

Infectious hepatitis and glandular fever

These conditions cause pain in the right hypochondrium. The pain is caused by swelling of the liver stretching the liver capsule. Jaundice usually develops within a few days.

Curtis–Fitz-Hugh syndrome

The pain of this syndrome is caused by a pericapsulitis around the liver that is related to pelvic inflammation with *Chlamydia*. A preceding vaginal discharge suggests the diagnosis, which has to be differentiated from acute cholecystitis.

Herpes zoster

This causes pain in the abdomen if an appropriate dermatome is involved (see Chapter 4). The diagnosis is only confirmed when the characteristic rash develops (see Fig. 4.38).

Diabetic ketoacidosis

This can cause marked abdominal pain. The diagnosis is confirmed by finding glycosuria and elevated blood glucose levels. Patients are often very thirsty and drowsy.

Syphilis

Syphilis can cause abdominal pain during a tabetic crisis, but tertiary syphilis is uncommon nowadays. Argyll Robertson pupils and evidence of destruction of the dorsal columns of the spinal cord causing loss of deep pain and proprioception indicate the diagnosis.

Henoch–Schönlein purpura

Purpura can present with intestinal colic (Fig. 15.10) The diagnosis should be suspected in children who have a purpuric rash over their thighs and buttocks.

Fig. 15.10 Henoch–Schönlein purpura. This shows haemorrhage under the serosa and in the mesentery of the upper segment of bowel wall caused by the Henoch–Schönlein purpura. The lower loops are normal. Apart from tenderness, this produces no physical signs in the abdomen.

CHAPTER 15 | THE ABDOMEN

Acquired immunodeficiency syndrome

Patients with AIDS have an increasing risk of developing abdominal lymphomas, which may perforate or obstruct. Because of the compromised state of the patient's immune system, appendicitis and other intra-abdominal infections can have a fulminating course.

Collagen diseases

A number of collagen diseases, especially systemic lupus erythematosus, are associated with abdominal pain with an increased risk of intestinal infarction secondary to small vessel obstruction.

Sickle-cell crisis

This can cause abdominal pain, usually from intestinal and splenic infarction.

Non-specific abdominal pain

In some patients, no cause for acute abdominal pain can be found, despite hospital admission, re-examination and special investigations. These patients are categorized as having non-specific abdominal pain, and account for nearly a third of the many patients admitted as acute surgical emergencies with abdominal pain. In the great majority, the pain disappears spontaneously and does not recur. In some, however, the cause eventually becomes apparent.

Munchausen's syndrome

A very small group of patients with Munchausen's syndrome invent abdominal pain for their own bizarre reasons. Many of these patients are psychiatrically disturbed. Some are attention-seekers, and some are drug addicts who bluff their way into being prescribed opiates. Beware the patient who has come from many miles away, or even a different country, whose abdomen bears the scars of many incisions (Fig. 15.11), especially if the pain is difficult to control and requires increasing quantities of analgesic drugs. The physical signs are often minimal, but some of these patients are very good at mimicking guarding and rebound tenderness. A phone call to a hospital that the patient claims to have previously visited reveals either that the patient has never been there or that the hospital also suspected the diagnosis of Munchausen's syndrome.

Fig. 15.11 Munchausen's syndrome. This is an abdomen showing many relatively recent laparotomy scars, which, in a newly presenting patient at a different hospital, should arouse suspicion.

Revision panel 15.8

The principal causes of abdominal pain

Inflammation/infection

Perforation of a viscus

Obstruction of a viscus

Infarction/strangulation

Intraperitoneal/retroperitoneal haemorrhage

Extra-abdominal and medical causes

CAUSES OF ACUTE UPPER ABDOMINAL PAIN

The common sites of inflammation and malignant disease in the upper abdomen causing upper abdominal pain are in the stomach and duodenum, gallbladder and pancreas.

The conditions causing acute upper abdominal pain are summarized in Revision panel 15.9.

Oesophagitis

This occurs when acid pepsin refluxes up out of the stomach into the oesophagus through the lower oesophageal sphincter onto the squamous epithelium lining the oesophagus, which is not able to resist these powerful chemicals. In many instances, the reflux occurs because of incompetence of the gastro-oesophageal junction caused by a hiatus hernia.

Patients complain of **heartburn**, which is a severe burning discomfort felt in the centre of the chest behind the heart, often experienced at night. The frequency and severity of the heartburn is made worse by lying flat, so patients sleep propped up on pillows to try to reduce its occurrence. Heartburn is often initiated by bending, stooping or heavy lifting. When reflux occurs, patients may experience a bitter taste developing in the mouth, which is often accompanied by flatulence and coughing if any of the refluxing acid spills over into the lungs. Sometimes the burning pain may only be experienced in the epigastrium.

After many years, patients may complain of difficulty with swallowing and of food sticking in their gullet. Although the presence of dysphagia suggests the development of a stricture caused by the acid reflux, achalasia or a carcinoma of the oesophagus or cardia must be excluded.

Examination

This rarely reveals any diagnostic signs. The diagnosis relies on endoscopy and other investigations.

Acute gastritis/duodenitis/peptic ulceration

Benign gastric and duodenal ulcers are classified together as *peptic ulceration*. Mucosal infection with *Helicobacter pylori* is a major factor in their development.

Gastric ulcers are now rare in the UK, so any patient presenting with indigestion, non-specific upper abdominal pain and a recent onset of weight loss should be suspected of having a gastric cancer.

Duodenal ulcers are still common throughout the world and affect both sexes in equal numbers. They can occur at any age, but most often arise in middle-aged patients.

History

Symptoms Patients with acute peptic ulceration present with acute pain of short duration, but may have had previous similar episodes interspersed with periods of relief lasting for many months or even years.

The main symptom of acute peptic ulceration is an epigastric discomfort or pain, which is related to meals and described as **indigestion** or **dyspepsia**. It can vary from a mild discomfort to a very severe pain that forces the patient to lie down. The severity and tenderness may equal those of a perforated peptic ulcer.

Patients with **gastric ulcers** are typically afraid to eat because the pain is induced by food. Vomiting often relieves the pain.

Patients with **duodenal ulcers** typically have a good appetite and rarely lose weight because they eat frequently to relieve their pain. Acid brash, water brash and heartburn are rare symptoms. They are more frequent in patients with duodenal than gastric ulceration.

Haematemesis and melaena may complicate all forms of peptic ulceration.

Drugs Many drugs, but especially aspirin and the non-steroidal anti-inflammatory drugs that are used to treat arthritis, irritate the gastric mucosa and cause ulceration, so it is essential to ascertain the precise details of any drug ingestion.

Social history Cigarette smoking and periods of stress may be important risk factors.

Examination

Abdominal examination often reveals epigastric tenderness, with guarding if the pain is severe. The patient may be anaemic if there has been chronic silent bleeding before the acute episode.

Perforated peptic ulcer

Acid gastric juice enters the peritoneal cavity if a peptic ulcer erodes the wall of the stomach or duodenum at a point where it is covered only by visceral peritoneum. This causes a chemical peritonitis, which later becomes infected with bacteria.

History

Age and sex Perforated peptic ulcers are most common between the ages of 40 and 60 years, but also occur in the very old because many old people are given non-steroidal anti-inflammatory drugs for joint disease. Males and females are equally affected.

Symptoms A perforation causes **sudden severe and constant pain**. This usually begins in the epigastrium, reaches its maximum intensity quickly and remains severe for many hours. It gradually extends to involve the whole of the abdomen. All movement, including respiration, makes the pain worse, causing the patient to lie immobile on the bed. Many patients give no history of previous dyspepsia, but it is important to ask if they have ever suffered from indigestion in the past.

Drug history It is important to enquire whether the patient has taken steroids, non-steroidal anti-inflammatory drugs or salicylates, because these dispose to perforation.

Examination

General appearance The patient looks ill and is obviously in pain, lying completely still.

A tachycardia is common and respiration is shallow, but the temperature is usually normal.

Abdomen Inspection. The abdomen is flat and does not rise and fall with respiration. The abdominal muscles can be seen to be tightly contracted.

Palpation. In the early stages, tenderness and guarding may be confined to the epigastrium and right side, but eventually, when the entire peritoneal cavity is contaminated, the whole abdomen becomes very tender, with intense guarding, often described as **board-like rigidity**. No intra-abdominal viscus or masses can be felt because the abdominal musculature is permanently contracted.

Percussion. This is usually painful. The liver dullness may be diminished or completely absent if a large quantity of air has escaped into the peritoneal cavity.

Auscultation. The bowel sounds disappear once generalized peritonitis is established.

Beware After 4–6 hours, the acid in the peritoneal cavity becomes diluted and the pain and guarding decrease. Patients think they are improving, but they are in fact getting worse. The peritonitis is progressing and hypervolaemia is developing. An increasing tachycardia and absent bowel sounds associated with increasing abdominal distension and sunken eyes indicate that the patient is becoming extremely ill.

Gallstone colic/biliary colic

There is an overlap between gallstone colic and acute cholecystitis. Gallstone colic is a severe pain caused by spasm of the gallbladder as it tries to force a gallstone down the cystic duct, which is why 'gallstone colic' is a preferable term to 'biliary colic'. About a fifth of patients who present in this way become jaundiced. Many cases of gallstone colic progress to acute cholecystitis.

History

Symptoms Gallstone colic begins suddenly across the upper abdomen. Patients are often unable to indicate which side is more affected. The pain is severe and constant with excruciating exacerbations. It is not a true colic because it does not remit between exacerbations. The severe pain seldom lasts longer than a few hours unless acute cholecystitis develops. It is usually accompanied by nausea and vomiting and is relieved only by strong analgesia.

Previous history Many patients give a history of flatulent dyspepsia and previous episodes of upper abdominal pain.

Examination

General appearance The patient is frightened and becomes restless as a consequence of the intensity of the pain. A mild tachycardia is often present in the early stages, but the temperature is usually normal. Jaundice may be present.

Abdomen The abdomen is often extremely tender, with intense guarding in the upper abdomen.

Acute cholecystitis

Acute inflammation of the gallbladder is commonly caused by obstruction of the cystic duct by a small stone causing gallbladder distension, chemical inflammation of its wall and, eventually, secondary infection.

History

Age Patients are commonly 30–60 years of age and female. Younger patients with sickle-cell disease often form pigment stones, which may precipitate an attack of acute cholecystitis.

Sex Acute cholecystitis is more common in females than in males.

Symptoms The main symptom is a sudden pain, often without any previous symptoms of chronic indigestion. It is felt in the right hypochondrium and often radiates through to the back close to the tip of the right scapula. The pain is continuous, lasting more than 6 hours, and is exacerbated by moving and breathing. Nothing except analgesic drugs brings relief. Some patients recognize the pain as a severe version of their chronic indigestion pain but, as stated above, it often occurs *de novo*. Patients nearly always feel nauseated and often vomit. The urine may be dark, the stools pale and the skin itchy, if there is an associated obstructive jaundice.

Previous history There may be a history of flatulent dyspepsia or previous attacks of gallstone colic.

Examination

General appearance The patient is distressed by the pain and lies still, breathing shallowly. There is usually a tachycardia and pyrexia, although in the early stages of the attack the temperature is often normal. **Jaundice** may be present and the patient may be sweating.

Abdomen Inspection. Rarely, there may be a fullness in the right hypochondrium in the early stages of the inflammation.

Palpation. There is almost always tenderness and guarding in the right hypochondrium. Palpate the abdomen just below the tip of the ninth costal cartilage and ask the patient to take a deep breath. When the liver and the attached gallbladder descend and strike the palpating hand, the patient will experience a sharp pain that prevents further inspiration. This is called *Murphy's sign.*

At an early stage before there is any guarding, an enlarged gallbladder may be palpable. At a later stage when the inflammation has been present for several days and the tenderness is beginning to subside, an inflammatory mass may become palpable (*Zackary Cope's sign*). This will still be very tender and moves little with respiration. It usually indicates that there is pus in the gallbladder (an *empyema*).

Occasionally, the contents of an obstructed gallbladder do not become infected, and a large **mucocele** may develop. This may reach down to the level of the umbilicus.

Because gallbladder pain often radiates through to the tip of the scapula, the affected dermatome may be hyperaesthetic, a change detected by lightly drawing a pin down the back of the patient's chest. This is called *Boas' sign.*

Percussion. A dull area just beneath the costal margin indicates the presence of an inflammatory mass.

Auscultation. The bowel sounds are normally present unless the gallbladder has infarcted or ruptured and caused biliary peritonitis. This complication is rare.

CHAPTER 15 | THE ABDOMEN

Acute pancreatitis

Acute pancreatitis is a condition in which activated pancreatic enzymes autodigest the pancreatic gland. It may be caused by obstruction of the pancreatic duct, usually by a small gallstone obstructing the ampulla of Vater. It can also be caused by a periampullary carcinoma or alcohol abuse. The mechanism by which alcohol abuse causes pancreatitis is not known.

Viral infections, trauma and a number of rarer conditions may also cause acute pancreatitis. In about one-third of cases, a cause is never discovered (Revision panel 15.10).

Pancreatitis can vary from a very mild inflammation to an acute haemorrhagic destruction of the whole gland – a condition with a high mortality.

Revision panel 15.10

The causes of acute pancreatitis

Gallstones

Alcohol

Metabolic (hypercalcaemia, hyperlipidaemia)

Endoscopic retrograde cholangiopancreatography

Trauma

Idiopathic

Autoimmune

Medication (thiazides, steroids)

Infections (mumps, Coxsackie virus)

Structural abnormalities (pancreatic divisum, choledochocele)

History

Age and sex Pancreatitis is equally common in males and females. The peak incidence is in the fourth and fifth decades of life, but it can occur at any age.

Symptoms The common presenting symptom is pain that begins suddenly, high in the epigastrium, and steadily increases in severity until it is very severe, causing the patient to lie still and breathe shallowly. It usually radiates through to the back. Nothing relieves the pain, which is exacerbated by movement. Frequent vomiting and retching are very common, and are an important pointer to the correct diagnosis. There is persistent nausea between the bouts of vomiting. Many patients have eaten an unusually large meal or drunk some alcohol before the pain began.

Previous history In Great Britain, nearly half the patients who present with acute pancreatitis have biliary tract disease. Many patients therefore have a previous history of indigestion.

Social history A careful history of the patient's alcohol intake is important. Relatives may have to be interviewed, as many alcoholics refuse to reveal the true extent of their drinking habits. Mumps is a very rare cause of pancreatitis, but ask about any recent contacts with children or the disease.

Examination

General appearance Patients lie still because the pain is severe, and, if they are pale and sweating, it is likely that they have become hypovolaemic. When respiration is impaired, they become grey, apprehensive, dyspnoeic and cyanosed. The sclerae may reveal a slight tinge of jaundice if the pancreatitis has been caused by a stone lodged in the lower end of the bile duct. Mild jaundice may also appear on the second or third day of the illness if oedema in the head of the pancreas causes compression of the bile duct. There is usually a tachycardia and, if the patient has become hypovolaemic, the jugular venous pressure and blood pressure may be low. Pyrexia is usually mild.

Abdomen Inspection. There is always tenderness and guarding in the upper abdomen but the signs may be mild. Any patient with severe pain but minimal abdominal signs may have acute pancreatitis.

If the pain is severe and the tone of the abdominal muscles is increased, the abdomen will not move with respiration. A paralytic ileus may develop, causing mild abdominal distension.

Bruising and discolouration in the left flank (*Grey Turner's sign*) and around the umbilicus (*Cullen's sign*) only develop in patients with very severe haemorrhagic pancreatitis. These are rare and late signs, and indicate extensive destruction of the gland. Remember that they may also occur after a large intraperitoneal or retroperitoneal haemorrhage from another cause, such as a leaking abdominal aortic aneurysm.

A number of patients develop a collection of inflammatory exudate in the lesser sac. This is initially suggested by fullness in the epigastrium, which may become a more prominent mass if a pseudocyst or abscess develops.

Percussion. Percussion may cause pain if there is peritonitis and be dull over any pseudocysts that are developing.

Auscultation. Bowel sounds are usually present in the first 12–24 hours but fade away if a paralytic ileus develops.

Note Acute pancreatitis can be extremely difficult to diagnose and, as it has no distinctive features, is often forgotten and missed. Whenever you examine an acute abdomen and cannot find a obvious cause, think 'Could this be acute pancreatitis?' 'Or a mesenteric vascular infarction?' 'Or a leaking abdominal aortic aneurysm?'

Gastric volvulus

Acute gastric volvulus is a rare condition and usually occurs in association with a giant hiatus hernia.

Age and sex It is equally common in males and females. The peak incidence is in elderly patients.

Symptoms Patients report a sudden onset of severe upper abdominal/chest pain in association with retching.

Previous history The pre-existing hiatus hernia may have caused a history of reflux, regurgitation, breathlessness, early satiety and upper abdominal discomfort.

Examination

General appearance The patient appears distressed with an increased respiratory rate and tachycardia. Cardiovascular collapse develops if the stomach becomes ischaemic.

Abdomen Inspection. There may be tenderness and guarding in the upper abdomen but often the abdominal signs are minimal.

Percussion. Percussion may cause pain if there is peritonitis from ischaemia or perforation.

Auscultation. Bowel sounds are usually present.

The lack of abdominal signs can often be misleading. A gastric volvulus should be suspected if a patient has sudden onset epigastric pain and intractable retching, and passing a nasogastric tube is difficult (*Borchardt's triad*).

Boerhaave's syndrome

This syndrome is caused by a full-thickness tear at the oesophagogastric junction, perhaps as a consequence of attempting to suppress a vomit.

The patient complains of the sudden onset of a severe pain in the upper abdomen or lower chest after a bout of vomiting. The condition should be suspected if, in addition to tenderness, guarding and rigidity in the upper abdomen, there is supraclavicular subcutaneous emphysema.

Subcutaneous bubbles of air – emphysema – feel like the little plastic air pockets in 'bubble wrap', which compress, crackle and pop beneath the fingers during gentle palpation. The triad of pain, vomiting and subcutaneous emphysema is known as *Mackler's triad*.

Haemorrhage/infarction

As previously mentioned, intra-abdominal or retroperitoneal haemorrhage can result in acute upper abdominal pain. Rupture of the spleen or a liver adenoma will result in upper abdominal pain. Pain from a ruptured aneurysm can be felt in any part of the abdomen or the back depending on the site of the rupture.

Extra-abdominal causes

Extra-abdominal causes such as pneumonia are often perceived to be arising in the upper abdomen and can mimic conditions such as acute cholecystitis. Splenic infarction is seen in patients with sickle-cell disease. This can cause acute left upper quadrant pain, which may radiate to the tip of the left shoulder.

ACUTE CENTRAL ABDOMINAL PAIN

Causes are listed in Revision panel 15.11.

Small bowel obstruction

Intestinal obstruction produces a severe central griping pain interspersed with periods of little or no pain. Small bowel colic is felt in the centre of the abdomen and is associated with vomiting (see page 489). The pain becomes more severe, is constant and will become more generalized if the bowel becomes ischaemic or perforates

Small bowel perforation

Small bowel perforation causes sudden onset central abdominal pain progressing to generalized peritonitis. It is usually the result of ischaemia from small bowel volvulus or a closed loop obstruction.

Mesenteric ischaemia

Infarction of the bowel caused by a sudden mesenteric artery occlusion causes acute abdominal pain. The patient is usually a middle-aged male smoker with other signs of arterial disease such as intermittent claudication, angina or a previous myocardial infarction. It can also be the result of a twist in the intestinal mesentery – *volvulus*. Venous occlusion can be seen in some prothrombotic conditions and presents in a similar manner.

The vasculitides such as systemic lupus erythematosus and conditions such as sickle-cell disease can also cause acute and chronic abdominal pain, which is thought to be related to mesenteric ischaemia.

Intussusception

Intussusception occurs as a segment of bowel invaginates and enters the bowel beyond it, and is driven on by peristalsis (Fig. 15.12). The apex of the intussusception can be an appendix, a Meckel's diverticulum, a polyp or a tumour.

Initially, pain may be similar to that of intestinal obstruction. The most common site is an ileocolic intussusception leading to small bowel obstruction. As the condition progresses, the bowel may become ischaemic and perforate. This will cause generalized peritonitis, and the abdominal signs will change accordingly. The intussusception can sometimes be felt as a sausage-shaped mass in the right iliac fossa. Patients occasionally pass '*redcurrant jelly*' stools. Rarely, the intussusception can be felt on rectal examination.

Fig. 15.12 This shows an intussucceped loop of small bowel arrowed. It may be palpable as a sausage-shaped mass.

Spontaneous bacterial peritonitis

This condition is seen in patients on peritoneal dialysis or with ascites (Fig. 15.13). Patients may have minimal tenderness until the later stages, but equally can present with generalized peritonitis. The dialysate or ascitic fluid is usually altered in appearance and can be tested for bacterial contamination and the presence of white cells.

Fig. 15.13 Patient on peritoneal dialysis or with ascites.

Acute Meckel's diverticulitis

Meckel's diverticulum is the remnant of the vittelo-intestinal duct. It contains all layers of the bowel wall, occurs in about 2 per cent of the population and causes abdominal pain if it becomes inflamed.

Inflammation of a Meckel's diverticulum produces symptoms and signs that are indistinguishable from those of acute appendicitis, although the pain and tenderness are generally felt more towards the centre of the abdomen than in the right iliac fossa.

A Meckel's diverticulum may give rise to central abdominal pain if any ectopic gastric or pancreatic mucosa within it becomes ulcerated or inflamed.

It may also cause colicky abdominal pain if it acts as the head of an intussusception or if a congenital band arising from its apex causes small bowel obstruction or a volvulus.

Acute gastroenteritis

Gastroenteritis is usually caused by a *Campylobacter* or viral infection, but must be differentiated from food poisoning. The symptoms of vomiting and diarrhoea usually predominate over the abdominal pain, which may be non-existent or very mild.

Occasionally, it causes severe colicky, cramping pains that must be differentiated from the colic of small bowel obstruction caused by diseases such as Crohn's disease (see pages 506, 514), *Yersinia* infections (see below) or acute appendicitis.

There are usually few signs on abdominal examination.

The stool should be cultured to exclude *Campylobacter*, *Giardia*, ova and parasites, particularly if the patient has recently travelled to a foreign country.

Inflammatory bowel disease

Crohn's disease and ulcerative colitis may present with acute or chronic central abdominal pain together with a variety of other gastrointestinal symptoms.

Acute Crohn's disease may present with central or right iliac fossa discomfort and signs similar to those of appendicitis. A thick and tender terminal ileum may be palpable in the right iliac fossa, and thickened ileum and jejunum may also be palpable in the umbilical region.

Acute fulminating ulcerative colitis may present with acute abdominal pain, especially when complicated by acute toxic dilatation or perforation of the colon. The abdominal pain is invariably preceded by severe incessant diarrhoea accompanied by the passage of blood, mucus and pus.

Acute *Yersinia* ileitis

This condition is indistinguishable from acute Crohn's disease and appendicitis on the history and physical signs. A mass is rarely palpable. It is usually incorrectly diagnosed as acute appendicitis.

Typhoid

Typhoid normally presents with toxaemia and diarrhoea. Severe abdominal pain and all the signs of peritonitis can be present if a typhoid ulcer perforates the small bowel.

Urinary tract infection (cystitis and pyelonephritis)

The symptoms and signs of urinary tract infections are discussed in Chapter 17. Pain from pyelonephritis is felt mainly in the lumbar region, but may spread to the centre of the abdomen. When patients are asked to describe the site of their renal pain, they usually put their hands on their waist with their thumbs pointing forwards and their fingers spread backwards between the 12th rib and the iliac crest. It is easier to detect tenderness in the renal angle if the patient is sitting up and leaning slightly forwards.

Deep abdominal palpation must be carried out to ensure that there is not an enlarged kidney caused by another pathology responsible for the infection, such as a hydronephrosis. The bladder may be enlarged and should be palpated and percussed. Examination of the external genitalia and a rectal examination are essential (see Chapters 16 and 18). The urine should be examined for red and white cells and organisms. The presence of red cells in the urine suggests that the pain is more likely to be coming from a calculus or a tumour than an infection.

Intra-abdominal or retroperitoneal haemorrhage

As previously mentioned, intra-abdominal or retroperitoneal haemorrhage, for example with a ruptured abdominal aortic aneurysm, can result in acute central abdominal pain.

Revision panel 15.11

The causes of acute central abdominal pain

- Small bowel obstruction
- Small bowel perforation
- Mesenteric infarction
- Intussusception
- Spontaneous bacterial peritonitis
- Meckel's diverticulitis
- Acute gastroenteritis
- Inflammatory bowel disease
- *Yersinia* ileitis
- Typhoid
- Tuberculosis
- Urinary tract infection
- Ruptured aortic aneurysm

ACUTE LOWER ABDOMINAL PAIN

Causes are listed in Revision panel 15.12.

Revision panel 15.12

The causes of acute lower abdominal pain

Acute appendicitis
Meckel's diverticulitis
Mesenteric adenitis
Crohn's disease
Diverticulitis
Salpingitis/pelvic inflammatory disease
Ectopic pregnancy
Twisting or degenerating fibroid
Acute urinary retention
Cystitis/pyelonephritis/renal colic
Colonic carcinoma/diverticulitis/perforation

Acute appendicitis

Acute appendicitis is the most common cause of acute abdominal pain in the Western world. The cause of appendicitis remains unknown, but obstruction of the lumen by a faecolith, swollen Peyer's patches, a stricture or a carcinoid tumour at its base all can play a part. Threadworms, which are often found in the appendix, may be an aetiological factor, as may diet and childhood infections.

History

Age and sex Appendicitis can and does occur at any age, but most often affects young adults or teenagers of either sex.

Symptoms The condition most often presents with a **vague often 'colicky' pain that begins in the centre of the abdomen**. At first, this is often thought to be indigestion and ignored, but after a varying period, usually a few hours but sometimes 2–3 days, the **pain shifts to the right iliac fossa** and becomes more severe. This 'typical' history is almost diagnostic of appendicitis but only occurs in about half the patients.

The remainder present with a variety of patterns of pain. It may begin and remain in the right iliac fossa, or only be felt in the centre of the abdomen.

There may be pain in both sites simultaneously, and a few patients have no pain at all.

The central pain is a referred pain. The normal visceral innervation of the appendix comes from the tenth thoracic spinal segment. The corresponding somatic dermatome encircles the abdomen at the level of the umbilicus. The midline pain is higher if the spinal segment visceral innervation is higher. Some patients have retrosternal pain that shifts to the right iliac fossa. Therefore, the important feature of the initial pain is its central location and not its precise level.

The inflamed appendix most commonly lies behind the caecum (retrocaecal) so causes pain in the lateral part of the right iliac fossa and the flank, but it may hang down into the pelvis and lie against the bladder or a loop of large bowel (Fig. 15.14). In these circumstances, the patient may present with misleading bladder or large bowel symptoms.

Acute appendicitis may also present with intestinal obstruction – colic and abdominal distension – if the appendix lies too close to and inflames the terminal ileum (preileal or postileal).

A loss of appetite usually precedes the onset of pain by a few hours, and most patients feel slightly nauseated. Many patients vomit once or twice. Most patients with appendicitis state that they had been constipated for a few days before the pain started,

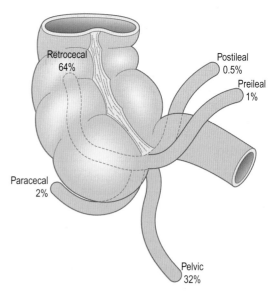

Fig. 15.14 This shows the different positions that the appendix may lie in relation to the caecum and terminal ileum.

but a few complain of diarrhoea, which may lead to a mistaken diagnosis of gastroenteritis, especially in children.

Some patients present with symptoms of generalized peritonitis – generalized abdominal pain, nausea and vomiting, sweating and sometimes rigors – especially if the initial stages of the disease are silent.

Atypical presentations are common in the very young, in pregnant females and in the very old, when the appendicitis may be related to obstruction of its ostium by a carcinoma of the caecum.

Examination

General appearance Patients often look unwell with flushed cheeks. A **low-grade pyrexia** is usually present, while a high temperature should suggest another cause for the pain, or general peritonitis associated with a ruptured appendix. The pulse rate is usually elevated and rises as the infection spreads.

Head and neck The tongue is usually furred, and most patients have a distinctive **fetor oris**. Palpable lymph glands in the neck and enlarged tonsils indicate that the patient may have mesenteric adenitis rather than appendicitis, but beware – acute appendicitis often follows a viral infection.

Chest The lung examination findings should be normal. It is important to exclude any signs of a right-sided basal pneumonia, because this can occasionally cause abdominal pain and mimic appendicitis, especially in children.

Abdomen Inspection. The abdomen, although it may be slightly distended, usually looks normal. The right hip may be kept slightly flexed if the appendix is lying against the psoas major muscle. Coughing and sudden movements cause pain if peritonitis has developed.

Palpation. **The right iliac fossa is tender, and the overlying muscles show guarding**. The maximum site of tenderness must be carefully assessed by gentle palpation. It is classically maximal over *McBurney's point*, one third of the way along a line joining the anterior superior iliac spine to the umbilicus. High or low tenderness may indicate that the appendix is lying in an unusual position. There may be release or rebound tenderness in the right iliac fossa. Pressure on the left iliac fossa may cause pain in the right iliac fossa (*Rovsing's sign*). Release of pressure on the left iliac fossa may cause pain on the right. All these manoeuvres cause pain because they move the inflamed appendix as it lies in the right iliac fossa against the overlying peritoneum, which contains many somatic pain fibres.

When the appendix is behind the caecum, the tenderness may be experienced in the lateral part of the lumbar region – the flank.

When a sub-hepatic appendix produces pain and tenderness below the right costal margin, it must be differentiated from acute cholecystitis.

A tender, indistinct mass may be felt in the right iliac fossa. It is usually impossible to feel below it because it is fixed posteriorly. It is dull to percussion. An appendix mass usually takes a few days to develop. An appendix abscess should be suspected if the temperature is high and the mass is very tender. The features of an appendix mass and abscess are described on pages 528–529.

Percussion. This causes pain if peritonitis is present. Dullness on percussion may suggest the presence of an underlying mass that is obscured by tenderness and guarding.

Auscultation. Bowel sounds are present unless perforation and general peritonitis have caused a paralytic ileus.

Rectal examination There is considerable debate about the usefulness of this examination, especially in young children, but the presence of tenderness high in the pelvis usually indicates an inflamed pelvic appendix.

Hip movement Extension of the right hip joint exacerbates the pain if the appendix is in a retrocaecal position lying against the psoas muscle. Pain on external and internal rotation of the hip indicates that the appendix is lying against the obturator internis muscle.

Meckel's diverticulitis

Inflammation of a Meckel's diverticulum produces symptoms and signs that are indistinguishable from those of acute appendicitis, although the pain and tenderness are generally felt more towards the centre of the abdomen.

Mesenteric adenitis

This condition is usually seen in children and is associated with a preceding upper respiratory tract infection and cervical lymphadenopathy. It often

CHAPTER 15 | THE ABDOMEN

causes a more central abdominal pain but can cause pain in the right iliac fossa mimicking appendicitis. The pain can sometimes be shown to be move when the patient is placed in the lateral decubitus position as the glands move over with the mesentery.

Crohn's disease

Acute Crohn's disease affecting the terminal ileum can present with symptoms and signs similar to those of appendicitis. Occasionally, a mass will be palpable and has to be differentiated from an intussusception or a tumour.

Acute diverticulitis of the colon

Acquired diverticula develop in the colon, especially the sigmoid colon, probably as a result of changes in bowel motility and the consistency of the faeces. The condition may be related to the low-roughage diet popular in the USA and Europe. Diverticula often cause no symptoms, but they may become obstructed and acutely inflamed – acute diverticulitis. This may progress to a pericolic abscess situated on the outside of the colon, which may then perforate, causing generalized peritonitis (see below).

When a solitary diverticulum of the caecum becomes inflamed, the signs are indistinguishable from those of acute appendicitis or a carcinoma of the colon.

History

Age, sex and ethnic group Patients with diverticulitis are commonly between the ages of 50 and 70 years. The condition is slightly more common in females than in males. Native Africans and Asians are rarely affected.

Symptoms The first symptom is often a mild intermittent lower abdominal pain that then shifts to the left iliac fossa (for the same reasons as appendicitis moves to the right), where it becomes a more constant ache. The pain begins gradually before becoming more severe and constant. It may become colicky if the large bowel becomes obstructed. The pain is often associated with nausea and a loss of appetite, but rarely vomiting. Most patients are constipated, but a few develop diarrhoea. If the colon lies against the vault of the bladder and the bladder wall becomes inflamed, there may be painful and increased frequency of micturition.

Some patients can relate their attacks to the type of food they have eaten.

Previous history Some patients give a history of chronic diverticular disease, flatulence, distension and left iliac fossa pain.

Examination

General appearance Patients lie still because of the pain and often look flushed. They are usually pyrexial and have a tachycardia.

Abdomen Inspection. If there is a generalized peritonitis or intestinal obstruction, the abdomen moves with respiration and may be distended.

Palpation. There is tenderness and guarding in the left iliac fossa, where there may be a palpable, tender, sausage-shaped mass. Pressure on the right side of the abdomen may induce pain on the left (*reversed Rovsing's sign*). Rebound tenderness will be present if generalized peritonitis has developed. In the latter stages of peritonitis or obstruction, there may be considerable abdominal distension.

Percussion. Any palpable mass in the left iliac fossa should be dull to percussion.

Auscultation. The bowel sounds may be normal, amphoric if there is intestinal obstruction, or absent if a generalized peritonitis develops causing a paralytic ileus.

Rectal examination Pain may be experienced when the finger is pushed high into the left side of the pelvis. Rectal examination is important to exclude a carcinoma of the rectosigmoid junction, which can perforate and cause similar symptoms. Sigmoidoscopy is indicated to exclude a carcinoma but often causes pain when attempting to negotiate the rectosigmoid junction. The findings are rarely diagnostic unless a carcinoma is seen.

Differential diagnoses Acute diverticulitis must be differentiated from carcinoma of the colon with a pericolic abscess, ischaemic colitis and occasionally acute appendicitis or Crohn's disease.

Acute salpingitis/pelvic inflammatory disease

Acute salpingitis is an infection in one or both Fallopian tubes, and is often associated with infection within the surrounding supporting tissues around the adnexae – hence the term 'pelvic inflammatory disease'. The common infecting organisms are

Gonococcus and *Streptococcus*. These organisms usually reach the Fallopian tubes by direct spread through the vagina and uterus, and rarely from the bloodstream. Salpingitis is a well-recognized complication of the puerperium and following abortion.

History

Age and sex Salpingitis usually occurs in sexually active females between the ages of 15 and 50 years.
Symptoms A purulent, yellow–white vaginal discharge usually precedes, by a few days, the gradual onset of lower abdominal pain. The pain is constant and can become severe. It may radiate to the lower part of the back. Sometimes the abdominal pain is preceded by a low backache. Menstruation may have been irregular over the previous months, and patients often give a history of dysmenorrhoea. Sweating and rigors are common, but there is usually no nausea, vomiting or change in bowel habit. By contrast, urinary tract symptoms, such as painful and frequent micturition, are common as the urinary tract is often also infected.
Previous history Patients may have had previous attacks of infection or know that they have had or have been exposed to gonorrhoea.

Examination

General appearance The patient looks flushed and feverish. There is no distinctive fetor oris, and the oral temperature is often higher than in appendicitis, being between 38°C and 39.5°C.
Abdomen Inspection. The abdomen moves normally and looks normal.

Palpation. Tenderness and some guarding are present across the lower abdomen. **The tenderness is often bilateral** as both Fallopian tubes may be infected, but can be asymmetrical if one tube is more inflamed than the other. It is usually lower and nearer to the midline than the tenderness of acute appendicitis. A huge pyosalpinx is occasionally palpable, but even large swollen tubes can often only be felt by manual examination (see below).

Percussion. This seldom causes pain, but may do so if there is associated peritonitis.

Auscultation. The bowel sounds are usually normal.
Vaginal examination Examination of the vaginal introitus may reveal a yellow–white discharge, a specimen of which should be sent for culture. The cervix and uterus should be of normal size, but

bimanual palpation of the adnexae will cause pain. Moving the cervix (cervical excitation) is also painful. Speculum examination may demonstrate pus coming from the cervical canal. If a pyosalpinx or tubo-ovarian abscess is present, a mass may be felt to one side of the uterus.

Ectopic pregnancy

A sudden onset of lower abdominal pain in a female of child-bearing age should be immediately treated as a suspected ectopic pregnancy. The patient usually gives a history of delayed menstruation followed by a few days history of mild abdominal pain or cramps. If it is associated with a major intra-abdominal bleed, the patient will be showing signs of haemorrhagic shock and will require immediate resuscitation. The pain initially arises in the lower abdomen on the side of the ectopic pregnancy. The pain becomes more generalized if there is significant bleeding, with shoulder tip pain if blood collects beneath the diaphragm.

Twisted/degenerating fibroids

Pedunculated fibroids can twist and infarct, leading to severe lower abdominal pain. Degeneration occurs when the fibroid reaches a size at which it can no longer maintain an adequate blood supply. This can result in acute lower abdominal pain, which can last for several weeks.

Urological causes

Acute urinary retention, cystitis, bladder colic, ureteric colic and pyelonephritis can all cause acute lower abdominal symptoms and are discussed in Chapter 17.

Uterine colic

This is always associated with pregnancy. The presence of a large pelvic mass should confirm the presence of a pregnant uterus.

Carcinoma of the colon

A carcinoma of the caecum may cause appendicitis. The physical signs are indistinguishable from those of simple acute appendicitis. Even when a mass is palpable, it is rarely possible to be certain that this is not an inflammatory mass, and even if the mass is very hard, discrete, knobbly and not very tender, it may simply be the result of inflammation. Consequently, the possibility of a cancer of the caecum must always be considered in a patient over 40 years old who presents with acute appendicitis. Other possible diagnoses include an inflamed solitary caecal diverticulum, Crohn's disease and ileocaecal tuberculosis. Localized perforation of the caecum can also occur, leading to initially localized and then generalized peritonitis.

Tumours in the left side of the colon can present with generalized peritonitis. In such cases, severe generalized abdominal pain develops, accompanied by signs of shock with tachycardia, hypotension, distension, tenderness, loss of liver dullness and absent bowel sounds. In many cases, the peritonitis is caused by a rupture of a distended caecum caused by an obstructing left-sided tumour.

CHRONIC ABDOMINAL PAIN

CHRONIC UPPER ABDOMINAL PAIN

Causes of chronic upper abdominal pain are listed in Revision panel 15.13.

Chronic peptic ulceration, gastritis and duodenitis

History

Age Peptic ulceration tends to occur between the ages of 20 and 60 years.

Sex Both gastric and duodenal ulcers are more common in males than females.

Occupation There is a higher incidence among those in the professions and those with executive appointments!

Symptoms Although a few patients present to hospital with an acute, sometimes very severe upper abdominal pain of short duration as described above, the great majority of patients with chronic peptic ulceration present with a chronic, less severe and more intermittent pain, which they usually call 'indigestion' or dyspepsia because it is directly related to the ingestion of food. Nevertheless, some experience continuous pain over many hours or days that is unaffected by food.

Night pain, which wakes the patient and seems to be unrelated to food, is a common symptom of duodenal ulceration. This is thought to be caused by the drop in pH in the stomach at night, when the acid secretions are no longer buffered by the presence of food. The pain is usually experienced in the epigastrium and may radiate into either the back or the right hypochondrium if the ulcer is situated in the posterior part of the stomach or the second part of the duodenum. The pain is usually described as a continuous gnawing or boring ache and is rarely very severe. It is usually episodic, occurring for 2 or 3 weeks at a time before resolving spontaneously, only to recur a few months later – a feature known as *periodicity*. The rapid onset of pain after food, causing food fear and loss of weight, suggests the presence of a gastric ulcer. Pain that is relieved by eating indicates the probability of a duodenal ulcer.

The pain is usually relieved by commercially available antacids, H2 receptor blockers and proton pump inhibitors.

Peptic ulcers commonly arise in middle-aged smokers, but are also common in middle-aged and elderly patients on long-term non-steroidal anti-inflammatory drugs.

Vomiting is rare unless a pyloric stenosis has developed.

Excessive salivation (*water brash*) and *acid brash* are highly suggestive of duodenal ulceration. Some patients develop heartburn.

Haematemesis and *melaena* are important complications that occur in a small proportion of patients with chronic, and acute, peptic ulceration. Chronic blood loss may cause an iron deficiency anaemia, which presents with tiredness and shortness of breath.

Chronic peptic ulceration must be differentiated from other causes of chronic abdominal pain. A clear history of weight loss suggests a gastric carcinoma, whereas acid heartburn and reflux (see below) suggest oesophagitis. Gallstones and chronic cholecystitis may coexist and are important differential diagnoses (see below).

Examination

General Anaemia and cervical lymphadenopathy with obvious cachexia should suggest the possibility of carcinoma of the stomach rather than peptic ulceration.

Abdomen Inspection. **Epigastric distension and visible peristalsis may be present if a pyloric stenosis has developed.**

Palpation. Minor tenderness in the epigastrium is often the only abnormality. The presence of a *succussion splash* indicates the presence of pyloric stenosis.

The diagnosis of chronic peptic ulcer is now almost exclusively made on flexible endoscopy and biopsy. The importance of *Helicobacter pylori* as a cause has already been described, and a breath test is available to confirm its involvement.

Percussion and auscultation. These should be normal.

Carcinoma of the stomach

Carcinoma of the stomach is a common cause of death in males. Pernicious anaemia, gastric polyps and chronic gastric ulcers are known to be premalignant conditions, but the majority of gastric cancers arise spontaneously. *Helicobacter pylori* is an important predisposing factor.

History

Age The incidence of gastric carcinoma reaches its peak between 50 and 70 years, but it can arise at an earlier age.

Sex Gastric cancer is two to three times more common in males than in females.

Geography There are unexplained variations in the incidence of this disease. It is very common in Japan, closely followed by Chile, Austria and Finland. In the UK, it affects approximately 20–30 per 100 000 of the population. Genetic and dietary factors may be important, as may be the ingestion of nitrites.

Symptoms **The onset of indigestion or epigastric pain, however vague, in a patient over 40 years of age should be treated very seriously.** The pain may be mild and related to food, but, unlike the indigestion associated with peptic ulcer, the pain of a gastric ulcer is constant and not solely brought on by eating. When patients have had symptoms of a peptic ulcer for many years, they are usually aware that the nature of the pain has changed. Often their periodic pain becomes constant.

Patients with stomach cancer do not want to eat, and **loss of appetite is a cardinal symptom**. The inevitable consequence of a loss of appetite is **loss of weight**. The patient may lose 10–20 kg in 1 or 2 months. The loss of appetite and weight often occur long before any other symptoms.

Tumours near the cardia may cause obstruction of the oesophagogastric junction and cause the patient to complain of difficulty swallowing (*dysphagia*). As the dysphagia increases, undigested food may be regurgitated from the oesophagus.

Cancers in the pyloric region often obstruct the outflow of food from the stomach. If so, the patient may vomit large quantities of *undigested food* (undigested because of the low acid production associated with the accompanying atrophic gastritis), and notice epigastric discomfort and distension. Some cancers grow to a considerable size without producing symptoms, apart from mild weight loss.

Systematic questions A systematic review of the other systems may reveal symptoms that suggest that the tumour has metastasized, such as weakness, tiredness or dyspnoea.

Previous history The patient may have a long history of peptic ulceration or have had an ulcer some years previously that was cured with medication. Pernicious anaemia and atrophic gastritis predispose to gastric cancers. The patient may have been taking vitamin B12 supplements for their anaemia.

Examination

General appearance The most noticeable features are *wasting* and *pallor*. The wasting is often most apparent in the face and hands. The pallor is usually caused by an iron deficiency anaemia that is the result of chronic bleeding and lack of iron in the diet. Many patients present at an advanced stage with multiple hepatic metastases or metastases in the lymph glands around the porta hepatis. Mild jaundice suggests the latter.

Neck **The supraclavicular fossa must be carefully examined**, as secondary deposits in the supraclavicular lymph glands are common. A palpable supraclavicular gland in a patient with a carcinoma of the stomach is called *Virchow's gland*, and its presence is referred to as *Troisier's sign*.

Lungs The presence of a pleural effusion suggests pulmonary metastases.

Abdomen Inspection. The abdomen is often scaphoid as a consequence of weight loss but, paradoxically, there may be generalized abdominal distension if ascites is present. Pyloric obstruction causes **epigastric distension and visible peristalsis**. These physical signs can only be seen in thin patients. In the majority, the primary tumour is too small, too high or too deep to be seen.

Palpation. In the majority of patients, the only physical sign is epigastric tenderness. Deep palpation on full inspiration may reveal an epigastric mass.

In a thin patient with advanced disease, there may be a hard, irregular, dull epigastric mass that moves with respiration. The liver may be palpable and its edge and surface knobbly and irregular. The epigastrium may be distended, and there may be a succussion splash if there is pyloric obstruction.

Percussion. Shifting dullness may be present if there is an associated ascites.

Auscultation. The bowel sounds should be normal.
Rectal examination Metastatic nodules may be felt in the pelvis and in the ovaries (*Krukenberg's tumours*).

Often physical signs are minimal, and endoscopy is required for diagnosis.

Lymphoma of the stomach

Lymphoma presents with symptoms and signs similar to those of a carcinoma of the stomach – vague epigastric pain and weight loss. It may arise in middle-aged patients. Endoscopic deep biopsy is required for diagnosis.

Chronic pancreatitis

Chronic pancreatitis progressively destroys the exocrine and endocrine tissues of the pancreatic gland.

History

Age and sex Many patients are middle-aged, and 80 per cent are males. It is a rare condition, affecting between three and ten patients per million in Western countries.
Symptoms Patients complain of severe, recurrent episodes of upper abdominal pain that usually radiates through to the back. The pain is a gnawing, dull, persistent ache. The pattern and periodicity of the attacks vary greatly, but they are often related to episodes of excessive alcohol drinking. The condition can develop after multiple attacks of acute pancreatitis (acute relapsing pancreatitis) but more often develops *de novo* in patients who subject themselves to chronic alcohol abuse.

Weight loss and nausea are common. Diabetes, steatorrhoea and jaundice develop in about 10 per cent of affected patients.

Drug addiction is common, as long-term opiate analgesics are often required to relieve the persistent, intolerably severe pain.

Examination

There are often few physical signs. Patients often look distraught and dishevelled. Weight loss and jaundice may be apparent. A mass (a pseudocyst) may be palpable in the epigastrium. The diagnosis ultimately relies on special tests.

Chronic pancreatitis can cause thrombosis of the portal vein, in which case the signs of portal hypertension will be present.

Carcinoma of the pancreas is the important differential diagnosis (see below).

Chronic cholecystitis

Chronic or recurrent infection in the gallbladder is almost always associated with gallstones. The combination of stones and infection may present various clinical pictures: indigestion, flatulent dyspepsia (chronic cholecystitis), acute pain (acute cholecystitis), gallstone colic, obstructive jaundice and, less commonly, ascending cholangitis, acute pancreatitis and intestinal obstruction. Most of these complications are associated with abdominal pain.

History

Age Gallstones can form at any age. The majority of patients with symptoms are between 30 and 60 years old, but a number of females between the ages of 15 and 25 years develop gallstones. Younger patients with sickle-cell disease develop pigment stones.
Sex Gallstones are far more common in females than in males.
Ethnic group North American Indians are particularly liable to develop gallstones.
Symptoms The common complaint is of an **upper abdominal indigestion-like pain after eating**. The pain normally begins gradually, 15–30 minutes after a meal, and lasts for 30–90 minutes. When it becomes severe, it tends to move over into the **right hypochondrium and may radiate through to the back**. It is not relieved by anything except analgesic drugs. Patients often notice that the pain is worse after eating a fatty meal, such as bacon and eggs or fish and chips. The attacks of pain are irregular, lasting for weeks or months, with pain-free intervals of varying length. There is often postprandial belching, hence the description *flatulent dyspepsia*. The patient's appetite remains good, and

their weight stays steady or increases. Nausea and vomiting can occur during acute exacerbations.

Previous history Apart from previous episodes of dyspepsia, the patient may have been jaundiced or noticed their stools were pale, offensive and floated on the water in the lavatory pan.

Examination

General appearance Medical students believe that almost every patient with gallstones is female, fair, fat, fertile and forty. Many are, but enough are male, thin, dark and of any age to make one pay scant attention to the 'five Fs' as an aid to diagnosis. The skin or sclerae may show signs of jaundice, indicating that there may be stones in the common bile duct.

Abdomen Inspection. The abdomen usually looks normal.

Palpation. The patient is **tender in the right hypochondrium just below the tip of the ninth rib**, the point where the edge of the rectus abdominis muscle crosses the costal margin. It may be necessary to palpate deeply behind the costal margin as the patient takes a deep breath to detect mild tenderness or a small mass. A mass present in the right hypochondrium suggests that a stone is obstructing the cystic duct and that a mucocele or empyema is developing.

Percussion, auscultation and rectal examination. These should be normal.

Carcinoma of the pancreas

Eighty-five per cent of pancreatic cancers arise in the head of the pancreas. Although many present with **jaundice and weight loss, abdominal pain** is the presenting symptom in more than half, and occurs at some stage in over 90 per cent.

The pain is usually a continuous, dull, boring pain, felt in the epigastrium and radiating through to the back. It is often worse at night and may be relieved by sitting forward.

Radiation of the pain to the right hypochondrium is common with tumours of the head of the pancreas, while radiation to the left hypochondrium indicates an infiltrating tumour of the tail of the gland.

Jaundice develops in almost 90 per cent of patients at some stage of the disease, and is characteristically progressive but rarely painless. Pale stools, dark urine and skin itching indicate obstructive jaundice. Weight loss is almost universal.

Steatorrhoea, epigastric bloating, flatulence, diarrhoea, vomiting and constipation may all occur in between 20 and 30 per cent of patients.

Ten per cent of patients present with thrombophlebitis migrans (see Chapter 10).

Examination

Obstructive jaundice, a palpable gallbladder and an enlarged liver indicate a carcinoma of the head of the pancreas, but in the early stages, physical signs are rarely present. Carcinomas of the tail or body of the pancreas often present late with the symptoms and signs of distant metastases.

Liver metastases/tumours

Distension of the liver capsule stimulates pain fibres. Liver metastases are a common complication of all intra-abdominal malignancies. A constant dull ache in the right hypochondrium, general malaise, weight loss and sometimes mild jaundice may be the first indication of their presence.

Patients with liver cirrhosis who develop a hepatoma often complain of epigastric or right hypochondrial pain. A hepatoma should be suspected when severe pain and weight loss develop in a patient who is known to have cirrhosis.

Splenomegaly

The causes of splenomegaly are given on page 522. A large spleen can cause dull, persistent left hypochondrial pain. Splenic infarction, which is often associated with sickle-cell disease, causes a more severe pain that may be exacerbated by deep respiration.

Revision panel 15.13

The common conditions that present with chronic upper abdominal pain

Chronic peptic ulceration
Carcinoma of the stomach
Chronic pancreatitis
Chronic cholecystitis
Carcinoma of the pancreas
Liver metastases
Splenomegaly

CHRONIC CENTRAL ABDOMINAL PAIN

See Revision panel 15.15.

Irritable bowel syndrome

The irritable bowel syndrome is a functional disorder of the bowel of unknown aetiology which causes chronic intermittent abdominal pain that may be associated with changes in bowel habit and abdominal distension. Combinations of these symptoms occur in at least 10 per cent of the population, suggesting the possibility that the syndrome is simply a variant of normality. Many aetiological factors have been proposed, including the quantity of fibre in the diet, food allergies, disorders of bowel motility, abnormalities of visceral autonomic nerve perception, psychological disorders and social and behavioural problems.

The diagnosis is based solely on the history, as there are no physical signs except for an indefinite, ill-localized abdominal sensitivity on palpation.

It is important to exclude all other causes of abdominal pain, so enquire about any symptoms or signs that might indicate the presence of organic disease, such as anaemia, bleeding, weight loss, fever or a change in bowel habit.

The following symptoms suggest the diagnosis of irritable bowel syndrome:

- continuous or recurrent abdominal pain or discomfort for at least 3 months that is relieved by defaecation; and/or
- a change in the frequency of defaecation; and/or
- a change in the consistency of the stool.

These symptoms are diagnostic when presenting together with two or more of the following complaints:

- an altered frequency of defaecation;
- an altered stool consistency;
- problems with defaecation (straining/incomplete evacuation);
- bloated feelings of abdominal distension;
- the passage of mucus.

Crohn's disease

Crohn's disease usually runs a chronic course. It generally presents with a long history of colicky central or lower abdominal pain coming on every 15–30 minutes, associated with diarrhoea. Thickened segments of small bowel may be palpable, but some patients have no detectable abdominal physical signs.

The patient may show other stigmas of a chronic inflammatory disease (Revision panel 15.14).

Revision panel 15.14
Extra-abdominal manifestations of Crohn's disease
Finger clubbing
Erythema nodosum
Arthritis – sacroiliitis
Aphthous ulceration
Episcleritis/uveitis
Pyoderma gangrenosum
Anal sepsis/fistulation
Sclerosing cholangitis
Gallstones
Renal stones
Anaemia
Osteoporosis
Hypoproteinaemia

Recurrent adhesive obstruction

Adhesive obstruction is suggested when the signs and symptoms of small bowel obstruction develop in a patient with an abdominal scar. Congenital bands and internal hernias may also cause recurrent episodes of small bowel obstruction.

Adhesive obstruction is a difficult diagnosis to make and is often applied incorrectly to any patient who experiences pain after abdominal surgery. The diagnosis can only be made with certainty when the obstruction becomes acute and laparotomy confirms the presence of adhesions obstructing the bowel.

Tumours of the small bowel

Small bowel tumours are rare and often found incidentally at autopsy. They present late with unexplained small bowel obstruction. Adenomas that occur in association with familial polyposis and Gardner's syndrome may cause intussusception and acute small bowel obstruction. Lipomas and hamartomas can also arise in the small bowel. The latter are known to occur in the *Peutz–Jeghers syndrome*, together with *circumoral pigmentation* (see Fig. 11.10).

Carcinoid tumours are common in the appendix, where they are usually benign, but they can also arise in the small bowel, where they are more likely to be malignant.

Lymphomas can occur anywhere in the intestine, but quite commonly arise in the small intestine.

Adenocarcinomas of the small bowel are extremely rare.

All these rare tumours can present with chronic subacute small bowel obstruction causing a central colicky abdominal pain, weight loss and a change in bowel habit. Acute obstruction may develop, and a mass may be palpable.

Mesenteric ischaemia

Less acute occlusions of the mesenteric vessels may cause chronic central or general abdominal pain. This pain is often brought on by eating and is called intestinal angina. It begins insidiously with umbilical epigastric cramping pains, vomiting and diarrhoea, which lead to 'food fear', anorexia and weight loss. An abdominal bruit from a stenosed mesenteric artery may be the only detectable physical sign, but is often not present. Chronic mesenteric ischaemia should be considered in all patients with unexplained abdominal pain associated with severe weight loss.

Mesenteric venous thrombosis can complicate abdominal trauma, portal vein thrombosis, splenectomy and other causes of a hypercoagulable state.

Radiation damage

Both the small and large bowel can be damaged by the external beam radiation used to treat pelvic malignancies such as cancer of the uterus, cervix and bladder. Most patients develop transient diarrhoea at the time of the radiation, but some present months or years later, when fibrosis and strictures form, with colicky or continuous pain, vomiting, weight loss, constipation or diarrhoea. Eventually, the endarteritis in the small mesenteric vessels, caused by the irradiation, may lead to ischaemia, necrosis and perforation of the bowel. Radiation bowel injury must be differentiated from a recurrence of the primary tumour and/or widespread metastatic spread throughout the abdominal cavity (see below).

Carcinomatosis

Patients with extensive 'seedling' metastases throughout the peritoneal cavity may develop a non-specific aching abdominal pain that they find difficult to describe and that may be associated with few physical signs. Eventually, clinical ascites, abdominal masses, evidence of tumour at other sites and generalized weight loss and cachexia make the diagnosis obvious. In the early stages, the nebulous nature of the pain and the lack of physical signs can lead the physician to give, mistakenly, calming reassurance or make an incorrect diagnosis of irritable bowel syndrome.

Retroperitoneal fibrosis

Retroperitoneal fibrosis not only obstructs the ureters, but may also involve the abdominal aorta and inferior vena cava. It often causes a vague central, persistent abdominal pain. The kidneys may be enlarged by a hydronephrosis, or there may be a tender abdominal aneurysm. If the fibrosis obstructs the vena cava, the patient may present with the symptoms of an acute deep vein thrombosis or oedema of the lower limbs (see Chapter 10).

Tuberculosis

Intra-abdominal tuberculosis is relatively rare in Western countries but is still quite common in India and Africa, where it may be associated with the increasing incidence of AIDS. Ileocaecal tuberculosis may cause colicky or continuous central abdominal pain, often associated with abdominal distension and weight loss. There may be a mass of matted glands in the right iliac fossa, a dough-like feeling to the abdomen, ascites or signs of chronic intestinal obstruction, together with evidence of tuberculous infection at other sites such as the lungs or cervical lymph glands.

Lumbar spine disorders

Pain caused by abnormalities in the spine may radiate from the back to the front of the abdomen and cause diagnostic difficulties. Any suggestion that an abdominal pain is affected by movement and position should indicate the possibility that the pain is arising in the back. This can sometimes be confirmed by careful examination of the spine.

CHAPTER 15 | THE ABDOMEN

Constipation

Severe chronic constipation may cause a rather indeterminate abdominal pain and general abdominal distension. In these cases there are hard faeces in the rectum and palpable, indentable masses in the abdomen.

Psychosomatic pain

This is a dangerous diagnosis to make, especially knowing how difficult it is to recognize the pain of widespread intra-abdominal malignancy. There are, however, some patients with profound psychological disturbances, severe anxiety or 'cancer phobia' who persistently present with abdominal pain for which no cause can be found.

Beware of adopting the 'cry wolf' attitude. Each new episode of pain requires an open-minded new history and examination.

Revision panel 15.15

The causes of chronic central abdominal pain

Irritable bowel syndrome
Inflammatory bowel disease
Recurrent adhesive obstruction
Small bowel tumours
Mesenteric ischaemia
Radiation damage
Carcinomatosis
Retroperitoneal fibrosis/tumours
Tuberculosis
Lumbar spine pain
Chronic constipation
Psychosomatic

CHRONIC LOWER ABDOMINAL PAIN

See Revision panel 15.16.

Chronic diverticular disease

Although diverticular disease may present with acute abdominal pain or large bowel obstruction as described above, it most commonly presents in middle-aged or elderly patients with episodes of central or lower left-sided abdominal pain, often associated with or preceded by constipation. The pain is dull or colicky and there may be weeks, months or years between attacks. The condition needs to be differentiated from carcinoma of the colon, irritable bowel syndrome and other causes of inflammatory bowel disease. Examination of the abdomen may reveal some tenderness in the left iliac fossa and, very occasionally, a palpable mass. Rectal examination and sigmoidoscopy are rarely helpful and the diagnosis is made by special investigations.

Crohn's disease

Crohn's disease usually presents with a long history of colicky central or lower abdominal pain associated with an altered bowel habit. Patients may also report the systemic manifestations of Crohn's disease (Revision panel 15.14).

Carcinoma of the caecum and right colon

Cancer of the caecum is often silent until it has grown to a considerable size.

History

Most right-sided colonic and caecal tumours present with symptoms of **anaemia** (tiredness and shortness of breath), **weight loss and a mass**. They can also present with a dull pain in the right iliac fossa or with the colicky pains of small bowel obstruction. Sometimes the symptoms closely mimic acute appendicitis.

Examination

General appearance Patients usually appear pale and thin.

Abdomen Inspection. The abdomen may be generally distended or full in the right iliac fossa. A mass may be visible in a thin patient.

Palpation. The right iliac fossa is often tender, with some guarding of the overlying muscles. A **firm, irregular mass** may be felt in the right iliac fossa or right lumbar region, which may be fixed or freely mobile (Fig. 15.15). The liver may be palpable, enlarged and irregular.

Percussion. The mass is usually dull to percussion.

Auscultation. Bowel sounds are normal unless obstruction or peritonitis is present.

Rectal examination This is usually normal, as is sigmoidoscopy, although the latter may show the presence of rectal polyps.

Fig. 15.15 A mass clearly visible in the right iliac fossa (arrowed).

Occult blood may be detected in the faeces with the appropriate test.

Cancer of the left colon

The symptoms of cancer of the left colon differ according to the part of the colon involved. The majority of colon cancers are found in the sigmoid colon and at the rectosigmoid junction, where they are usually small, annular and ulcerated. They usually present with a **change in bowel habit**, often with variable periods of constipation interspersed with episodes of explosive diarrhoea and the passage of a number of loose stools.

History

Age The majority of patients are over 50 years old, but colon cancer can occur in young adults with ulcerative colitis or familial polyposis.

Sex Both sexes are equally affected.

Symptoms Pain is a rare symptom and, when it is present, it is usually a mild lower abdominal colic or ache. After some weeks or months, it usually becomes a persistent pain in the left lower abdomen. **Alternating constipation and diarrhoea** is typical of the annular variety of carcinoma of the left colon. The constipation is caused by the intestinal obstruction, and the diarrhoea by liquefaction of faeces above the obstruction. The diarrhoea may be increased by inflammation of the colonic mucosa and an excessive secretion of mucus. The episodes of colicky abdominal pain are accompanied by distension, but early loss of weight and appetite is uncommon. The weight loss often precedes the anorexia.

Thin patients may feel a lump in their abdomen.

Rectal bleeding is not a common symptom of a tumour of the sigmoid or descending colon but, when it occurs, the blood is dark and plum-coloured, sometimes with clots of blood interspersed among the faeces. When the tumour is at the rectosigmoid junction or within the rectum, it is more likely to cause bleeding and it may prolapse, causing tenesmus.

Rectal tumours usually present with bleeding rather than abdominal pain or large bowel obstruction. Painful frequent micturition indicates involvement of the bladder.

Examination

General appearance Weight loss may be apparent.

Abdomen Inspection. In thin patients, there may be swelling in the left iliac fossa. The colon, especially the caecum, may be visibly distended with faeces.

Palpation. A large tumour may be palpable, often in the left lumbar region or iliac fossa. Part of the mass may be hard faeces above the tumour rather than the tumour itself, in which case the mass is indentable. The mass is tender if there is any surrounding inflammation or a pericolic abscess associated with a perforation.

The liver may be palpable with an irregular knobbly surface and edge.

Percussion. A mass in the left iliac fossa will be dull to percussion.

Auscultation. Loud, high-pitched continuous gurglings can be heard during the attacks of colic, but if the colon perforates, the abdomen becomes silent and, of course, tender.

Rectal examination A tumour in the apex of a loop of the sigmoid colon hanging down into the pelvis may be palpable on bimanual examination. Secondary nodules may be felt within the pelvis, and blood may be visible on the fingerstall. Rectal and rectosigmoid tumours should be visible on rigid sigmoidoscopy

Tumours in the left side of the colon can present with generalized peritonitis if the patient has ignored the symptoms described above. In such cases, severe generalized abdominal pain develops accompanied by signs of shock with tachycardia, hypotension, distension, tenderness, loss of liver dullness and absent bowel sounds. In many cases, the peritonitis is caused by a rupture of a distended caecum, not a rupture at the site of the cancer.

Gynaecological malignancy

Signs and symptoms of gynaecological malignancy are insidious and often absent early in the disease. Patients can report abdominal pain, bloating, weight loss, urinary urgency and fatigue. Ovarian malignancy should be suspected and investigated before a diagnosis of irritable bowel syndrome is given.

Chronic infections

- *Tuberculosis*. Ileocaecal tuberculosis can lead to chronic lower abdominal pain. Fistulation of the small bowel can lead to chronic abdominal pain, but may present acutely if associated with abscess formation or cellulitis.
- *Actinomycosis*. Abscesses form in the gastrointestinal tract. They are painful and enlarge before discharging, commonly in the right iliac fossa.
- *Yersinia pseudotuberculosis*. This causes a short-lived terminal ileitis similar to Crohn's disease.
- *Enterobius vermicularis*. These are small threadworms, often found in the appendix, and may cause right lower abdominal pain.
- *Ascaris lumbricoides*. These worms can form a tangled mass resulting in intestinal obstruction.

'Chronic' appendicitis

Two forms of chronic inflammation may develop in the appendix: the mucocele and the empyema. Both follow an attack of acute inflammation, and both may cause recurrent pain in the right iliac fossa that is sometimes colicky in nature. Worms and faecoliths may produce similar symptoms.

Recurrent episodes of mild acute infection, commonly classified as a 'grumbling' appendix, are extremely rare. Do not make that diagnosis; look for another cause for the patient's pain.

Chronic pelvic sepsis

A number of patients with acute pelvic inflammatory disease develop lower abdominal pain, which is often related to the menstrual cycle. Adnexal tenderness on bimanual examination in association with a low-grade fever and a continuing vaginal discharge indicates the diagnosis. There may be associated urinary frequency and dysuria. Gonococci and other pathogens found on a high vaginal swab confirm the diagnosis.

Endometriosis

This is a condition in which ectopic endometrial tissue is present in sites in the abdomen other than the uterus, such as the large and small bowel and the lining of the abdominal cavity. It causes abdominal pain at the time of menstruation.

Degenerating fibroids

The pain is initially acute, but can last up to a number of weeks.

Urological causes

Urinary retention, cystitis, bladder colic, ureteric colic and pyelonephritis can all cause chronic lower abdominal symptoms and are discussed in Chapter 17.

Uterine colic

Abdominal pain during pregnancy is always concerning. It is important to exclude other causes as they can be difficult to differentiate.

Revision panel 15.16
The causes of chronic lower abdominal pain
Diverticular disease
Crohn's disease
Carcinoma of the colon
Gynaecological malignancy
Chronic infections
Chronic appendicitis
Chronic pelvic sepsis
Endometriosis
Degenerating fibroid
Urological causes
Uterine colic

CONDITIONS PRESENTING WITH DYSPHAGIA

Some serious alimentary diseases do not cause abdominal pain, but do affect swallowing and may cause retrosternal pain.

Foreign body

A swallowed foreign body can become impacted in the oesophagus, leading to obstruction and complete dysphagia. An underlying stricture or malignancy should be ruled out by endoscopic examination.

Motility disorders

The common forms of dysmotility are diffuse oesophageal spasm, non-specific motility disorder and achalasia. All of these can present with dysphagia with or without pain.

The connective tissue disorder systemic sclerosis also causes poor oesophageal motility. This can lead to a failure of acid clearance from the oesophagus, resulting in stricture formation.

Neurological diseases

Conditions such as myasthenia gravis, multiple sclerosis and cerebrovascular disease can lead to oropharyngeal dysmotility.

Reflux oesophagitis

This causes a retrosternal burning sensation, described by the patient as heartburn. Patients may also develop dysphagia. Apart from the nature of the pain, the clue to the diagnosis of reflux oesophagitis is its relationship to posture. Bending, stooping, heavy lifting and tight clothes all force acid up into the oesophagus and cause heartburn. It is often worse at night if the patient slips off their pillow. This is often the only symptom of a hiatus hernia. Recurrent or persistent reflux can result in a peptic stricture or a Schatzki ring, causing dysphagia. Strictures can also be the result of ingestion of a corrosive substance.

Oesophageal webs

A postcricoid web is found in patients with Plummer–Vinson syndrome, which is associated with iron deficiency anaemia. Other causes include bullous diseases such as pemphigus.

Pharyngeal pouch

This conditions leads to regurgitation, aspiration and dysphagia as the pouch enlarges (see Chapter 12).

Oesophageal carcinoma

The diagnosis is suspected when the patient complains of dysphagia and weight loss. Palpable supraclavicular lymph glands often develop. At first, large pieces of food stick, but ultimately fluids cannot be swallowed. Benign neoplasms of the oesophagus can occur, but are rare.

CONDITIONS PRESENTING WITH VOMITING

Acute gastroenteritis

Symptoms usually begin 12–72 hours after infection. Patients may present predominantly with either diarrhoea or vomiting. Bacterial infections are associated with severe abdominal cramps and blood in the stool.

Pyloric stenosis or obstruction

This occurs in neonates with congenital hypertrophic pyloric stenosis, and in adults with either a cicatrizing peptic ulceration of their pylorus or duodenum, or a carcinoma of the antrum of the stomach.

Neonates, with congenital *hypertrophic pyloric stenosis*, usually present between 2 and 6 weeks after birth. After feeding, they vomit large quantities of curdled and unpleasant-smelling milk. The vomit is forcefully ejected, justifying the adjective '**projectile**'. The child becomes thin and dehydrated, but retains its appetite. Careful abdominal examination shortly after a feed may reveal a **smooth ovoid mass just below the right costal margin**, sometimes called a pyloric 'tumour'. This is the hypertrophied pylorus, and is a diagnostic physical sign.

Adults with pyloric stenosis present with vomiting. The vomit is usually large in volume, not bile stained and, when the condition is long-standing, not acidic because the chronic gastric retention causes achlorhydria. The stomach contents are, therefore, not digested, and the patient may notice that their vomit contains food that was eaten 24 or 48 hours previously. Epigastric distension, visible gastric peristalsis and a succussion splash may be present.

Small bowel obstruction

As previously described in this chapter, small bowel obstruction presents with vomiting as one of the main symptoms.

Gastric volvulus

Patients report severe epigastric or retrosternal pain. They are unable to tolerate liquids and suffer from continuous retching.

CHAPTER 15 | THE ABDOMEN

Acute gastric dilatation

This condition can occur after surgery or in association with metabolic disturbances such as hyperglycaemia. The abdomen is distended and tender. There may be a succussion splash. Vomiting places the patient at risk of aspiration pneumonia.

Meconium ileus

Meconium ileus is often the presenting symptom in children with either cystic fibrosis or Hirschsprung's disease. Vomiting and abdominal distension occur soon after birth as a result of thickened meconium impacted within the bowel lumen causing bowel obstruction.

Duodenal atresia

This presents with bilious vomiting that occurs soon after birth. The diagnosis may have been detected during antenatal checks and is often associated with other congenital abnormalities.

Medical causes

Medical causes of vomiting are listed in Revision panel 15.17.

Revision panel 15.17

Medical causes of vomiting

Medications, e.g. opioids
Alcohol
Chemotherapy
Pregnancy
Uraemia
Hyper/hypoglycaemia
Cerebrovascular accident
Migraine
Brain neoplasm
Concussion
Adrenal insufficiency
Ménière's disease

CONDITIONS PRESENTING WITH HAEMATEMESIS OR MELAENA

Haematemesis is the vomiting of blood. This must be differentiated from haemoptysis, when the blood is coughed up and originates from the respiratory tract.

Patients describe vomit that resembles coffee grounds. This is the result of the blood becoming altered by the acid present within the stomach.

Melaena refers to the black, tarry stool produced in the presence of upper gastrointestinal haemorrhage. The black appearance of the stool is caused by oxidation of iron in the haemoglobin as it passes through the ileum and colon. The causes are listed in the Revision panel 15.18.

Revision panel 15.18

The causes of haematemesis and melaena

Peptic ulceration:

Spontaneous
Steroid ingestion

Acute gastric erosions:

Aspirin
Non-steroidal anti-inflammatory drugs
Steroids
Trauma
Burns

Carcinoma:

Stomach
Oesophagus

Oesophageal varices

CONDITIONS PRESENTING WITH JAUNDICE

The term 'jaundice' is derived from the French word *jaune*, meaning yellow. The yellow discolouration of the skin is caused by an excess of bile pigments in the plasma. This is initially visible against the white background of the sclerae, and then becomes more obvious as the skin turns yellow with elevation of the serum levels. The conditions which cause jaundice can be subdivided as below:

- *Haemolytic jaundice* (prehepatic) is associated with increased red cell fragility and high levels of *unconjugated bilirubin* in the bloodstream, which does not enter the urine (acholuric). Causes include sickle-cell anaemia, spherocytosis, thalassaemia and glucose 6-phosphate dehydrogenase deficiency.
- *Hepatocellular jaundice* is due to parenchymal liver abnormalities, leading to a mixed picture of *elevated unconjugated and conjugated bilirubin.*

Causes include chronic active hepatitis, cirrhosis, drug-induced hepatitis and alcohol-induced liver disease.

- *Obstructive jaundice* (posthepatic) is associated with pruritis, pale stools and dark urine. This is as a result of obstruction of the biliary tree, leading to a systemic absorption and *elevation of conjugated bilirubin*. In extrahepatic cholestasis, Courvoisier's Law holds that the presence of a palpable gallbladder suggest that the cause is likely to be carcinoma of the head of the pancreas. Causes include choledocholithiasis, cholangitis, pancreatic malignancy, Mirizzi's syndrome (see below), bile duct strictures, choledochal cyst and biliary atresia.

Causes of obstructive jaundice

Choledocholithiasis

Gallstones can pass from the gallbladder into the common bile duct. Obstructive jaundice occurs when the stone becomes impacted within the duct. This often occurs at the ampulla, where the stone can also cause acute pancreatitis by obstructing the pancreatic duct. The jaundice is often fluctuating, and the gallbladder is not palpable.

Cholangitis

Cholangitis is an ascending infection as a result of a poorly draining or obstructed biliary tree. This is most commonly caused by bile duct stones, but is also caused by malignancy of the pancreas, bile duct, ampulla or bile duct strictures. The classic Charcot's triad of symptoms include pain, obstructive jaundice and fever (often with rigors).

Pancreatic malignancy

The jaundice is usually painless and progressive. It is often associated with weight loss and pruritis. The gallbladder maybe palpable.

Mirizzi's syndrome

Obstruction of the hepatic duct can be caused by a stone impacted in the cystic duct leading to oedema and direct compression of the extrahepatic biliary tree.

Bile duct strictures

Benign causes include primary sclerosing cholangitis, iatrogenic injury from previous biliary surgery and fibrosis secondary to choledocholithiasis. Malignant causes include cholangiocarcinoma, adenocarcinoma of the pancreas and ampullary tumours.

Choledochal cyst

This condition usually presents in childhood and can manifest as one or all of the following: jaundice, pain and an upper abdominal mass. It is most commonly the result of a fusiform dilatation of the common bile duct. The condition carries an increased risk of cholangiocarcinoma.

Biliary atresia

Presentation is usually in the early neonatal period with persistent neonatal jaundice. It occurs in approximately 1 per 10 000 live births, and the cause is unknown.

CONDITIONS PRESENTING WITH DIARRHOEA

This is defined as the frequent passage of loose or liquid stool exceeding three or more bowel actions per day. Some diseases of the large bowel cause diarrhoea without any other symptoms. The nature of the diarrhoea may suggest the diagnosis, but it often relies on the results of investigations such as flexible sigmoidoscopy, biopsy, colonoscopy, barium enema or stool cultures.

Infections of the gastrointestinal tract

Infections from food, such as *Salmonella* and staphylococcal toxins, are called food poisoning. The stools are watery, brown and passed with great frequency. Abdominal colic is common and may be associated with nausea, vomiting and thirst.

In tropical countries, the most common causes of diarrhoea are bacillary dysentery and amoebic dysentery. The diagnosis is confirmed on stool culture.

Cholera presents with vomiting, cramps and severe diarrhoea. The diarrhoea lasts for up to 3 or 4 days. The patient passes colourless, watery stools (known as rice-water stools), which consist of an inflammatory exudate, mucus, flakes of epithelium, the casts of villi and the infecting organism.

CHAPTER 15 | THE ABDOMEN

Salmonella can present with abdominal pain if ulcers in the small bowel perforate.

Giardia and *Campylobacter* are also common infections causing abdominal pain and diarrhoea, and will be differentiated by stool culture.

Norovirus is a common viral cause in institutions and *rotavirus* is commonly seen in children.

Clostridium difficile is an important infection that can occur in patients on broad-spectrum antibiotics. The toxins produced can lead to a condition known as *pseudomembranous colitis*. White plaques can be seen over the mucosa when performing sigmoidoscopy. Severe infections can result in a life-threatening condition known as *toxic megacolon*.

Small bowel and pancreatic disorders

Pancreatic damage as a consequence of *cystic fibrosis* or *chronic pancreatitis* leads to a loss of pancreatic digestive enzyme production (i.e. lipases and amylases), and this in turn causes pale frothy and offensive stools, known as *steatorrhoea*.

Small bowel infiltration, infestation or fistulation can also cause diarrhoea. *Tropical sprue* and *coeliac disease* can also present with loose or frequent stools.

Patients who have had extensive previous bowel resections may have *short bowel syndrome*, leading to a rapid bowel transit time.

Ulcerative colitis and Crohn's disease

Patients with these conditions develop chronic frequent diarrhoea often associated with diffuse intermittent abdominal pain. They sometimes pass a watery brown fluid, while at other times they pass just mucus containing red flecks of blood or dark, altered blood. Patients may have 20–30 bowel actions a day.

Associated colicky abdominal pain suggests a diagnosis of Crohn's disease.

Persistent pain may be the result of *acute toxic dilatation* of the colon, especially if this is complicated by bowel perforation. The patient is dehydrated, thin, ill and feverish, with signs of abdominal distension and acute peritonitis, i.e. tenderness and guarding with a loss of liver dullness and an absence of bowel sounds.

Carcinoma of the colon and rectum

Most cancers of the left-hand side of the colon cause a *change in bowel habit*, which may be associated with pain and bleeding. Persistent copious diarrhoea is not usually a prominent feature.

A villous papilloma is a benign or malignant rectal tumour that causes excessive mucus secretion. Patients frequently pass stools of pure mucus. This may cause dehydration and the loss of large quantities of sodium and potassium.

Spurious (overflow) diarrhoea occurs when a very constipated patient passes loose, watery stools around a mass of faeces impacted in the rectum. Diagnosis is by rectal examination.

Cancers of the rectum can present with diarrhoea, especially if they are locally advanced, when a frequent and sometimes painful urge to defaecate (*tenesmus*) may develop.

Drugs

Medications are a common cause of diarrhoea, and a complete drug history including non-prescribed medications should be established. Drugs such as orlistat (which inhibits the absorption of fat), chemotherapy agents, antibiotics and overuse of laxatives can all lead to increased bowel frequency.

Endocrine causes

Hormone-secreting tumours (VIPomas, glucagon-omas, Zollinger–Ellison syndrome) and conditions such as hyperthyroidism and Addison's disease can also cause increased bowel frequency.

ABDOMINAL MASSES: CAUSES AND SIGNS

The techniques for palpating the liver, spleen and kidneys are described on pages 483, 484.

Hepatomegaly

The causes of enlargement of the liver, (Fig. 15.16, Revision panel 15.19) classified according to their clinical presentation, are listed below.

Fig. 15.16 Hepatomegaly.

Smooth generalized enlargement, without jaundice

- Congestion from heart failure.
- Cirrhosis.
- Lymphoma.
- Hepatic vein obstruction (Budd–Chiari syndrome).
- Amyloid disease.
- Kala-azar.
- Gaucher's disease.

Smooth generalized enlargement, with jaundice

- Infective hepatitis.
- Biliary tract obstruction (gallstones, carcinoma of pancreas, atresia).
- Cholangitis.
- Portal pyaemia.
- Chronic active hepatitis.

Knobbly generalized enlargement, without jaundice

- Metastatic deposits.
- Cirrhosis.
- Polycystic disease.
- Primary liver carcinoma (hepatocellular and cholangiocarcinoma).

Knobbly generalized enlargement, with jaundice

- Metastatic deposits.
- Cirrhosis.

Localized swellings

- Riedel's lobe.
- Secondary carcinoma.
- Hydatid cyst.
- Liver abscess.
- Primary liver carcinoma.
- Cholangiocarcinoma.
- Benign liver adenoma.

Revision panel 15.19
Causes of hepatomegaly
Infection
Congestion
Bile duct obstruction
Cellular infiltration
Cellular proliferation
Space-occupying lesions

The physical signs of an enlarged liver are as follows:

- It descends below the right costal margin.
- You cannot feel its upper limit.
- It moves with respiration.
- It is dull to percussion up to the level of the eighth rib in the mid-axillary line.
- It may have a sharp or rounded edge with a smooth or irregular surface.

Remember Riedel's lobe. This is an extension of the right lobe of the liver below the costal margin, along the anterior axillary line. It is often mistaken for a pathological enlargement of the liver or a gallbladder. It is a normal anatomical variation.

Splenomegaly

The spleen is almost always uniformly enlarged (Figs 15.17–15.19). The causes of splenomegaly are classified according to the underlying disease (see Revision panel 15.20).

Infection
Bacterial

- Typhoid.
- Typhus.

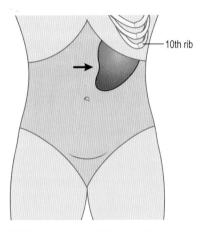

Fig. 15.17 Splenomegaly. The notch is not always palpable.

Fig. 15.18 Patient with splenomegaly; swelling outlined on surface with felt-tip pen.

Fig. 15.19 Massive hepatosplenomegaly in a patient with lymphoma.

- Tuberculosis.
- Brucellosis.
- General septicaemia.

Viral

- Glandular fever.
- Epstein–Barr virus.

Spirochaetal

- Syphilis.
- Leptospirosis (Weil's disease).

Protozoal

- Malaria.
- Kala-azar (leishmaniasis).
- Schistosomiasis.

Cellular proliferation

- Myeloid and lymphatic leukaemia.
- Lymphomas.
- Pernicious anaemia.
- Polycythaemia rubra vera.
- Spherocytosis and other haemolytic anaemias, for example elliptocytosis, autoimmune haemolytic anaemia and thalassaemia.
- Thrombocytopenic purpura.
- Myelofibrosis.
- Sarcoidosis.

Congestion

- Portal hypertension (cirrhosis, portal vein thrombosis).
- Hepatic vein obstruction.
- Congestive heart failure.

Infarction and injury

- Emboli from bacterial endocarditis.
- Splenic artery or vein thrombosis caused by polycythaemia or sickle-cell disease.
- Haematoma.

Cellular infiltration

- Amyloidosis.
- Gaucher's disease.

Collagen diseases

- Felty's syndrome.
- Still's disease.

Space-occupying lesions

- True solitary cysts.
- Polycystic disease.
- Hydatid cysts.
- Angioma.
- Lymphomas.
- Secondary tumours (very rare).

The physical signs of an enlarged spleen are:

- It appears from below the tip of the left tenth rib and enlarges along the line of the rib towards the umbilicus.
- It is firm, smooth and usually spleen shaped; it often has a definite notch on its upper edge.
- You cannot get above it.
- It moves with respiration.
- It is dull to percussion.
- Although it may be possible to bring it forwards by lifting the left lower ribs forwards, it cannot be felt bimanually or be balloted.

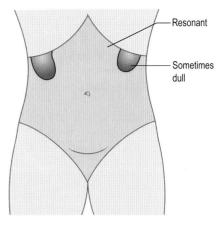

Fig. 15.20 Bilateral enlargement of the kidneys.

Revision panel 15.20

Causes of splenomegaly

Infection

Cellular proliferation

Congestion

Infarction

Cellular infiltration

Collagen diseases

Space-occupying lesions

Enlargement of the kidney

One or both kidneys may be enlarged (Fig. 15.20, Revision panel 15.21). The common causes of renal enlargement are:

- hydronephrosis;
- pyonephrosis;
- malignant disease: carcinoma of the kidney and nephroblastoma;
- solitary cysts;
- polycystic disease;
- perinephric abscess.

A mobile or low-lying kidney may be easily palpable and seem to be enlarged, especially if the patient is thin.

Revision panel 15.21

Causes of enlargement of the kidney

Distension of the pelvi-calyceal system

Space-occupying lesions

Single:

Cyst

Abscess

Tumour

Multiple:

Polycystic disease

Compensatory hypertrophy

Hydronephrosis may be bilateral if the obstructing lesion is in or distal to the neck of the bladder.

Nephroblastoma is occasionally bilateral.

Polycystic disease is very likely to affect both kidneys.

The physical signs of an enlarged kidney are as follows:

- It lies in the paracolic gutter or can be pushed back into this gutter – that is to say, it can be reduced into the loin.
- It is usually only possible to feel the lower pole, which is smooth and hemiovoid.
- It moves with respiration.
- It is not dull to percussion because it is covered by the colon; even when a large kidney reaches the anterior abdominal wall, it has a band of resonance across it.
- It can be felt bimanually.
- It can be balloted (see page 484).

Pancreatic pseudocysts

This is a collection of pancreatic juice and inflammatory exudate, usually associated with acute pancreatitis, which forms on the surface of the pancreatic gland and may bulge forwards, filling the lesser sac. The patient is usually known to have had an attack of acute pancreatitis (see page 500). They may then develop epigastric fullness, pain, nausea and vomiting. If the cyst becomes infected, the patient develops severe pain, sweating and rigors.

The physical characteristics of a pancreatic pseudocyst are the following:

- The epigastrium contains a firm, sometimes tender, mass with an indistinct lower edge; the upper limit is rarely palpable (Fig. 15.21).
- It is usually resonant to percussion because it is covered by the stomach.
- It moves very slightly with respiration.
- It is not possible to elicit fluctuation or a fluid thrill.

These swellings can be very difficult to feel as most of their bulk is beneath the costal margin.

Fig. 15.21 A pancreatic, lesser sac, pseudocyst.

Mesenteric cysts

These are cysts containing clear fluid that develop in the mesentery. They arise from the vestigial remnants of reduplicated bowel and are usually found by chance. They can, rarely, cause abdominal distension or recurrent colicky pain. Like all cysts, they can rupture, twist and bleed from their lining. Twisting is rare because they are fixed within the small bowel mesentery.

The physical characteristics of a mesenteric cyst are as follows:

- It forms a smooth, mobile, spherical swelling in the centre of the abdomen (Fig. 15.22).
- It moves freely at right angles to the line of the root of the mesentery, but only slightly along a line parallel to the root of the mesentery.
- It is dull to percussion.
- Large cysts may be felt to fluctuate and have a fluid thrill.

It is difficult to discriminate between a very large cyst and tense ascites.

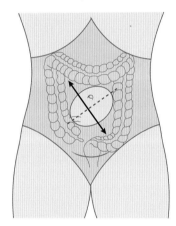

Fig. 15.22 A mesenteric cyst.

Retroperitoneal tumours

Apart from primary and secondary tumours of the lymph glands, retroperitoneal tumours are rare. The most common variety is the *liposarcoma*. They grow slowly and silently and usually become quite large before they are noticed by the patient or become palpable. The patient complains of distension, a vague abdominal pain and sometimes anorexia and weight loss.

They produce the following physical signs:

- abdominal distension;
- a smooth or bosselated mass with an indistinct edge and a soft to firm consistency;

- resonance while they are covered with bowel, but when they reach the anterior abdominal wall and push the bowel out to the flanks, they become dull to percussion (Fig. 15.23).
- very little movement with respiration;
- possible transmission of aortic pulsation.

Fig. 15.23 Abdominal distension caused by a retroperitoneal liposarcoma in a young male.

Carcinoma of the stomach

The symptoms of carcinoma of the stomach are described on page 509. Although stomach cancers can become large, hard masses, they are notoriously difficult to feel because they are situated high in the abdomen beneath the costal margin. A palpable tumour is hard and irregular, disappearing beneath the costal margin (Fig. 15.24). It is rarely possible to feel its upper edge. The symptoms of abdominal pain or indigestion with loss of appetite and weight are far more significant than the physical signs. Do not expect to feel a mass in a patient with carcinoma of the stomach.

Fig. 15.24 Stomach mass.

Gallbladder

An enlarged gallbladder is usually easy to recognize from its shape and position (Fig. 15.25). The causes of enlargement of the gallbladder are:

- obstruction of the cystic duct, usually by a gallstone, and rarely by an intrinsic or extrinsic carcinoma – the patient is not jaundiced and the gallbladder often contains bile, mucus (a mucocele) or pus (an empyema);
- obstruction of the common bile duct, usually by a stone or a carcinoma of the head of the pancreas – the patient will be jaundiced.

Courvoisier's law states that 'When the gallbladder is palpable and the patient is jaundiced, the bile duct is unlikely to be obstructed by a stone because

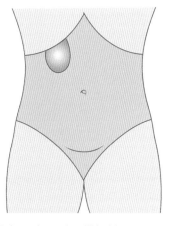

Fig. 15.25 An enlarged gallbladder.

previous attacks of inflammation result in a thick-walled, fibrotic and non-distensible gallbladder'.

This is a useful clinical rule but there are a number of exceptions:

- Stones that form in the bile duct rather than in the gallbladder may obstruct the duct in the presence of a normal distensible gallbladder.
- There may be double pathology – a stone in the cystic duct causing gallbladder distension, and a carcinoma or a stone blocking the lower end of the bile duct.
- The converse of the law, jaundice without a palpable gallbladder, does not mean that jaundice is caused by stones. In such cases, the obstruction may be caused by a cancer of the head of the pancreas, but the gallbladder distension is minimal. Alternatively, the jaundice may be caused by a carcinoma of the bile or hepatic ducts above the entry of the cystic duct into the bile duct.
- *Mirizzi's syndrome*: when the cystic duct is closely applied to the common hepatic duct or is very short, a stone impacted in it can inflame and obstruct the bile duct and cause jaundice. The gallbladder is often distended.

The physical features of an enlarged gallbladder are as follows:

- It appears from beneath the tip of the right ninth rib.
- It is smooth and hemiovoid.
- It moves with respiration.
- There is no space between the lump and the edge of the liver.
- It is dull to percussion.

When an acutely inflamed gallbladder becomes surrounded by adherent omentum and bowel, it loses some of its characteristics. A gallbladder mass is diffuse and tender, lies in the right hypochondrium, and does not move much with respiration. As the infection subsides, it becomes more discrete and mobile, and less tender.

Faeces

The colon can become grossly distended with faeces as a result of a mechanical obstruction or chronic constipation. The patient may complain of diarrhoea,

but this is actually mucus and a little watery faeces leaking out around the main mass of faeces (spurious diarrhoea).

The physical characteristics of faeces are as follows:

- The masses lie in that part of the abdomen occupied by the colon – the flanks and across the lower part of the epigastrium (Fig. 15.26).
- They feel firm or hard but are indentable. This means that they can be dented by firm pressure with the fingers, and this dent persists after releasing the pressure.
- There may be multiple separate masses in the line of the colon, but in gross cases the faeces coalesce to form one vast mass that is easy to mistake for a tumour.
- When there is no mechanical obstruction, rectal examination confirms a rectum full of very hard faeces, but if there is a blockage in the lower colon, the rectum will be empty.

Do not forget that faecal masses can form above an annular stenosing carcinoma of the colon.

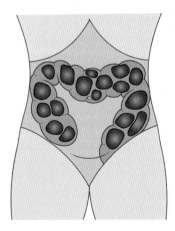

Fig. 15.26 A colon distended with faeces. The masses are indentable. Faecal impaction of this degree is likely to be caused by Hirschsprung's disease or gross constipation.

Urinary bladder

The causes of retention of urine are listed in Revision panel 17.4, page 568. The bladder may be tense and painful (acute retention) or enlarged and painless (chronic retention) (see Fig. 17.3).

The physical features of an enlarged bladder are the following:

- It arises out of the pelvis so has no lower edge (Fig. 15.27).
- It is hemiovoid in shape, usually deviated a little to one side.
- It may vary in size: a very large bladder can extend up to and above the umbilicus.
- It is not mobile.
- It is dull to percussion.
- If it is large enough to permit the necessary simultaneous percussion and palpation, it will have a fluid thrill.
- Direct pressure on the swelling often produces a desire to micturate.
- It does not bulge into the pelvis and can only be felt indistinctly on bimanual (combined rectal and abdominal) examination.

Fig. 15.27 A distended urinary bladder.

Ovarian cyst

Small ovarian cysts are common and are impalpable. When they enlarge, they rise up out of the pelvis into the lower abdomen and become palpable.

The physical features of a large ovarian cyst are as follows:

- It is smooth and spherical with a distinct outline.
- It arises from the pelvis, so its lower limit is not palpable; i.e. you cannot 'get below it' (Fig. 15.28).

- It may be mobile from side to side but cannot be moved up and down.
- It is dull to percussion.
- It has a fluid thrill.
- Its lower extremity may be palpable in the pelvis during rectal or vaginal examination, and movement of the cyst may produce some movement of the uterus.

Fig. 15.28 A large ovarian cyst.

Pregnant uterus

Never forget that pregnancy is the most common cause of enlargement of the uterus, and of abdominal distension.

The diagnosis of pregnancy is more difficult in the first 20 weeks, when the uterus is still relatively small and there are no fetal movements.

A pregnant uterus is a smooth, firm, dull swelling arising out of the pelvis.

The uterus enlarges to the xiphisternum by the 36th week of pregnancy. At this stage, the fetus is palpable (ballotable), moves and has a heart beat.

The diagnosis of pregnancy is confirmed if bimanual examination reveals that the mass cannot be moved independently of the cervix and that the cervix is soft and patulous.

Note An enlarged uterus must not be squeezed during a bimanual examination, as this can theoretically cause the patient to go into labour and abort the fetus.

Fibroids

Fibroids are benign fibromyomatous uterine tumours that can grow to an enormous size and fill the whole abdomen. They are usually multiple. They can cause irregular and heavy periods, disturbed micturition, lower abdominal pain and backache.

The physical signs of a fibroid uterus are the following:

● It arises out of the pelvis, so its lower edge is not palpable (Fig. 15.29).
● It is firm or hard, bosselated or distinctly knobbly, each knob corresponding to a fibroid.
● It moves slightly in a transverse direction, and any movement of the abdominal mass moves the cervix.
● It is dull to percussion,
● It is palpable bimanually: a moderately enlarged uterus can be pushed down into the pelvis.

Fig. 15.29 A large fibroid uterus.

CAUSES OF A MASS IN THE RIGHT ILIAC FOSSA

A mass in the right iliac fossa is a common physical finding (Figs 15.30 and 15.15, Revision panel 15.22). There are a number of conditions that may be responsible. This section describes the important features in the history and examination of each cause.

Appendix mass

History

The patient usually complains of a period of central abdominal pain followed by a pain in the right iliac

Fig. 15.30 A common diagnostic problem: a mass in the right iliac fossa.

fossa. The pain often persists for several days, and is usually accompanied by malaise, loss of appetite and pyrexia.

Examination

There is a tender, indistinct mass, which is dull to percussion, fixed to the iliac fossa posteriorly, and accompanied by a persistent low fever and tachycardia. An appendix mass must be differentiated from carcinoma of the caecum.

Revision panel 15.22

The causes of a mass in the right iliac fossa

Appendix mass
Appendix abscess
Tuberculosis
Carcinoma of the caecum
Crohn's disease (terminal ileitis)
Iliac lymphadenopathy
Iliac artery aneurysm
Psoas abscess
Chondrosarcoma or osteosarcoma of the ilium
Actinomycosis
Spigelian hernia
Ruptured epigastric artery
Kidney transplant
Ovarian cyst/tumour
Fibroid
Malignant change in an undescended testis

Appendix abscess

History

This is the same as for an appendix mass, with the additional symptoms of an abscess, namely, fever, rigors, sweating and increased local pain.

Examination

There is a tender mass that, in its late stages, may be associated with oedema and reddening of the overlying skin. The patient will have a swinging, intermittent fever and an increasing tachycardia.

Tuberculosis

In many parts of the world, tuberculosis is more often the cause of an inflammatory mass in the right iliac fossa than is appendicitis. The mass consists of the inflamed ileocaecal lymph glands and parts of the caecum and terminal ileum that are also inflamed.

History

The patient has often had a vague central pain for months, with general ill-health, loss of weight and changes in bowel habit. The pain then becomes intense and settles in the iliac fossa. An acute episode of central abdominal pain moving to the right iliac fossa, similar to appendicitis, is uncommon.

Examination

The mass is firm, tender and very indistinct. The surface and the edge are difficult to define. If there is a tuberculous peritonitis, the abdomen will be swollen and less pliable – often described as a 'doughy' abdomen.

Carcinoma of the caecum

History

Often there is no acute pain, just a dull discomfort in the right iliac fossa. Some patients present with anaemia, diarrhoea or intestinal obstruction.

Examination

The mass is firm, distinct and hard. It is usually fixed to the posterior abdominal wall, but is sometimes mobile. It is not tender and does not resolve with observation. The patient's temperature and pulse are normal unless there is an associated pericolic abscess.

Crohn's disease

(Terminal ileitis)

History

The patient will have experienced recurrent episodes of pain in the right iliac fossa, general malaise, weight loss and episodes of diarrhoea.

Examination

The swollen terminal ileum forms an elongated sausage-shaped mass that usually lies transversely in the right iliac fossa and feels rubbery and tender.

Iliac lymph glands

History

The symptoms depend on the cause of the lymphadenopathy. There may be a generalized disease, or local disease in the limb, perineum or genitalia.

Examination

Enlarged iliac lymph glands form an indistinct mass with no clear contours. The mass follows the line of the iliac vessels and may bulge forwards just above the inguinal ligament. It can be easy to feel, or be no more than a fullness in the depths of the iliac fossa.

All the other lymph glands must be examined, as must the lower limb, to try to find the cause of the lymphadenopathy.

Iliac artery aneurysm

History

The patient may have noticed a pulsating mass or felt an aching pain in the right iliac fossa.

Examination

The common iliac artery dilates more often than the external iliac artery, so the smooth, distinct mass with an expansile pulsation is usually in the upper medial corner of the iliac fossa.

Psoas abscess

History

The patient is likely to have felt ill for some months, with night sweats and loss of weight. Back pain and abdominal pain can also occur.

Examination

The iliac fossa is filled with a soft, tender, dull, compressible mass. There may be a fullness in the lumbar region that is accentuated by pressing on the mass in the iliac fossa. The swelling may extend below the groin, and it may be possible to empty the swelling below the groin into the swelling above, and vice versa.

Back movements may be painful and limited.

Chondroma and sarcoma of the ilium

Rarely, chondromas and chondrosarcomas arise in the iliac bones. They grow slowly and may bulge into the iliac fossa. They are large, hard, non-tender and clearly fixed to the skeleton. They usually lie in the lateral part of the iliac fossa. Osteomas and osteosarcomas of the ileum are equally rare.

Actinomycosis

This invariably develops as a complication of appendicitis, but may present *de novo* as a mass in the iliac fossa with a number of discharging sinuses that produce characteristic '*sulphur granules*'. It is a rare condition.

Spigelian hernia

These hernias appear at the outer edge of the rectus abdominis muscle along the linea semilunaris. The lump is still palpable when the abdominal wall muscles are contracted, and it is felt to lie above them.

Ruptured inferior epigastric artery

This occurs as a result of straining or coughing. The haematoma tracks beneath the abdominal wall, extraperitoneally, to produce a mass in the iliac fossa. It is diffuse, and there may be discolouration of the skin. It is attached to the anterior abdominal wall but, as it is on its deep surface, it becomes impalpable when the muscles contract. Contraction of the abdominal muscles is usually painful.

Transplanted kidney

The mass is situated beneath the transplant scar and a history of transplantation makes the diagnosis easy. The lump is smooth, kidney shaped and rubbery.

Ovarian cysts and fibroids

These can fall to the right into the right iliac fossa. They will be felt to be connected to the uterus on bimanual examination. A huge pyosalpinx may occasionally be palpable in the right iliac fossa.

Malignant change in an undescended testis

This is a rarity but is easily suspected provided you remember always to examine the scrotum as part of the abdominal examination.

CAUSES OF A MASS IN THE LEFT ILIAC FOSSA

Diverticulitis and carcinoma of the colon are the common causes of a mass in the left iliac fossa. It must be remembered that the normal sigmoid colon is palpable in one out of three patients. An appendix mass on the left side only occurs if the patient has *situs inversus*. Tuberculosis and Crohn's disease only cause masses in the right iliac fossa. All the other causes of a mass in the right iliac fossa mentioned above can also cause a mass in the left iliac fossa (Revision panel 15.23).

Diverticulitis

When sigmoid diverticula become inflamed, the swollen colon and surrounding pericolic abscess may be palpable.

History

The patient may have suffered from recurrent lower abdominal pains and chronic constipation for years. The acute episode starts suddenly with a severe left iliac fossa pain, nausea, loss of appetite and constipation.

be confused with iliac fossa masses (see Revision panels 15.23 and 15.24).

The diagnosis is made from the site and shape of the lump and, if present, its reducibility and an expansile cough impulse.

Examination

The left iliac fossa contains a tender, indistinct mass whose long axis lies parallel to the inguinal ligament. There may be signs of general or local peritonitis and intestinal obstruction. The diagnosis depends upon the site of the tenderness. There are very few other acute inflammatory conditions that present with a mass in the left iliac fossa.

Carcinoma of the sigmoid colon

History

The patient may present with lower abdominal pain, abdominal colic, intestinal obstruction, a change in bowel habit, rectal bleeding and general cachexia.

Examination

The mass is hard, easily palpable and not tender. It may be mobile or fixed. The colon above the mass may be distended with indentable faeces. The tumour can perforate locally and cause a 'pericolic' abscess similar to that of diverticular disease.

CAUSES OF A LUMP IN THE GROIN

The inguinal region is part of the iliac fossa and swellings within it and just below it in the groin can

ABDOMINAL DISTENSION

The causes of abdominal distension can be remembered by repeating the letter 'F' six times: fetus, flatus, faeces, fat, fluid (free and encysted), and fibroids and other solid tumours (Revision panel 15.25).

Fetus

Pregnancy is the most common cause of abdominal distension. The features of a pregnant uterus have already been described on page 527.

Flatus

(Tympanites)

Gas in the intestine can cause considerable abdominal distension.

In the early stages, the distension may be localized to that part of the abdomen containing the distended bowel, such as the epigastrium when the stomach is distended, or the right iliac fossa when the caecum is distended, but as the distension affects the whole bowel, the whole abdomen swells.

The distension remains localized if the bowel twists into a volvulus. This is a common complication of a long sigmoid colon combined with a narrow base of the mesocolon.

Distended bowel has no palpable surface or edge. The only diagnostic features are hyper-resonance and, when there is obstruction, visible peristalsis. The bowel sounds may be hyperactive. Shaking the patient causes a splashing sound as the thin layer of fluid in the distended bowel splashes about. This is known as a succussion splash and is particularly common when there is gastric distension caused by pyloric stenosis.

Acute dilatation of the stomach, mechanical intestinal obstruction, paralytic ileus, aerophagy (air swallowing) and massive amounts of free gas from a perforation all cause hyper-resonance on abdominal percussion.

Faeces

Faecal impaction may present as abdominal distension or an abdominal mass. The physical features of faecal masses in the abdomen are described on page 526. The diagnosis can usually be suspected from a history of the patient's bowel habits. The common causes are Hirschsprung's disease, chronic intestinal obstruction, chronic constipation and antidepressant drugs.

Fat

Fat rarely causes distension, but frequently makes the patient pot-bellied. A large fat abdomen may be caused by a thick layer of subcutaneous fat or by excess fat in the omentum and mesentery. These two sites of fat deposition do not necessarily enlarge together. A protuberant, round abdomen often has a thin layer of subcutaneous fat but contains a heavy, thick omentum.

Fluid: ascites

Free fluid in the peritoneal cavity is called ascites. It is caused by a variety of conditions, but they all fall into one of four groups: those which raise the portal venous pressure, those which lower the plasma proteins, those which cause peritonitis, and those which allow a direct leak of lymph into the peritoneal cavity (Revision panel 15.26).

Revision panel 15.26

Aetiology of ascites

Raised portal venous pressure
Prehepatic, intrahepatic and posthepatic
Cardiac
Pulmonary

Hypoproteinaemia
Renal
Hepatic
General

Peritonitis
Acute and chronic
Traumatic, chemical, infective, neoplastic

Lymphatic obstruction (chylous ascites)

Causes of an increased portal venous pressure

Prehepatic

- Portal vein thrombosis.
- Compression of the portal vein by lymph glands.

Hepatic

- Cirrhosis.

Posthepatic

- Budd–Chiari syndrome.

Cardiac

- Constrictive pericarditis.
- Right heart failure caused by mitral stenosis, tricuspid incompetence and pulmonary hypertension.

Pulmonary

- Pulmonary hypertension and right heart failure.

Causes of hypoproteinaemia

- Kidney disease associated with albuminuria.
- Cirrhosis of the liver.
- The cachexia of wasting diseases, malignancy and starvation.
- Protein-losing enteropathies.
- Malnutrition.

Causes of chronic peritonitis

Physical

- Postirradiation
- Starch granuloma.

Infection

- Tuberculous peritonitis.

Neoplasms

- Secondary peritoneal deposits of carcinoma.
- 'Mucus'-forming tumours (pseudomyxoma peritonei).

Causes of chylous ascites

Chylous ascites is caused by the leakage of lymph from the lacteals or the cisterna chyli as a result of congenital abnormalities, trauma and primary or secondary lymph gland disease.

Physical signs of ascites

- A fluid thrill.
- Shifting dullness.

A *fluid thrill* is elicited by flicking one side of the abdomen with the index or middle finger, and feeling the vibrations when they reach the other side of the abdomen with your other hand. Before doing this, you must place the edge of the patient's (or an assistant's) hand on the abdomen at the umbilicus to prevent the percussion wave being transmitted through the fat in the abdominal wall. A fluid thrill is present in any fluid-filled cavity, so that the difference between free and encysted fluid depends upon the recognition of shifting dullness.

Shifting dullness is a dull area that moves or changes shape when the patient changes position. The dullness of ascites is found in the flanks and

across the lower abdomen. Percuss the medial limits of the flank dullness carefully, and place vertical marks on the abdomen with a felt-tipped pen. Then ask the patient to turn onto one side to an angle of approximately 45°. Wait a few seconds and percuss again. If there is free fluid moving under the influence of gravity, the medial limits of dullness will have moved towards the midline on the lower side of the abdomen and away from it on the upper side.

Fluid: encysted

Fluid trapped in a cyst, in the renal pelvis or between adhesions has a fluid thrill, is dull to percussion, but does not shift.

The position and features of a cyst depend upon its anatomical origin. The following cysts or fluid-filled swellings may become large enough to present as abdominal distension:

- Ovarian cysts.
- Hydronephrosis.
- Urinary bladder.
- Pancreatic pseudocysts.
- Mesenteric cysts.
- Hydatid cysts.

A large aortic aneurysm can also distend the abdomen. It is distinguished by the presence of an expansile pulsation.

Fibroids and other solid tumours

Solid tumours that can become very large and cause abdominal distension are, in approximate order of frequency:

- Hepatomegaly (Budd–Chiari syndrome or metastatic liver tumours).
- Fibroids.
- Splenomegaly (myelofibrosis).
- Large cancers of the colon.
- Polycystic kidneys.
- Primary carcinoma of the liver.
- Retroperitoneal sarcoma and lymphadenopathy.
- Ganglioneuroma (in children).
- Nephroblastoma (in children).
- Neurofibroma/schwannoma.

The physical signs of most of these tumours are described in the preceding parts of this chapter.

16 The rectum and anal canal

APPLIED ANATOMY

The rectum has a continuous layer of longitudinal muscle outside the inner circular muscle, unlike the sigmoid colon where the longitudinal muscle is in three bands, the taeniae. The ano-rectal junction forms a right angle, held in this position by the puborectalis muscle.

At the anus, the gut joins the skin. The anus is lined by squamous epithelium, while the rectum is lined by columnar epithelium. The location where the epithelium changes is known as the mucocutaneous junction, and is visible as a wavy white line in the lower third of the anal canal (sometimes called *Hilton's white line*).

Above this junction is the rectum, which:

- has autonomic sensation and is sensitive only to stretching;
- receives its arterial blood supply from the mesenteric vessels;
- drains venous blood into the portal circulation;
- drains lymph into the mesocolic and eventually into the preaortic lymph nodes.

Below the mucocutaneous junction is anal skin, which:

- has somatic sensation and is as sensitive as skin;
- receives its arterial blood supply from the iliac vessels;
- drains venous blood into the iliac veins;
- drains lymph into the inguinal lymph glands.

This differentiation explains the way in which cancers spread and the genesis of many symptoms.

SYMPTOMS OF ANO-RECTAL DISEASE

Embarrassment often inhibits patients from describing their 'ano-rectal' symptoms in precise detail, although as ever the history is often crucial in making the correct diagnosis. The principal symptoms include bleeding, pain, pruritus, incontinence, prolapse, tenesmus and a change of bowel habit, mentioned in Chapter 1, but now discussed in detail.

Bleeding

Blood passed per rectum may be fresh or altered. When blood is degraded by intestinal enzymes and bacteria, it becomes black and acquires a characteristic smell. Such a black, tarry stool is called **melaena** (see Chapter 15). To have time to turn black before it reaches the rectum, the blood has usually come from the stomach or duodenum.

Recognizable blood may appear in four ways:

- mixed in with the faeces;
- on the surface of the faeces;
- separate from the faeces, either after or unrelated to defaecation;
- on the toilet paper after wiping.

Blood mixed with the faeces or on the surface of the faeces

These are difficult to differentiate. Blood 'mixed in' with the faeces should theoretically have come from above the sigmoid colon to give sufficient time for mixing, while blood 'on' the faeces has usually come from the rectum or anal canal.

Blood separate from the faeces

An anal condition such as haemorrhoids is usually responsible for bleeding following defaecation.

When blood is passed by itself, it has accumulated rapidly, causing a strong desire to defaecate. Causes include diverticular disease and angiodysplasia.

Note Bleeding from the upper gastrointestinal tract is occasionally sufficiently rapid to be passed as recognizable blood and not melaena, but usually the brighter red the blood is, the lower down is its source.

Blood on the toilet paper

This is usually the result of minor bleeding from conditions close to the anal margin, such as haemorrhoids or a fissure.

Pain

Pain from the anal canal is felt principally on defaecation, and is often protracted, cramp-like and distressing. There may be a background ache. Excessive stretching of the anal canal may cause a sharp, splitting pain, sometimes described as if something is tearing. This is true if the patient has a fissure!

Uncomplicated haemorrhoids and rectal cancer (see below) are not usually painful, while fissures, abscesses and perianal haematomas always are.

Pruritus

Perianal itching is a common symptom and may be accompanied by a burning discomfort, which can be severe if the enzyme-rich small bowel contents make prolonged contact with the perianal skin. Itching occurs in those perianal conditions that produce leakage of mucus, liquid faeces or purulent discharge onto the perianal skin, but may also be caused by a primary skin disease. In children, the most common cause is a worm infestation.

The symptom is frequently worse at night, perhaps because there are no other sensory distractions.

Incontinence and soiling

Incontinence may be caused by sphincter failure, impaction with overflow, extreme urgency or neurological impairment. A fistula connecting the small bowel or colon with the vagina will cause leakage of either small bowel content or stool. The symptom may be concealed by an embarrassed patient. The nature of the leakage should be recorded as gas, liquid or solid. The amount of leakage and the frequency of its occurrence must be ascertained. Questions on 'staining on the underclothes', the need for pads and the passage of a full bowel motion will reveal the extent of the problem. It is important to establish whether the patient has an awareness of the need to 'open the bowels'.

A defective external anal sphincter (voluntary muscle) is associated with a feeling of urgency with inability to retain the stool, while internal anal sphincter dysfunction (of smooth muscle, which is autonomically innervated) is associated with the unconscious passage of small amounts of stool between bowel actions.

Difficulty in defaecation

This should be differentiated from the infrequent passage of hard stool. Here, the patient strains to pass stool and may utilize a variety of body positions or local finger pressure around or in the anal canal to aid defaecation. This may even occur when the stool is loose.

Prolapse

The patient may notice something 'coming down' from either the vagina or the rectum. This may occur sporadically with a bowel action or during walking or standing. Faecal and urinary incontinence commonly coexist.

Tenesmus

This is defined as a constant intense desire to defaecate. When the patient tries to evacuate the rectum, either nothing or just a small amount of mucus and loose faeces appears. Tenesmus should always be taken seriously as it may indicate a space-occupying lesion mimicking the presence of faeces, often a carcinoma of the rectum or anus. It can, however, be caused by benign conditions including inflammatory bowel disease and even irritable bowel syndrome.

Change in bowel habit

Beware of the terms 'diarrhoea' and 'constipation'. When patients use the word constipation, some mean that their bowels are opening less frequently than usual, while others feel that their motions are harder. Diarrhoea has a similar double meaning, either frequent defaecation or loose motions. Make sure that you find out what the patient means. It is better to record the frequency of bowel action and the consistency of the stool than to use these lay terms.

Many patients, particularly the elderly, complain of a change in bowel habit – some of these patients feel that daily defaecation is a basic human right! However, all individuals with this symptom must be taken seriously as bowel cancer frequently presents in this way. A change to a looser stool is generally more worrying than the development of constipation.

TECHNIQUE FOR DIGITAL ANO-RECTAL EXAMINATION

This is commonly called a rectal examination but is actually an examination of the anus and lower rectum. The patient should give clear verbal consent.

Preparation (Fig. 16.1)

Position of the patient

Ensure adequate privacy and uncover the patient from the waist to the middle of the thighs.

The patient should lie in the left lateral position with the neck and shoulders rounded so that the chin rests on the chest, with the hips flexed to 90° or more, and the knees flexed to slightly less than 90°.

(b) Part the buttocks, and inspect the anus and perineum.

(c) Place the pulp of your finger on the anus.

(d) As you insert your finger, pull backwards to counteract the tone in the puborectalis muscle.

(a) Place the patient in the left lateral position, with the hips flexed to 90° and the knees less flexed to 100°.

(e) After examining the anal canal and rectum, place your hand on the abdomen and examine the contents of the pelvis bimanually.

Fig. 16.1 THE TECHNIQUE OF ANO-RECTAL EXAMINATION

CHAPTER 16 | THE RECTUM AND ANAL CANAL

If the knees are flexed to more than 90°, the patient's ankles will get in your way. If the bed is soft, ask the patient to bring their buttocks to its edge. This makes inspection easier and tips its abdominal contents forwards, which helps bimanual examination.

Equipment

You need a plastic glove, some inert lubricating jelly and a good light. Tissues must be available for cleansing afterwards.

Tell the patient what you are going to do. Explain that you are going to feel inside their 'back passage', which will be uncomfortable but not painful. Ask the patient to relax by breathing deeply and letting their knees go loose.

Inspection

Lift the uppermost buttock with your left hand so that you can see clearly the anus, perianal skin and perineum. Look for:

- skin rashes and excoriation;
- faecal soiling, blood or mucus;
- scarring, or the opening of a fistula;
- lumps and bumps (e.g. polyps, papillomas, condylomas, perianal haematoma, prolapsed piles, rectal prolapse or even a visible carcinoma);
- ulcers;
- distortion of the anal canal by an underlying muscular defect;
- whether the anus appears to gape;
- whether a fissure is visible on parting the buttocks.

The patient should be asked to cough, which causes the normal anal sphincter to contract. They should then be asked to 'bear down' as if to open their bowels. This tests for prolapse of the bowel wall and for prolapsing piles.

Palpation

Before carrying out a digital examination, the anus should be inspected, particularly if there is a history of pain on defaecation. This demonstrates whether there is any spasm associated with a fissure, which may be visible. In no circumstances carry out instrumentation if there is any spasm or a fissure, as this could cause severe pain.

Place the pulp of your gloved right index finger on the centre of the anus, with the finger parallel to the skin of the perineum and in the midline. Press gently into the anal canal, but at the same time press backwards against the skin of the posterior wall of the anal canal and the underlying sling of the puborectalis muscle. This overcomes most of the tone in the anal sphincter and allows the finger to straighten and slip into the rectum. Never thrust the tip of your finger straight in.

The anal canal

As the finger passes through the anal canal, note the tone of the sphincter, any pain or tenderness and any thickening or masses.

Patients with fissures or abscesses may have so much spasm that rectal examination is extremely painful. Do not continue in these circumstances. General anaesthetic may be needed for adequate assessment.

The rectum

Feel all around the rectum as high as possible. You may have to push quite hard in a fat patient, and in some it is difficult to feel much beyond the anal canal. The mucosa of the anus and rectum should feel smooth, and it is important to elicit the presence of any masses or ulcers. The site of any abnormality should be noted for its level above the anal verge and its position.

If you feel a mass, try to decide if it is:

- ulcerated or polypoid;
- within or outside the wall – test the mobility of the mucosa over the mass, which provides a vital distinction;
- mobile or fixed to other structures, for example the sacrum.

Do not forget to feel the lower rectum, just above the anal canal. Posteriorly, the rectum turns away at a right angle, and it is easy to miss a small abnormality in this area (as it also is at sigmoidoscopy).

Note the contents of the rectum. The rectum may be:

- full of faeces (hard or soft);
- empty and collapsed;
- empty but 'ballooned out'.

Faeces may feel like a tumour but are indentable, the only rectal mass that is.

When you can just detect a possible abnormality at your fingertip, ask the patient to strain or 'bear down'. This will often move the mass down 1–2 cm or so and bring it within your reach.

The recto-vesico/recto-uterine pouch

Turn your finger to feel forwards to detect any masses outside the rectum in the peritoneal pouch between the rectum and the bladder or uterus. This is the pouch of Douglas (between the rectum and vaginal vault) in the female, and the recto-vesical pouch in the male. Pelvic abscesses are tender and boggy, while malignant pelvic deposits are hard and craggy.

Bimanual examination

Examination of the contents of the pelvis is helped if you feel 'bimanually' between the left hand on the abdomen and the right index finger in the rectum. This gives a much better idea of the size, shape and nature of any pelvic mass. This examination is much more difficult in an obese patient.

The cervix and uterus

These structures are easy to feel per rectum, and on bimanual palpation you should be able to define the shape and size of the uterus and any adnexal masses.

Note **A tampon, palpable as a firm mass, can be mistaken for the cervix.**

The prostate and seminal vesicles (Fig. 16.2)

It takes practice to be able to tell the normal prostate and cervix from an abnormal mass, so do not be downhearted if you get it wrong at first.

The normal prostate gland is firm, rubbery, bilobed and 2–3 cm across. Its surface should be smooth, with a shallow central sulcus (median groove), and the rectal mucosa should move freely over it. The seminal vesicles may occasionally be palpable just above the upper lateral edges of the gland.

Benign hypertrophy of the prostate produces enlargement of the whole gland, which bulges backwards into the rectum. The central sulcus is palpable unless the gland is very large. It may feel lobulated, and the overlying rectal mucosa remains mobile.

Carcinoma of the prostate causes an irregular, hard enlargement of the gland, which is often unilateral or

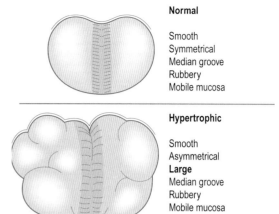

Normal

Smooth
Symmetrical
Median groove
Rubbery
Mobile mucosa

Hypertrophic

Smooth
Asymmetrical
Large
Median groove
Rubbery
Mobile mucosa

Malignant

Irregular
Asymmetrical
Loss of median groove
Hard
Mucosa may be fixed
Lateral extension

Fig. 16.2 The prostate gland.

asymmetrical. The edge of the enlarged area is usually indistinct. Thickening can often be felt either side of the gland, and in advanced cases can encircle the rectum. The central sulcus is distorted or obliterated at an early stage of the disease, and the rectal mucosa becomes fixed to the underlying gland.

Note When assessing the prostate, beware of the incompletely emptied bladder, which pushes the prostate downwards and makes it feel bigger than it actually is.

The anal sphincter

The anal sphincter may be assessed for strength at rest and by asking the patient to squeeze the examining finger. In females, the vaginal septum is easily felt anteriorly.

The rectal contents

Hard, packed stool is indicative of 'faecal impaction', which often presents with anal discomfort and leakage. An empty ballooned rectum is found in large bowel obstruction.

On completion of the examination always inspect the glove for the presence of blood or mucus, and note the colour of the faeces.

SIGMOIDOSCOPY AND PROCTOSCOPY

Sigmoidoscopy and proctoscopy using simple rigid instruments are part of the routine clinical examination of every patient with bowel symptoms.

Sigmoidoscopy

The sigmoidoscope should really be called a rectoscope. It is an illuminated tube, 30 cm in length, that is passed through the anus to inspect the rectum and its lining. It has an obturator with a rounded end to allow introduction, and a sealed lens with a bellows attachment that fits into the end of the tube when the obturator has been removed. Insufflation of air allows the rectal lining to be inspected. It can usually be passed as far as the recto-sigmoid junction or just beyond. Many patients experience significant discomfort when the sigmoid colon is entered.

Technique of rigid sigmoidoscopy (Fig. 16.3)

- No bowel preparation is necessary.
- Position the patient as for a rectal examination, making sure that they are lying as transversely as possible on the couch, with their buttocks at the edge or slightly overhanging. Elderly patients may feel they are going to fall off, and need reassurance.

(a) Position the patient with the body as near transverse as possible, with the legs drawn up and the buttocks at the edge of the couch. Insert the well-lubricated instrument along the axis of the anal canal by aiming it in the direction of the umbilicus.

(b) Point the sigmoidoscope backwards to follow the course of the rectum into the sacral hollow.

(c) Under direct vision, insufflating air as you go, pass the instrument up the rectosigmoid junction.

(d) Carefully inspect the lining of the rectum as you withdraw the instrument.

Fig. 16.3 SIGMOIDOSCOPY

- Explain to the patient what you are going to do. Tell them that they will experience discomfort and a feeling of fullness as air is 'pumped in', that you will release this pressure at the end to the examination, and that you will stop at once if there is any pain.
- Check the anus again to make sure there is no fissure or other painful condition.
- Warm the instrument if it is metal, and apply adequate amounts of lubricating jelly.
- Insert the instrument in the direction of the anal canal. This is achieved by pointing it towards the umbilicus.
- Once you have entered the rectum, remove the obturator and attach the light source and bellows. At this point, change the angle of insertion backwards, to follow the course of the rectum into the sacral hollow.
- Under direct vision, insufflating enough air to separate the rectal walls, negotiate the instrument to the recto-sigmoid junction. You will see and work around the three semi-circular folds known as *Houston's valves*.
- At the recto-sigmoid junction, you will see the rectum narrowing down to the diameter of the colon, which is similar in calibre to the instrument you are using. You will occasionally find a wide-open recto-sigmoid junction, which allows you to pass the instrument to its full length without any problem.
- Any gross pathology will be evident as soon as the rectum is entered, but it is best first to advance the sigmoidoscope to the recto-sigmoid junction, and inspect the contents and lining during withdrawal.
- A variable amount of faeces will be present, but in most cases a reasonable assessment of the rectum and its contents can be made. Are the faeces solid or liquid? Is there any obvious blood or melaena? Is there blood coming through the recto-sigmoid junction? Is there an excess of mucus?
- Look at the whole lining of the rectum, searching for tumours or polyps. Is the mucosa shiny, smooth and of normal colour, or is it velvety, granular and reddened, as in proctitis?
- Carefully inspect the posterior area just above the anal canal. This is a potential blind spot on sigmoidoscopy where it is easy to miss a small polyp. (The same applies to rectal examination.)
- On completion of the examination, make sure all the air is released, and wipe away any lubricating jelly from around the anus.
- Remember that sigmoidoscopy only demonstrates pathology in the lumen or wall of the rectum, and does not show lesions outside the wall or in the pelvis.

Flexible sigmoidoscopy (Fig. 16.4)

Most conditions of the rectum and some of the lower sigmoid colon can be diagnosed by the rigid sigmoidoscope. The flexible sigmoidoscope has increased the detection rate, as it can be passed further into the sigmoid colon. Bowel preparation is required.

(a) A flexible sigmoidoscope, rigid proctoscope and rigid sigmoidoscope.

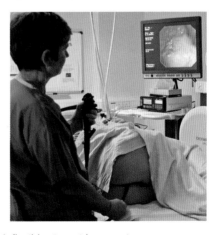

(b) A flexible sigmoidoscope in use.

Fig. 16.4 SIGMOIDOSCOPES

CHAPTER 16 | THE RECTUM AND ANAL CANAL

Proctoscopy (Fig. 16.5)

The proctoscope is a short illuminated tube, employed to inspect the anal canal. Its principal use is for the diagnosis and treatment of haemorrhoids. It should really be called an anoscope, but is always called a proctoscope. Proctoscopy usually follows immediately after sigmoidoscopy.

Technique of proctoscopy

- Position the patient as for sigmoidoscopy.
- No bowel preparation is necessary, and only gross faecal loading prevents adequate assessment of the anal canal.
- Confirm that there is no painful external pathology.

- Insert the instrument in the direction of the anal canal, pointing at the patient's umbilicus.
- Remove the obturator, and inspect the anal canal as you withdraw the instrument.
- Before removing the instrument, ask the patient to push down, which may cause haemorrhoids to swell and prolapse into view

Note Every patient with any rectal complaint must have a proper examination, with either sigmoidoscopy or simple digital examination. You will be considered negligent if you fail to perform a rectal examination on a patient complaining of rectal bleeding.

(a) Insert the proctoscope as you would the finger for a rectal examination, obliquely and from behind, pulling backwards against the puborectalis muscle.

(b) Pass the instrument along the axis of the anal canal.

(c) Inspect the anal canal as you slowly withdraw the proctoscope.

Fig. 16.5 PROCTOSCOPY

(d) A large haemorrhoid will fall into the lumen of the proctoscope; smaller ones just bulge over its end, an appearance that can be enhanced by advancing the scope 5 mm.

CONDITIONS PRESENTING WITH RECTAL BLEEDING (SEE REVISION PANEL 16.1)

Haemorrhoids

The mucosa and submucosa of the anal canal fall into three anal cushions that help to provide an efficient gas- and fluid-proof seal. The submucosa of the anal canal has a rich blood supply with a cavernous and capillary network of blood vessels covered by a thin epithelium, These highly vascular cushions can become congested, enlarge, bleed, prolapse and even become pedunculated. Abnormal enlargements of the anal cushions are called haemorrhoids (Fig. 16.6). They are *not* varicose veins of the anus.

The process of prolapse eventually stretches the overlying perianal skin, often producing an external skin tag. The two together are sometimes termed a *pile mass*. Skin tags may occur in isolation. The general public uses the term 'piles' for any swelling near the anus, and sometimes for anal pain – remember this when taking a history.

History

Age Piles occur at all ages but are uncommon below the age of 20 years. They are extremely rare in children.

Symptoms **Uncomplicated piles do not cause pain.** The two common symptoms are bleeding and a palpable lump or a sensation of 'something coming out' of the anus (prolapse) after defaecation. They may also cause perianal discomfort and a mucous discharge that leads to pruritus.

The bleeding, which is bright red, usually occurs after defaecation. It may just streak the faeces or be noticed on the toilet paper. When it is copious, it may splash into the lavatory pan and even result in iron-deficiency anaemia.

If the piles prolapse out of the anus after defaecation, a swelling is noticed on wiping, which may return to the rectum spontaneously or may need to be pushed back. If the prolapse becomes permanent, the skin tags often hypertrophy as well forming a major component of the pile mass.

Pruritus is commonly associated with piles; this is caused by the leakage of mucus from the exposed mucosa onto the perianal skin.

The vascular pads which become haemorrhoids close the anorectal junction

During defaecation the sphincter relaxes, the anal canal everts and the haemorrhoids are compressed by the faeces. The faeces scratch the mucosa

After the faeces have passed, the haemorrhoids are left scratched and unsupported so they drip blood onto the faeces

If they do not retract when the sphincter begins to close, their venous drainage is obstructed and the bleeding is made worse so that it splashes into the pan

Fig. 16.6 The way in which haemorrrhoids are caused to bleed.

Classification

Piles are categorized into three degrees by the history:

- *First-degree* piles bleed but do not prolapse.
- *Second-degree* piles prolapse but reduce spontaneously.
- *Third-degree* piles prolapse and need reduction, or may not go back at all.

Although this distinction is artificial, it does help to guide treatment.

Cause

The geographical incidence of haemorrhoids is inversely proportional to the stool volume, which depends on the amount of fibre in the diet. Piles are rare in Africa, and common in the industrialized developed nations. The lower volume of stool may lead to more straining on defaecation, which leads to congestion and enlargement of the cushions, although some patients with piles never have any difficulty defaecating and do not complain of straining.

Examination

First- and second-degree piles

After a full examination of the abdomen, you should then carry out an external inspection of the anus and perianal skin and perform a digital rectal examination to exclude other rectal conditions.

External skin tags will be immediately visible.

After the digital rectal examination, all patients with rectal bleeding must be sigmoidoscoped to make sure there is no other serious coexisting pathology.

A proctoscope is then inserted. On withdrawal through the anal canal, pale pink mucosa can be seen collapsing over its end (see Fig. 16.5d). Piles are darker bluish-red, and bulge into the end of the instrument. The multiple longitudinal corrugations are lost, and three deep clefts appear between the bulging piles.

The three 'primary' positions for haemorrhoids are at 3, 7 and 11 o'clock (with the patient in the lithotomy position), corresponding to the most common sites of the three anal cushions (which are associated with the arterial supply). 'Secondary' piles seen at other positions in the anal canal are usually smaller and appear between the primary piles.

Note Do not confuse degree with position, and remember that you cannot palpate haemorrhoids with your finger.

Third-degree piles (Fig. 16.7)

These are bluish-purple, permanently prolapsed swellings, in the 3, 7 and 11 o'clock positions. Their distinguishing feature is their mucosal covering, recognized by its soft, smooth, mucus-exuding surface. They are usually associated with skin tags,

Fig. 16.7 Third-degree (prolapsed) haemorrhoids. The epithelium covering the 3 o'clock pile is becoming thick and white. The 7 o'clock pile is bleeding.

which lie over the true haemorrhoid. If piles remain prolapsed, they ulcerate and bleed.

Thrombosed prolapsed piles

Piles are painful only when complications develop. A pile becomes tense, hard and oedematous if the submucosal vessels thrombose. Defaecation is then painful.

Inspection reveals one to three red–purple dark swellings protruding from the anus with oedematous skin tags (Fig. 16.8). The pile mass can eventually become ulcerated, resembling an anal tumour.

Fig. 16.8 Prolapsed, strangulated, thrombosed haemorrhoids. Note the bloody serous discharge.

In these circumstances, sigmoidoscopy and proper assessment may require a general anaesthetic.

The other common cause of a localized painful anal swelling is a perianal haematoma (see below). This can be distinguished from a mucosa-covered prolapsed haemorrhoid because it is covered by skin.

Revision panel 16.1

Possible diagnoses of conditions that present with rectal bleeding

Bleeding but no anal pain

Blood and looser stool = Colorectal carcinoma

Blood after defaecation = Haemorrhoids

Blood and mucus = Colitis

Bleeding and pain = Fissure (or carcinoma of the anal canal)

Blood alone = Diverticular disease or angiodysplasia

Melaena = Peptic ulceration

Carcinoma of the rectum

Most rectal cancers occur in the lower part of the rectal ampulla, where they tend to be papilliferous or ulcerated with an everted edge. Cancers in the upper part of the rectum and at the rectosigmoid junction are often annular in shape. The vast majority are adenocarcinomas.

History

Age Rectal carcinoma usually develops in middle and old age, but can occur in young adults.
Sex It is equally common in both sexes.
Symptoms **Many patients present with rectal bleeding**, usually a small amount of dark red blood streaked onto the surface of the stool. Very occasionally, enough blood accumulates in the rectum to be passed without faeces.

There is usually an associated change in bowel habit. The surface of the tumour produces excessive amounts of mucus, causing liquid motions, often described as 'diarrhoea'. Patients who complain of 'passing water through the back passage' either have a rectal cancer or a villous adenoma (see below) until proved otherwise.

High cancers of the annular variety at the recto-sigmoid junction may cause partial obstruction, presenting as alternating episodes of diarrhoea and constipation. This is because initial obstruction causes true constipation, followed by irritation of the colon above the tumour by impacted faeces, which liquefy before passing through the carcinomatous stenosis as loose stool.

Tenesmus occurs when a tumour in the lower part of the rectum becomes large enough to be mistaken for faeces. The persistent desire to empty the rectum is often accompanied by the passage of mucus, called 'slime' by the patient.

Small primary cancers may not cause symptoms but can metastasize to the liver. The patient then presents with upper abdominal pain and/or malaise, and has a palpably enlarged liver.

Pain is an uncommon symptom of carcinoma of the rectum, but three types can occur:

- *colic*, with distension, caused by high annular tumours obstructing the lumen of the bowel;
- *local pain* in the rectum, perineum or lower abdomen, caused by direct spread of the tumour to the surrounding structures, especially the sacral nerves;
- *pain on defaecation*, which occurs if the tumour has spread downwards below the mucocutaneous junction into the sensitive anal canal.

Previous history Always ask about any previous large bowel symptoms, particularly recurrent episodes of diarrhoea associated with the passage of mucus and blood. Long-standing inflammatory bowel disease increases the risk of malignant change in the colon and rectum after 10 or more years of the disease. The fact that the colitis has been quiescent for many years does not reduce the risk of malignancy. The symptoms of a cancer may be passed off as a recurrence of the colitis and lead to a late presentation.
Family history **Familial adenomatous polyposis** is a rare inherited condition in which the entire colon and rectum are carpeted with adenomatous polyps, one or more of which inevitably becomes malignant. Twenty-five per cent of cases arise as new mutations, so there is no family history. The family history may be denied out of fear of cancer.

Examination

Rectal examination When the tumour is low in the ampulla, the whole lesion is palpable. More commonly, however, only the lower edge of a malignant ulcer is palpable.

A carcinomatous ulcer feels hard, and the raised, rolled, everted edge bulges into the lumen of the rectum. The base is irregular and friable. Record the site of the tumour (anterior, posterior or lateral), and estimate its distance from the anal verge. Try to decide if the tumour is fixed or mobile.

Blood and mucus are commonly seen on the glove after the finger has been withdrawn.

When the cancer is in the upper part of the rectum, only its lower edge may be palpable. It may be difficult to determine whether a tumour is inside or outside the rectum on digital examination, but this can be easily elucidated by sigmoidoscopy, which should be carried out in all cases.

General examination **The liver is by far the most common site of distant metastase**s from rectal cancer and must always be palpated. Every patient should also have staging investigations (see *Investigation and Management*, Chapter 19).

Lymph from the rectum drains to the mesenteric and then to the preaortic lymph glands, which are rarely palpable.

Rare rectal tumours

These include carcinoid tumours, lymphomas and secondary malignant melanomas. The symptoms are similar to those of carcinoma.

Malignant pelvic tumours

Bladder carcinomas, carcinomas of gynaecological or prostatic origin and any intraperitoneal malignancy with spread to the pelvis may present with rectal symptoms of a change in bowel habit or bleeding. The extrarectal deposits can cause a stricture presenting as constipation, or the tumour mass can cause tenesmus.

Digital examination reveals a hard, craggy mass in the pelvis.

Adenomas of the rectum

Benign adenomas of the rectum may be solitary or multiple throughout the colon and rectum, and are sometimes of the familial variety. They are *villous* or *polypoid* in shape. In narrow parts of the bowel such as the sigmoid colon, peristalsis draws the adenomas down on a stalk. In the wider rectum, they are usually sessile.

Adenomas that are initially benign can develop dysplasia and undergo malignant change to invasive cancer. This is unusual if the adenoma is less than 3 cm in diameter, but eventually most true adenomas will turn into carcinomas.

The *villous adenoma* is a distinct clinical variety of rectal adenoma, more common in the elderly. There is a broad base with a frondular (lots of villi) surface that exudes large quantities of mucus. Growth is slow, and the onset of symptoms is often so gradual that presentation is late. Frail patients with large villous adenomas lose vast amounts of potassium with the mucus and can present with hypokalaemia. Malignant change in the base of the papilloma is common.

History

A large adenoma produces mucous discharge and diarrhoea with a variable degree of bleeding. A small adenoma may bleed or prolapse.

Examination

Adenomas are soft and sometimes difficult to feel on rectal examination, but are always visible on sigmoidoscopy as dark pink, frond-covered tumours.

Not all polyps in the rectum are true adenomas. *Hyperplastic polyps* are most common in the recto-sigmoid colon, and are usually less than 5 mm in diameter. On histology, these have long crypts with excess proliferation in the base. Biopsy confirms the diagnosis.

Pseudopolyps are islands of normal mucosa in patients with severe ulcerative colitis. The rolled-up edge of the mucosa appears 'polypoid'.

Rare *hamartomatous polyps* are found in children and can cause intussusception or rectal bleeding. They also occur in *Peutz–Jeghers syndrome* (see Chapter 15).

Solitary rectal ulcer

This is a rare condition of young adults, with a peak age of between 30 and 40 years, although all ages can be affected. It is linked to rectal prolapse in nearly two-thirds of those affected, and is thought to be caused by repeated episodes of intussusception, difficulty in defaecation and straining at stool. The majority of ulcers lie anteriorly about 10 cm from the anal verge.

Symptoms include rectal bleeding, the passage of mucus, anal discomfort and occasionally incontinence. There is almost always some difficulty in evacuation.

The mucosa is usually reddened and oedematous with ulceration in more than half the cases. In half the ulcers, the edge is raised and polypoid, and **it can be easily mistaken for a carcinoma.**

Diverticular disease

Diverticular disease is often an incidental finding in patients with other colorectal disease (see Chapter 15). It can, however, present with rectal bleeding, which can be acute, massive and fresh. The usually elderly patient feels a little faint, gets lower abdominal pain and then has a desire to defaecate. When they empty the rectum, they pass a large volume of fresh blood and clots.

This is a fairly common reason for emergency admission. Fortunately, most such bleeds stop spontaneously, but occasionally the patient may be shocked, and the bleeding can be life-threatening. The bleeding usually comes from an eroded artery in the mouth of a diverticulum, but in many patients the diverticular disease is incidental, and the bleeding is caused by *angiodysplasia* of the colonic mucosa. This can only be diagnosed by colonoscopy or angiography (see *Investigation and Management*, Chapter 18, pages 463–467).

CONDITIONS PRESENTING WITH ANAL PAIN (REVISION PANEL 16.2)

Perianal haematoma

(Thrombosed perianal varix)
The name of this condition is well established, even though it is not a true haematoma but a thrombosis of a vein in the subcutaneous plexus, probably caused by an injury to the vein wall during defaecation. It also occurs after childbirth, from stretching of the perineum.

The thrombus/haematoma causes an inflammatory reaction with pain and oedema.

History

Age and sex Perianal haematomas occur at all ages and are equally common in both sexes.
Symptoms The main symptoms are of **pain and a swelling at the anal margin**. The pain is of sudden onset and subsides gradually over a few days. It is a continuous discomfort, made worse by sitting, moving and defaecation, and is clearly localized to the lump.

The swelling is small and spherical, but may gradually enlarge and become more painful.

Bleeding occurs if the skin over the lump ulcerates.

Perianal haematomas may recur.

Examination

Position The lump (occasionally multiple) may be anywhere around the anal margin.
Colour The lump is deep blue–purple.
Tenderness The lump is tender.
Shape and size It is initially spherical, and up to 1 cm in diameter.
Surface It is a smooth lump covered by skin, which may be normal or oedematous.
Composition The lump feels rubbery or firm.
Relations It is directly under the perianal skin, and superficial to the external sphincter.

Revision panel 16.2

Possible diagnoses of anal conditions that present with pain

Pain alone
Fissure (pain after defaecation)
Proctalgia fugax (spontaneous pain at night)
Ano-rectal abscess

Pain and bleeding
Fissure
Crohn's disease

Pain and a lump
Perianal haematoma
Ano-rectal abscess

Pain, a lump and bleeding
Thrombosed prolapsed haemorrhoids
Carcinoma of the anal canal
Prolapsed rectal polyp or carcinoma
Prolapsed rectum

CHAPTER 16 | THE RECTUM AND ANAL CANAL

Fissure-in-ano

An anal fissure is a longitudinal split (ulcer) in the skin of the anal canal.

An acute tear is quite a common event in patients with constipation and usually heals quickly. Reopening of the tear when the patient next defaecates causes further pain, leading to an increase in anal sphincter tone that progresses to spasm. This makes the tear more likely to reopen at each subsequent episode of defaecation, and leads to a vicious circle of tearing–pain–spasm and more tearing. The base then becomes fibrous and does not heal. It effectively becomes a chronic ulcer of the anal verge.

History

Age and sex Most fissures develop in young males, and in females after childbirth. They are quite common in children, who often pass bulky stools very quickly.

Symptoms Both acute and chronic fissures are **very painful**. The pain begins during defaecation and is often described as a tearing sensation. With a chronic fissure, pain persists for hours and can be so severe that the patient becomes afraid to defaecate. This results in large, hard, masses of faeces, which make the pain worse when the next defaecation occurs. It also becomes more difficult to pass a stool, because of the spasm.

Fissures streak the stool with blood and stain the toilet paper. When parents notice rectal bleeding in children, it always causes great alarm. The child rarely complains of the pain, unless questioned directly.

Persistence There may be periods of remission, and eventually the condition either heals or becomes chronic.

Examination

Position The majority of fissures, especially in males, are in the midline posteriorly, but some, particularly in females, are anterior. A few are lateral, and both anterior and posterior fissures can coexist.

The diagnosis is made by gently parting the skin of the anus and looking for a split in the anal skin. This may be all that is possible, because further examination is prevented by pain. A small skin tag, often called incorrectly a *sentinel pile*, may be visible at the lower end of the fissure.

Tenderness The anal sphincter is usually in spasm and exquisitely tender. A careful rectal examination is possible in a few patients, but is mainly of value in excluding alternative pathology.

Sigmoidoscopy and proctoscopy **Never attempt either of these examinations in a conscious patient with a fissure** – they would be much too painful. Proctoscopy under general anaesthesia displays the raw base of the fissure.

Ano-rectal abscess

There are two distinct varieties of ano-rectal abscess:

- In a *perianal abscess*, the swelling is clearly at the anal margin, which it distorts.
- An *ischio-rectal abscess* lies lateral to the anus, occupies a much larger space and can track round behind the anus to the opposite side.

The infection that causes both types of abscess probably begins in an anal gland. From here, the pus either tracks down to the perineum between the sphincters to form a perianal abscess, or penetrates the external sphincter to reach the ischio-rectal fossa. The anal gland is usually destroyed if the abscess is drained externally or bursts quickly, but if it continues to secrete, a fistula will develop. This can then be associated with further episodes of infection.

Abscesses can also form in the intersphincteric space and in the submucosa of the anus. Abscesses in these positions can led to severe pain with very few external signs.

History

Age Ano-rectal abscess is most common in patients between 20 and 50 years old, but occurs at all ages, rarely in childhood.

Sex It is more common in males.

Symptoms **There is a gradual (often over several days) onset of severe, throbbing pain, which makes sitting, moving and defaecation painful.**

A tender swelling close to the anus will become apparent to the patient, who may have had previous episodes of infection. If left untreated, the abscess will eventually point and burst.

Systemic effects A patient with an ischio-rectal abscess is more likely to be systemically unwell with the general symptoms of an abscess – malaise, loss of appetite, sweating and even rigors. Pain and tenderness tend to be greater with a perianal abscess, as the space in which it can expand is confined.

Examination

General examination The patient tries not to move, and lies on their side. There is likely to be tachycardia, pyrexia, sweating, a dry, furred tongue and fetor oris.

Position **A tender red mass** is usually obvious lateral to the anus in the soft tissues between the anus and the ischial tuberosity, although this is less obvious with an ischio-rectal abscess. A perianal abscess may develop anywhere around the anal margin. The distinction between the physical signs of the two types of is often blurred.

Tenderness The whole area is usually exquisitely tender.

Colour and temperature The overlying skin eventually becomes hot and red.

Shape, size and composition The surface of the abscess is often indistinct, and its size may be difficult to assess. Tenderness makes testing for fluctuation impossible.

Rectal examination This is best deferred until the patient is anaesthetized prior to drainage. The abscess can then be felt to bulge into the side of the lower part of the rectum. Fluctuation and the size of the abscess can then be determined.

Lymph drainage The inguinal lymph glands are sometimes enlarged and tender.

Local tissues There may be scarring from previous abscesses and fistulas. Cellulitis and, very occasionally, necrotizing fasciitis may occur.

Pelvic sepsis

Infection in the abdominal cavity (see Chapter 15) can result in pus collecting in the pelvis, its most dependent part, particularly after acute appendicitis, salpingitis (pelvic inflammatory disease) and diverticulitis. It can also occur after operations, especially after anastomotic dehiscence.

Patients complain of **pelvic discomfort, diarrhoea and tenesmus**. There are general signs of sepsis such as fever, malaise, lassitude, sweats, rigors and pyrexia.

Digital rectal examination may demonstrate a tender, hot boggy swelling high in the pelvis.

Fistula-in-ano

A fistula is a pathological track, lined with epithelium or granulation tissue, that connects two epithelial surfaces. A fistula-in-ano connects the lumen of the rectum or anal canal with the external perianal skin. It is caused by an abscess developing in an anal crypt gland in the intersphincteric space that bursts in two directions – internally into the anal canal, and externally through the skin. Mucus is forced through the fistulous tract as stool is expelled, and this is the mechanism that stops a fistula from ever healing.

Fistulae-in-ano may also be associated with Crohn's disease or ulcerative colitis. Rarely, a fistula can be caused by direct infiltration and necrosis of a low rectal carcinoma.

Classification

A fistula-in-ano can run through a variety of anatomical planes, illustrated in Fig. 16.9. The important distinction is between low and high fistulas, as the subsequent surgical management is completely different.

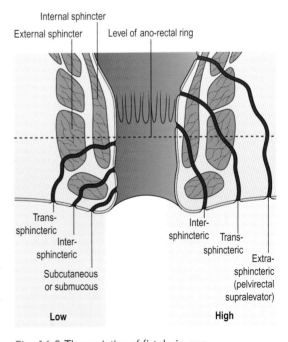

Fig. 16.9 The varieties of fistula-in-ano.

A *low fistula-in-ano* has its internal opening below the ano-rectal ring. This is the point where the puborectalis muscle sling fuses with the external sphincter, and is the major muscle involved in maintaining continence. It is more likely that a fistula at this level can be laid open without significant impairment of continence, although there will virtually always be some change in control if enquiry afterwards is careful enough. Particular caution should be employed in females with anterior fistulas as the sphincter is smaller anteriorly.

A *high fistula-in-ano* joins the rectum above the ano-rectal ring. Laying this open would divide the ring and render the patient incontinent.

History

Age A fistula-in-ano can occur at any time during adult life, and rarely in children.

Symptoms There may be a history of a perianal abscess that has spontaneously burst or has been drained surgically. Some patients with a fistula have never had an abscess but notice a small tender lump in the perineum that discharges pus.

The most common symptom is a watery or purulent discharge from the external opening of the fistula. There may be recurrent episodes of pain if pus collects in the fistulous track. The fistula may appear to heal, but then becomes painful and discharges again, with relief of the discomfort.

The discharge, which can on occasion be bloodstained, may cause pruritus ani.

Other symptoms (direct questions) Up to 70 per cent of patients with rectal Crohn's disease develop a fistula, and it is important to enquire about any bowel or abdominal symptoms or systemic upset.

Examination

Position The external opening(s) of the fistula is usually visible as a puckered scar or a small tuft of granulation tissue anywhere around the anus (Fig. 16.10), usually close to the anal verge, although it is sometimes several centimetres away.

Goodsall's rule states that the internal opening of an anterior fistula lies along a radial line drawn from the external opening to the anus, but the internal opening of a posterior fistula always lies in the midline posteriorly. Although things are rarely certain in medicine, this rule is reliable.

Fig. 16.10 An anterior low-level fistula, obeying Goodsall's rule.

There may be more than one opening, particularly if the patient has Crohn's disease.

Tenderness The external opening of the fistula is not usually painful, but the tissues around it may be thickened and tender.

Discharge The discharge, usually purulent, may be visible on the skin or the underclothes.

Rectal examination The internal opening of the fistula can sometimes be felt as an area of induration or a small nodule beneath the mucosa. If you can feel it, try to decide if the internal opening of the fistula is below or above the ano-rectal junction, i.e. at the low level or high level.

The indurated track of the fistula between the internal and external openings is sometimes palpable beneath the perianal skin but is easier to define under anaesthesia. The track may be palpable between a gloved index finger in the rectum and the thumb of the same hand. Look for coexistent pathology, such as a carcinoma.

Sigmoidoscopy and proctoscopy These are essential to exclude Crohn's disease, ulcerative colitis, a carcinoma of the anus and even tuberculosis. Disappointingly, the internal opening of the fistula is rarely visible.

Local lymph glands The inguinal lymph glands are not enlarged.

Local tissues These are indurated and 'violacious' if the patient has Crohn's disease.

General examination Many of the diseases mentioned above have associated abdominal and general clinical signs, so never confine your examination to the patient's perineum. Examine the abdomen carefully.

Perianal Crohn's disease

Perianal disease can occur in isolation, but many patients are already known to have Crohn's disease elsewhere in the intestine, especially the colon. Bleeding, discharge, pain and faecal leakage can all occur, and fistulas and fissures are also common.

The appearances are protean, with abscesses, complex fistulas and indolent fissures predominating in an indurated perianal region that looks inflamed and 'sore'.

Pilonidal sinus

The word *pilonidal* means a nest of hairs. A pilonidal sinus usually, but not always, contains hair. They are found commonly in the midline skin of the natal cleft, between the coccyx and the anus. They sometimes develop between the fingers of hairdressers, and occasionally at the umbilicus.

A pilonidal sinus is lined by granulation tissue, not skin, and hair does not grow within it. The hairs in the sinus have often come from the scalp. The midline skin in the natal cleft is tethered, and during walking the motion of the buttocks rubbing together causes shed hairs that are covered in small barbs to be driven into a pre-existing dimple, or to pierce normal skin. When an infection develops, the hairs act as foreign bodies, preventing clearance of infection. The end result is a chronic abscess that periodically flares up into an acute abscess.

History

Age Pilonidal sinus is rare before puberty and over the age of 40 years.

Sex This condition is far more common in males than in females, and most often develops in dark-haired, hirsute males.

Symptoms The common symptoms are **pain and a swelling in the natal cleft**, often associated with a purulent discharge if the sinus becomes infected. Local discomfort sometimes leads the patient to discover the openings. The pain varies between a dull ache and an acute throbbing pain. An abscess may be the first event. A patient with a pilonidal abscess finds some relief from the throbbing pain by lying prone, in contrast to patients with ano-rectal abscesses who usually prefer to lie on their side.

Chronic discharge indicates chronic low-grade infection, but between acute exacerbations patients often think the sinus has disappeared.

Examination (Fig. 16.11)

Position Pilonidal sinuses arise in the midline of the natal cleft between the coccyx and the anus. They are usually closer to the tip of the coccyx than the anus.

(a) The patient is lying on his right side with his buttocks held apart to expose the bottom of the natal cleft. The sinus, which is difficult to see, is the small, pale, central pit. The stiff black hair that commonly covers the buttocks of these patients has been shaved off.

(b) The hairs that were removed from the sinus shown in (a).

Fig. 16.11 PILONIDAL SINUS

Temperature and tenderness The skin over a pilonidal abscess is red and tender.

The sinus **The sinus openings are usually easy to see as small midline pits** with epithelialized edges. Protruding hairs are rarely seen, but **pouting granulation tissue and purulent discharge are common**. Pressure may produce a small quantity of serous discharge. When the sinus becomes infected, it is indistinguishable from any other type of subcutaneous abscess.

There is palpable subcutaneous induration, corresponding to the extent of the granulation tissue beneath the skin. There may be scars well away from the midline, where previous abscesses have discharged or been incised.

Lymph drainage The inguinal lymph glands are not enlarged.

Local tissues The local tissues are normal.

Proctalgia fugax

This condition is thought to be caused by a spontaneous spasm (cramp) in the muscles of the pelvic floor, or possibly by a spasm at the recto-sigmoid junction. It is often associated with the irritable bowel syndrome.

It presents with sudden, severe, cramp-like rectal pain experienced within the rectum or pelvis rather than the anal canal, which comes on suddenly, often at night. It is of short duration, sometimes lasting just a few seconds and rarely longer than 5 minutes. Nothing relieves the pain, but it passes off spontaneously. There may be associated symptoms of a functional bowel disorder (see Chapter 15).

General and rectal examination are normal. The patient may experience the same pain on sigmoidoscopy as air is insufflated at the recto-sigmoid junction.

CONDITIONS PRESENTING AS AN ANAL LUMP WITH OR WITHOUT PAIN

The following conditions are not necessarily 'painless', but the lump is the dominant symptom (Revision panel 16.3).

Revision panel 16.3
Possible diagnoses of anal conditions that present with a lump

A lump and no other symptoms
Anal warts
Skin tags

A lump and pain
Perianal haematoma

A lump, pain and bleeding
Prolapsed haemorrhoids
Carcinoma of anal canal
Prolapsed rectal polyp or carcinoma
Prolapsed rectum

Prolapsed thrombosed strangulated haemorrhoids

These are very painful and tender (see above).

Two or three tense, tender, red–purple mucosa-covered swellings protrude from the anal canal at the 3, 7 and 11 o'clock positions, often associated with oedematous skin tags (see Fig. 16.8). They may eventually become so ulcerated and infected that they resemble a prolapsing carcinoma.

Anal skin tags

Tags of skin, of varying size and shape, are commonly found in the perianal area. They represent an exaggeration of the normal wrinkling of the lax anal skin, which stretches during defaecation (Fig. 16.12). They are usually symptomless, but may rub, catch or itch. A fastidious patient may complain that skin tags prevent proper cleaning of the perianal area.

Skin tags in the 3, 7, and 11 o'clock positions are normally part of a pile mass, but quite large skin tags can occur without piles and, of course, quite large piles can be present without skin tags.

A tag may develop at the lower end of an anal fissure, called a *sentinel tag* (see above).

Anal skin tags may become polypoid in shape, and are called fibroepithelial anal polyps. They must not be confused with adenomatous polyps (Fig. 16.13).

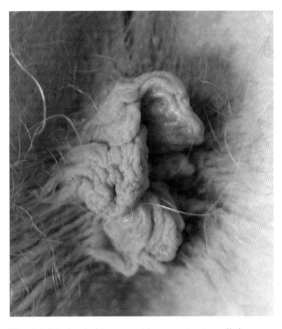

Fig. 16.12 Anal skin tags. Many patients call these tags 'piles', but they are not haemorrhoids.

(a)

Fig. 16.13 An anal polyp. This is clearly fibrous and quite different from an adenomatous polyp, in both level and appearance.

(b)

Fig. 16.14 TWO EXAMPLES OF MULTIPLE PERIANAL WARTS

Anal warts

(Condylomata acuminata)

These are multiple, pedunculated, papilliferous skin excrescences that resemble warts elsewhere in the body (Fig. 16.14). They may spread over the whole perineum and are caused by the human papilloma virus (subtypes 6 and 11), which is carried by 20 per cent of the population and is transmitted by sexual contact. They are therefore often associated with other sexually transmitted diseases. They also develop in patients whose immune response has been depressed with steroids or cancer chemotherapy, and in acquired immunodeficiency syndrome.

Condylomata lata are a nowadays rarely seen manifestation of secondary syphilis. They are broad-based, flat-topped papules that are highly contagious.

All condylomas cause irritation, discomfort and pain from rubbing, and may ulcerate, bleed and become infected. Intra-anal warts can only be seen on proctoscopy.

Squamous cell carcinoma of the anus

This is a carcinoma of the anal or perianal skin, and is identical to the squamous cell carcinoma found elsewhere in the body. It may follow precancerous changes in the local skin known as anal intraepithelial neoplasia. Human papilloma virus (subtypes 16 and 18) can cause dysplasia of the anal skin and eventually lead to anal cancer. This occurs more frequently in men who have sex with men, and suspicious lesions should be biopsied.

The presenting symptoms depend on how close the cancer is to the anal verge. If it is in the anal canal, it presents with **pain on defaecation and bleeding, or the patient notices a lump** (Fig. 16.15). A squamous cell carcinoma does not exude mucus.

On examination, the tumour often has the appearance of a skin cancer. It can be an ulcer with a raised everted edge, or a plaque, and occasionally it can be circumferential and stenosing.

The lesion is likely to be an anal squamous carcinoma if there are enlarged inguinal glands, as a rectal adenocarcinoma spreads to the abdominal lymph glands.

Fig. 16.15 A carcinoma of the anal canal that has spread into the skin of the perineum. The patient was still able to defaecate. The patient is in the lithotomy position.

PROLAPSE OF THE RECTUM

This is an eversion of the lower part of the rectum through the anal canal. There are two varieties.

Full-thickness prolapse

With a full-thickness prolapse, the entire rectal wall, muscle and mucosa become displaced through the anus. This occurs when the structures in the floor of the pelvis that normally hold the rectum in the curve of the sacrum become weak and lax. Chronic constipation and prolonged straining at stool are other aetiological factors. It is always associated with impaired continence because of weakness and stretching of the anal sphincter. Continence problems precede the prolapse, often for many years.

History

Age Prolapse of the rectum is primarily a disease of the elderly, although it does occur in infants and children.

Sex It is 20 times more common in females than males. Normal anal sphincters are thin anteriorly behind the vagina, and the anal canal may be stretched and damaged during childbirth.

Symptoms The patient complains of a **large lump that appears at the anus after defaecation**, or sometimes spontaneously when standing, walking or coughing. **The lump can usually be pushed back into the rectum** or may reduce spontaneously when the patient lies down.

A prolapsed rectum is uncomfortable, and causes a persistent desire to defaecate. The prolapsed rectal mucosa secretes mucus and, if it remains prolapsed, ulcerates and bleeds.

Examination

Colour and shape The prolapsed rectum, which may be up to 20 cm in length, forms **a long tubular mass protruding symmetrically through the anus**. The bowel is not tender and can be handled without causing the patient discomfort. The exposed mucosa is red and thrown into circumferential concentric folds around a central orifice, which is the lumen of the rectum (Fig. 16.16).

Note **Sometimes you need to ask the patient to strain down to produce the prolapse, and the diagnosis may be missed if this manoeuvre is omitted.**

Fig. 16.16 A rectal prolapse.

Reducibility It is usually possible to reduce a prolapse with gentle compression and cephalad pressure.
Local tissues The anal sphincter is very lax when it is contracted on the examining finger.

Partial-thickness or mucosal prolapse

The history is very similar to that of prolapsing piles, and the two conditions do overlap. However, instead of there being purplish anal cushions, pink folds of anal mucosa are seen, with a less circular appearance than a full-thickness prolapse. A mucosal prolapse may not reach the anal verge.

On examination, a soft painless mass is visible and palpable at the anal margin; this consists of two thin mucosal layers. A mucous discharge is often the main symptom, and the redundant mucosa is visible on proctoscopy.

Mucosal rectal prolapse in children

In children, the mucosa of the bowel is more loosely attached to the muscle layer than in adults. In addition, there is often hypertrophy of the submucosal lymphoid aggregates known as *Peyer's patches*. This may result in prolapse of the anal mucosa.

History

Age The condition usually presents at potty training, but occurs up to puberty.
Symptoms The parents notice a smooth, soft swelling coming out of the anal margin after defaecation. The child may complain of discomfort, and older children may become frightened. Mucous discharge is common, but bleeding is rare. The frightened child may try to avoid defaecation, and the rectum then becomes impacted with hard faeces.

Examination The swelling is rarely reproducible in the clinic, and the diagnosis must be made on the history. The only differential diagnosis is the very rare juvenile polyp, which usually presents with bleeding. *Note* The condition often cures itself over time (see *Investigation and Management*, Chapter 19).

CONDITIONS PRESENTING WITH PRURITUS ANI

This is a symptom rather than a condition. Many people experience an idiopathic perianal itch, worse overnight. It is, however, important to seek a cause (Revision panel 16.4).

Associated prolapse or bleeding suggest the presence of haemorrhoids, one of the most common

---

Revision panel 16.4

The causes of pruritus ani

Mucous discharge from the anus caused by:

Haemorrhoids

Polyps

Skin tags

Condylomas

Fissure

Fistula

Carcinoma of the anus

Vaginal discharge caused by:

Trichomonas vaginitis

Monilia vaginitis

Cervicitis

Gonorrhoea

Skin diseases

Tinea cruris

Fungal infections, especially monilial infections in diabetes

Parasites

Threadworms

Faecal soiling

Poor hygiene

Incontinence

Diarrhoea

Psychoneuroses

---

causes of pruritis. Other intra-anal conditions that cause the leakage of small amounts of liquid faeces or mucus cause itching. Contact with the perianal skin produces maceration and excoriation, which leads to 'scratching'. A vaginal discharge may be responsible, for example from *Trichomonas* or *Monilia* infection.

A few patients have a sensitivity to washing powder or other allergens, and some have a high intake of coffee or fizzy drinks.

On examination, there may be evidence of perianal redness and excoriation (Fig. 16.17), as well as the presence of piles or the opening of a fistula. A primary skin disorders may be responsible, and plaques of psoriasis may be visible. Fungal infection usually has a very distinctive edge, and microscopy of skin scrapings can be diagnostic.

In children, threadworms are a common cause of itching, and may be visible or detected on a stool swab. Generalized causes of itching such as obstructive jaundice should not be forgotten.

Fig. 16.17 Severe pruritis caused by the leakage of mucus from large second-degree haemorrhoids. There is a small skin tag.

CONDITIONS PRESENTING WITH FAECAL INCONTINENCE

This is defined as an involuntary loss of control of flatus, fluid motions or solid faeces.

Normal continence depends on maintenance of the anorectal angle at rest by the puborectalis muscle, and closure of the anal canal by the internal and external sphincters. The presence of functioning sensory receptors in the anal canal is also important.

The problem is particularly common in older females who have had children, as is prolapse.

Causes of faecal incontinence are:

- diarrhoea – infective or inflammatory;
- reduced rectal compliance caused by inflammation, tumour or surgery, for example low anterior resection or severe irritable bowel syndrome;
- neurological – multiple sclerosis, dementia, spinal trauma, pudendal neuropathy;
- damage to the anal sphincter from childbirth, anal surgery or other trauma;
- fistula to the vagina from small bowel (entero-vaginal), colon (colo-vaginal) or rectum (recto-vaginal);
- connective tissue disease, which causes fibrosis and thinning of the internal anal sphincter;
- autonomic neuropathy, for example associated with diabetes, which causes weakness of the internal sphincter.

Many patients have more than one of the above factors impacting on their continence.

Some patients have uncontrollable passage of an entire bowel action, often associated with severe urgency of defaecation. This is usually the result of an inability to contract the external sphincter. Others report a more constant leakage of smaller quantities of liquid or solid stool of which they are unaware. This is the result of a defective action of the autonomically innervated internal sphincter. Some patients have a combination of both problems.

Patients with loose stools may be incontinent despite a normal sphincter mechanism. Incontinence can occur in patients with inflamed or irritable bowels, when excessive peristalsis overcomes the anal sphincter in a very 'sensitive' rectum.

When taking the patient's past medical history, ask specifically about surgery on the anus, pelvic radiotherapy and local or spinal trauma. A detailed obstetric history should also be documented.

Inspection may demonstrate an excoriated perineum because of the leakage of loose stool.

When there is a large defect in the anal sphincter from an obstetric injury, the pelvic floor usually appears very attenuated. The perineum may appear flat, with the anal verge at the same level as the buttocks. This becomes even more pronounced if the patient is asked to 'bear down', which may reveal a prolapse. The anal canal often gapes.

There may be evidence of the opening of a fistula, or of bowel content leaking from the vagina.

The sphincter pressure may be found to be reduced if the patient is asked to 'squeeze' the examining finger. This requires experience to assess.

Hirschsprung's disease

This inherited condition affects one in 5000 infants. There is an absence of ganglia in Auerbach's plexus in the colonic wall. This produces an abnormal segment of variable length in the large bowel, and results in a functional obstruction.

It is four times more common in males than females, and usually presents in childhood. There is an adult form of the disease, presenting with chronic constipation.

In this condition, neonates fail to pass meconium in the first 24–48 hours of life, and the abdomen becomes distended. The infants develop feeding difficulties, and eventually vomit if left untreated. Older children develop chronic constipation and fail to thrive.

The abdomen is usually markedly distended, and a mucus plug is often present on rectal examination.

The dislodgement of this plug is often followed by a dramatic decompression of the abdomen. Older children usually have a chronically distended abdomen with an empty rectum.

Ano-rectal anomalies

(Imperforate anus)

These occur in approximately 1 in 5000 live births, and the cause is unknown. They can be classified as either 'low' or 'high' defects, with or without an associated fistula to the genitourinary tract. They vary from simple to complex, with the simplest being an anterior anal displacement or the presence of an anal membrane. The most complex include a persistent cloaca in a female, or in either sex a very high rectal agenesis with defective anal innervation.

Neonates present with a failure to pass meconium; this may leak from the vagina or be present in the urine if a fistula is present.

An absent or 'covered' anus should be obvious on careful inspection of the perineum at the routine postnatal examination. The fistula may be visible. Other malformations commonly coexist.

CHAPTER 16 | THE RECTUM AND ANAL CANAL

The kidneys, urinary tract and prostate

SYMPTOMS OF RENAL AND URINARY TRACT DISEASE

It is very important to obtain an exact history of the symptoms of renal and urinary tract disease because the kidney, ureter and bladder are not readily accessible for physical examination.

Renal pain

Site Pain from the kidney is typically felt in the:

- loin – the space below the 12th rib and the iliac crest;
- renal angle – the angle between the 12th rib and the edge of the erector spinae muscle (Fig. 17.1).

When asked to show you the site of renal pain, the patient usually spreads a hand around his waist with fingers covering the renal angle and thumb above the anterior superior iliac spine.

Nature **Renal pain can be a continuous dull ache or be sharp and very severe. Do not use the term 'renal colic'.** True colic is autonomically modulated and can only come from distension of the smooth muscle wall of a conducting tube such as the ureter. Because the intensity of renal pain often fluctuates rapidly, it gets called renal colic, but patients rarely describe it as spasmodic, and it does not usually disappear completely between exacerbations.

Ureteric colic

Site Pain from the ureter is felt along the line of the ureter (Fig. 17.2). The point where it begins is a reliable indicator of the level of the obstruction.

Fig. 17.1 The renal angle is the area in the loin between the 12th rib and the edge of the erector spinae muscle.

Fig. 17.2 Ureteric colic radiates down from the renal angle, along a line parallel to the inguinal ligament, and into the base of the penis, the scrotum or the labium majus.

In most cases, the pain starts in the loin and then radiates downwards, around the waist, obliquely across the abdomen just above the inguinal ligament, and to the base of the penis, the testes or the labia.

Severity Ureteric colic is severe. The patient tries to relieve the pain by rolling around the bed or walking about. Patients often say it is the worst pain they have ever experienced, and females may say it is as bad as labour pains. It is accompanied by sweating, and often by nausea and vomiting.

Nature It is a true colic, griping in nature and coming in waves, with pain-free periods between attacks.

Haematuria (Revision panel 17.1)

Blood may be noticed during or after micturition. Modest bleeding may not affect the colour of the urine, or may make it look darker than usual. With heavy bleeding, the urine may be bright red. Old blood or clot in the bladder is usually very dark.

If the blood is coming from the bladder neck or the lower part of the urinary tract, it may appear only at the end of micturition.

Make sure that female patients have not mistaken menstrual bleeding for haematuria, and remember that there are other rare causes of a red/brown discolouration of the urine, such as:

Revision panel 17.1

The causes of haematuria

Kidney
Congenital
Polycystic kidney
Traumatic
Blunt or penetrating injury
Stone
Inflammatory:
  Pyelonephritis
  Tuberculosis
Neoplastic:
  Carcinoma of the kidney
  Carcinoma of the renal pelvis
  Angiomyolipoma
Blood disorders:
  Anticoagulant drugs
  Purpura
  Sickle-cell disease
  Haemophilia
  Scurvy
  Malaria
Congestion:
  Right heart failure
  Renal vein thrombosis
Infarction:
  Arterial emboli from:
    Myocardial infarct
    Subacute bacterial endocarditis

Ureter
Stone
Neoplasm
Trauma (often iatrogenic)

Bladder
Stone
Blunt or penetrating trauma
Iatrogenic (after endoscopic surgery)
Inflammatory:
  Bacterial cystitis
  Non-specific cystitis or ulceration
  Tuberculosis
  Schistosomiasis (bilharzia)
Neoplastic:
  Carcinoma
  After radiotherapy to pelvis or bladder

Prostate
Benign and malignant enlargement
Acute prostatitis
Post transurethral resection

Urethra
Traumatic:
  Rupture
  Stone
  Foreign body
Inflammatory:
  Acute urethritis
Neoplastic:
  Squamous cell carcinoma

- eating large amounts of beetroot;
- paroxysmal haemoglobinuria;
- porphyria;
- medications (e.g. rifampicin).

Vesical pain

This is usually a dull, suprapubic ache, made worse by micturition.

Strangury (literally, squeezing urine) is a term used by some to describe a painful desire to micturate, which starts in the bladder and radiates into the urethra. Others use it to describe pain felt at the end of micturition as the patient squeezes out the last few drops of urine. To avoid confusion, do not use it at all.

Frequency of micturition

Increased frequency of micturition may be caused by a reduction in functioning bladder capacity following incomplete emptying, or by irritation of the bladder mucosa. It is of greater significance if it wakes the patient from sleep, so remember to ask about frequency by day and night.

Dysuria should be used to describe pain (often burning or stinging) that originates from the urethra during urination. Do not confuse it with, for example, the abdominal pain experienced on micturition by a patient with appendicitis, which has a totally different cause.

Prostatic pain

Pain from the prostate gland is felt deep inside the pelvis, between the legs, in the perineum and sometimes in the lower back. It is poorly localized, and patients may think it is coming from the rectum or the penile tip.

DISEASES OF THE URINARY TRACT

Congenital anomalies of the renal tract

There are a large number of congenital anomalies of the urinary tract, many of which are asymptomatic and insignificant. Only some of the more common ones are considered here.

Horseshoe kidney

The incidence of horseshoe kidney is 1 in 400, males being affected twice as often as females.

The kidneys are joined at their lower poles by an isthmus, which is under the inferior mesenteric artery. This prevents them rising to the normal position, and pulls the pelves and ureters to face anteriorly, with the ureters passing in front of the isthmus.

The condition is associated with Turner's syndrome, trisomy 18 and other genitourinary abnormalities.

Although impalpable, horseshoe kidneys are at increased risk of injury from abdominal trauma due to their reduced mobility. They are usually asymptomatic, but there is an increased risk of renal calculi, pelvi-ureteric junction (PUJ) obstruction and infection because of impaired drainage of the collecting systems.

Pelvic kidney

The incidence of pelvic kidney is 1 in 2000.

One kidney (usually the left) fails to ascend normally and remains in the pelvis. There may be contralateral renal agenesis or other anomalies. The condition is very rarely bilateral. The ectopic kidney is usually malrotated, with an anteriorly facing renal pelvis and a short ureter, although the ureteric orifice in the bladder is normal. Most cases are asymptomatic, but, as with horseshoe kidneys, the impaired drainage can cause problems.

Malrotation may occur in normally placed kidneys, when the renal shape may also be abnormal. Again, the complications of impaired drainage may occur.

Duplex kidney/ureter

The incidence of duplex kidney is 1 in 125, with females being affected twice as often as males. The condition is usually unilateral.

There are two separate renal collecting systems draining into two ureters, which may join at the level of the kidney (a bifid collecting system) or at some point in their descent (partial duplication), or may remain separate all the way to the bladder, giving two ureteric orifices (full duplication).

The presentation can be with flank pain, loin mass and urinary infection, but most are asymptomatic.

CHAPTER 17 | THE KIDNEYS, URINARY TRACT AND PROSTATE

In a complete duplex, the upper pole ureter enters the bladder below and medial to the lower-pole ureter, giving it a longer intramural course. The lower-pole ureter is shorter and enters the bladder more directly. The upper pole of the kidney is thus prone to obstruction, and the lower to reflux.

Cross-fused renal ectopia

The incidence is 1 in 1000 births, males being affected twice as often as females.

The kidneys are fused and located on the same side. Complications include infection and obstruction causing hydronephrosis and calculi.

Hydronephrosis

Hydronephrosis is distension of the calyces and pelvis of the kidney (Revision panel 17.2).

Hydronephrosis is often symptomless, but it may produce renal pain, may present as renal failure or may be detected when investigating the symptoms of the disease causing it.

History

Age Hydronephrosis occurs at all ages.

Symptoms The most common symptom is pain in the loin. This is a dull, persistent ache that can be so mild that it is accepted by the patient as backache and ignored, but which gets worse as the hydronephrosis enlarges. If a sudden enlargement occurs, the pain can be severe. As it is autonomic pain, it is poorly localized and occasionally felt in unexpected sites such as the epigastrium. A patient with this sort of pain will never be able to localize the exact site with a finger, but will place their hand over quite a wide area.

The pain associated with hydronephrosis may be initiated or exacerbated by an increased urine flow. Alcohol and caffeinated drinks are diuretics and may exacerbate the pain.

Pain is less frequent in bilateral hydronephrosis as the cause usually lies in the lower urinary tract, and distension of the renal pelvis tends to develop slowly.

Congenital PUJ obstruction is often intermittent and associated with more severe pain.

Only a very large hydronephrosis will cause abdominal distension.

Revision panel 17.2

The causes of hydronephrosis

Unilateral hydronephrosis

Pelvi-ureteric obstruction:

> Congenital PUJ stenosis
> Pressure from aberrant vessels crossing the PUJ
> Stones and tumours in the renal pelvis, occluding the opening into the ureter

Ureteric obstruction:

> Stones
> Tumour compressing or infiltrating the ureter from the cervix, rectum, colon or prostate
> Tumours of the ureter
> Ureterocele
> Schistosomiasis
> Bladder tumour

Reflux

Bilateral hydronephrosis

Bladder outflow obstruction:

> Benign prostatic enlargement
> Urethral strictures and valves
> Phimosis (causing chronic retention)

Malignant invasion of the bladder trigone:

> Carcinoma of the bladder
> Carcinoma of the prostate

External compression from malignant pelvic lymphadenopathy

Retroperitoneal fibrosis

Schistosomiasis

There are usually no general symptoms unless the back pressure damages both kidneys so severely that renal failure and uraemia result.

Examination

The kidney is well hidden in the back wall of the abdomen (retroperitoneum), and only a large hydronephrosis will be palpable. However, the kidney may be tender, especially if there is coexisting infection. The features of a palpable kidney are described in detail in Chapter 15.

An enlarged palpable hydronephrosis should:

- arise from the loin;
- be reducible into the loin;
- be palpable bimanually;
- be ballotable.

Acute pyelonephritis

Acute pyelonephritis (pyelitis) is an infection in the upper part of the urinary tract caused by bacteria that have come from the bloodstream or up the ureter from the urethra or bladder. It is more common in females because the shorter length of their urethra makes the entry of bacteria into the lower urinary tract more likely.

History

Sex Pyelonephritis is much more common in females than in males.

Age It occurs in children, in females soon after the initiation of sexual activity (honeymoon cystitis) and during pregnancy.

Symptoms The patient complains of a sudden onset of severe pain in one or both loins. It may occasionally be felt anteriorly, and on the right-hand side can be mistaken for biliary pain.

Either simultaneously with or before the onset of the loin pain, micturition becomes frequent and painful. Although there may be a vague suprapubic ache, the main pain during micturition is felt as a burning sensation along the length of the urethra. The patient may also complain of a painful desire to micturate, with only small volumes of urine produced.

Headache, malaise, nausea and vomiting often begin a few hours before the loin pain.

The urine may become cloudy and even bloodstained. The patient feels ill, hot and sweaty and may, in severe cases, suffer rigors and be clinically septic.

Cause The patient may have had similar attacks and be aware of their relationship to sexual intercourse or pregnancy.

Examination

General features The patient looks ill and may be flushed and sweating with fever and tachycardia. The tongue is dry and furred.

Abdomen One or both kidneys are moderately tender when palpated through the abdomen, and the renal angle is very tender. Guarding and peritonism will not be found. There may be mild suprapubic tenderness.

The kidneys are not clinically enlarged unless the infection has arisen in a previously hydronephrotic kidney.

Urine The urine may look cloudy and bloodstained. Red blood cells and pus cells will be seen on microscopy.

Genitourinary tuberculosis

Tuberculosis of the urinary tract is a rare condition in the Western world, although it has been becoming less so in recent years. It produces fibrosis, scarring, calcification and strictures. Presentation is often late, when chronic damage has already been done.

History

Age It can occur at any age, but is most common in the fourth decade.

Sex It is twice as common in males.

Travel The patient may have travelled to areas where tuberculosis is endemic, but infection can occur from exposure to infected individuals anywhere.

General Patients may complain of weight loss, night sweats or chronic chest symptoms.

Urological symptoms Tuberculosis can affect anywhere in the urogenital tract, so the range of symptoms is wide. There may be loin pain (from ureteric obstruction), haematuria or lower urinary tract symptoms (from bladder inflammation, fibrosis and scarring).

A history of chronic recurrent urinary tract infection, usually with negative bacterial cultures, should raise a suspicion of tuberculosis.

The symptoms of genitourinary tuberculosis are non-specific. Therefore, the condition should be borne in mind in any patient with recurrent unexplained urological symptoms or failure to respond to treatment.

Examination

General There will rarely be any physical signs, but there may be evidence of weight loss. The prostate should be examined as prostatic tuberculosis may mimic malignancy, with a firm or hard prostate on palpation.

External genitalia Tuberculous epididymitis is described in Chapter 18.

CHAPTER 17 | THE KIDNEYS, URINARY TRACT AND PROSTATE

Carcinoma of the kidney

Correctly called a renal cell carcinoma, and usually of clear cell, papillary or chromophobe subtypes, this tumour was previously called a hypernephroma because of its macroscopic appearance and site of occurrence. It can present in a huge variety of ways due to local, metastatic, general and paraneoplastic effects.

History

Age Carcinoma of the kidney is uncommon below the age of 50 years.

Sex It is twice as common in males as it is in females.

Symptoms

- **Haematuria.** This is the most common symptom. The bleeding is usually intermittent, macroscopic and sufficient to stain the urine a pale red colour. Occasionally, the bleeding is heavy, and causes ureteric colic as blood clots obstruct the ureter (clot colic).
- **General debility.** Many patients with renal carcinoma have no symptoms until secondary deposits or the burden of the primary tumour cause general malaise, loss of energy and loss of weight.
- Carcinoma of the kidney is one of the cancers that metastasizes to bone, and some patients present with bone pain and pathological fractures.
- **Pain in the loin.** When this occurs, it usually signifies advanced disease.
- **A mass.** A mass may be felt by chance at a routine examination or by the patient, or it may cause abdominal distension.

    Less common symptoms include:

- **Pyrexia of unknown origin** (PUO). Carcinoma of the kidney should be excluded in every patient who presents with a PUO.
- **Polycythaemia.** The tumour cells produce erythropoietin, resulting in polycythaemia. This causes redness of the face and hands, and spontaneous venous and arterial thromboses. To emphasize the multiplicity of symptoms of renal cancer, other patients present with anaemia from their haematuria.
- **Varicocele.** Occlusion of the left renal and testicular veins by direct spread of the tumour along the renal vein can cause an acute-onset varicocele (see Chapter 18). There may even be inferior vena caval obstruction, producing oedema of both legs and the abdominal wall.
- Sudden severe **abdominal pain** may indicate acute haemorrhage into the tumour or even spontaneous rupture, with collapse caused by massive intraperitoneal bleeding.
- **Hypertension** of renal origin is a rare complication of renal carcinoma.
- **Incidental finding.** As a result of the increase in the number of imaging studies being performed, small incidental renal masses are increasingly and commonly discovered.

Examination

General features The patient may show signs of recent weight loss.

Abdomen Large tumours are palpable, and demonstrate the physical signs of an enlarged kidney. There is no tenderness.

Skeleton There may be areas of swelling and tenderness in the bones, at the sites of secondary deposits. Very rarely, such deposits of renal carcinoma are vascular and feel soft with an audible bruit.

Chest There may be a pleural effusion on the side of the tumour if it has spread through the diaphragm.

The usual type of lung metastasis, sometimes solitary, from carcinoma of the kidney has a 'cannon ball' appearance on chest X-ray.

Childhood renal tumours

Although rare, renal tumours are among the most common causes of an abdominal mass in children, accounting for 7 per cent of malignancies.

Symptoms There may be abdominal pain and bloating, as well as macroscopic haematuria, usually painless but sometimes producing clot colic. Pressure effects include anorexia, malaise, lethargy, nausea and vomiting.

Signs An abdominal mass is seen, perhaps with evidence of disseminated malignancy.

Wilms tumour/nephroblastoma

Incidence The most common childhood renal tumour occurring in one in 125 000 individuals. A total of 5 per cent of cases are bilateral (either synchronous or metachronous).

Age Peak age is 3–4 years.

Race There is a preponderance of Afro-Caribbean children.

Associated conditions A quarter of children affected have another congenital anomaly, including hemihypertrophy, cryptorchidism and hypospadias. In some rare syndromes, there is a role for screening for renal masses.

In addition to the symptoms listed above, there may be fever, and occasionally hypertension. The tumours are encapsulated, vascular and generally do not cross the midline, but they may metastasize widely.

Other childhood renal tumours

There are a number of extremely rare kidney tumours that present in the same way as a Wilms tumour, and the diagnosis is often not made until after resection. These tumours usually have a higher rate of relapse and death than classical Wilms tumours.

Renal cell carcinoma can be seen in children and adolescents, often related to von Hippel–Lindau disease, familial renal cell carcinoma or sickle-cell disease.

Carcinoma of the renal pelvis

This is a transitional cell carcinoma of the urothelium, and is identical to the type commonly found in the bladder. It is often associated with tumours elsewhere in the urinary tract, but may be the only manifestation of uroepithelial malignant change.

The condition presents with haematuria and occasionally with clot colic, with clots described as 'stringy'. There are no physical signs.

Renal and ureteric calculi

Stones in renal calyces may lie silent for years and not present until complications such as infection occur. Stones in the ureter usually cause pain.

History

Age Renal and ureteric calculi are found most often between the ages of 30 and 50 years.

Sex They are more common in males than in females.

Occupation They are more common in professionals and manual workers.

Season Urinary calculi develop more frequently in the summer, perhaps initiated by the lower urine flow in warm, dry weather, and an abundance of soft fruits, which are rich in oxalates, an important constituent of calculi.

Symptoms The principal symptoms are **pain and haematuria.**

The pain depends on the site of the stone. A dull ache in the loin is typical of a renal stone. A stone in the ureter produces ureteric colic (described above), which moves down along the line of the ureter as the stone makes its way to the bladder. All stones start in the kidney. A large stone will not pass the PUJ. A stone small enough to enter the ureter will normally pass through to the bladder, with much patient discomfort as it intermittently becomes jammed and causes colic.

Ninety per cent of patients with ureteric colic have microscopic haematuria. Visible haematuria is unusual.

The first indication of the presence of a stone may be acute pyelonephritis, or if the calculous disease has damaged renal function, symptoms of uraemia.

Examination

Abdomen Abdominal examination is difficult during an attack of ureteric colic because the patient is rolling around with tense muscles. There may be secondary abdominal distension, as with other problems that arise in the posterior abdominal wall.

Investigation is needed to make the diagnosis, but 90 per cent of urinary calculi show up on a plain abdominal X-ray.

Some metabolic disorders predispose to the formation of urinary calculi. The least rare (1 in 300) is *hyperparathyroidism*. There may be symptoms of hypercalcaemia (thirst, polydypsia, nausea, vomiting and eventually drowsiness). All patients with stone disease should have their serum calcium measured.

Bladder calculi

Stones may form in the bladder in association with stasis, infection or tumour, or enter from the ureter. There is always a degree of bladder outflow obstruction, otherwise the stone would have been rapidly voided.

CHAPTER 17 | THE KIDNEYS, URINARY TRACT AND PROSTATE

History

Age Bladder stones are rare in Western countries, except in middle-aged and elderly males with prostatic problems.

Symptoms The most common symptom is increased frequency of micturition, sometimes related to posture. When the patient stands up, the stone falls onto the trigone, causing a stabbing pain and initiating a desire to micturate. During the night, the stone rolls away and the problem resolves.

There is sometimes a history of a sudden cessation of urinary flow, which is relieved by lying down.

There may be suprapubic stabbing pain, exacerbated by standing.

Haematuria, particularly at the end of micturition, also occurs.

Many patients have chronic infection, with the symptoms of cystitis.

The symptoms caused by the stone are often preceded by the symptoms of its cause, namely bladder outflow obstruction, recurrent infections and bladder tumours.

Examination

There are rarely any physical signs, although very large stones can sometimes be felt on bimanual examination of the pelvis.

Sounding the bladder Bladder stones were common in past centuries and were diagnosed, before X-rays, by passing a metal instrument into the bladder via the urethra and listening to the sound made as it tapped on the stone. The legacy of this is the name urethral 'sound'.

Cystitis

Cystitis is infection of the urine within the bladder, with a concomitant inflammatory reaction in the bladder wall. The common predisposing factors for cystitis are incomplete emptying of the bladder, abnormalities within the bladder and, in females, bacteria migrating up the urethra. In females, there is often a clear relationship with sexual activity.

History

Age Cystitis occurs often in young and middle-aged females, in young males with urethritis and in elderly males with benign prostatic enlargement and bladder tumours.

Symptoms The usual symptoms are **increased frequency and urgency of micturition**, which begin suddenly and persist through the night as well as the day. The patient often wants to micturate every few minutes.

Passing urine causes a burning or scalding pain along the length of the urethra. It is often so bad that the patient tries to avoid passing urine. There may be a mild suprapubic ache.

Haematuria is common, with a few drops of bloody urine at the end of micturition. The urine may be cloudy and malodorous.

Examination

Mild suprapubic tenderness is the only physical sign. Remember to look at and dipstick-test the urine, and to send it for culture.

Urethral syndrome

Many females with the symptoms of recurrent cystitis never have bacteria demonstrated in the urine. This collection of symptoms is termed the urethral syndrome. Its cause is unknown and its management difficult.

Carcinoma of the bladder

Bladder cancer is nearly always a transitional cell carcinoma, although there are other rare types (squamous cell and adenocarcinoma). It rarely produces any physical signs, so the diagnosis must be suspected from the history.

History

Age Bladder cancer occurs throughout adult life, with a peak incidence between 60 and 70 years.
Sex Males are afflicted more often than females, and smoking is the main risk factor.
Occupation Some industrial chemicals are excreted in the urine and can stimulate malignant change in the uroepithelium (Revision panel 17.3). The better known ones are alpha- and beta-naphthylamine, benzidine and xylenamine, and artificial sweeteners such as cyclamates. The industries that use these chemicals (the rubber and cable industries, printing and dyeing) are well aware of the relationship, and chemically induced bladder cancer is now rare.

Revision panel 17.3

Risk factors for bladder cancer

Bladder carcinogens

Smoking

Aniline dyes

Alpha- and beta-naphthylamine

Xylenamine

Benzidine

Occupations associated with exposure to bladder carcinogens

Dry cleaners

Hairdressers

Leather workers

Painters and decorators

Paper and rubber manufacturers

Dental technicians

Predisposing conditions Squamous cell carcinoma may be induced by the chronic irritation caused by schistosomiasis, bladder calculi or recurrent infections.

Symptoms In 95 per cent of cases, carcinoma of the bladder presents with **bright red haematuria**, which may be intermittent or occur every time the bladder is emptied. The passage of blood clots may cause pain and difficulty with micturition.

If the urine becomes infected, the patient will experience a suprapubic ache and burning micturition.

Pain in the loin may occur, as bladder tumours often begin near the ureteric orifice and obstruct the lower end of the ureter.

Pain in the pelvis and lower abdomen, and nerve root pain down the legs, can occur if the tumour spreads through the wall of the bladder into the pelvis.

A small group of patients with bladder cancer present with frequent and painful micturition, without visible haematuria, but there will be microscopic haematuria.

Never forget that symptoms of cystitis may indicate a bladder tumour, particularly when they persist after treatment.

Examination

It is unusual to find any abnormality. If the tumour is large, it may be felt bimanually or on rectal examination alone, and if it has spread beyond the bladder, the floor of the pelvis may be indurated. Examination under anaesthetic is an important part of staging a bladder tumour.

RETENTION OF URINE

There are two classic forms of retention of urine, acute and chronic, which are usually easily distinguished. Acute retention is painful and sudden. Chronic retention is painless, and there is a chronically distended bladder.

As ever in medicine, things are rarely black and white. Acute retention may develop in the presence of chronic retention, when the expression *acute-on-chronic retention* is sometimes used.

Acute retention in the absence of bladder outlet obstruction is rare, and occurs only after a surgical operation, anaesthesia or an injury to the urethra. Most patients with acute retention give a history of progressive slowing of the urinary stream caused by narrowing of the bladder outlet or urethra. This is termed *bladder outlet obstruction*.

Patients with chronic retention may be symptom-free except for the abdominal swelling produced by the large bladder (Fig. 17.3).

Photo Researchers

Fig. 17.3 Bladder distension.

Thus:

- *acute retention* is the sudden, painful inability to micturate;
- *chronic retention* is an enlarged, painless bladder, whether or not the patient is having difficulty micturating.

The causes of retention are listed in Revision panel 17.4. It is a long list, but the most common cause by far is prostatic obstruction (benign or malignant) in middle-aged and elderly males. In

---

Revision panel 17.4

The causes of retention of urine

Mechanical

In the lumen of the urethra, or overlying the internal urethral orifice:

> Blood clot
> Stones
> Tumour
> Foreign bodies
> Congenital valves

In the wall of the bladder or the urethra:

> Prostatic enlargement (benign and malignant)
> Trauma (rupture of the urethra)
> Urethral stricture
> Urethritis
> Meatal ulcer
> Tumour

Outside the wall:

> Pregnancy (retroverted gravid uterus)
> Fibroids
> Ovarian cyst
> Faecal impaction
> Phimosis or paraphimosis

Neurogenic

Denervation of bladder (e.g. after rectal resection)

Diabetes

Postoperative retention

Spinal cord injuries

Spinal cord disease

Multiple sclerosis

Psychogenic

Drugs:

> Alcohol
> Anticholinergics
> Antihistamines
> Smooth muscle relaxants
> Some tranquillizers

---

hospitals, an operation under general anaesthesia is a common precipitating factor.

Acute retention

History

Symptoms The patient is likely to have symptoms related to one of the causes listed in Revision panel 17.4, as well as suprapubic pain and an inability to pass urine. **The pain is severe and is described as a gross exaggeration of the normal desire to micturate.** The patient is aware that the bladder is overdistended.

Examination

The bladder has usually enlarged sufficiently to become **a palpable, tense, dull, rounded, tender mass arising out of the pelvis** to a point a few centimetres above the pubis. Gentle pressure on the swelling exacerbates the patient's desire to micturate. However, it may be too tender to palpate, particularly when the abdominal wall is tense or the patient is overweight.

Percussion is useful in deciding whether a patient is in acute retention, as the bladder is always dull.

If the patient has had chronic retention before the acute episode, the bladder may reach up to, or above, the umbilicus. A large bladder of this size indicates acute-on-chronic retention.

Rectal examination, if the patient is not too distressed, will reveal that the prostate or uterus is pushed backwards and downwards, with the cystic mass of the bladder filling the front half of the pelvis.

You cannot assess the size of the prostate gland, or the pelvis, when the bladder is full.

It is better to defer the rectal examination for prostate assessment until after the retention has been relieved with a catheter.

Remember to examine not only the prostate, the urethra and the contents of the pelvis, but also the central and peripheral nervous systems to exclude a neurological cause.

Chronic retention

There are two varieties of chronic retention – high pressure and low pressure.

In the *high-pressure* type, the cause is obstruction of the bladder outlet. Bladder pressure builds up and, in a proportion of cases, produces dilatation of the ureters and the renal collection systems as well as the bladder. This ultimately results in renal failure, of the postrenal type.

In the *low-pressure* type, the fault seems to lie with the bladder muscle, which is atonic. The vesico-ureteric junctions remain competent, and there is no back-pressure effect on the kidneys.

If a patient in chronic retention has the symptoms and signs of renal failure, the retention is of the high-pressure type.

History

Age and sex Chronic retention is most common in elderly males.

Symptoms The patient may be unaware of his chronic retention, but complains of symptoms related to bladder outflow obstruction, such as hesitancy, poor and intermittent flow, nocturia and postmicturition dribbling.

Chronic retention is painless.

Many patients with chronic retention have dribbling overflow incontinence, particularly at night. This is not nocturia but leakage while asleep, and is pathognomonic of chronic retention.

Examination

The bladder will be palpable. It is likely to reach at least half way up to the umbilicus. It is not tense or tender, and suprapubic pressure may not always induce a desire to micturate.

The palpable bladder of chronic retention is dull to percussion, will fluctuate and has a fluid thrill.

Look for signs of the cause of the retention in the pelvis, prostate, urethra and nervous system.

Bladder diverticula

A bladder diverticulum is an outpouching of bladder mucosa through a defect in all layers of the muscle in the bladder wall.

Diverticula usually occur just above one or both ureteric orifices. They are caused by outflow obstruction.

Bladder diverticula are rarely palpable because of their position, but they may give rise to a peculiar symptom. When the patient needs to pass urine, the muscle contracts and empties the bladder, but the diverticulum does not empty because its orifice closes as the bladder shrinks. When the patient has finished and the detrusor muscle relaxes, the urine in the diverticulum passes into the bladder, and within minutes the patient feels the need to micturate again (*pis en deux*).

THE PROSTATE GLAND

Benign enlargement (hyperplasia) of the prostate gland

The inner portion (*transitional zone*) of the prostate gland enlarges during late adult life. As it grows, it compresses the outer layers into a false capsule, and bulges centrally into the urethra and the base of the bladder. The cause of this hyperplasia is not known, but it is probably in response to a changing hormonal environment.

The voiding symptoms of prostatic obstruction result from either mechanical obstruction or secondary overactivity of the bladder detrusor muscle (storage symptoms). They are summarized in Revision panel 17.5.

History

Age The prostate starts enlarging at the age of 40 years, but symptoms commonly appear between the ages of 50 and 70 years.

Symptoms **Poor stream.** The cardinal symptom of prostatic obstruction is a reduced rate of urine flow during micturition, that is, a poor stream. However, the condition develops slowly and intermittently, and the bladder compensates by muscular hypertrophy of its wall, which initially overcomes the increased outflow resistance. In consequence, the reduced rate

Revision panel 17.5
Symptoms of hypertrophy of the prostate gland
Symptoms of bladder outflow obstruction (voiding symptoms)

Hesitancy
Poor flow
Intermittent flow
Postmicturition dribbling
Sensation of incomplete emptying
Double micturition

Symptoms of bladder and bladder neck irritation (storage symptoms)
Increased frequency of micturition
Urgency
Nocturia
Urge incontinence

of flow comes on gradually, and you must enquire about this. Ask whether the flow is as good as it was 20 years earlier.

Hesitancy. Associated with the reduced urinary flow are two other symptoms, hesitancy and dribbling. Hesitancy is the inability to start to pass urine. Straining does not help; it actually prolongs the waiting time before the urine starts to flow.

Dribbling. Dribbling is the inability to finish cleanly. A few drops continue to appear for some time after the main stream has ceased. This goes on until patience is lost, resulting in staining of the underclothing.

Increased frequency. What the patient complains of most is increased frequency of micturition, often first noticed when it is necessary to pass urine during the night (*nocturia*). Inadequate emptying of the bladder, and therefore a reduction in functional volume (the additional volume needed to trigger the desire to micturate), is the cause of the frequency.

Urgency. In addition to increased frequency of micturition, the patient reports an urgent need to start passing urine as soon as the desire arises. This is called urgency, and is caused by increased bladder pressure.

Haematuria, in the form of a little dark blood at the end of micturition, is a not uncommon symptom, but should be investigated appropriately to rule out bladder or renal malignancy.

A proportion of patients first present with acute or chronic retention, described above.

Examination

Abdomen The bladder will be palpable if there is acute or chronic retention.

Rectal examination Benign hyperplasia causes a diffuse enlargement. The gland bulges into the rectum, its surface is smooth, but the enlargement is often slightly asymmetrical and the surface bosselated. The consistency of the gland is firm, rubbery and homogeneous.

The median sulcus usually remains palpable, even when the gland is grossly enlarged, and the rectal mucosa moves freely over the gland. It is not tender.

Note that there may be quite significant prostatic obstruction without gross enlargement of the gland. The key factor in the generation of symptoms is the compression of the prostatic urethra, which may occur with quite modest enlargement.

Remember that a full bladder pushes the prostate downwards and makes it feel bigger.

Carcinoma of the prostate

Adenocarcinoma of the prostate gland begins in its outer part (the peripheral zone), which permits easy spread into the seminal vesicles and floor of the pelvis. It is commonly quite locally advanced before it causes lower urinary tract symptoms.

History

Age Carcinoma of the prostate is predominantly a disease of the elderly. Its incidence increases from the fifties onwards. By the late eighties and nineties, it can be found in nearly all males, but in the vast majority it produces no symptoms or signs.

Symptoms The most common presentation is with symptoms similar to those caused by benign prostatic hypertrophy and collectively called voiding symptoms, namely **hesitancy, poor stream, incomplete emptying, coupled with urgency and frequency.** With prostatic cancer, these symptoms tend to progress more rapidly and do not fluctuate in severity, as is so often the case with benign hypertrophy.

A proportion of patients with carcinoma of the prostate present with some form of retention of urine.

If the tumour spreads outside the gland, it may cause pain in the lower abdomen and perineum.

Presentation with secondary deposits is common, with local symptoms that are absent or ignored. There may be debility and loss of weight.

Prostatic cancer metastasizes to bone, particularly the pelvis and lumbar spine. These bone deposits are nearly always osteosclerotic and osteoblastic, so tend to produce bone pain rather than pathological fractures.

Note **Do not forget to consider prostatic bone metastases in any elderly male with skeletal pain.**

Screening Prostatic cancer may be detected by measuring the serum levels of **prostate-specific antigen** (PSA). There is controversy over the value of this investigation as a screening tool, as it has been estimated that, on the basis of this test, there are approximately 1 million males with occult prostatic cancer in the UK, but only 10 000 die from the disease each year. However, an elevated PSA is a mode of presentation that is becoming increasingly common.

Examination

The bladder will be palpable if there is retention of urine.

Rectal examination The prostate gland may be asymmetrically enlarged or distorted. It is **irregular in contour and heterogeneous in texture.** Some areas are hard and knobbly; others are soft. The median sulcus may be absent, and the rectal mucosa may be tethered to the gland. However, if the presentation is through a raised PSA level, the prostate often does not feel malignant.

The tissues of the pelvis, lateral to the gland and around the rectum, may be infiltrated by tumour, and it may be possible to feel seminal vesical involvement. Other physical signs will be those caused by metastases. Carcinoma of the prostate gland sometimes gives rise to metastases in the skin and other unusual sites, as well as in bone. Presentation is occasionally with symptoms of renal impairment, either from retention of urine or direct invasion of the bladder base and obstruction of the ureters.

THE URETHRA

Urethritis (Revision panel 17.6)

This produces symptoms of painful micturition, with a purulent discharge from the external meatus, which is easier to notice in males than in females. It is usually caused by a sexually transmitted disease, commonly *Gonococcus* and *Chlamydia*. If not properly and promptly treated, it heals with a scar, producing a urethral stricture.

Urethral stricture

Urethral strictures occur as a result of the damage or destruction of the urethral mucosa followed by healing with fibrous scar tissue (Revision panel 17.7).

History

Age Urethral strictures occur at all ages. The most common cause used to be gonorrhoea, which is a disease of the sexually active, so the strictures that follow it appeared in young and middle-aged males. Better and quicker treatment of the infection has reduced the incidence of postgonorrhoeal strictures, and the most common cause nowadays is

---

> **Revision panel 17.6**
>
> ## Causes of a urethral discharge
>
> Infection (urethritis)
> Gonococcus
> *Chlamydia*
> Coliforms
> *Trichomonas*
> *Candida*
>
> Lesions in the urethra
> Warts
> Herpes
>
> Foreign bodies

> **Revision panel 17.7**
>
> ## The causes of urethral stricture
>
> Congenital
> Pinhole meatus
> Urethral valves (not a true stricture)
>
> Traumatic
> Instrumentation (catheterization)
> Foreign bodies
> Prostatectomy (transurethral or radical prostatectomy)
> Amputation of the penis
> Direct perineal injuries
>
> Inflammatory
> Gonorrhoea/non-specific urethritis/*Chlamydia*
> Meatal ulceration/balanitis
> Balanitis xerotica obliterans
>
> Neoplastic
> Primary and secondary neoplasms

---

probably catheterization or surgical instrumentation of the urethra.

Symptoms The key symptom is **poor urinary flow**, with a classical flat and prolonged trace on flow rate measurements. The stream is prolonged, thin and dribbles at its end. Attacks of cystitis are common, but retention of urine is rare unless there is added pathology such as a bladder calculus.

There may be a urethral discharge, which is particularly noticeable in the morning.

Increasing frequency of micturition indicates that the bladder is not emptying completely.

Examination

The bladder is sometimes palpable. Renal failure is occasionally seen.

The penis and urethra usually feel normal because the most common site for stricture is where the urethra passes through the perineal membrane. A stricture caused by scarring of the penile urethra can sometimes be felt as an area of induration.

Meatal strictures, common following transurethral operations, are usually visible if the edges of the meatus are gently retracted.

TRAUMA TO THE URINARY TRACT

Renal trauma

The kidneys are protected by the rib cage and are mobile, so injury from blunt trauma is relatively unlikely.

There may be flank pain and tenderness, or bruising and haematuria. The patient may be shocked and haemodynamically unstable. The diagnosis can be made only with computed tomography imaging, and occasionally at urgent laparotomy. Simultaneous injury to other viscera is common.

Bladder trauma

Usually only a full bladder will be ruptured in abdominal trauma. The tear is usually intraperitoneal, so urine collects in the abdominal cavity where it does not produce significant peritoneal irritation. The diagnosis is suggested when the (sometimes inebriated) patient does not pass urine and does not feel the need.

Urethral trauma

The site of injury may be suspected from the history:

- The penile urethra is occasionally injured during sexual intercourse.
- The bulbar urethra may be injured by falling astride a fairly narrow object.
- The membranous urethra may be damaged and even transected by a pelvic fracture.

Urethral injury is suspected if the patient is unable to pass urine, or there is blood at the external meatus.

The findings depend on the site of the injury:

- There will be **tenderness and bruising** at the site of injury to the penile urethra.
- **Bruising and extravasated urine** are seen if the rupture (total or partial) of the bulbar urethra is deep to the membranous layer of the superficial fascia. In this situation, the blood tracks to the perineum, scrotum, lower abdomen and the upper thighs, but only as far as the attachment of the fascia.
- Rupture of the membranous urethra allows the bladder and prostate to float upwards. This is theoretically palpable on rectal examination, but this is likely to be impossible in a patient with a fractured pelvis.

Penetrating trauma of the urinary tract is unusual. The history and site of the entrance wound will suggest the diagnosis, which is usually confirmed on surgical exploration.

The external genitalia

EXAMINATION OF THE MALE GENITALIA

Remember to wear protective gloves and take care to be gentle, especially if the testes are tender.

The penis

Inspection (Fig. 18.1)

Note the size and shape of the penis, the colour of the skin, the presence or absence of the foreskin, scarring and the position and patency of the urethral meatus.

Palpation

Assess the texture of the body of the penis and the whole length of the urethra, right down to the perineal membrane.

Ask the patient to retract the prepuce to examine the skin on its inner aspect, the glans penis and the external urethral meatus (Fig. 18.2).

At birth, the foreskin is tethered to the glans penis with only a small opening, so do not try to retract the foreskin of a small child (less than 4 years of age).

(a) **Always look at the ventral surface of the penis.**

(b) In this patient, this revealed a hypospadias.

Fig. 18.1 EXAMINATION OF THE PENIS

Phimosis is a narrowing of the distal rim of the prepuce, which prevents retraction. This occurs in all age groups.

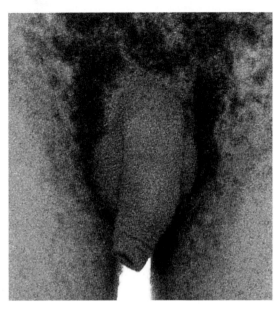

(a) **Always retract the prepuce** and inspect its inner surface, and the glans penis.

(b) In this patient, this revealed a carcinoma.

Fig. 18.2 EXAMINATION OF THE PENIS

The scrotal skin

The skin of the scrotum is usually wrinkled and freely mobile over the testes. If it is reddened, tethered or fixed, there is probably a deep abnormality. Do not forget that the conditions which affect hair-bearing skin on any other part of the body – sebaceous cyst, infected hair follicle and squamous carcinoma – may affect the scrotal skin.

Remember that the scrotum has a back and front, and do not forget to examine its posterior aspect (Fig. 18.3).

Should you find a lesion in the scrotal skin, proceed methodically through your examination of any lump or ulcer found elsewhere (see Chapter 1).

The scrotal contents

The shape of the scrotum and the position of the testes within it can only be observed properly when the patient is standing up, but it is more comfortable for patient and student to perform the major part of the examination with the patient lying supine.

Inspection

Note the size and shape of the scrotum, particularly any asymmetry, erythema, discharge and scarring.

Palpation

First, is there a testicle on each side?

The scrotal contents are examined by gently supporting the scrotum on the fingers of one or both hands, while feeling the testis and any other lumps between your index finger, which is behind the scrotum, and your thumb, which is in front. Do not squeeze the testis or a lump between your thumb and index finger – let it slip from side to side so that you can feel its shape and surface.

Decide the position and nature of the body of each testis, epididymis and spermatic cords. If you are unsure if what you are feeling is the testis, ask the patient. The testis has unique sensation.

With knowledge of the anatomy and the pathology of scrotal conditions, it is possible to make an accurate clinical diagnosis in most cases.

(a) **Always look at the posterior surface** of the scrotum.

(b) In this patient, this revealed a squamous carcinoma.

Fig. 18.3 EXAMINATION OF THE SCROTUM

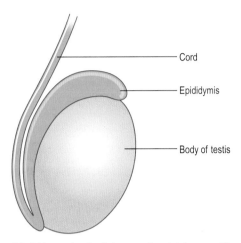

Fig. 18.4 If you think of the way in which you will draw the testes, and any abnormality you find, in your notes, it will help you to define the anatomy. Define the cord, the epididymis and the body of the testes.

There are several characteristics of any scrotal lump that must be determined for all scrotal lumps:

- Can you get above it? (Is the lump confined to the scrotum?)
- Does the lump transilluminate?
- Does the lump have an expansile cough impulse?
- Is the lump separate from the body of the testis?

When you have established the answers to these questions, and have defined the physical characteristics of the lump and its relations to each testis and epididymis, you will be able to make the diagnosis. Record your findings on a diagram similar to that shown in Fig. 18.4.

The perineum and rectum

Examination of the perineum and rectal examination to feel the prostate and seminal vesicles is obligatory (see Chapter 16).

Lymph drainage (Fig. 18.5)

The skin of the external genitalia drains to the inguinal lymph glands. The scrotal contents, however, develop in the para-aortic area in the back wall of the abdomen. During the descent into the scrotum,

CHAPTER 18 | THE EXTERNAL GENITALIA

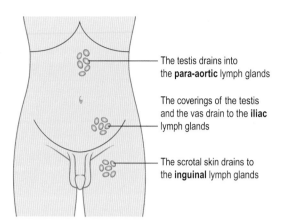

Fig. 18.5 The lymph drainage of the testis, its coverings and the scrotum.

- The testis drains into the **para-aortic** lymph glands
- The coverings of the testis and the vas drain to the **iliac** lymph glands
- The scrotal skin drains to the **inguinal** lymph glands

the arterial blood supply and venous and lymphatic drainage follow the testis. In consequence:

- lymph from the skin of the penis and scrotum drains to the inguinal glands;
- lymph from the coverings of the testis and spermatic cord (i.e. the tunica vaginalis and the cremasteric and spermatic fasciae) drains to the iliac glands;
- lymph from the body of the testis drains to the para-aortic glands.

THE PENIS

Phimosis

Phimosis is a narrowing of the end of the prepuce (foreskin), which prevents its retraction over the glans penis. It may be congenital, or it may develop due to scarring of the skin following infection or trauma.

Natural history of the foreskin

At birth, the foreskin covers and is adherent to the glans penis. The opening may initially be very narrow, like a pinhole. In the first few years of life, the foreskin gradually separates and widens so that, by the age of 5 years, approximately 90 per cent of males are able to retract it freely and easily. The mechanism by which this happens is uncertain. Certainly, the normal skin secretions that build up between the foreskin and the glans (smegma) play a part, and there is also stretching from erections and patient self-curiosity.

It is normal to have a non-retractile foreskin in early childhood. Even when the foreskin retracts, adhesions between the foreskin and glans may persist into the early teens. There is no 'normal' age beyond which failure to be able to retract the prepuce may be termed abnormal and require treatment, but full retraction should be possible in all adults. So when does failure to be able to retract become a disease? This is a grey area, and can cause considerable parental concern.

There is one variety of phimosis that is clearly pathological from the beginning, and that is balanitis xerotica obliterans (BXO). In this condition, there is scarring of the tip of the foreskin, presumably due to minor tearing and healing with scarring. The appearance is characteristic (Fig. 18.6). On gently

(a) Phimosis in a child with a ring of BXO. Note the white scar tissue that is made prominent as the patient tries to retract his foreskin.

(b) Phimosis and BXO in an adult.

Fig. 18.6 TWO EXAMPLES OF BALANITIS XEROTICA OBLITERANS (BXO) AND PHIMOSIS attempting retraction, whitish, irregular scarring is seen. The process usually begins at the tip of the foreskin, but may spread on to the glans and even narrow the urethral meatus.

Symptoms **Ballooning of the prepuce on micturition** is usually not abnormal in a young child. It can only occur when there are no preputial adhesions.

Recurrent balanitis (see below) causing pain and a purulent discharge may occur, but actual urinary tract infection is uncommon, although it is sometimes attributed to phimosis.

Similar symptoms may occur in the adult, but the most common complaint is of discomfort with erection and during sexual intercourse. If a tight foreskin gets retracted, it may not be possible to pull it forwards again; the patient then has a paraphimosis (see below).

Examination

In a child, gently draw back the foreskin and look at the tip. In a normal but narrow foreskin in a small child, the orifice will be small, but the skin will appear normal. As you continue to retract it, the foreskin will not come back completely, but skin on the inside of the prepuce will 'flower' outwards. It is pinker and more delicate than the exposed skin on the outside. If there is any BXO, you will see a narrow ring of white scar tissue (Fig. 18.6) and will be unable to retract the skin at all.

In children, smegma may build up as yellow masses visible and palpable through the foreskin. This appearance may alarm both parents and referring physicians.

Paraphimosis

This occurs when the narrowing of the prepuce is just sufficiently tight for it to get stuck behind the glans penis, often during an erection. In this position, it impedes venous blood flow and causes oedema and congestion of the glans, which in turn makes reduction of the prepuce more difficult.

History

Age Paraphimosis usually occurs in young males and sometimes in children. It is a common complication of urethral catheterization at any age. It is preventable by ensuring that the foreskin is always pulled forward after catheter insertion.

Symptoms There is swelling and discomfort of the glans penis, with a tender, tight band at the coronal sulcus. It is uncommon for the urethra to be obstructed.

Past history The patient will not usually have been circumcised, but note that in some religious circumcisions the whole of the prepuce is not removed, so recurrent phimosis and hence paraphimosis may occur.

Examination

The diagnosis is usually obvious (Fig. 18.7). The glans penis is swollen and oedematous, and there is a deep groove just below the corona where the skin looks tight, and may be split and ulcerated.

The condition may be chronic, in which case there may be superficial ulceration and infection of the skin of the glans penis.

Fig. 18.7 Paraphimosis. The retracted, tight, constricting ring of preputial skin is causing oedema of the skin distal to it, and congestion of the glans penis.

Hypospadias

Hypospadias is a congenital abnormality in which the urethra opens on the ventral surface of the penis, proximal to its usual position (Fig. 18.8).

The opening may be anywhere along the line of the urethra, from the tip of the penis to the perineum. If the urethral opening is in the perineum,

(a) Glandular hypospadias. The urethral opening is on the edge of the glans penis. The pit where the opening should be is also visible.

(b) Penile hypospadias. The urethral opening is 1 cm below the edge of the glans.

(c) Scrotal hypospadias. The urethra opens in the scrotum with the penile urethra deficient ventrally.

(d) Perineal hypospadias. The urethral opening is in the perineum. The scrotum is bifid.

Fig. 18.8 HYPOSPADIAS
Note that the external urethral meatus may be on the glans penis, the shaft of the penis or the perineum.

the scrotum is *bifid*. The site of the opening may be classified as glandular (on the glans), penile (on the shaft) or perineal.

Glandular hypospadias is easy to miss because it causes no symptoms and there is a deceptive vertical slit at the normal site of the urethral opening. The actual meatus may be quite small, and a common site is in the coronal sulcus.

The prepuce has a hooded appearance in proximal hypospadias, because it is deficient ventrally where the urethra emerges. It is vital never to carry out circumcision in a child with any degree of

hypospadias, as the preputial skin may be needed for corrective surgery.

Chordee is a descriptive term for a curved penis, commonly associated with hypospadias. The curvature is convex dorsally and is more pronounced the further the urethral meatus is away from the end of the penis. It is caused by the corpus spongiosum being shorter than the corpora cavernosa when the urethral opening fails to reach the end of the penis. It may only be visible on erection.

Chordee in the other direction, convex ventrally, is seen in adults with Peyronie's disease (see below).

Epispadias

Epispadias is the opposite of hypospadias. The urethral opening is on the dorsal surface of the glans penis (Fig. 18.9). It is extremely rare and is part of a spectrum of deficiencies with abdominal and pelvic fusion in the first months of embryogenesis known as the *exstrophy–epispadias complex*.

Fig. 18.9 Epispadias. The urethra opens on the dorsum of the glans penis, almost on the dorsal aspect of the shaft of the penis.

Balanitis

Strictly speaking, this is inflammation of the prepuce, and the term for inflammation of the glans is *posthitis*. It is usually caused by bacterial and sexually transmitted infections. Most patients have inflammation of both prepuce and glans, and therefore have balanoposthitis, but in practice the only term used is balanitis. It may be caused by poor personal hygiene and smegma/debris accumulating beneath the prepuce.

Symptoms The patient may complain of itching, pain or discharge, almost invariably with difficulty retracting the foreskin.

Examination

The foreskin appears reddened and oedematous, and there may be a purulent discharge. Patients are occasionally febrile and systemically unwell. In children, there will usually be collections of smegma, which may be visible. Look for signs of BXO.

In elderly males, remember the possibility that balanitis may be caused by a carcinoma hidden beneath the prepuce, so retract it if possible.

Palpate the glans and the inguinal lymph glands.

Other causes of balanitis

Candidal balanitis is seen particularly in those with diabetes and immunosuppressed patients. The glans penis will show itchy red patches. The foreskin has a white appearance with longitudinal fissuring, particularly at the tip (Fig. 18.10).

Fig. 18.10 Monilial balanoposthitis.

Genital herpes can involve the shaft, glans or foreskin. The vesicles, initially itchy, are soon replaced by shallow, painful erosions. There may be painful inguinal lymphadenopathy.

Drug eruptions are usually painless discolourations, most often seen on the glans penis, and are sometimes the only manifestation of drug hypersensitivity (Fig. 18.11).

Fig. 18.11 A drug eruption. This ulcer was part of a reaction to co-trimoxazole.

Fig. 18.12 Penile warts.

Zoon's balanitis, also known as *plasma cell balanitis*, is a rare, idiopathic, benign, penile dermatosis. There are discrete plaques on both the glans and inner prepuce, which appear moist and erythematous.

Penile warts are viral in origin and sexually transmitted (Fig. 18.12).

Syphilitic chancre

In many parts of the developed world, syphilis is now rare. The primary sore, known as a *chancre*, is solitary and always painless. It usually occurs in the coronal sinus, the prepuce or the frenulum, and produces a serosanguinous discharge.

Beneath an area of superficial ulceration is an indistinct, indurated lump, 5–10 mm in diameter. The ulcer is covered with a slough and has a sloping, indolent edge (see Chapter 1) (Fig. 18.13). It is not fixed to deeper structures.

The inguinal lymph glands are invariably enlarged, often mainly on one side. They are rubbery and discrete, but not tender.

General examination may reveal no other abnormalities, but a primary sore may still be present should the patient present with the secondary manifestations of the disease 4–6 weeks after the appearance of the chancre.

Fig. 18.13 A syphilitic chancre on the inner surface of the prepuce.

Carcinoma of the penis

Carcinoma of the penis is a squamous cell carcinoma. It is exceedingly rare in males who have been circumcised at birth or in adolescence, as in Jewish and Muslim communities.

It may be preceded by a number of premalignant conditions described below. It invades from the penile skin into the tissues of the shaft of the penis and spreads via the lymphatics.

History

Age Carcinoma of the penis presents in middle or old age, and rarely in young males.

Ethnic group Carcinoma of the penis occurs in cultures that do not practise ritual circumcision.

Symptoms Most patients present with a lump or an ulcer that may be painful, especially if infected.

There is usually a **purulent discharge, which may be bloodstained**.

The patient may have a phimosis if the primary lesion has become quite advanced before detection.

The **inguinal lymph glands may be enlarged** by secondary infection or secondary deposits, and may be the first abnormality noticed by the patient. Presentation with distant metastases is rare.

The occasional patient ignores his symptoms until the tumour compresses or invades the urethra and urinary retention occurs.

Examination

Prepuce The patient is usually uncircumcised, and in the UK is commonly elderly and self-neglected. There may be a serous, purulent or sanguineous discharge coming from beneath the prepuce. If the foreskin cannot be retracted, full examination of its inner surface and the glans penis may require a surgical dorsal slit.

Deformity The penis may be swollen at its tip owing to the mass beneath the prepuce. In the advanced stages, the tumour may appear through the opening in the prepuce or erode through the preputial skin.

Position The lesion may be anywhere on the skin of the prepuce or the glans penis.

Tenderness **The lump or ulcer is not usually tender**, except with concomitant infection.

Shape Carcinoma of the penis tends to adopt one of two macroscopic forms: a classic carcinomatous ulcer with a raised everted edge and necrotic base, or a papilliferous tumour with a wide sessile pedicle and an indurated base (Fig. 18.14). The microscopic pathology is the same.

(a) An early carcinomatous ulcer on the glans penis, exposed by a circumcision.

(b) A papilliferous carcinoma arising in the coronal sulcus.

Fig. 18.14 CARCINOMA OF THE PENIS

CHAPTER 18 | THE EXTERNAL GENITALIA

(c) An advanced infiltrating carcinoma that has invaded the whole thickness of the prepuce.

(d) An ulcerating carcinoma that has destroyed half of the glans penis.

Fig. 18.14 CARCINOMA OF THE PENIS (CONTINUED)

The shape reflects the degree of tumour necrosis.

Size Patients who can retract their foreskin present earlier.

Composition The tumour is hard, especially at its base. Any part of the penis that is infiltrated also feels hard. The surface of the papilliferous variety is soft and friable. It resembles granulation tissue, and bleeds easily.

Relations At first, the tumour is confined to the skin, but it may invade and spread through the whole corpus cavernosum, making it indurated and hard. If it begins on the inner side of the prepuce, it may spread to and through the outer layer of skin.

Lymph drainage The inguinal lymph glands of both groins may be enlarged by infection or metastatic deposits.

Skin conditions of the penis

Various skin conditions are associated with an increased incidence of carcinoma of the penis, and the underlying pathological condition is called *intraepithelial neoplasia* (Fig. 18.15). This is the same as that seen in the female genital tract in the cervix and vulva, and in the perianal skin.

It is now appreciated that various clinical appearances, often classified by their colour (e.g. leukoplakia) or eponymously (e.g. Paget's disease and erythroplasia of Querat), have essentially the same pathology. Any chronic skin eruption on the penis might be penile intraepithelial neoplasia and should be assessed and treated accordingly.

Clinical diagnosis is difficult because any skin disease may occur on the skin of the penis.

Fig. 18.15 An example of penile intraepithelial neoplasia. This variety is commonly called leukoplakia.

Lichen sclerosis (BXO) particularly mimics intraepithelial neoplasia.

Viral warts are common (see Fig. 18.12) and sexually transmitted.

Priapism

Priapism is a persistent, usually painful erection. There are two varieties, low-flow (ischaemic) and high-flow.

Low-flow priapism is seen in previously fit males after sexual activity. It is caused by a failure of the venular spasm that sustains erection to relax, often triggered by intracavernosal injections or oral agents. Because of embarrassment, presentation may be late. It may also be caused by haematological disorders such as leukaemia or sickle-cell disease, which cause thrombosis of the corpora cavernosa, or by obstruction of the venous and lymphatic drainage of the penis by pelvic malignancy.

The erection seen in priapism is not of the normal pattern and shape. The corpus spongiosum remains soft. Without immediate surgical treatment, irreversible impotence may result.

High-flow priapism is not painful or ischaemic and usually results from an arteriovenous fistula following pelvic trauma.

Peyronie's disease

This is an idiopathic plaque of fibrosis in one or both of the corpora cavernosa, usually on the dorsal side. It occurs in middle-aged males. The symptoms are pain and a curvature of the penis when erect, which can interfere with sexual intercourse. The plaque may be palpable when the penis is flaccid, and in the first 6 months the plaques are tender.

The differential diagnosis includes metastatic tumour deposits and sarcomatous soft tissue tumours, but these are rare.

THE SCROTAL SKIN

Sebaceous cysts

Sebaceous cysts are common in the scrotal skin and are often multiple (Fig. 18.16). They have all the features described in Chapter 4. They occasionally become infected, discharge and produce so much granulation tissue that they look like a carcinoma.

Fig. 18.16 Sebaceous cyst.

Carcinoma of the scrotal skin

This is a squamous carcinoma caused by chronic irritation. Historically, it was caused by frequent contact with soot (Pott's chimney sweep's cancer). The skin must be exposed to these irritants for many years before a cancer develops.

History

Occupation The patient's occupation may be responsible for frequent soiling of the scrotal skin with oil and other carcinogenic hydrocarbons, and should be documented.

Symptoms Presentation is with a lump or an ulcer. A purulent discharge may be present. The patient may notice lumps in the groin if the inguinal lymph glands are involved.

Examination

Position A carcinomatous ulcer can occur on any part of the scrotal skin (Fig. 18.17). Industrial cancers are often located high up in the cleft between the leg and the scrotum, where there is friction and persistent traces of oil.

Tenderness The ulcer is usually painless and not tender.

Shape In its early stages, the ulcer is small and circular, but it enlarges in an irregular fashion with an irregular outline.

Edge The edge is reddish, friable and typically everted.

Base The base is covered with yellow–grey, infected, necrotic tumour.

Relations In the early stages, the ulcer is freely mobile, but with deep spread to the skin it may become tethered to the underlying testis.

Lymph drainage The inguinal lymph glands may be enlarged by tumour metastases or secondary infection.

Fig. 18.17 A carcinoma of the scrotal skin. Note that it is on the posteromedial surface of the scrotum.

Lymphoedema

Swelling of the penis and scrotum caused by excess fluid in the subcutaneous tissue (oedema) is seen in patients confined to bed with heart failure or fluid retention. It also occurs after surgery in the groin or pelvis.

True lymphoedema of the genitalia – oedema caused by the retention of protein-rich lymph in the subcutaneous tissues – is uncommon. It may be associated with lymphoedema of one or both limbs.

Fig. 18.18 Lymphoedema of the penis.

The cause is obstruction of the inguinal and iliac lymph pathways by secondary or primary malignant disease or, in tropical areas, by worms (*Wuchereria bancrofti*, which causes filariasis)(Fig. 18.18).

Primary genital lymphoedema is very rare, and is caused by hypoplastic lymphatics.

Sinuses of the scrotum

Advanced disease of the testis or epididymis occasionally spreads to and erodes through the scrotal skin to create a sinus between the primary lesion and the skin surface.

Provided the testis is lying in the normal position, disease of the body of the testis tends to spread to the anterolateral surface of the scrotum, whereas disease of the epididymis spreads to the posterior surface.

The most common sinus in the scrotal area is a discharging cutaneous sebaceous cyst.

Fournier's gangrene

(Necrotizing fasciitis)

This highly lethal condition, an example of synergistic gangrene, is a disease of the scrotal skin and subcutaneous tissues, and not of the testicles themselves, which are unaffected, protected by the external spermatic fascia. It primarily affects older patients who are immunocompromised from a wide variety of causes.

There is infection with a combination of aerobic organisms (e.g. *Escherichia coli*, enterococcus) and anaerobic organisms such as *Bacteroides* and *Clostridium*. The combined infection produces toxins that cause tissue necrosis, in which the bacteria can flourish and spread.

The prominent feature is an acutely unwell patient with septic shock. The scrotal skin shows dusky erythema, which progresses to a purple blotchy appearance with rapidly spreading black patches of obvious skin gangrene (Fig. 18.19). There is often gas in the subcutaneous tissues, and there is a crackling sensation on gentle palpation (*crepitus*).

The mortality is as high as 80 per cent, because of the comorbidity of the sufferers. Urgent treatment is essential (see *Investigation and Management*, Chapter 3).

Fig. 18.19 Fournier's gangrene.

THE TESTES

Failure of normal testicular descent

(Cryptorchidism)

The testis develops *in utero* in the posterior abdominal wall. Its blood supply comes from the aorta, and its veins drain into the inferior vena cava, on the left via the renal vein. Lymph drainage is to the para-aortic glands.

Guided by the gubernaculum, the testis descends into the scrotum at between 25 and 30 weeks' gestation. Most testes have reached the scrotum by full term. In premature males, testicular descent may occur during the first 3 months of life.

Examination of the scrotum and groin can be difficult in small babies.

You can only confirm the presence or absence of the testes by careful palpation. A quick glance at the scrotum is not good enough.

By 3 months, only 1–2 per cent of testes cannot be found by an experienced examiner.

If the testis has never been in the scrotum, the scrotal skin on that side will be underdeveloped.

If a testis is not in the scrotum, it may either have found its way to an abnormal site or have stopped somewhere along the route of normal descent:

- A testis that has descended to an abnormal site is an *ectopic testis*. The testis may be in the superficial inguinal pouch, the femoral triangle or the perineum (Fig. 18.20). The mechanism causing descent is normal, but the guidance system has gone wrong. The testis itself is normal.
- A testis that is in its correct anatomical path but has failed to reach the scrotum is a truly *undescended testis* (Fig. 18.21).

The truly undescended testis is small and abnormal, with a separated epididymis and often an associated indirect inguinal hernial sac. The absence of both testes from the scrotum may prompt further genetic investigation to exclude intersex conditions.

True congenital absence of a testis is rare. The testis is sometimes missing because it has met with a vascular accident, usually torsion (see below) in early or even intrauterine life.

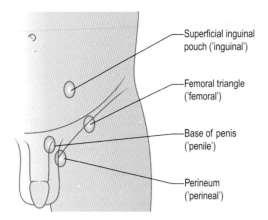

Fig. 18.20 The sites where you may find an ectopic testis.

- Superficial inguinal pouch ('inguinal')
- Femoral triangle ('femoral')
- Base of penis ('penile')
- Perineum ('perineal')

Fig. 18.22 This baby has a truly undescended and impalpable left testis. The scrotal skin is very poorly developed compared with the right side, where the testis has fully descended.

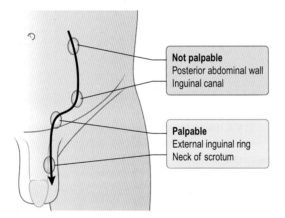

Not palpable
Posterior abdominal wall
Inguinal canal

Palpable
External inguinal ring
Neck of scrotum

Fig. 18.21 The line of normal testicular descent. A truly undescended testis may be found anywhere on this line. If it is above the external inguinal ring, it will be impalpable.

Examination of a child with a missing testis

This can be difficult with a child who does not want to be examined and anxious parents. Make sure that the room and your hands are both warm. The child has to be persuaded to lie down.

Inspection The child must be undressed from the waist downwards in a good light. An empty scrotum, with very little development of the scrotal skin because it has never had the testis within it, is usually obvious (Fig. 18.22). If the testes are visible in the scrotum, a retractile testis is the likely diagnosis.

If the testis is in the superficial inguinal pouch, it may be visible in a thin patient.

Palpation Try to get the child to relax, as muscular activity makes the dartos muscle contract and draw the testis up towards the groin.

Examine the groin before palpating the scrotum. If you cannot see or feel the testis in the subcutaneous tissues, find out if it is in the inguinal canal by gently sweeping your fingers from the anterior superior iliac spine obliquely across the groin to the pubis, along the line of the inguinal canal and towards the neck of the scrotum; this will 'milk' the testis, if present, through the external ring. If the testis becomes palpable, catch it gently with the thumb and index finger of your other hand and draw it down to the scrotum. If it is a retractile testis, it will move down easily.

Should you get the testis down into the scrotum, show it to the parents before you remove your fingers and the testis retracts!

Ectopic testis

History

Age Children in developed countries will usually be routinely examined at birth and again in the first year of life. The patient may not discover the abnormality himself until adolescence.

Symptoms Absence of a testis is the common presenting symptom, but the child may complain of pain or discomfort if the testis is in a site such as the superficial inguinal pouch, where it is likely to be rubbed or compressed during normal physical activity. Note that the pain pathway is via the autonomic afferent nerves so, for developmental reasons, pain may be experienced in the groin or even loin.

Systemic effects If both testes are ectopic, the patient may be subfertile, but he rarely lacks secondary sexual characteristics.

Examination

The side of the scrotum without the testis may be poorly developed, but not as obviously as with a truly undescended testis.

Site An ectopic testis is nearly always palpable, although with difficulty in a fat child. A truly undescended testis lying in the inguinal canal or abdomen is not palpable. If the testis is not in the scrotum, you must carefully examine those sites where ectopic testes are known to settle:

- **Superficial inguinal pouch.** This is by far the most common site in which to find an ectopic testis. It is also the place to which the retractile testis retreats. An ectopic testis in this site has emerged through the external ring but, having failed to enter the scrotum, turns upwards and laterally to lie in a pouch deep to the superficial fascia. This may be caused by some obstruction at the neck of the scrotum from tight fascia. The testis can be palpated in the subcutaneous tissue just above and lateral to the crest of the pubis and the pubic tubercle.
- **Femoral triangle.** If the testis moves laterally after leaving the external inguinal ring, it can come to rest in the upper medial corner of the femoral triangle. A testis in this site is easy to feel, and is easily misdiagnosed as a lymph gland or even a femoral hernia, although the latter is very rare in children. This variety is sometimes termed **crural**, as it lies in the thigh.
- **Base of the penis.** If the testis moves medially, it will lie at the base of the penis, where it can be easily felt against the underlying pubic bone.
- **Perineum.** Occasionally, the testis passes over the pubis and then backwards, instead of downwards, to lie in the perineum just to one side of the corpus cavernosum of the penis (Fig. 18.23). An ectopic testis cannot be manipulated into the scrotum.

It is unusual to be able to define the separate features of the body of the testis and the epididymis.

Fig. **18.23** Perineal ectopic testicle.

Any enlargement, irregularity or immobility should make you suspect the presence of malignant change in the testis, or make you look for another diagnosis.

Truly undescended testis

History

Age Truly undescended testes are usually noticed in early life at postnatal check-ups, but occasionally not until adolescence.

Symptoms **An absence of one or both testes from the scrotum is the presenting symptom.** The parents may notice that the scrotum has not developed – unaware of the absence of the testes. A small proportion of patients present in adult life with infertility. Although failure of testicular descent is invariably associated with abnormal spermatogenesis, the hormone-producing cells are usually normal, so the male has a normal puberty and secondary sexual characteristics.

Truly undescended testes are associated with an indirect inguinal hernia, and a groin swelling may be the presenting complaint.

Examination

The scrotum When both testes are undescended, the scrotum is small and hypoplastic. If only one testis has descended, it is markedly asymmetrical (see Fig. 18.22).

Site A truly undescended testis lies somewhere in the line of normal descent but only becomes palpable when it reaches, or is outside, the external inguinal ring.

It cannot be felt within the inguinal canal because the tense overlying external oblique aponeurosis conceals it, and it tends to slip back through the internal ring into the abdomen. Thus, if you can feel a testis lateral to the external inguinal ring, it must be superficial to the external oblique, and is therefore an ectopic testis in the superficial inguinal pouch rather than a truly undescended testis.

Some testes that lie in the inguinal canal can be milked down to the external ring by gently stroking along the line of the canal, as described above.

The lump A truly undescended testis is usually smaller than normal.

In an adult, the appearance of a mass in the line of testicular descent, whether within the abdomen or the inguinal canal, and an empty scrotum should make you suspect malignant change in a truly undescended testis. The risk of malignant change is many times greater than in a normally descended or ectopic testis. Fixing the testis in the scrotum (orchidopexy) does not eliminate this risk.

The truly undescended testis is also more likely to undergo torsion than a normally descended testis.

Retractile testes

The cremaster is a strong active muscle during childhood, and the testes of many young children (commonly 2–7 years of age) move freely up and down between the scrotum and the inguinal canal or the superficial inguinal pouch. A cold examining hand may be sufficient stimulus to cause retraction. If the patient is seen when the testis is retracted, it may be misdiagnosed as a truly undescended testis and surgical treatment advised. This will be an unnecessary operation because all retractile testes ultimately descend properly, either before or at puberty.

History

The parents notice that the testis (frequently both) is absent from the scrotum. This situation is often intermittent, and it may be noticed that everything appears normal when the child is warm and relaxed, typically in the bath.

The testis may have been reported in the scrotum at previous routine examinations.

Examination

When the testes are retractile, the scrotum is normally developed.

You should always attempt to manipulate the testis into the scrotum, as described above. If the testis can be persuaded into the scrotum and it rests there when you let go, it is a retractile testis. A testis should only be classified as truly undescended or ectopic if you cannot manipulate it into the scrotum.

The ascending testis

There is also a group of patients in whom the testis has been found and placed in the scrotum to the satisfaction of all, but some while later the parents notice that it is no longer visible and seek further advice. On this occasion, the testis may be palpable in the superficial inguinal pouch and cannot be persuaded into the scrotum. This is termed the 'ascending testis' and may require surgery.

Hydrocele

A hydrocele is an abnormal quantity of fluid within the tunica vaginalis (Revision panel 18.1). There are two varieties:

- **primary**, of unknown cause;
- **secondary**, caused by trauma, infection or neoplasm.

Most secondary hydroceles appear rapidly in the presence of other symptoms associated with their cause, are lax and may contain altered blood. They are much less common than primary (idiopathic) hydroceles, which develop slowly and progressively and become large and tense.

History

Age Primary hydroceles are most common over the age of 40 years. In children, the swelling may be intermittent, and the condition is always associated with a patent processus vaginalis and is a variety of inguinal hernia (see Chapter 14). It occurs in 2–5 per cent of newborn males, and 90 per cent of cases resolve within 1 year.

Secondary hydroceles occur in an older age group because trauma, infection and testicular neoplasms are more common in this period.

Symptoms The patient complains of an **increase in the size of the testis, or a swelling in the scrotum.** There may be pain and discomfort if there is underlying testicular disease, but idiopathic hydroceles reach a considerable size without causing pain. The patient may complain of the social embarrassment of his large scrotum, which shows through his trousers.

(a) A large hydrocele. The swelling is confined to the scrotum, is not tender, and is fluctuant and translucent, and the testis is not palpable.

> ### Revision panel 18.1
> ## The causes of hydrocele
> **Primary**
> Idiopathic
>
> **Secondary**
> Trauma
> Epididymo-orchitis
> Tumour
> Lymphatic obstruction

Hydroceles do not affect fertility, although a large one may cause problems during sexual intercourse.

Examination

Position The swelling fills one side of the scrotum but is within the scrotum, and the spermatic cord can be felt above the lump. The testis cannot be palpated separately because it is within the swelling. This is the cardinal physical sign that distinguishes a hydrocele from an epididymal cyst (Fig. 18.24).

Hydroceles may be bilateral.

Colour and temperature The colour and temperature of the overlying scrotal skin are normal.

Tenderness Primary hydroceles are not tender. Secondary hydroceles may be tender if the underlying testis is tender.

Shape and size Hydroceles can be enormous and contain as much as 500 mL of fluid. They are ovoid in shape.

Surface The surface is always smooth and well defined. Occasionally, a weak spot in the wall gives way to form a small, fluctuant bump – a hernia of the hydrocele fluid through its coverings.

Composition Hydroceles contain a clear, straw-coloured fluid that is rich in protein. They are fluctuant, have a fluid thrill if they are large enough, are dull to percussion and usually **transilluminate** (Fig. 18.24b).

They may be tense or lax, depending on the cause.

(b) A transilluminated hydrocele.

Fig. 18.24 HYDROCELES

The wall of a long-standing hydrocele may become calcified, making the mass hard and opaque.

Reducibility Hydroceles cannot be reduced.

Relations The fluid of a hydrocele surrounds the body of the testis, usually making the testis impalpable. If you can feel the testis separate from a scrotal swelling, the swelling cannot be a hydrocele.

When a hydrocele is lax, which is seen only in secondary hydroceles, it may be possible to feel the surface of the testis through the fluid.

The spermatic cord can be felt coming down to and running into the swelling. The skin of the scrotum is freely mobile over the swelling.

Lymph drainage If you think the swelling is a secondary hydrocele, you should palpate the para-aortic lymph glands in the epigastrium. This is the area of lymphatic drainage of a testicular tumour.

Epididymal cyst

Epididymal cysts are fluid-filled swellings arising from the epididymis. Their aetiology has not been satisfactorily explained, but they are derived from the collecting tubules.

An epididymal cyst usually contains clear fluid. The variety that contains slightly grey, opaque, 'barley water'-like fluid and a few spermatozoa is sometimes termed a *spermatocele*, and may occur following a vasectomy operation (Fig. 18.25). As the large majority of cysts connected with the epididymis contain clear fluid, it is usual to call them all *epididymal cysts* and not use the term 'spermatocele'.

History

Age Most epididymal cysts occur in males over the age of 40 years, but they are occasionally seen in children and adolescents.

Fig. 18.25 Large epididymal cyst (arrow: cyst; arrowhead: testis).

Symptoms The main complaint is of **swelling in the scrotum**, with the occasional patient believing that he has developed a tumour or a third testis.

In older age groups, the swelling is usually painless.

Small epididymal cysts in males in their thirties and forties may be painful and tender.

Development Epididymal cysts enlarge very slowly, but rarely become enormous, unlike primary hydroceles.

Multiplicity They are often multiple or multilocular, and are frequently bilateral.

Fertility Epididymal cysts do not interfere with fertility, but surgery to remove such cysts may do so.

Examination

Position The swelling lies within the scrotum, usually above and slightly behind the testis. **The testis can be felt separately from the swelling**. If the swelling is similar in size to a testis, the patient may identify which of the lumps is which.

The spermatic cord can be felt above it.

Tenderness Small cysts of the epididymis in younger males may be tender, but larger cysts in older males are not.

Shape Because the cysts are usually multilocular, the swelling is rarely a perfect sphere. It is usually elongated and bosselated, and individual loculi may be palpable.

Size Epididymal cysts may vary in size from a few millimetres to 5–10 cm in diameter. They rarely reach the size of the large hydroceles.

Surface The surface is smooth but the contours of individual loculi may be palpable.

Composition These swellings are fluctuant, have a fluid thrill, are translucent if large enough to transilluminate, and are dull to percussion.

Epididymal cysts cannot be reduced.

All the signs mentioned in this section on composition are identical to those for hydrocele. The difference between a hydrocele and an epididymal cyst lies in the relation of the swelling to the testis.

Relations Epididymal cysts are separate from the testis, and therefore the testis remains palpable.

Most epididymal cysts are connected to the head of the epididymis, so lie above the testis, with the spermatic cord descending into or behind them. They occasionally lie at the lower pole.

Lymph drainage The regional lymph glands should not be palpable.

Differential diagnosis

The normal epididymis is usually palpable and may be noticed by concerned young males who think they have a testicular tumour. It may on occasion be difficult to say if a swelling is a normal palpable organ or a small cyst.

Tumours of the epididymis itself are so rare as to be virtually non-existent. Any swelling that is clearly in the epididymis is therefore benign.

Varicocele

A varicocele is a collection of dilated and tortuous veins in the pampiniform plexus. The condition could be renamed varicose veins of the spermatic cord. It is much more common on the left. The right testicular veins drain into the inferior vena cava, but on the left they drain into the renal vein. The left testicular vein (or veins) is a much longer vessel, and it is hardly surprising that its valves can fail and cause a varicocele.

Small symptomless varicoceles occur in 25 per cent of healthy males, on the left side. When the veins become large, they may cause a vague, dragging sensation and aching pain in the scrotum or groin. The appearance may embarrass adolescents and young males.

The sudden appearance of a varicocele in middle or old age may be caused by a renal neoplasm spreading along the renal vein and obstructing the testicular vein. This is a very rare presentation of carcinoma of the kidney but should not be forgotten, particularly if there are other urinary tract symptoms, especially haematuria.

A varicocele can be difficult to palpate when the patient is lying down because the veins are empty. This is one of the reasons why you must always examine the scrotum with the patient standing up (Fig. 18.26). The dilated, compressible veins above the testis are then palpable and often visible. They feel like a '**bag of worms**', an accurate description.

Fig. 18.26 A varicocele (arrow). When the patient is standing, the tense, tortuous, distended veins are said to feel like a 'bag of worms'. When the patient is supine, they collapse and are almost impalpable.

The testis below a large varicocele may be smaller and softer than the testis on the normal side. The effect of a varicocele on spermatogenesis is controversial.

Haematocele

A haematocele is a collection of blood within the tunica vaginalis. The bleeding is usually caused by trauma or underlying malignant disease.

In the acute phase, the mass has the same physical signs as a hydrocele, except that it is not translucent and may be tender. When the blood clots, it contracts and forms a small, hard mass, which can cause diagnostic problems.

Acute haematocele

The patient usually but not always gives a clear history of an injury, or of vague discomfort in the testis, followed by a painful, rapid swelling of the scrotum. It is a condition particularly associated with cricket, rugby and cycling.

The unilateral swelling is tense, tender and fluctuant, but does not transilluminate. The testis cannot be felt separate from the swelling.

Chronic haematocele

If the acute episode is managed conservatively or not recognized, the blood in the tunica vaginalis will clot. As time passes, the clot that surrounds the testis contracts and hardens. This may result in a hard mass, which is no longer tender and is not fluctuant. Normal testicular sensation may be lost if the contracting clot causes ischaemic necrosis of the testis.

These changes make a chronic haematocele difficult to distinguish from a testicular tumour, and investigation or even exploration may be needed.

Torsion of the testis

Testicular torsion can occur at any age, and is of two distinct types, intra- and extravaginal.

- *Intravaginal torsion.* The testis twists within the tunica vaginalis itself. This is the most common type, predisposed to by the 'bell clapper' abnormality in which the testis lies horizontally (Fig. 18.27) and is more mobile because of a longer length of the vessels. This process can be aided by contraction of the spiral fibres of the cremaster muscle.
- *Extravaginal torsion.* The entire testis and tunica vaginalis twists on the spermatic cord itself. This is seen rarely in neonates and infants.

Fig. 18.27 A testis hanging horizontally and susceptible to torsion.

The anatomical abnormality that allows torsion is invariably bilateral.

The condition may resolve spontaneously, or may progress to testicular infarction.

History

Age Torsion presents most commonly in teenagers between 14 and 16 years of age, but as the cause is a congenital abnormality, it can occur in young children, in neonates and even *in utero*. It is uncommon in males over 25 years of age.

Symptoms The initial symptom is **acute severe scrotal pain**, which may be poorly localized, and may radiate to or only be felt in the lower abdomen, loin or groin. This is because it is autonomically modulated, so is referred to the embryological site of origin of the testis. Nausea and vomiting are common. In a baby, there may be restlessness and a failure to eat.

Previous attacks The patient may have had similar mild attacks of pain that subsided spontaneously, or an episode on the other side that required surgery. Recurrent torsion is possible if the testis has not been appropriately fixed.

Cause Although the majority of torsions seem to occur spontaneously, often in the early hours of the morning, some follow minor trauma.

Examination

Position The swelling is confined to the scrotum. The affected testis lies higher in the scrotum than the normal testis. This is a most important physical sign.

Colour The scrotal skin may be red and oedematous. Although the latter changes are more commonly associated with epididymo-orchitis, their presence must not dissuade you from making a diagnosis of torsion.

Temperature The skin will feel hot if it is red and hyperaemic.

Tenderness **The testis is exquisitely tender, making palpation very difficult.**

Shape The whole of the testis is swollen, and it is usually impossible to distinguish the contours of the epididymis from those of the body of the testis.

Surface The surface of the testis is smooth, but may be obscured by scrotal oedema.

Composition Because of tenderness, it is usually impossible to elicit the signs that will reveal the composition of the mass in the scrotum. The mass may be the testis, or the testis surrounded by an acute secondary hydrocele.

Surrounding tissues Apart from the scrotal skin, which may be red and oedematous, the other nearby tissues, including the other testis, will be normal.

Differential diagnosis

Torsion of a testis within the scrotum may be indistinguishable from acute epididymo-orchitis, particularly if there are no urinary symptoms. However, epididymo-orchitis usually occurs in an older age group. Torsion of an undescended testis in the groin may be indistinguishable from a strangulated inguinal hernia.

- *Torsion of a testicular appendage* is the most common condition mimicking torsion. There are two appendages (the appendix of the testis and the appendix of the epididymis), and either may tort. The initial symptoms may be identical. The testis is not usually as tender, and sometimes the torted appendage is palpable as a tender nodule, or is visible through the scrotal skin as the 'blue dot sign'. However, a secondary hydrocele may obscure this.
- *Idiopathic scrotal oedema* is a condition in which the skin and subcutaneous tissues of the scrotum become oedematous, red and inflamed, in most cases as the result of a streptococcal infection. The swelling is confined by the attachments of the scrotal fascia (Fig. 18.28). A clinical diagnosis can usually be made, as the testis itself is not tender.

Fig. 18.28 A very severe case of idiopathic scrotal oedema. The scrotal skin has lost its wrinkled appearance. Unusually, the oedema has tracked into the groin, the perineum and the other side of the scrotum. The attachment of Scarpa's fascia in the thigh is clearly visible.

Warning When in doubt about a painful scrotal or testicular swelling, make a diagnosis of torsion, because failure to explore the scrotum within 6 hours and reduce the torsion will result in the death of the testis. If the diagnosis turns out to be wrong and the patient has epididymo-orchitis, the surgical exploration will have done no harm, and decompression of the tunica vaginalis may relieve the painful pressure from the secondary hydrocele.

There are occasional reports of manual external detorsion. Although possibly successful at times, this does not replace surgical exploration.

Orchitis

Acute orchitis, in the absence of epididymitis, is invariably caused by a virus infection, commonly mumps. The damage caused by orchitis may leave the patient with a painful testis or render him subfertile, especially if the condition is bilateral. Mumps orchitis may occur without enlargement of the salivary glands, but there is usually a history of contact.

Acute epididymo-orchitis

This is primarily an infection of the epididymis, but oedema and inflammatory changes spread into the testis. There is usually an associated urinary tract or sexually transmitted infection.

The common infecting organisms in patients under 40 years old are *Chlamydia trachomatis* and *Neisseria gonorrhoeae*. In older patients, *Escherichia coli* is common.

History

Age This condition can affect all age groups, but is most common in young and middle-aged males. It is rare in children.

Symptoms There is often an initial flu-like illness, with malaise and fever, and sometimes deep-seated pelvic pain caused by inflammation of the prostate. The patient then **develops severe pain and swelling in one side of the scrotum**, which usually comes on quite quickly over 30–60 minutes and is sometimes relieved by supporting the scrotum. Frequency of micturition and painful micturition may indicate the presence of a urinary tract infection.

Examination

Position The swelling is confined to one side of the scrotum (Revision panel 18.2).

Colour The scrotal skin is red and shiny. After a few days, it turns a bronze colour, and the superficial layers of skin desquamate.

Temperature The scrotal skin is hot.

Revision panel 18.2

The causes of a unilateral scrotal swelling

Hydrocele

Epididymal cyst

Varicocele

Haematocele

Orchitis (mumps)

Epididymo-orchitis

Testicular tumour

Tenderness The testis and epididymis are extremely tender, but the scrotal skin is not. Careful palpation will reveal that the tenderness is in the swollen epididymis, and that the body of the testis itself is not so tender.

Shape and size The whole testicle may be enlarged and tender, and **you may be unable to distinguish the epididymis from testis**. This is more likely in the presence of a small secondary hydrocele. If a hydrocele does not form, you should be able to distinguish the testis from the epididymis, which is commonly enlarged to a centimetre or so in width.

In mild cases, the inflammation may be localized to the head or tail of the epididymis.

Surface The surface of the epididymis remains smooth, but will probably be too tender for this to be obvious.

Composition If there is a small hydrocele, the swelling may be fluctuant, with the testis palpable through the fluid.

If there is no hydrocele, you may be able to detect that the body of the testis feels a little more tense than normal. The epididymis is initially soft, but as the inflammation subsides, it becomes hard and craggy.

Relations and local tissues The skin over the involved testis is oedematous but mobile. Untreated, the infection may spread beyond the epididymis to the surrounding tissues, and the skin then becomes fixed. If an abscess develops in the epididymis, it may point and discharge through the area of skin fixation. As the epididymis normally lies behind the testis, epididymal disease involves the skin of the back of the scrotum, so always remember to look at its posterior aspect.

The spermatic cord is always thickened and tender because epididymal infection spreads distally from the urinary tract along the vas deferens.

The other testis should feel normal.

General examination Pay particular attention to the lower urinary tract. Rectal examination may reveal tenderness of the prostate and seminal vesicles, and there may be a palpable bladder. There may also be a fever and a tachycardia.

Tuberculous epididymo-orchitis

History

This condition is now uncommon in the UK, but is still seen in many other parts of the world. The tubercle bacillus reaches the epididymis via the bloodstream or by travelling along the vas from the lower urinary tract. The infection develops slowly, without causing severe or acute pain or tenderness. There may be systemic symptoms of tuberculosis, or only the urinary tract may be clinically involved, with a prior history of tuberculous exposure.

Most patients complain of a lump in the scrotum, and an associated dull, aching pain.

Examination

On examination, the epididymis is hard, irregular and two or three times its normal size. A secondary hydrocele is unusual. The spermatic cord is thickened as far as you can feel. The vas deferens is often irregular and swollen, and feels like a string of beads. This physical sign is rare, but is diagnostic of tuberculosis.

Tumours of the testis

There are several varieties of testicular tumour. Around 90 per cent are *germ cell* in origin, including seminoma and non-seminomatous germ cell tumours, comprising teratoma, yolk sack tumour and choriocarcinoma. The rest are *tumours of the sex cord and stromal structures*, such as Leydig and Sertoli cell tumours. Rarely, *lymphoma* and *metastases* present in the testes.

History

Age Non-seminomatous germ cell tumours commonly occur between the ages of 20 and 35 years, but seminomas often occur a few years later (age 35–45 years). Both are very rare in childhood and the teenage years.

Symptoms The most common presentation is a **swelling arising from the body of the testis, which is not usually painful**. However, the occasional patient presents acutely with a painful, tender testis, and the diagnosis is not always straightforward, especially if there is a history of minor testicular trauma.

Dull, aching, dragging pains in the scrotum and groin occur in some patients, particularly if the testis is significantly enlarged. Many patients complain that the affected testicle feels heavy.

Presentation with distant metastases may occur in many different ways, such as general malaise, loss of appetite, wasting, abdominal pains and dyspnoea. Rarely, there may be generalized lymphadenopathy, haemoptysis and headache. Presentation may be with an abdominal mass.

There is a considerably higher incidence of malignant change in the incompletely descended testis. As the testis is not in the scrotum, diagnosis will be difficult and may be delayed.

Examination

Position The swelling is confined to the scrotum.

Temperature and colour The scrotal skin should be normal, except in the extremely rare circumstance in which the tumour has invaded and ulcerated through it.

Tenderness Testicular tumours are not tender except in the unusual acute presentation. Normal testicular sensation may be lost. Ask the patient about this, as it is an important symptom of a testicular tumour and rarely associated with other conditions.

Shape The majority of testicular tumours are not noticed until they occupy the whole testis. Rarely, you may be able to feel a nodule that is clearly in the testis and not in the epididymis. A nodule that is in the epididymis is almost never a tumour. Testicular tumours are irregular and variable in shape, but are basically spherical.

Size Tumours are noticed by the patient when the testis is clearly larger than its companion. Large swellings are now uncommon in the UK because of heightened public awareness.

Surface This is usually smooth, but can be irregular or nodular.

Composition Testicular tumours feel harder than a normal testis, and are not fluctuant or translucent.

Heaviness is an important physical sign. With the patient lying down, lift the testis with your fingers. Compare with the normal side. A feeling of heaviness is characteristic of a tumour.

Relations to surrounding tissues The other testis should be normal, but tumours are bilateral in 1–2 per cent of cases. The spermatic cord and the vas deferens should be normal. A very advanced tumour may infiltrate the skin of the scrotum.

Lymph drainage Lymph from the testis drains to the para-aortic lymph glands. Remember that these glands lie in the abdomen above the level of the umbilicus.

The inguinal glands will only be enlarged if the tumour has spread to the scrotal skin, a rare event.

General examination **Pay particular attention to all the lymph glands, especially the para-aortic and supraclavicular groups.**

Testicular tumours may metastasize anywhere in the body. Unusual swellings may be detected on general examination. Lung metastases are not usually detectable on clinical examination, but are readily visible on a chest X-ray or computed tomography scan.

CHAPTER 18 | THE EXTERNAL GENITALIA

First decide the answers to these four questions:

1 Can you get above the swelling?   **2** Can you identify the testis and epididymis?   **3** Is the swelling translucent?   **4** Is the swelling tender?

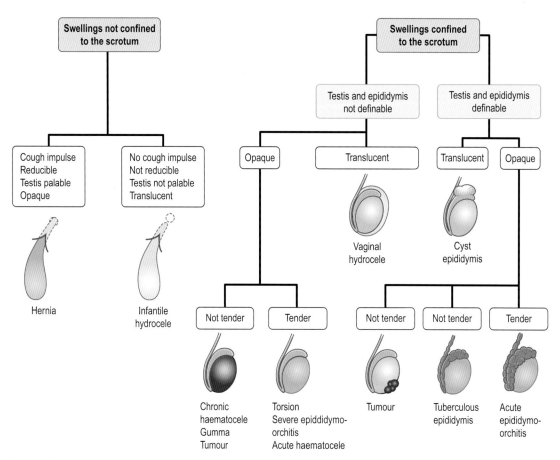

Fig. 18.29 A plan for the diagnosis of scrotal swellings.

Differential diagnosis

The testicular swellings likely to be confused with tumours are acute and chronic epididymo-orchitis, and haematocele. Worried well patients often present wanting reassurance regarding simple epididymal cysts.

Figure 18.29 outlines a plan for diagnosis of scrotal swellings (see also Fig. 18.30).

Chronic testicular pain

This is a common reason for referral to a surgical clinic. The patient is a young or middle-aged male. The pain may be localized to the testis, or it may radiate to the groin. It may be associated with exercise and movement, or with sitting in certain positions.

Common findings are:

- a mildly tender but otherwise normal epididymis, occasionally associated with a chlamydial urinary tract infection;
- a small epididymal cyst – differentiation from a normal epididymis may be difficult;
- an inguinal hernia – the skin of the scrotum is supplied by the genitofemoral nerve, which may be compressed in the groin by a hernia, causing discomfort referred to the testis;
- rarely, but significantly, a testicular tumour;
- nothing abnormal.

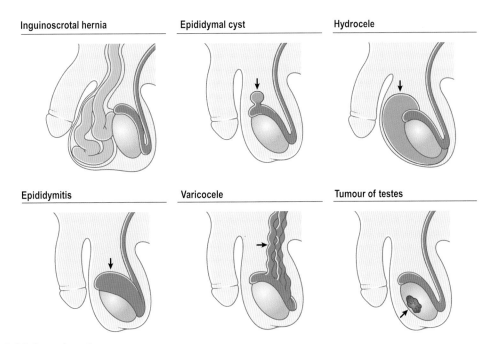

Fig. 18.30 Scrotal swellings.

The possibilities are many, but, frustratingly for both patient and doctor, there may be no physical signs, and a diagnosis cannot be made. Patients can often be reassured that there is no physical abnormality, and the symptoms usually settle with time.

Erectile dysfunction

The condition is defined as the persistent inability to achieve or maintain an erection sufficient for intercourse. This definition is necessarily loose, as what is normal for one may be abnormal for another.

Studies have suggested that as many as a fifth of males are affected. Psychogenic factors (performance anxiety) are common in the young. Diabetes, cardiovascular disease, obesity and prostatic problems are factors in older males.

History

Age The incidence increases with age.

Symptoms Inquiry should be made into how long there has been a problem and the suddenness of its onset. Are there early morning erections, and is it better with masturbation? Is there any loss of libido, and did the problem occur with previous partners?

General Specific enquiry should be made about hypertension, diabetes, previous endocrine or neurological problems, and pelvic surgery or trauma. A full drug history is essential, including alcohol, smoking and prescription, over-the-counter and recreational drug use.

Psychosocial A psychosocial history is vital. Is there occupational stress or financial insecurity? Is the relationship happy, and do both partners want children?

Questionnaire Questionnaires and sexual function scores assess the severity of the condition and monitor the response to treatment. An example is the International Index of Erectile Function.

Examination

General Note factors such as obesity, the condition of the cardiovascular system and the abdomen. An appropriate neurological examination is essential – test the genital and perineal sensation, and elicit the bulbocavernosus reflex.

Assess secondary sexual characteristics. Is there any gynaecomastia or any other signs of hypogonadism? Is there evidence of an intersex condition (see below)?

Genital The penis should be inspected for signs of deformity, curvature, chordae or phimosis. Are the testes of normal size? Assess the prostate by digital rectal examination.

Male infertility

Definition This is defined as failure to conceive after a year of unprotected intercourse.

Approximately 90 per cent of couples will conceive within 1 year. Approximately 20 per cent of infertility is a result of pathology in the male, with 30–40 per cent from combined male and female factors. Infertile females are usually seen and treated by a gynaecologically trained infertility specialist. It is, however, important to take a history from the female partner.

History

Age Fertility declines with the age of both partners.
Reproductive history Inquiry should be made into previous fertility, erectile and ejaculatory function, frequency of intercourse and other factors such as contraception and the use of spermicidal lubricants.
Development The age at puberty should be documented. Early (precocious) or delayed puberty may be a sign of an underlying endocrinological disorder such as Kallmann's syndrome or congenital adrenal hyperplasia.
Full medical history Any history of an undescended testicle or corrective surgery is important, as is any previous testicular problem such as torsion, varicocele, tumour, orchitis or sexually transmitted disease. Ask about any previous radiotherapy or chemotherapy, and diabetes. A recent viral or febrile illness may temporarily impair spermatogenesis. A full drug history should also be taken.

Examination

Carry out a full examination as described above for the patient with erectile dysfunction. In addition, examine the patient when he is standing to look for a varicocele. Note the size and consistency of the testes. Feel the vasa, which may be absent or nodular due to previous infection.

THE FEMALE EXTERNAL GENITALIA

Most complaints about the external genitalia are referred to gynaecologists, but there are two common conditions that quite often appear in a general surgical clinic.

Bartholin's cyst

The Bartholin's glands are a pair of small glands that lie at the sides of the lower end of the vagina, and whose ducts open on to the inner side of the posterior part of the labium minus. They are normally impalpable. When the duct of a gland is distended by obstruction or infection, it forms a cystic swelling in the posterior part of the labia majora.

Urethral caruncle

This is a bright red, polypoid granuloma that arises from the mucosa of the urethral orifice in postmenopausal females. It is very tender and causes painful micturition, dyspareunia and occasional bleeding.

The differential diagnosis is urethral mucosal prolapse, which is purple in colour and not so tender, and rarely urethral carcinoma.

INTERSEX CONDITIONS

An in-depth description of the intersex conditions is beyond the scope of this book. It is a topic that confuses most!

Intersex is divided into:

- Female (46XX) with inappropriate virilization (*female pseudohermaphrodite*). The most common example is congenital adrenal hyperplasia, which accounts for 85 per cent of all ambiguous genitalia.
- Incomplete virilization of a male (46XY) – a *male pseudohermaphrodite.*
- *Gonadal dysgenesis with abnormal sex chromosomes*, e.g. Turner's syndrome (45X0) and Klinefelter'ssyndrome (47XXY).
- *True hermaphrodites*, where both ovarian and testicular tissue coexist. This is very rare.

Investigation of a newborn with ambiguous genitalia should take place at a specialist unit. However, it is important to recognize life-threatening conditions such as salt-losing aldosterone deficiency in congenital adrenal hypoplasia.

It is important to recognize the general appearance of older children or adults who may present with related (e.g. infertility) or unrelated problems. Two such disorders are Klinefelter's and Turner's syndromes.

Klinefelter's syndrome

Klinefelter's syndrome is a congenital abnormality in which a male has an extra female (X) chromosome. Thus, instead of being a normal XY male, he is XXY, and testosterone production is subnormal.

The patients are tall, with a female distribution of fat around the breast and pelvis, but normal male hair growth on the face and pubis.

The testes are very small and soft, and do not produce spermatozoa, so the patients are sterile.

Turner's syndrome

Turner's syndrome is a congenital abnormality in which a female has only one female (X) chromosome. Thus, instead of being a normal XX female, she is X0.

There are no skeletal abnormalities, but the patient has a masculine shape – wide shoulders and narrow pelvis – and is invariably shorter than average for a female.

The most distinctive feature, when present, is 'webbing' of the shoulders. This is a thickening of the neck and a prominence of the skin folds that run from the neck to the shoulders.

The breasts and pubic hair are usually underdeveloped.

CHAPTER 18 | THE EXTERNAL GENITALIA

Index